WN 17 POP 2014

WN 17 POP 2014

*Aunt Minnie's Atlas and*
*Imaging-Specific Diagnosis*

# Aunt Minnie's Atlas and *Imaging-Specific Diagnosis*

**FOURTH EDITION**

## Thomas L. Pope Jr., MD, FACR

Formerly:
Professor of Radiology and Orthopaedics
University of Virginia
Charlottesville, Virginia

Professor of Radiology and Orthopaedics
Associate Dean for Continuing Medical Education
Wake Forest University School of Medicine
Wake Forest/Baptist Medical Center
Winston-Salem, North Carolina

Professor of Radiology and Orthopaedics and
    Chair of Radiology
Medical University of South Carolina
Charleston, South Carolina

Presently:
Vice Chairman of Radiology
Director of Women's Imaging
Clinical Advisory Board
Radisphere National Radiology Group
Beachwood, Ohio and Westport, Connecticut

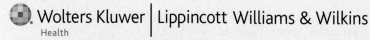

Wolters Kluwer | Lippincott Williams & Wilkins
Health

Philadelphia · Baltimore · New York · London
Buenos Aires · Hong Kong · Sydney · Tokyo

*Senior Executive Editor:* Jonathan W. Pine, Jr.
*Product Manager:* Amy G. Dinkel
*Production Project Manager:* Alicia Jackson
*Senior Manufacturing Coordinator:* Beth Welsh
*Senior Marketing Manager:* Kimberly Schonberger
*Design Coordinator:* Holly McLaughlin
*Production Service:* S4Carlisle Publishing Services

© 2014 by LIPPINCOTT WILLIAMS & WILKINS, a WOLTERS KLUWER business
Two Commerce Square
2001 Market Street
Philadelphia, PA 19103 USA
LWW.com

Third Edition © 2009 by Lippincott Williams & Wilkins
Second Edition © 2003 by Lippincott Williams & Wilkins
First Edition © 1997 by Williams & Wilkins

Printed in China

**Library of Congress Cataloging-in-Publication Data**

Aunt Minnie's atlas and imaging-specific diagnosis/[edited by] Thomas L. Pope Jr.—Fourth edition.
     p. ; cm.
  Atlas and imaging-specific diagnosis
  Includes bibliographical references and index.
  ISBN 978-1-4511-7215-7 (hardback : alk. paper)
  I. Pope, Thomas Lee, Jr., editor of compilation.   II. Title: Atlas and imaging-specific diagnosis.
  [DNLM: 1. Diagnostic Imaging—Atlases.   2. Diagnosis, Differential—Atlases.   3. Radiography—methods—Atlases.   WN 17]
  RC78.7.D53
  616.07'54—dc23

                                                                      2013017934

Care has been taken to confirm the accuracy of the information presented and to describe generally accepted practices. However, the authors, editors, and publisher are not responsible for errors or omissions or for any consequences from application of the information in this book and make no warranty, expressed or implied, with respect to the currency, completeness, or accuracy of the contents of the publication. Application of the information in a particular situation remains the professional responsibility of the practitioner.

The authors, editors, and publisher have exerted every effort to ensure that drug selection and dosage set forth in this text are in accordance with current recommendations and practice at the time of publication. However, in view of ongoing research, changes in government regulations, and the constant flow of information relating to drug therapy and drug reactions, the reader is urged to check the package insert for each drug for any change in indications and dosage and for added warnings and precautions. This is particularly important when the recommended agent is a new or infrequently employed drug.

Some drugs and medical devices presented in the publication have Food and Drug Administration (FDA) clearance for limited use in restricted research settings. It is the responsibility of the health care provider to ascertain the FDA status of each drug or device planned for use in their clinical practice.

To purchase additional copies of this book, call our customer service department at (800) 638-3030 or fax orders to (301) 223-2320. International customers should call (301) 223-2300.

Visit Lippincott Williams & Wilkins on the Internet: at LWW.com. Lippincott Williams & Wilkins customer service representatives are available from 8:30 am to 6 pm, EST.

10 9 8 7 6 5 4 3 2 1

CCS0913

# DEDICATION

Only the first of the three previous editions of Aunt Minnie's Atlas had a dedication. Even I, as the editor, don't know exactly why we neglected acknowledgements in the latter two editions, as this is a common practice in medical books. I considered not having one for Aunt Minnie 4, but after further consideration I decided that there were two people who should be acknowledged and to whom this fourth edition should be dedicated.

The first of these individuals is the first author of Aunt Minnie 1, Dr. Ken Ford, of Dallas, Texas. This was a very easy choice, from my perspective. Simply put, without Ken, this series of books would never have existed. He created the idea of an "Aunt Minnie's Atlas" when one of his fellow residents missed a "classic case" of Trevor's disease at a visiting professor's conference way back in the early 1990's, at Wake Forest University/Baptist Medical Center. Ken's resident class was the brightest single group of radiology residents whom I have ever had the honor of teaching. He discussed his idea for this new book with a few other faculty members before walking into my office to test my appreciation for the concept. I immediately liked it and within a few days, we had written our book proposal and we were "on our way." Fortunately, we had no difficulties finding a publishing company or recruiting friends and colleagues to write the initial chapters for Aunt Minnie 1....and this first edition became a big success. The book engendered a "must read" attitude for those residents preparing for the annual "Louisville pilgrimage" and the ongoing success of the book has lead to a successful fourth iteration. So, Ken, this fourth edition is dedicated to you. Thank you so much for your original idea and for including me in the first edition!

The second individual deserving of acknowledgement was also very easy to choose. He wrote the Foreword for Aunt Minnie 3 and met an untimely passing between the publication of Aunt Minnie 3 and this release of Aunt Minnie 4. As Dr. George Bisset noted in the Foreword for this edition, Dr. Jerome Wiot was actually the reason George finds himself in Radiology instead of Cardiology today. I know there are many others who might be reading this who owe their choice of radiology as a career to this icon of our specialty. "Jerry," as he was affectionately called by all who knew him and as George so eloquently describes in the Foreward, was the penultimate individual and physician. I first met him in Louisville at the ABR oral examinations in the mid 80's when I served as a first time examiner in the musculoskeletal section. Dr. Paul Capp introduced me to him at the nightly gathering of ABR examiners from all subspecialties. As a young academician, I was in awe of him and all of the other "rock stars" in radiology about whom I had read and studied, who were assembled in that room each night. Most of my "heroes" whom I met that year did not remember me the June when I returned. But Jerry approached me immediately at the first nightly gathering and said, "Hey, Tommy, how are you?" I was dumbfounded that he remembered my name from the year before, but when I asked George about this, he said, "typical of Jerry!" And every year I went back to Louisville, I was amazed and inspired by Dr. Wiot's boundless energy, sense of humor and kind consideration of fellow man and woman. I asked him to write the Foreword to Aunt Minnie 3 since he was at Cincinnati with Dr. Ben Felson, who legend tells us coined the phrase, "Aunt Minnie." He immediately accepted this thankless task, and wrote a wonderful Foreword for that book with a tremendous tribute to his close friend and colleague. So, Jerry, we dedicate this book to you in appreciation and celebration for your life as a mentor, teacher, colleague and superb radiologist who advanced our specialty more than we likely will ever know!

*Thomas L. Pope, MD, FACR*

# CONTRIBUTING AUTHORS

**Susan J. Ackerman, MD**
Professor
Department of Radiology and Radiological Science
Medical University of South Carolina
Charleston, South Carolina

**Lejla Aganovic, MD**
Assistant Professor of Radiology
VA Hospital
University of California San Diego
San Diego, California

**Timothy J. Amrhein, MD**
Assistant Professor
Division of Neuroradiology
Department of Radiology and Radiological Sciences
Medical University of South Carolina
Charleston, South Carolina

**Laura W. Bancroft, MD**
Program Director–Diagnostic Radiology Residency,
    Florida Hospital
Chief of Musculoskeletal Radiology–Florida Hospital
Adjunct Professor–University of Central Florida
    College of Medicine
Clinical Professor–Florida State University College
    of Medicine

**Marques Bradshaw, MD**
Assistant Professor of Radiology
Medical University of South Carolina
Charleston, South Carolina

**Amy S. Campbell, MD**
Assistant Professor
Radiology
Medical University of South Carolina
Charleston, South Carolina

**Melanie P. Caserta, MD**
Assistant Professor
Department of Radiology
Wake Forest Baptist Health
Winston Salem, North Carolina

**Matthew S. Chin, MD**
Resident Physician in Radiology
University of North Carolina
Chapel Hill, North Carolina

**Abbie Cluver, MD**
Assistant Professor
Radiology
Medical University of South Carolina
Charleston, South Carolina

**Jennifer Cranny, MD**
Radisphere National Radiology Group
Medical Director, East Cooper Medical Center
Mount Pleasant, South Carolina

**Brian Dupree, MD**
Radiology Resident
Department of Radiology
University of Tennessee
Knoxville, Tennessee

**Judson R. Gash, MD**
Professor of Radiology
Department of Radiology
University of Tennessee
Knoxville, Tennessee

**Jeanne G. Hill, MD**
Professor of Radiology and Pediatrics
Department of Radiology and
    Radiological Science
Medical University of South Carolina
Charleston, South Carolina

**Abid Irshad, MD**
Professor of Radiology
Medical University of South Carolina
Charleston, South Carolina

**Yeong Shyan Lee, MD**
Professor of Radiology, Medicine and
    Pediatrics
Director of Division of Cardiovascular Imaging
Department of Radiology and
    Radiological Science
Medical University of South Carolina
Charleston, South Carolina

**Stephen P. Loehr, MD**
Medical Director
Vascular and Interventional Radiology
Triangle Vascular Associates
Cary, North Carolina

Usman Manzoor, MBBS
Fellow, Interventional Radiology
Department of Radiology and
    Radiological Sciences
Medical University of South Carolina
Charleston, South Carolina

Michelle McDonough, MD
Assistant Professor of Radiology
Section Chief of Breast Imaging
Diagnostic Radiology
Mayo Clinic Florida
Jacksonville, Florida

Blaine Mischen, MD
Resident
Department of Nuclear Medicine
Medical University of South Carolina
Charleston, South Carolina

Daniel B. Nissman, MD, MPH, MSEE
Assistant Professor of Radiology
Musculoskeletal Imaging
University of North Carolina
Chapel Hill, North Carolina

Samuel Porter, MD
Professor of Radiology
Department of Radiology
University of Tennessee
Knoxville, Tennessee

Anil G. Rao, MD
Assistant Professor of Radiology
Medical University of South Carolina
Charleston, South Carolina

James G. Ravenel, MD
Associate Professor of Radiology
Chief, Thoracic Imaging
Medical University of South Carolina
Charleston, South Carolina

Catherine C. Roberts, MD
Assistant Professor
Department of Radiology
Mayo Clinic
Phoenix, Arizona

Zoran Rumboldt, MD, PhD
Professor
Neuroradiology Chief & Fellowship Program Director
Department of Radiology and Radiological Science
Medical University of South Carolina
Charleston, South Carolina

U. Joseph Schoepf, MD
Professor of Radiology, Medicine and Pediatrics
Director of Division of Cardiovascular Imaging
Department of Radiology and Radiological Science
Medical University of South Carolina
Charleston, South Carolina

Lubdha M. Shah, MD
Associate Professor
Director of Spine Imaging
Departments of Radiology and Neurosurgery
University of Utah Health Sciences Center
Salt Lake City, Utah

Timothy Singewald, MD
MD, Diagnostic Radiology Resident
University of California, San Diego
San Diego, California

Pal Suranyi, MD, PhD
Professor of Radiology, Medicine and Pediatrics
Director of Division of Cardiovascular Imaging
Department of Radiology and Radiological Science
Medical University of South Carolina
Charleston, South Carolina

Paul Thacker, MD
Assistant Professor
Radiology and Radiological Science
Medical University of South Carolina
Charleston, South Carolina

Richard H. Wiggins, MD
Director of Imaging Informatics
Director of Head and Neck Imaging
Professor, Departments of Radiology,
    Otolaryngology, Head and Neck Surgery,
    and BioMedical Informatics
University of Utah Health Sciences Center
Salt Lake City, Utah

# FOREWORD

When I was asked to write the Foreword for this book, my attention was immediately drawn to the title, "Aunt Minnie's Atlas and Imaging-Specific Diagnosis." It brought back memories of my residency at the University of Cincinnati, where Drs. Ben Felson and Jerry Wiot consistently conjured up visions of a legendary aunt who everyone recognized. During my training we heard the term "Aunt Minnie" countless times, describing a radiographic pattern that was instantly recognizable and diagnostic. I remember being shown cases by Dr. Felson when, after I struggled for a minute or so, he would sit back in his chair and say, "Dr. Bisset, this is an 'Aunt Minnie'." I recall responding (in a sometimes irreverent fashion) that I hadn't seen Aunt Minnie yet, and he said . . . "Well, you have now. The next time you won't miss this diagnosis." Although even Dr. Felson was not exactly sure where the phrase came from, he was certainly charismatic enough to bear the weighty responsibility for having popularized the term.

Dr. Thomas Pope took this "Aunt Minnie" concept and ran with it. "Tommy," as he is known by friends, has a unique background in radiology. He is recognized as a jack-of-all-trades when it comes to radiology expertise. Some know him as a breast imager, some as a musculoskeletal radiologist, and others consider him a generalist. This diverse expertise gives him the credibility and breadth of knowledge to make him the perfect editor of a case-based book. I have had the pleasure of knowing Tommy for probably 25 years, and his enthusiasm and intellectual curiosity never seem to wane. He has been an avid teacher, and for those who have seen him lecture you can readily understand how his passion could translate to a textbook. However, Tommy doesn't spend too much time doing any one thing—his rapid-fire approach to life is epitomized in his book. Each case is illustrated, the appropriate teaching points are made, and it's on to the next. As I indicated earlier, a case-based book is the ideal model for a book from Dr. Pope.

So, the chemistry is perfect—the combination of an "Aunt Minnie Atlas" and Tommy Pope is a match that is tough to duplicate. Dr. Felson passed away in 1988 and Dr. Wiot died in 2010, but I am sure that they would have been proud to know that the legacy of "Aunt Minnie" lives on in the Fourth Edition of this book.

*George Bisset, MD*

# FOREWORD TO THE THIRD EDITION

It gives me great pleasure to write a Foreword to the text, *Aunt Minnie*, because it brings back many fond memories of working with Ben Felson for 34 years prior to his death in 1988.

Ben Felson, an outstanding diagnostic radiologist, was primarily a teacher who devoted his entire career to his residents and medical students and the education of radiologists throughout the world. He began his academic career while still in the US Army during World War II. He was assigned to reviewing hundreds of chest x-rays for young men entering active duty. As testimony to his inquisitive and resourceful nature, Ben took the opportunity to record and tabulate the normal findings and variants on PA chest x-rays of 30,000 individuals, both those in service and, later, miners ranging in age from 17 to 55. To my knowledge, this remains the largest description of the spectrum of normal chest radiographic findings recorded to date.

Dr. Felson came to the Department of Radiology at the University of Cincinnati in 1945, when it was known as the Cincinnati General Hospital. He served as acting director until 1951, when he was officially appointed Professor and Director of Radiology.

Ben is best known for the Silhouette Sign. This sign evolved, in part, from the financial status of the hospital at that time. The hospital budget was very limited, and in order to have adequate funds to purchase film through July 1, the end of the fiscal year, only PA films were obtained. Only with approval of faculty or residents was a lateral film obtained. His prior experience with the 30,000 normal PA chest x-rays was invaluable in demonstrating that in the right hands, one view could be adequate to fully characterize radiographic findings for most patients.

Ben coined the term "Aunt Minnie" to describe his approach of pattern recognition. You know it's your Aunt Minnie because that's what she looks like. It was his premise that familiarity with the radiographic findings of a disease would guarantee recognition the next time you "met up" with it in the reading room.

Dr. Felson loved teaching. His conferences were always educational and filled with jokes and anecdotes. Ben Felson died in 1988 at his desk while preparing a lecture. He would be proud to know that the "Aunt Minnie" legacy he started lives on in this book.

*Jerome F. Wiot, MD*
*Professor Emeritus*
*University of Cincinnati*

It is hard for me to believe that the first edition of "Aunt Minnie's Atlas" was published over 18 years ago. At that time, the concept was innovative and the format compelling. Dr. Ken Ford and I wanted the book to make only a point about the importance of recognizing cases that have "classic" appearances. In the preface to the second edition, I commented on how lucky we were to have "survived" the first edition and to be able to do a second one. Now almost two decades later, I am privileged enough to yet again have an opportunity to compose a preface for this fourth edition.

For historical interest we have included the First Edition Preface and the Third edition Foreword by Jerry Wiott, which explain the origin of the term "Aunt Minnie." Jerry Wiott, a longtime faculty member at the University of Cincinnati, who was a close personal and professional colleague of Dr. Ben Felson, the originator of term *Aunt Minnie*. Dr. Wiott commented that he was sure that Dr. Felson would have been happy to know the concept of the "Aunt Minnie's case" will be continued by our book. Moreover, we are all very honored that we can continue this tradition. Dr. George Bisset, a close friend for more than 20 years, a former University of Cincinnati trainee and faculty member, and now Professor and Chair of the Department of Pediatrics at Texas Children's Hospital in Houston, Texas, kindly agreed to write the Foreword for this fourth edition and we are indebted to him for taking his valuable time to do this for us.

This fourth edition is "new and improved" with revisions of the chapter discussions, an update of the figures for the third edition cases continued, the addition of many new cases, overhaul of the "Aunt Minnie's Pearls" for many of the cases and an update of the reference material. The references have purposely been kept to a minimum as it is so easy today to use the various internet search engines to find material on the web.

I would like to personally thank the Chapter 10 authors of Aunt Minnie, Chapter 3 authors who could no longer participate in Aunt Minnie, and Chapter 4 authors for their hard work on that very successful product. To the Aunt Minnie Chapter 4 authors who stayed with this project, I extend my deepest appreciation for their loyalty and

commitment in completing this textbook. To the Chapter 6 authors new to AM 4, I extend my kindest regards for joining this successful endeavor and to what hopefully will be a long-term commitment for future editions—if we are fortunate enough to have an Aunt Minnie's Atlas 5. All of the time and effort in writing and mentoring for AM4 has been "above and beyond the call of duty," especially in what is a changing academic and private practice environment. Today academic chairs at many institutions require more RVU production from their faculty to keep salaries competitive, and this emphasis leaves less time for all academic pursuits. I know that many chairs consider chapter-writing the least important and rewarding of all academic endeavors. Private practice groups are also requiring more daily "output" in our ever-decreasing reimbursement environment. Most, if not all of our chapter authors have done their writing and editing at nights and weekends taking time off from personal pursuits and family and friends, and I cannot thank them enough for their efforts.

Our graduating radiology residents' yearly "Louisville ABR experience" will basically come to an end in 2013. Traditionally, according to the residents with whom I talk when I give my ACR-AIRP talks and participate in visiting professorships, these seniors almost always use "Aunt Minnie's Atlas" to help study for "the Boards." However, just because the Louisville trip no longer exists, it doesn't mean that there is no longer a role for this textbook. In our practice of image interpretation, the concept of recognizing the "Aunt Minnie" case will always be required and rewarded. In fact, it is far more embarrassing to miss an "Aunt Minnie" case than to not recognize an unusual and rare entity! So, we are confident that the original reason this book was conceived will continue to be a draw for medical students interested in a career in radiology, all levels of radiology residents, fellows in any subspecialty, and even academic and private practice radiologists who want an overall review of some of the most common and most recognizable entities in our subspecialty.

Finally, as any editor or author knows all too well, the publisher's contact editors are the "glue" that holds any project together, no matter what. Many thanks to LWW for initially providing Charley

Mitchell for the first edition of this book, Lisa McAllister and Ryan Shaw for editions two and three, and Amy Dinkel assisted by Mary Beth Murphy for this fourth revision. All of them have been a pleasure to work with and have the utmost in professional and personal attributes for the success of any project. Thank you all very, very much!

So, to our potential readers we say: Take a look at this fourth edition of Aunt Minnie's Atlas, browse the cases and figures, read a couple of chapters and attempt to grasp the concept of "Aunt Minnie." As always, if you see an error or omission, let us know as no human endeavor is perfect. We are all very proud of this product and hope that you will also be pleased with what you see and experience. Most important, however, just enjoy the learning experience, something that Dr. Felson and Dr. Wiot affirmed in their incredible academic careers and would have certainly wanted for you from this work. This is also precisely what I and all of our chapter authors' hope will be the end result of your interaction with Aunt Minnie 4.

ENJOY!!

*Thomas L. Pope, Jr., MD, FACR*

The idea to create this atlas was formed during a noon conference that I (K.F.) attended during the spring of my third year of radiology residency at the Bowman Gray School of Medicine. A visiting professor was conducting a didactic teaching conference and called on one of our brightest seniors to "take a case," proclaiming that the diagnosis was "somewhat of an Aunt Minnie." An audible groan erupted in the audience because we all understood what that statement meant. The senior resident would either "hit a home run" or "strike out" miserably in his interpretation of the case. All the residents had been introduced to the term Aunt Minnie during their training and knew the unwritten definition: a disease or condition that cannot be correctly diagnosed unless you have seen the case before. The resident looked carefully at the case and said: "I've never seen anything like this before, so I might as well take my seat." All of us felt sorry for the senior, because the visiting professor had no idea that this particular fourth year resident was one of the best in our program and rarely missed a case. It was this experience that planted the seed that a collection of Aunt Minnie's could be put into an imaging atlas format so that residents and practicing radiologist could be exposed to these unique cases in one easily obtainable source before they are encountered in conference or daily practice (or worse, in a visiting professor's teaching session!).

The concept, Aunt Minnie, is well known in North America and is practiced in every radiology department to some degree. The term was popularized by Ben Felson in the introduction of the first edition of his book, Fundamentals of Chest Roentgenology: "As she enters the room you say, 'Hello, Aunt Minnie.' But how do you know it's Aunt Minnie? 'Well,' you shrug, 'well—look at her. It's Aunt Minnie all right!'" (Felson B. Fundamentals of Chest Roentgenology, Philadelphia: Saunders, 1960). Thus, just as one would easily recognize his or her favorite aunt, the term refers to diseases or conditions that are diagnosed because of the specificity of the imaging findings.

The editors encountered many personal and regional variations in the definition of Aunt Minnie in preparing this text. The conservative school of thought believes that this diagnostic process can be applied only to plain films. The more liberal definition of the Aunt Minnie approach also includes cases where the imaging findings are correlated in a multimodality manner and interpreted in the context of the patient's clinical presentation to reach a specific diagnosis. To broaden the educational message of this text, we have chosen the liberal interpretation of Aunt Minnie in preparing this atlas (and this does not necessarily reflect the political leanings of either editor!). The inclusion of some cases that require historical information to appreciate the specificity of the imaging findings closely reflects the clinical practice of radiology and in no way artificially enhances the specificity of the diagnosis. These cases also emphasize to radiology trainees the importance of obtaining clinical information before rendering a final interpretation. To underscore the educational message contained in this text, the editors have chosen the title, Aunt Minnie's Atlas and Imaging-Specific Diagnosis, to encompass both the conservative and liberal definitions of the term. Thus if a specific case does not fit the reader's personal definition of an Aunt Minnie, the editors hope that the case can still be enjoyed as a nice example of an imaging-specific diagnosis.

Generating a table of contents was a big challenge for the editors, and we purposely recruited experienced academic radiologists as senior authors for each chapter to ensure credibility in case selection. Newer imaging modalities have greatly increased the number of diseases that radiologist confidently diagnose, and every effort has been made to include contemporary imaging without excluding plain-film Aunt Minnies. The atlas also emphasizes diagnoses that are encountered in everyday clinical practice and attempts to exclude obscure or clinically impractical cases. The text and the references that accompany each case are intentionally concise and include the essential and distinguishing features of each disease or condition. Diagnostic pitfalls are also discussed when appropriate, so the reader might avoid Aunt Minnie impostors.

At the end of each case are "Aunt Minnie's Pearls." These short vignettes are intended to emphasize the key features and "take home messages" of each case and also provide a mechanism for quick review of the atlas. All images were reproduced from original x-rays by computer digitization, ensuring the best quality and resolution. No image is altered or computer enhanced.

Finally, the editors realize that nothing in medicine is absolute, and many instances exist where an apparent Aunt Minnie diagnosis is shown to be incorrect. The reader should therefore not assume that most cases in radiology are amenable to the Aunt Minnie approach to diagnosis. Each case that one encounters should be systematically analyzed for diagnostic possibilities and potential pitfalls, and only after this careful process can the radiologist render an imaging-specific diagnosis.

The major educational objective of this book is to introduce the reader to a compilation of disease or conditions in which a confident diagnosis can be rendered based on the imaging findings and interpreted in the context of the patient's clinical presentation. Aunt Minnie's Atlas and Imaging-Specific Diagnosis is intended as a fun and informative educational tool that exposes readers to cases that would remain perplexing to all but the initiated. We hope you will enjoy the book and the experience.

Thanks to Sharon Meister, Nancy Ragland, and Donna Garrison at Bowman Gray for their excellent work editing the manuscript. Also, thanks to the numerous individuals at Bowman Gray and Mallinckrodt Institute of Radiology who unselfishly donated their favorite cases and time, and, finally, thanks to the Mallinckrodt Abdominal Imaging Section for supporting me (K.F.) fully in the preparation of this text.

*Kenneth L. Ford, iii*
*Thomas L. Pope, Jr.*

# CONTENTS

# CHAPTER 1

# PEDIATRICS

**Jeanne G. Hill / Paul Thacker / Anil G. Rao**

*The authors and editors acknowledge the contribution of the Chapter 1 author from the third edition: Paula Keslar, MD.*

HISTORY: A 3-day-old infant with acute onset of bilious vomiting

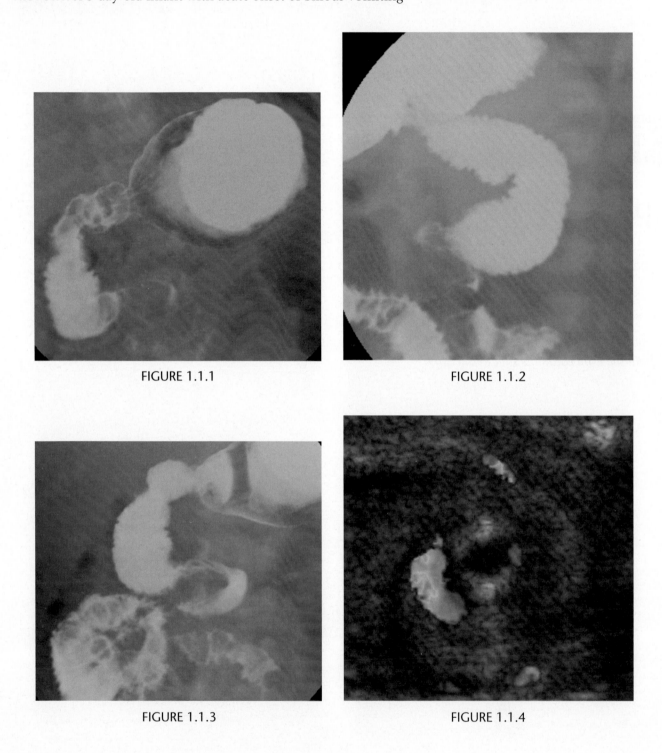

FIGURE 1.1.1

FIGURE 1.1.2

FIGURE 1.1.3

FIGURE 1.1.4

**FINDINGS:** Anteroposterior (AP; Fig. 1.1.1) and lateral (Fig. 1.1.2) views from an upper gastrointestinal series reveal partial duodenal obstruction, abnormal position of duodenal–jejunal junction (DJJ), and proximal small bowel in the right abdomen. A spiral or corkscrew configuration of the distal duodenum and proximal jejunum is also seen (Fig. 1.1.3). A sonographic image (Fig. 1.1.4) of the superior mesenteric artery (SMA) and vein (SMV) at the base of the small-bowel mesentery reveals a "whirlpool" pattern in which the SMV swirls around the SMA in a clockwise pattern.

**DIAGNOSIS:** Malrotation with midgut volvulus

**DISCUSSION:** Midgut malrotation complicated by midgut volvulus presents most frequently in the first month of life and is a true pediatric surgical emergency because of potential bowel ischemia and infarction. As plain films are unreliable for diagnosis or exclusion of midgut volvulus, an emergent upper gastrointestinal series with barium or nonionic water-soluble contrast medium is indicated to diagnose the duodenal obstruction and the abnormally positioned duodenal–jejunal junction (i.e., DJJ should be to the left of the spine and at the level of the bulb). The diagnosis of midgut volvulus may be made on ultrasound or computed tomography (CT) by identifying the characteristic "whirlpool sign" of the SMV wrapping around the SMA in a clockwise fashion. A Ladd's operation is performed to diagnose and reduce the volvulus, resect any dead bowel, and lyse dense, aberrant peritoneal bands, also known as Ladd's bands (1,2).

## Aunt Minnie's Pearls

Bilious vomiting in a newborn is malrotation with midgut volvulus until proven otherwise.

Check for abnormal position and appearance of the DJJ and proximal small bowel on upper gastrointestinal series, which is the gold standard for diagnosis.

"Whirlpool sign" of twisted mesenteric vessels on sonography or CT indicates a midgut volvulus.

**HISTORY:** Newborn with bilious vomiting, Down syndrome, and maternal polyhydramnios

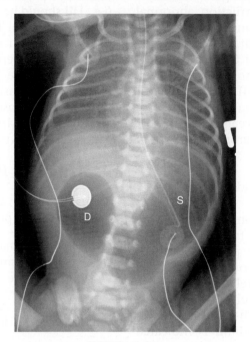

FIGURE 1.2.1

**FINDINGS:** The anteroposterior supine view of the chest and abdomen (Fig. 1.2.1) demonstrates a classic "double-bubble" sign: gaseous distention of the stomach (*S*) and an enlarged duodenal bulb or *mega bulb* (*D*). No intestinal gas is seen distal to the duodenum.

**DIAGNOSIS:** Duodenal atresia

**DISCUSSION:** Duodenal atresia is complete congenital intrinsic obstruction of the duodenum and is thought to result from failed recanalization. Approximately 30% of affected infants have Down syndrome (i.e., trisomy 21), 40% have maternal polyhydramnios, and 50% have some type of associated anomaly. Plain-film demonstration of the double-bubble sign is diagnostic and may be aided by injection of air through a nasogastric tube, as in the case presented. Upper gastrointestinal series is *not* indicated unless distal gas is present (i.e., partial duodenal obstruction exists). Distal gas requires further investigation for other etiologies of neonatal duodenal obstruction, such as duodenal stenosis or web, malrotation with Ladd's bands or volvulus, annular pancreas, or duplication cyst (3).

## Aunt Minnie's Pearl

A double-bubble sign without distal bowel gas is diagnostic of duodenal atresia.

**HISTORY:** A 3-month-old infant with altered mental status

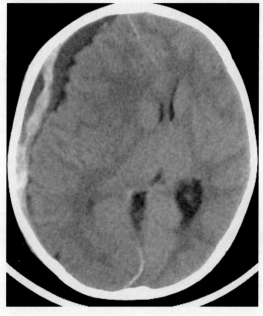

FIGURE 1.3.1

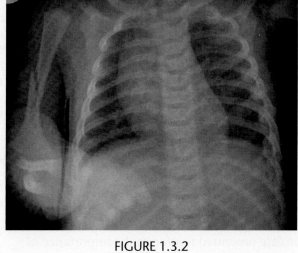

FIGURE 1.3.2

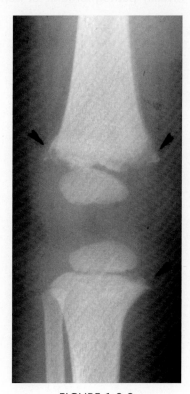

FIGURE 1.3.3

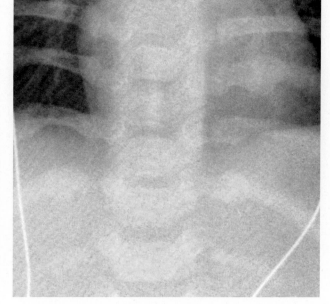

FIGURE 1.3.4

**FINDINGS:** An unenhanced axial CT reveals a right mixed-density subdural hematoma consistent with blood of varying ages (Fig. 1.3.1). The AP view of the chest reveals an acute spiral fracture of the right humerus, subacute fractures of the clavicles, and multiple healing rib fractures on the left (Fig. 1.3.2). Images from a skeletal survey reveal classic metaphyseal "corner" fractures of the medial proximal tibia (Fig. 1.3.3, *arrowheads*) as well as a "bucket-handle" fracture of the distal femoral metaphysis (Fig. 1.3.3, *arrowheads*). A coned down view of a follow-up chest x-ray (Fig. 1.3.4) obtained 2 weeks later reveals multiple healing posterior rib fractures that were not evident on the initial examination.

**DIAGNOSIS:** Non-accidental trauma

**DISCUSSION:** The classic metaphyseal corner and bucket-handle fractures are considered virtually pathognomonic of nonaccidental trauma (NAT) and result from indirectly applied shearing forces during shaking. These fractures are often subtle, and the case presented reinforces the importance of following suspicious areas on skeletal surveys with dedicated high-quality radiographs. On follow-up chest film (Fig. 1.3.4), multiple healing posterior rib fractures were identified in addition to the lateral fractures on the initial survey. Fractures of the posterior ribs at the junction of the transverse process of the vertebral body with the rib are highly specific for child abuse. It is thought that the forces generated by squeezing the chest of an infant while shaking are transferred along the course of the ribs, producing fractures in their lateral and posterior aspects. Shaken infants commonly present with seizures, lethargy, coma, retinal hemorrhages on funduscopic exam, and subdural hematomas caused by rupture of bridging veins from the cerebral cortex. All potentially abused infants with neurologic signs or symptoms should undergo an unenhanced CT of the brain (4,5).

## Aunt Minnie's Pearls

Metaphyseal corner and bucket-handle fractures are virtually pathognomonic of nonaccidental trauma.

Fractures of the posterior ribs at the junction of the transverse process of the adjacent vertebral body with the rib are virtually pathognomonic of nonaccidental trauma.

**HISTORY:** Newborn male infant with bilateral hydronephrosis detected in utero

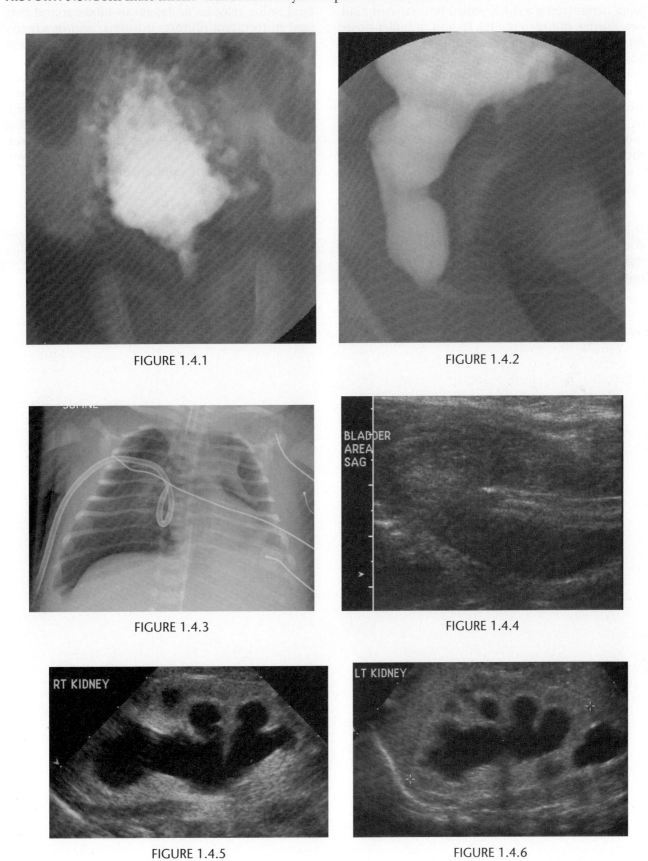

FIGURE 1.4.1

FIGURE 1.4.2

FIGURE 1.4.3

FIGURE 1.4.4

FIGURE 1.4.5

FIGURE 1.4.6

**FINDINGS:** Images during a voiding cystourethrogram demonstrate a thick-walled trabeculated bladder during filling (Fig. 1.4.1) and a bullet-nosed dilation of the posterior urethra (Fig. 1.4.2) with voiding. Shortly after birth, the patient had bilateral pneumothoraces and pulmonary hypoplasia (Fig. 1.4.3). Ultrasound examination reveals a markedly thickened bladder wall with a central catheter in place (Fig. 1.4.4) and bilateral hydronephrosis (Figs. 1.4.5 and 1.4.6) with loss of normal corticomedullary differentiation and cortical cysts.

**DIAGNOSIS:** Posterior urethral valves

**DISCUSSION:** Posterior urethral valves are the most common cause of bilateral hydronephrosis in a male infant. Affected infants may present with pulmonary hypoplasia and cystic renal dysplasia and a history of maternal oligohydramnios. Vesicoureteral reflux may be unilateral or bilateral and may lead to forniceal rupture, urinoma, and/or urinary ascites. Older children or adolescents may present with urinary tract infections, voiding difficulty, or end-stage renal disease. Type I valves are the most common and extend from the verumontanum distally, leaving a small eccentric opening posteriorly (Fig. 1.4.2) for the passage of urine. A voiding cystourethrogram is the test of choice for diagnosis. Treatment frequently involves early urinary diversion and subsequent valve ablation (6).

## Aunt Minnie's Pearls

Bullet-nosed dilatation of the posterior urethra and bilateral hydronephrosis in a male infant = posterior urethral valves.

# Case 1.5

**HISTORY:** A 1-year-old child with an abdominal mass, focal swelling of the right temple, anemia, and elevated urinary catecholamines

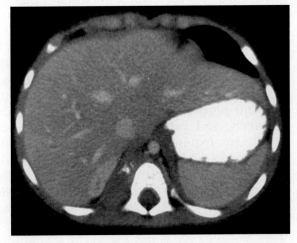

FIGURE 1.5.1

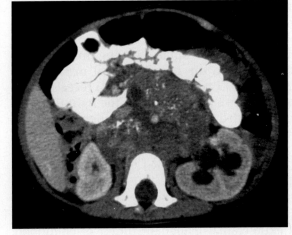

FIGURE 1.5.2

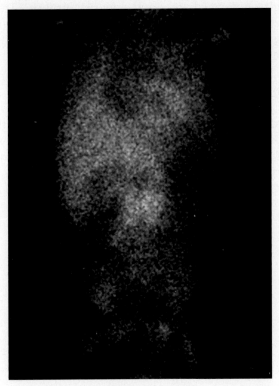

FIGURE 1.5.3

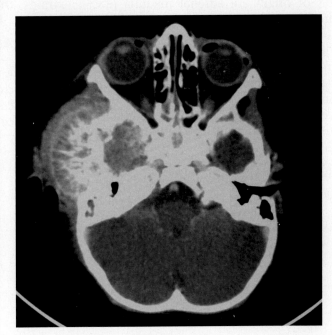

FIGURE 1.5.4

**FINDINGS:** IV contrast-enhanced CT images (Figs. 1.5.1 and 1.5.2) through the abdomen demonstrate a calcified right paraspinal mass; a large calcified retroperitoneal mass that crosses the midline, encasing the aorta and SMA; and left hydronephrosis. A delayed image from an meta-iodobenzylguanidine (MIBG) scan (Fig. 1.5.3) demonstrates increased uptake in the midabdomen corresponding to the retroperitoneal mass on CT. Head CT with IV contrast (Fig. 1.5.4) reveals a soft-tissue mass, with an epicenter in the right temporal bone, associated with bone destruction and a sunburst periosteal reaction.

**DIAGNOSIS:** Retroperitoneal neuroblastoma with skull metastases

**DISCUSSION:** Neuroblastoma is the most common solid extra-cranial malignant tumor of childhood. It is derived from primitive neural crest cells and, therefore, originates in the sympathetic chain ganglia and adrenal medulla. Two-thirds of cases arise in the abdomen, and two-thirds of abdominal tumors arise in the adrenal medulla. The most common sites of origin are adrenal medulla (35%), extra-adrenal retroperitoneum (30%–35%), and posterior mediastinum (20%). Tumors in the neck and pelvis (3%–8%) are much less common. Peak age of presentation is 22 months. At diagnosis, 60% to 70% of patients have metastatic disease with spread to cortical bone (in particular the skull), bone marrow, liver, and lymph nodes. The main challenge in imaging these tumors is differentiating neuroblastoma from Wilms tumor. Calcification, suprarenal location with a displaced but normal ipsilateral kidney, vessel encasement, retrocrural adenopathy, and extension across the midline are features that allow a confident diagnosis of neuroblastoma. Paraspinal tumor may invade the spinal canal via extension through adjacent neural foramina and is best evaluated with CT or magnetic resonance imaging (MRI). Although initial diagnosis is suspected when a calcified adrenal or paraspinal mass is identified on plain films and ultrasonography, CT of chest, abdomen, and pelvis, bone scans, MIBG scans, ± MRI are required for complete staging. MIBG (labeled with iodine-123) scintigraphy is sensitive and specific for catecholamine-secreting tumors; however, only 70% of neuroblastomas are MIBG-positive; therefore, normal results of MIBG do not exclude the diagnosis of neuroblastoma. Age and stage at diagnosis, *N-myc* oncogene amplification, DNA content, and Shimada histology are important prognostically and are used to stratify patients into high-, intermediate-, and low-risk groups. Treatment consists of chemotherapy and surgical debulking. Despite continued advancements in therapy, the prognosis remains poor (7).

## Aunt Minnie's Pearl

A childhood suprarenal mass with calcification that crosses the midline and encases the mesenteric vasculature and/or invades the neural foramina is almost certainly a neuroblastoma.

**HISTORY:** Newborn with respiratory distress during feedings and failure to pass a nasogastric tube

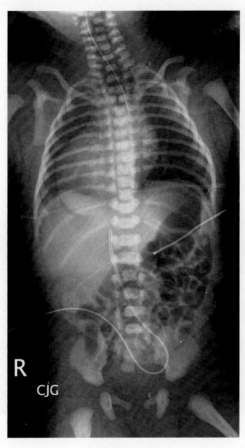

FIGURE 1.6.1

**FINDINGS:** Anteroposterior supine "babygram" (Fig. 1.6.1) reveals that the nasogastric tube terminates in a gas-filled proximal esophageal pouch. Bowel gas is present in the abdomen. The cardiac apex is in the right chest consistent with dextrocardia, and there are vertebral anomalies in the upper thoracic and sacral spine.

**DIAGNOSIS:** Esophageal atresia with tracheoesophageal fistula and vertebral and cardiac anomalies (VATER association)

**DISCUSSION:** The VATER association includes *ver*tebral and cardiovascular anomalies, *a*norectal malformations, *t*racheo*e*sophageal fistula, and *r*enal and *r*adial ray anomalies. The most common type of tracheoesophageal fistula is proximal esophageal atresia with a distal tracheoesophageal fistula, which is diagnosed on the basis of plain-radiographs demonstrating a feeding tube coiled in the proximal pouch with gas present distally. A barium "pouchogram" is not indicated, but the esophageal pouch can be made more conspicuous by injecting air through the nasogastric tube. Echocardiography and renal sonography are indicated to screen for congenital heart disease and renal anomalies, most commonly patent ductus arteriosus, ventricular septal defect, and renal agenesis. Complications of esophageal atresia with tracheoesophageal fistula include aspiration pneumonia, postoperative leak and stricture, recurrent fistula, disordered esophageal motility, gastroesophageal reflux, congenital esophageal stenosis, and tracheomalacia (8).

## Aunt Minnie's Pearls

In the proper clinical setting, esophageal atresia is diagnosed by failure to pass a nasogastric tube and visualization of an air-containing proximal esophageal pouch.

Always look for the VATER association in patients with esophageal atresia.

# Case 1.7

**HISTORY:** A 5-year-old child with a lap belt ecchymosis after a motor vehicle accident

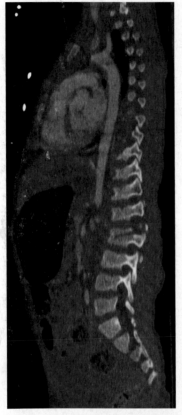

FIGURE 1.7.1

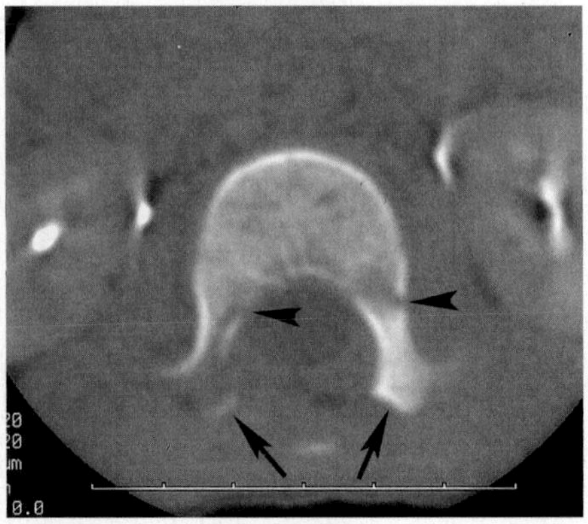

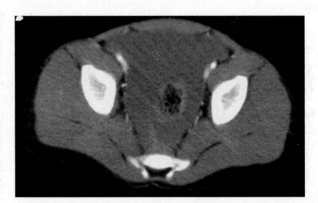

FIGURE 1.7.2

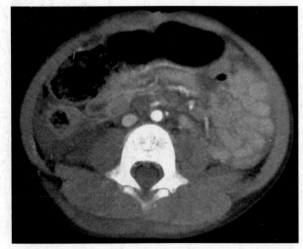

FIGURE 1.7.3

FIGURE 1.7.4

**FINDINGS:** A transverse fracture through the body and posterior elements as well as distraction and separation of the posterior elements of L2 vertebra without anterior compression are seen on a lateral reconstructed CT image of the thoracolumbar spine (Fig. 1.7.1). Axial CT of L2 (Fig. 1.7.2) demonstrates the "naked facet" sign or lack of opposing facets at L2 (*arrows*) and bilateral pedicle fractures (*arrowheads*). Contrast-enhanced abdominal and pelvic CT reveals bowel-wall thickening and retroperitoneal fluid (Fig. 1.7.3) as well as extensive free intraperitoneal fluid in the pelvis (Fig. 1.7.4).

**DIAGNOSIS:** Lap belt injury complex (lap belt ecchymosis, distraction fracture of the lumbar spine, and bowel injury)

**DISCUSSION:** In a sudden-deceleration accident, hyperflexion around the axis of a lap belt disrupts the posterior spinal ligaments and distracts the posterior elements, resulting in the "naked facet" sign. The anterior vertebral body is not compressed, but a horizontal fracture through the vertebral body (i.e., Chance fracture) may also occur as in this case. Injuries to bowel and abdominal viscera may dominate the clinical picture, and the unstable spine injury may be overlooked without lateral radiography. Manifestations of bowel injury on CT scans include bowel-wall enhancement, bowel-wall thickening, free fluid, free air, and extraluminal oral contrast. In this clinical setting, unexplained intraperitoneal fluid on CT is a bowel injury until proven otherwise (9).

## *Aunt Minnie's Pearls*

Lap belt injury complex = lap belt ecchymosis, distraction fracture of the lumbar spine, and bowel injury.

HISTORY: Newborn infant with acute decompensation

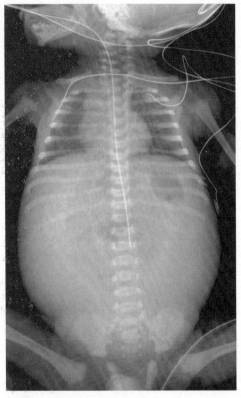

FIGURE 1.8.1

FINDINGS: Frontal supine radiograph of the chest and abdomen (Fig. 1.8.1) reveals a large oval-shaped lucency overlying the epigastrium. There is a vertical soft-tissue density running through the lucency.

DIAGNOSIS: Pneumoperitoneum

DISCUSSION: A large amount of free intraperitoneal gas on a supine radiograph of the abdomen is manifested by an oval radiolucency in the epigastrium, reminiscent of an American football. The reflections of the parietal peritoneum demarcate the edges of the football. As air rises to the most anterior portion of the abdominal cavity, it surrounds the falciform ligament and may form a vertical line within the lucency in the upper abdomen. Similarly, the median umbilical fold containing the urachal remnant and the medial and lateral umbilical folds containing the umbilical arteries and inferior epigastric vessels, respectively, may produce additional caudal vertical lines. Although these vertical lines were not included in the original description, other authors have described them as the "laces" or "seams" of the football and thus, an integral part of the "football sign." Typically, the football sign is seen in neonates and infants. The most common cause is spontaneous or iatrogenic gastric perforation, although it may be the consequence of a congenital bowel obstruction or necrotizing enterocolitis (10).

## Aunt Minnie's Pearls

The football sign, seen on a supine abdominal radiograph, is indicative of a massive pneumoperitoneum.

# Case 1.9

**HISTORY:** A 6-month-old with fever, stridor, and dysphagia

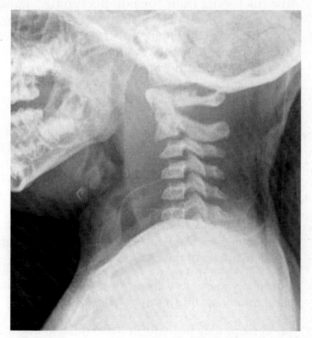

FIGURE 1.9.1

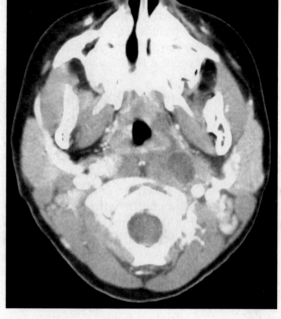

FIGURE 1.9.2

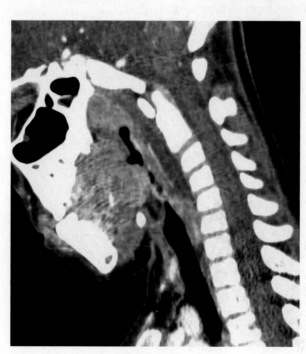

FIGURE 1.9.3

**FINDINGS:** Lateral radiograph of the neck reveals marked thickening of the retropharyngeal soft tissues with a convex anterior border (Fig. 1.9.1). Contrast-enhanced axial CT of the neck reveals a low-density, rim-enhancing region in the left lateral retropharyngeal soft tissues (Fig. 1.9.2) and a low-density region in the retropharyngeal soft tissues on the sagittal reconstruction (Fig. 1.9.3).

**DIAGNOSIS:** Retropharyngeal abscess and cellulitis

**DISCUSSION:** Typically, a retropharyngeal abscess is the sequela of a recent upper respiratory infection, most commonly *Staphylococcus aureus or Group A beta-hemolytic Streptococcus*. Less commonly, it may be caused by a foreign body. On lateral views of the neck, there is thickening of the retropharyngeal soft tissues and reversal of the normal cervical lordosis. The presence of gas in those tissues is diagnostic of an abscess; however, this is infrequent. The thickness of the soft tissues between the anterior edge of the cervical spine and the posterior aspect of the aerated pharynx should be no more than the AP diameter of the cervical vertebral bodies. Unfortunately, expiration and lack of extension can produce the appearance of thickening of the retropharyngeal soft tissues. Although repeat radiographs in full extension and inspiration can be helpful in differentiating true thickening from "pseudo-thickening," fluoroscopy of the lateral neck definitively clarifies the difficult cases as pathologic soft-tissue thickening will persist throughout the respiratory cycle, and in all patient positions; however, pseudo-thickening will not. CT is used to differentiate cellulitis, characterized by soft-tissue swelling, from an abscess, characterized by a discrete, focal fluid collection with rim enhancement. CT also defines the extent of disease and involvement of adjacent structures, such as the airway and mediastinum, and enables localization of a fluid collection for subsequent drainage (11).

## Aunt Minnie's Pearls

Retropharyngeal soft tissues should be no thicker than the AP diameter of the cervical vertebral bodies.

Retropharyngeal soft-tissue thickening with gas is pathognomonic of a retropharyngeal abscess.

Fluoroscopy may be useful in differentiating true thickening from "pseudo-thickening" of the retropharyngeal soft tissues.

**HISTORY:** A 32-week-old, 1,500 g premature infant with abdominal distension, increased gastric residuals, and thrombocytopenia on day 6 of life

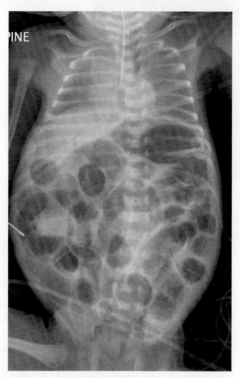

FIGURE 1.10.1

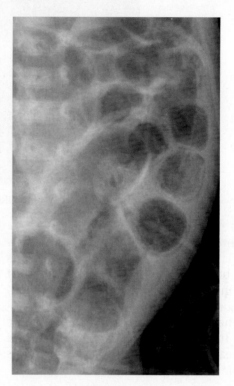

FIGURE 1.10.2

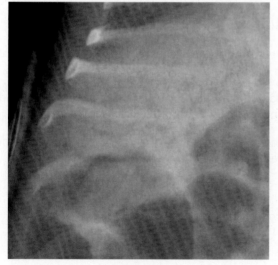

FIGURE 1.10.3

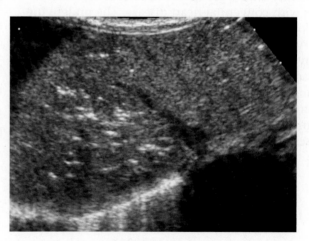

FIGURE 1.10.4

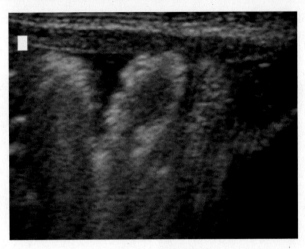

FIGURE 1.10.5

**FINDINGS:** Anteroposterior supine film of the abdomen (Fig. 1.10.1) demonstrates diffuse gaseous distention of bowel, linear and crescentic areas of pneumatosis intestinalis (Fig. 1.10.2), and branching lucencies of portal venous gas (Fig. 1.10.3). Sonography of the liver (Fig. 1.10.4) reveals echogenic foci bubbling through the liver. Sonography of the abdomen reveals free fluid between bowel loops with echogenic walls (Fig. 1.10.5).

**DIAGNOSIS:** Necrotizing enterocolitis

**DISCUSSION:** Necrotizing enterocolitis (NEC) most frequently affects premature infants or full-term infants with congenital heart disease. The underlying pathophysiology is multifactorial, but the mucosal injury probably results from ischemia compounded by hyperosmolar feedings and infection. The earliest radiographic signs are nonspecific dilatation and separation of loops. Pneumatosis and portal venous gas indicating severe disease appear subsequently. Submucosal air demonstrates a bubbly appearance. Subserosal pneumatosis manifests as crescentic rings and linear lucencies paralleling the bowel lumen. Sonographically, one may see thick-walled fluid-filled aperistaltic loops. Pneumatosis demonstrates intense intramural echoes with acoustic shadowing. Punctate echogenicities moving through the portal vein and its branches in the direction of blood flow are characteristic of portal venous gas. Pneumoperitoneum, ascites, or both signal perforation and the need for surgical intervention. The mortality rate in children with NEC approaches 40%. Colonic strictures, typically in the left colon, are a common late complication in survivors (12,13).

## Aunt Minnie's Pearls

Necrotizing enterocolitis occurs in premature infants or full-term infants with congenital heart disease.

Plain-film findings of NEC are dilated bowel loops, pneumatosis, and portal venous gas.

Pneumoperitoneum, ascites, or both indicate bowel perforation and the need for immediate surgery.

**HISTORY:** Full-term infant with progressive respiratory distress

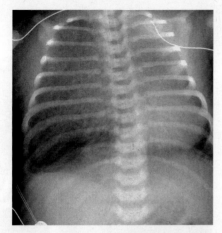

FIGURE 1.11.1

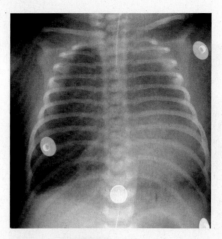

FIGURE 1.11.2

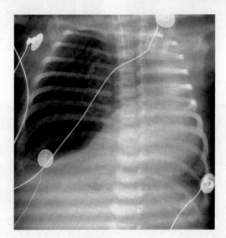

FIGURE 1.11.3

**FINDINGS:** A series of chest films obtained from day 1 to day 4 of life demonstrate initial opacification of the right upper lobe (Fig. 1.11.1), which subsequently becomes interstitial or reticular (Fig. 1.11.2) and finally hyperlucent (Fig. 1.11.3). Right-to-left mediastinal shift and progressive right middle and lower lobe collapse are also identified.

**DIAGNOSIS:** Congenital lobar emphysema of right upper lobe

**DISCUSSION:** Mediastinal shift is the hallmark of "surgical" causes of neonatal respiratory distress. The etiology of congenital lobar emphysema remains unclear. In most cases, congenital lobar emphysema is associated with an intrinsic ball-valve obstruction in the affected bronchus. The result is progressive air trapping with mediastinal shift and compressive atelectasis of adjacent lobes. The initial opacification of the affected lobe results from impaired drainage of fetal lung fluid. The upper lobes and the right middle lobe are most frequently affected. Differentiation of congenital lobar emphysema from other surgical lesions of the lung in newborns (sequestration and cystic adenomatoid malformation) requires recognition of the characteristic location and temporal evolution of this abnormality. Infants with severe respiratory distress are treated by lobectomy, whereas functional assessment with ventilation–perfusion scanning and nonsurgical management may be indicated in less severely affected infants (14).

## Aunt Minnie's Pearls

Progressive air trapping in the middle or either upper lobe in a newborn = congenital lobar emphysema.

Although it will become hyperlucent within days, the affected lobe may initially be opacified owing to retained fetal lung fluid.

# Case 1.12

**HISTORY:** An 8-year-old female with history of recurrent right lung pneumonias that does not ever clear completely.

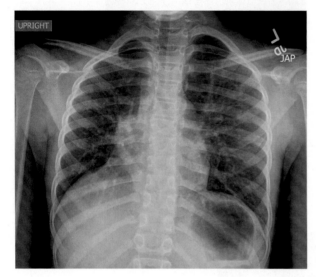

FIGURE 1.12.1

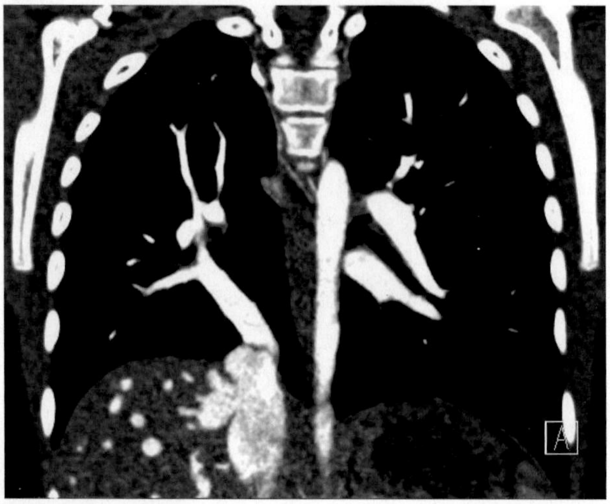

FIGURE 1.12.2

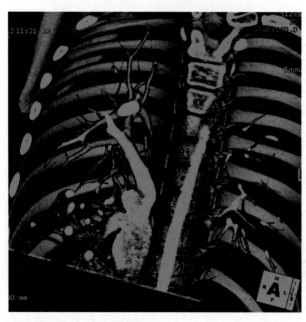

FIGURE 1.12.3

**FINDINGS:** Frontal radiograph of the chest (Fig. 1.12.1) reveals the heart to be shifted to the right, the right hemidiaphragm to be elevated, and the right heart border to be indistinct. There is a linear density pointing inferomedially in the right hemithorax to the medial right hemidiaphragm. Coronal (Fig. 1.12.2) and 3D reconstructions of chest CT with IV contrast (Fig. 1.12.3) reveal a large vessel draining the right pulmonary veins into the inferior vena cava (IVC) just below the hemidiaphragm.

**DIAGNOSIS:** Scimitar syndrome

**DISCUSSION:** Scimitar, or congenital venolobar, syndrome is a rare congenital anomaly classically characterized by right-sided anomalous pulmonary venous return below the diaphragm, right pulmonary hypoplasia, and dextroposition of the heart secondary to shift of the heart and mediastinum toward the hypoplastic lung. The eponym "scimitar" refers to the shape of the anomalous pulmonary vein on the frontal chest radiograph, which is reminiscent of the curved Turkish scimitar sword. In the majority of the patients with scimitar syndrome, the unilateral anomalous pulmonary venous drainage is total, whereas in approximately one-third, the anomalous vein drains only the lower portion of the lung. Typically, the anomalous vein drains into the subdiaphragmatic IVC, as in this example, but may drain into an hepatic vein, low in the right atrium, or even the portal vein. Seldom has the scimitar vein been described in the left lung.

Presentation is highly variable but has a bimodal distribution in infancy and later pediatric or adult life. The incidence is 2 per 100,000, and females are more commonly affected (2:1) than males. The infant with scimitar syndrome may present with tachypnea, recurrent pneumonia, failure to thrive, or heart failure. The infantile form has a higher incidence of morbidity and mortality secondary to numerous associated reported cardiovascular abnormalities (75% incidence in neonates as opposed to 36% in the older pediatric age group). The following cardiovascular anomalies in addition to the scimitar vein in order of descending frequency have been commonly reported: hypoplasia of the right pulmonary artery, systemic arterial supply to the right lung from infradiaphragmatic aorta, and secundum atrial septal defect. Noncardiovascular anomalies include pulmonary sequestration, right-sided diaphragmatic hernia, and horseshoe lung. The older child or adult may be relatively asymptomatic and the diagnosis made incidentally, have milder pulmonary symptoms or, as in this case, have a history of recurrent pneumonias.

Diagnosis is typically made by the characteristic plain-film findings. In cases with marked dextroposition of the heart, the scimitar vein, however, may be obscured or misinterpreted. CT is very helpful in delineating the anomalous venous drainage and other associated anomalies. In the symptomatic patients, cardiac catheterization is utilized to evaluate venous and arterial anatomy, potential areas of stenosis, and to measure pulmonary pressures.

For patients who are asymptomatic or only mildly symptomatic, conservative medical management is appropriate. Patients with infantile scimitar syndrome, heart failure, or pulmonary hypertension may require surgical intervention, typically consisting of redirection of the scimitar vein to the left atrium. The presence of pulmonary hypertension may necessitate embolization or surgical ligation of anomalous systemic arteries, and, in the setting of recurrent pulmonary infections, resection of the affected portions of the right lung (15,16).

## Aunt Minnie's Pearls

Scimitar syndrome is characterized by anomalous right pulmonary venous drainage (the scimitar vein), right pulmonary hypoplasia, and dextroposition of the heart.

The sine qua non of scimitar syndrome is the scimitar vein, which passes from superolateral position to inferomedial position in the right chest.

In general, the prognosis of the infantile form of scimitar syndrome is much poorer than that of patients who present in later childhood or even adulthood because of the increased incidence and severity of associated anomalies in the infantile form.

**HISTORY:** Full-term neonate with the classic obstructive triad of bilious vomiting, abdominal distention, and failure to pass meconium.

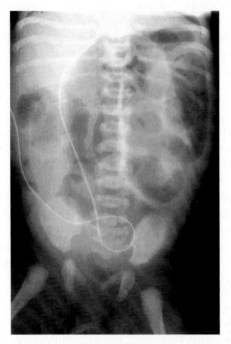

FIGURE 1.13.1

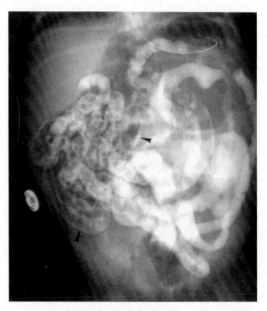

FIGURE 1.13.2

**FINDINGS:** Anteroposterior supine (Fig. 1.13.1) view of the abdomen demonstrates numerous dilated loops of bowel. A contrast enema (Fig. 1.13.2) reveals a microcolon and numerous filling defects in the ileum (*arrows*).

**DIAGNOSIS:** Meconium ileus

**DISCUSSION:** Meconium ileus is the neonatal presentation of cystic fibrosis. Hydramnios and a family history of cystic fibrosis may be present. With simple meconium ileus, abnormally viscid meconium obstructs the ileum, and a water-soluble contrast enema with ileal reflux to the level of the dilated loops can relieve the impaction. This disorder is said to produce the smallest of all microcolons because the obstructing meconium causes the colon to be completely unused. In nearly half of cases, meconium ileus may be complicated by volvulus, atresia, stenosis, perforation, peritonitis, or pseudocyst formation. Complicated meconium ileus may present early, and severe abdominal distension and respiratory distress may require corrective surgery (17). A similar diagnosis may be made in older children with cystic fibrosis where viscid stool obstructs the ileum and cecum. This disorder is known as *meconium ileus equivalent*.

## Aunt Minnie's Pearls

Meconium ileus is diagnostic of cystic fibrosis.

Meconium ileus produces the smallest of all microcolons.

A water-soluble contrast enema is diagnostic and therapeutic in uncomplicated cases.

HISTORY: Newborn with abdominal distension

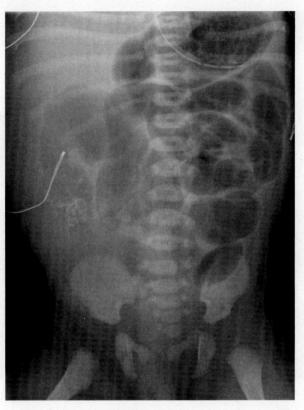

FIGURE 1.14.1

FINDINGS: AP supine radiograph of the abdomen (Fig. 1.14.1) reveals a collection of calcifications in the right lower quadrant and multiple dilated air-filled loops of bowel without definite gas in rectum, consistent with a distal bowel obstruction.

DIAGNOSIS: Meconium peritonitis

DISCUSSION: Meconium peritonitis is the result of in utero perforation and prenatal leak of meconium into the peritoneal cavity. The underlying etiology varies but includes obstruction or malformation, although obstructive lesions are identified in only 50% of the cases. Meconium peritonitis usually results in intraperitoneal calcification that may be focal or scattered, diffuse or punctuate, or may outline the walls of a pseudocyst, which contains meconium. Additional findings vary with the underlying cause but include bowel obstruction, mass, or distension. Sonographically, meconium peritonitis may be diagnosed prenatally or postnatally by the presence of focal or scattered areas of hyperechogenicity consistent with calcifications or of a cystic mass containing echogenic meconium with hyperechoic rim. Treatment and prognosis depend on the etiology. Calcification will gradually disappear over months or years (18).

## Aunt Minnie's Pearl

Scattered or focal, punctuate peritoneal calcifications or a calcified pseudocyst in a newborn = *shape in utero* bowel perforation and meconium peritonitis.

HISTORY: A 1-year-old immigrant child with growth failure

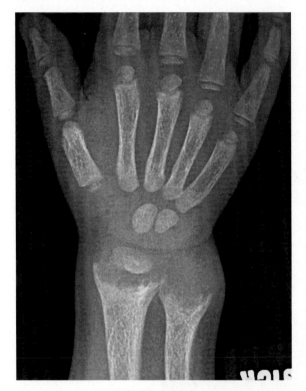

FIGURE 1.15.1

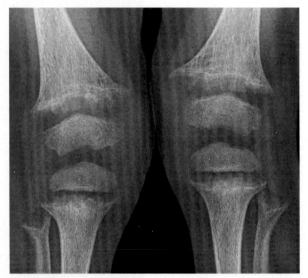

FIGURE 1.15.2

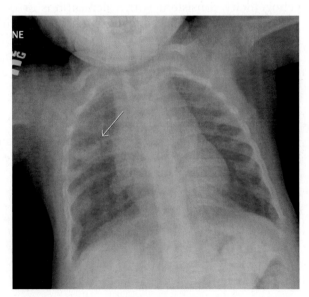

FIGURE 1.15.3

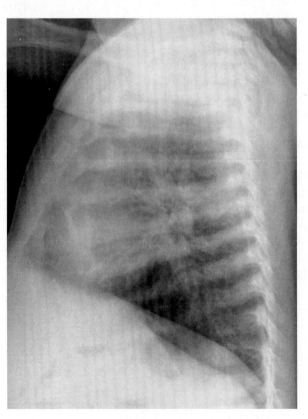

FIGURE 1.15.4

**FINDINGS:** Metaphyseal cupping, fraying, and splaying are demonstrated on AP views of the wrist (Fig. 1.15.1) and knees (Fig. 1.15.2). Also apparent is loss of the zone of provisional calcification—seen radiographically as widening of the physes and loss of the epiphyseal and metaphyseal margins. The visualized skeleton shows diffuse coarse demineralization. AP (Fig. 1.15.3) and lateral (Fig. 1.15.4) views of the chest reveal cupping and fraying of the costochondral junctions and proximal humeral metaphyses.

**DIAGNOSIS:** Rickets

**DISCUSSION:** Deficient mineralization of osteoid in children is known as *rickets*, whereas in adults the same pathologic process is osteomalacia. Many types and causes of rickets result in this classic Aunt Minnie appearance. Rachitic changes on radiographs reflect a relative or absolute deficiency of vitamin D or its hormonally active derivative 1,25-dihydroxycholecalciferol. Remembering that the biosynthetic pathway of vitamin D involves skin, gut, liver, and kidney assists formulation of a basic differential diagnosis. Other pathologic processes in the gut or kidneys that result in calcium or phosphorus wasting can also result in rickets.

Because rachitic changes are best visualized at the ends of the most rapidly growing bones, a rickets survey routinely includes views of the wrists and knees. In addition to the metaphyseal cupping and fraying and loss of the zone of provisional calcification producing widened physes, long bones may demonstrate bowing deformities as well. Cupping and fraying of the costochondral junctions, which are metaphyseal equivalents, create palpable masses on the anterior chest wall likened to the beads of a rosary. Rickets is seldom encountered before 6 months of age in full-term infants, and most cases are diagnosed before the patient is 2 years old (19).

## Aunt Minnie's Pearls

In rickets, the metaphyses are cupped, frayed, and splayed.

Vitamin D deficiency causes poor osteoid mineralization and widening of the physes.

HISTORY: Obese black male adolescent with pain in the right hip

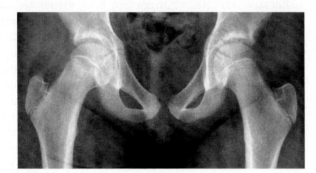

FIGURE 1.16.1

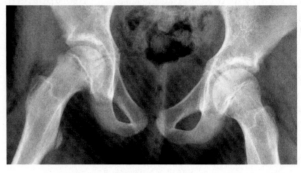

FIGURE 1.16.2

FINDINGS: An AP view of the pelvis (Fig. 1.16.1) shows widening of the right proximal femoral physis, metaphyseal irregularity, and regional osteopenia. Lines drawn along the lateral femoral necks would intersect less femoral epiphysis on the right than on the left. The frog-leg lateral view (Fig. 1.16.2) reveals posterior and medial displacement of the epiphysis relative to the metaphysis, producing the classic appearance of "ice cream falling off the cone."

DIAGNOSIS: Slipped capital femoral epiphysis (SCFE)

DISCUSSION: SCFE, a Salter–Harris type I fracture of the proximal growth plate of the femur, is usually encountered during the adolescent growth spurt. Black (male or female) and male (of any race) patients are most commonly affected. Children with SCFE are usually overweight and present with hip pain, limp, or referred knee pain. Younger and older presentations suggest hypothyroidism, hypopituitarism, and prior radiotherapy. Both hips are affected in approximately 25% of patients.

Anteroposterior and frog-leg lateral radiographs of the hips should be obtained in suspected cases of SCFE. A line, also known as Klein's line, drawn along the lateral edge of the femoral neck should bisect at least one-sixth of the femoral epiphysis on an AP view. If the line intersects less than this amount, SCFE should be suspected. As the primary direction of slippage is posterior and medial, the frog-leg lateral view may show the epiphyseal displacement to best advantage.

SCFE is a true orthopedic emergency, and the goal of treatment is to prevent further slippage by internal fixation. Complications of SCFE include avascular necrosis, chondrolysis, varus deformity with femoral neck shortening, and early degenerative osteoarthritis. The epiphysis is fixated in the position it is found in because attempts to reduce the epiphysis increase the risk of avascular necrosis (20).

## Aunt Minnie's Pearls

SCFE occurs most frequently in adolescent males, and 25% of cases are bilateral.

SCFE is an orthopedic emergency, and the epiphysis is pinned "as is" to prevent further slippage.

**HISTORY:** A 1-year-old with acute onset of wheezing

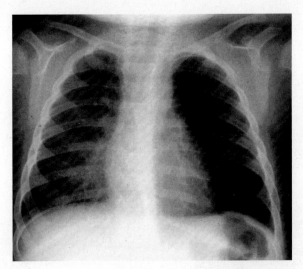

FIGURE 1.17.1

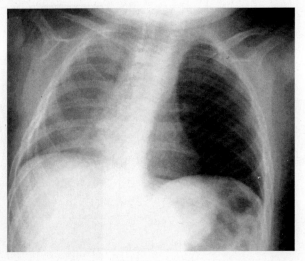

FIGURE 1.17.2

**FINDINGS:** AP chest radiograph (Fig. 1.17.1) demonstrates slight increased lucency of the left hemithorax. A film obtained during expiration (Fig. 1.17.2) shows impressive left-to-right mediastinal shift and unilateral left-sided air trapping.

**DIAGNOSIS:** Foreign body (Palmetto bug) in the left main stem bronchus

**DISCUSSION:** Foreign bodies in the lower airway are a commonly encountered pediatric problem, particularly in children younger than 3 years. The child may present acutely with cough, respiratory distress, and wheezing or more insidiously with fever, cough, recurrent pneumonia, pneumomediastinum, or pneumothorax. Peanuts are the most common foreign body to be aspirated, and bronchial impaction occurs more frequently on the right than on the left. The affected lung may be collapsed, normally aerated, or emphysematous. Inspiratory views alone have a normal appearance in 20% of patients, necessitating an expiratory view of the chest or chest fluoroscopy. Decubitus views in the uncooperative child may replace inspiratory/expiratory views. In the presence of an obstructing foreign body, the dependent lung fails to collapse. Routine radiologic evaluation can still be normal in up to 30% of children with proven lower-airway foreign bodies, hence the need for bronchoscopy in any child with strong clinical suspicion and negative films. CT may reveal the presence and location of an aspirated foreign body when initial imaging studies and bronchoscopy are negative (21).

## Aunt Minnie's Pearls

Foreign-body aspiration is most common in children younger than 3 years.

Unilateral air trapping during expiration is diagnostic in the appropriate clinical setting.

Chest fluoroscopy or decubitus views may be very useful in identifying air trapping in the uncooperative child.

Even in the absence of radiologic findings, bronchoscopy is recommended when there is a strong clinical suspicion of foreign-body aspiration.

HISTORY: Newborn with severe respiratory distress

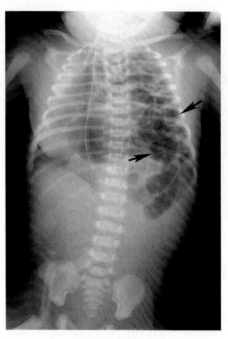

FIGURE 1.18.1

FINDINGS: AP chest and abdomen film (Fig. 1.18.1) shows marked left-to-right shift of the heart, mediastinum, and support apparatus. The left side of the chest contains multiple tubular radiolucencies (*arrows*), and the abdomen is gasless.

DIAGNOSIS: Congenital diaphragmatic hernia, Bochdalek type

DISCUSSION: Congenital Bochdalek-type diaphragmatic hernia is a common surgical cause of neonatal respiratory distress. Herniation of abdominal contents occurs through a posterolateral diaphragmatic defect or persistent pleuroperitoneal canal. It is convenient to remember that *Bochdalek* hernias occur in the *back*, are more common on the left than right, and are associated with a scaphoid, gasless abdomen. Intestinal malrotation is present in all cases. The degree of associated pulmonary hypoplasia and persistent fetal circulation from pulmonary hypertension determines prognosis and management. Delayed appearance of diaphragmatic hernias is often right-sided and may be idiopathic or may be associated with previous group B streptococcal pneumonia. Sonography is useful for both prenatal and postnatal diagnosis of diaphragmatic hernia. On prenatal sonograms, the presence of the stomach bubble adjacent to the heart on a true transverse image should alert the radiologist to this diagnosis (22).

## Aunt Minnie's Pearls

The presence of bowel in the left chest in a newborn is diagnostic of a congenital diaphragmatic hernia.

Older infants with right-sided hernias often have a history of previous group B streptococcal pneumonia.

On a transverse obstetrical ultrasound image, look for the stomach bubble adjacent to the heart to suggest this diagnosis.

HISTORY: One-hour-old newborn with abnormal prenatal ultrasound

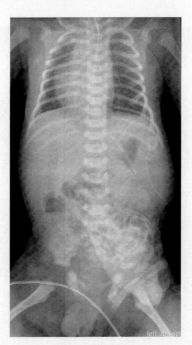

FIGURE 1.19.1

FINDINGS: AP chest and abdomen radiograph (Fig. 1.19.1) reveals an endotracheal tube and enteric tube to be in appropriate position. The apex of the cardiothymic silhouette is on the right. The stomach is noted to be on the left. There is a soft-tissue mass overlying the mid abdomen with indistinct superior margins and sharply defined inferior and lateral margins. The mass appears to contain bowel gas. An umbilical clip is noted at the inferior extent of the mass. The bowel gas pattern is not distended, and there is no evidence of free intraperitoneal air.

DIAGNOSIS: Omphalocele

DISCUSSION: Omphalocele is a congenital ventral abdominal defect in which abdominal contents, primarily bowel and sometimes liver, are herniated outside the abdominal wall and are covered by a sac. The defect is in the midline and invariably the umbilical cord inserts into the omphalocele sac as this anomaly is the result of failure of bowel to return to the abdomen after its normal developmental herniation into the umbilical cord during gestation from 6th to 10th weeks . Although maternal serum alpha fetoprotein levels may be elevated, omphalocele is most commonly diagnosed by prenatal ultrasound. The incidence is 1 in 4,000 live births. There is a high association (50%–70%) of structural or chromosomal abnormalities, primarily trisomies. The most commonly associated structural abnormalities are cardiac (30%–50%) but other VATERL anomalies and the potentially life-threatening anomalies of the central nervous system—hydrancephaly and holoprosencephaly—have been reported. Omphaloceles may be small or gigantic, and they may occur in the setting of syndromes, the most common one being Beckwith Weideman syndrome, comprising macroglossia, organomegaly, and hypoglycemia in addition to the omphalocele. These patients are also at increased risk for Wilm's, hepatoblastoma, and neuroblastoma in later childhood.

Surgical correction may be accomplished with primary (if small) or staged closure of the abdominal wall defect. Flaps, tissue expanders, and mesh patches have been utilized to achieve closure of the defect. The long-term outcome of the child with omphalocele is dependent on the type and severity of the associated anomalies (23,24).

## Aunt Minnie's Pearls

Omphalocele is a midline ventral abdominal wall defect in which abdominal contents are herniated into the base of the umbilical cord.

Associated anomalies (both structural and chromosomal anomalies) are extremely common (50%–70%) and are the primary determinant of prognosis and outcome in patients with omphalocele.

HISTORY: One-hour-old newborn with abnormal prenatal ultrasound

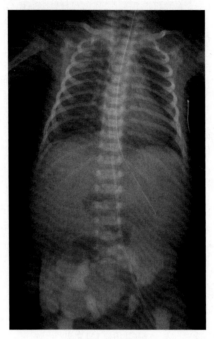

FIGURE 1.20.1

FINDINGS: AP chest and abdomen radiograph (Fig. 1.20.1) reveals an umbilical venous catheter with the tip overlying the right atrium and an enteric tube in the stomach. There is paucity of bowel gas in nondistended loops overlying the midabdomen. There is no evidence of free intraperitoneal air. There are well-circumscribed fingerlike masses overlying the right lower quadrant and pelvis.

DIAGNOSIS: Gastroschisis

DISCUSSION: Gastroschisis is a defect in the anterior abdominal wall typically located to the right of a normal umbilicus consisting of variable amounts of eviscerated bowel that is not contained within a sac or membrane. Although multiple theories have been proposed, the etiology of gastroschisis remains unclear. There is an association with young maternal age, <20 years of age. In addition, the incidence of gastroschisis—3 to 4 per 10,000 births—is increasing without identifiable cause. As in most newborns with congenital anomalies there is an increased incidence of other anomalies, typically of bowel. Approximately 10% of patients with gastroschisis have bowel atresia or stenosis secondary to vascular insufficiency. In contrast with omphalocele, chromosomal anomalies are uncommon (Table 1.20.1).

The diagnosis of gastroschisis may be made prenatally by ultrasound when loops of bowel are identified floating in the amniotic fluid after the 10th week of gestation. Maternal serum alpha fetoprotein, better known as a screening test for chromosomal abnormalities and neural tube defects, is commonly elevated in this disorder and therefore, may be the first indication of gastroschisis.

Treatment consists of surgical closure of the abdominal wall defect without injury to the herniated bowel. It may be performed immediately after delivery or delayed, and abdominal wall closure achieved primarily or in stages.

Prognosis is ultimately determined by the amount of in utero damage to the intestine but overall survival is 90% to 95%. Patients with gastroschisis are typically slow to tolerate feeds and may develop long-term feeding intolerance owing to dysmotility and impaired mucosal absorption. It is interesting to note that term infants with gastroschisis are at increased risk for the development of necrotizing enterocolitis, manifested by pneumatosis intestinalis, which tends to have an uncomplicated outcome. In the long term, children with gastroschisis are at risk for adhesive bowel obstruction, but most of them ultimately enjoy normal growth and development (23,24).

Table 1.20.1 Abdominal Wall Defects: Omphalocele versus Gastroschisis

|  | Omphalocele | Gastroschisis |
| --- | --- | --- |
| Peritoneal sac | Present | Absent |
| Location of defect | Midline | Right of midline |
| Involvement of umbilical cord (UC) | Yes, UC inserts into omphalocele membrane | No, UC inserts normally |
| Herniated organs | Bowel and sometimes liver | Bowel only |
| Associated anomalies | Common | Uncommon |
| Maternal age | Average | Young (teenagers) |
| Prognostic factors | Associated anomalies | Condition of bowel |

## Aunt Minnie's Pearl

Gastroschisis is a defect in the abdominal wall typically to the right of a normal umbilicus consisting of variable amounts of herniated bowel.

The bowel loops in gastroschisis are not contained in a peritoneal sac.

Prognosis depends on the condition of the herniated bowel.

HISTORY: A 6-week-old full-term infant with constipation

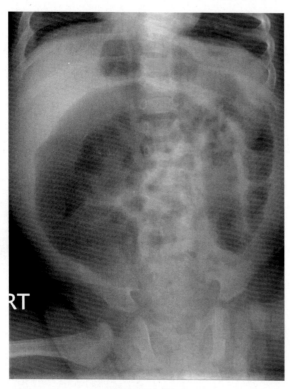

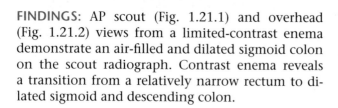

FIGURE 1.21.1

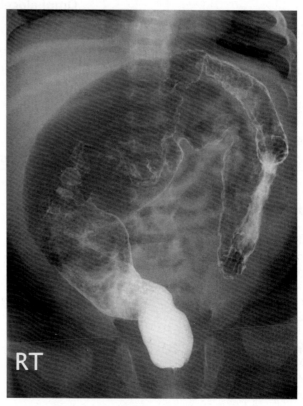

FIGURE 1.21.2

FINDINGS: AP scout (Fig. 1.21.1) and overhead (Fig. 1.21.2) views from a limited-contrast enema demonstrate an air-filled and dilated sigmoid colon on the scout radiograph. Contrast enema reveals a transition from a relatively narrow rectum to dilated sigmoid and descending colon.

DIAGNOSIS: Hirschsprung disease

DISCUSSION: Hirschsprung disease is a functional colonic obstruction characterized by an aganglionic hypertonic distal segment of bowel with associated proximal dilation. Radiographic demonstration of the transition zone between the dilated proximal ganglionic bowel and the nondilated distal aganglionic bowel is the most reliable diagnostic finding of Hirschsprung disease. Other roentgen findings include an abnormal rectosigmoid index (a fancy term to signify that the sigmoid should not be bigger than the rectum), a corrugated or saw-toothed rectosigmoid, and delayed evacuation of contrast medium. Enemas in these patients should be performed without bowel preparation to prevent false-negative studies.

Eighty percent of patients with Hirschsprung disease present during the first 6 weeks of life, and these patients account for 20% of all cases of neonatal bowel obstruction. Short-segment disease accounts for 80% of cases, has a rectosigmoid transition zone, and exhibits a male predominance. Long-segment disease accounts for 15% of cases and mimics small left colon meconium plug syndrome (therefore this variant is not an Aunt Minnie). Total colonic aganglionosis accounts for 5% of cases, can be familial, and has no sex predilection. Uncommon but severe complications of Hirschsprung disease include fulminant enterocolitis and bowel perforation (25).

## Aunt Minnie's Pearls

Eighty percent of patients with Hirschsprung disease present in the first 6 weeks of life.

Contrast enemas reveal the transition point between the aganglionic distal segment and the dilated proximal bowel.

Perform enemas without bowel preparation to diagnose this disorder.

# Case 1.22

**HISTORY:** A 10-month-old boy evaluated in the emergency room for abdominal distention and bilious vomiting

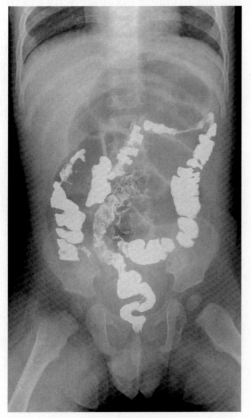

FIGURE 1.22.1

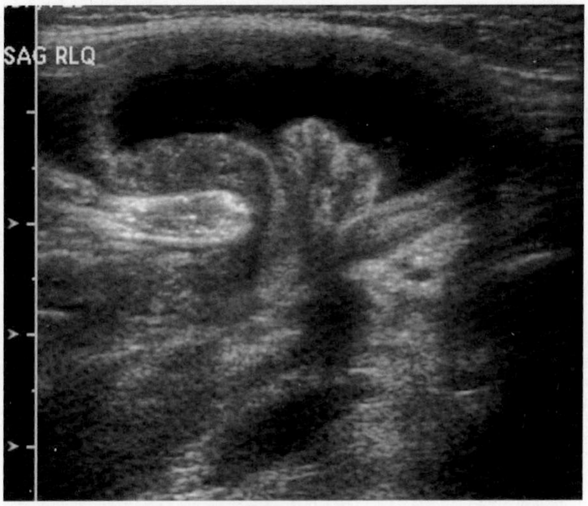

FIGURE 1.22.2

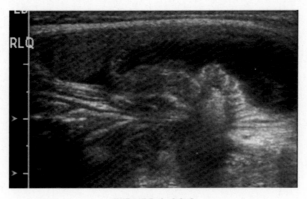

FIGURE 1.22.3

FINDINGS: This film was obtained after an enema at an outside hospital failed to identify a suspected intussusception. The supine AP view of the abdomen (Fig. 1.22.1) reveals distended small-bowel loops with residual contrast in a nondilated colon. Sonography reveals a fluid-filled structure herniating through an abdominal wall defect (Fig. 1.22.2) and displacing the testicle superiorly (Fig. 1.22.3).

DIAGNOSIS: Small-bowel obstruction resulting from an incarcerated right inguinal hernia

DISCUSSION: The embryologic connection between the celomic cavity and the scrotum is known as the *processus vaginalis*. When the processus remains patent during the first year of life, small bowel may descend into the inguinal canal and scrotum, resulting in the indirect inguinal hernia of childhood.

Inguinal hernias are more common in infant boys and more frequently right-sided. After the immediate newborn period and until the fourth month of life, incarcerated inguinal hernia is the most common cause of small-bowel obstruction. Besides small-bowel obstruction, plain films may show gas in the scrotum or inguinal canal, but more often a widened inguinoscrotal fold is the only clue to the diagnosis. Both plain films and sonography may be used to diagnose inguinal hernias, but physical examination is usually sufficient for diagnosis (26).

## Aunt Minnie's Pearl

Look for a small-bowel dilatation with a thickened inguinoscrotal fold or inguinal bowel gas to diagnose an incarcerated inguinal hernia in children.

HISTORY: A 10-year-old African American boy with fever and chest pain

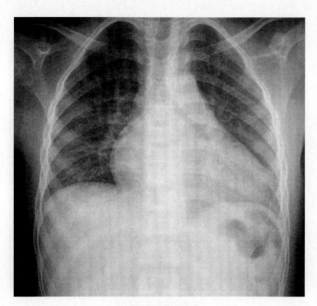

FIGURE 1.23.1

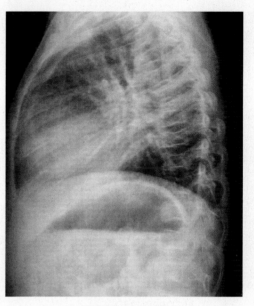

FIGURE 1.23.2

FINDINGS: Posteroanterior (Fig. 1.23.1) and lateral (Fig. 1.23.2) views of the chest reveal multiple findings, cardiomegaly, H-shaped or "Lincoln log" vertebrae with central endplate depressions, and absent splenic shadow.

DIAGNOSIS: Sickle cell disease

DISCUSSION: Children homozygous for hemoglobin S have the classic severe chronic hemolytic anemia known as *sickle cell anemia* or sickle cell disease. Sickle cell disease exhibits many abnormalities on chest films, including a small, absent, or calcified splenic shadow resulting from progressive splenic infarction, pulmonary opacities caused by pneumonia or infarction, pigment gallstones from hemolysis, and cardiomegaly from the high-output state induced by anemia. Sludging of sickled erythrocytes in bone leads to infarction or avascular necrosis.

Typical areas of involvement include the spine as well as humeral and femoral heads. In the spine, the "Lincoln log" or H-shaped vertebra caused by central microvascular endplate occlusion and relative overgrowth of the remaining endplate, is seen in approximately 10% of sickle cell patients but is virtually pathognomonic of the disease. Bone infarction may be complicated by or difficult to differentiate from *Salmonella* osteomyelitis in patients with sickle cell disease (27,28).

## Aunt Minnie's Pearls

To diagnose sickle cell disease based on a chest film, look for H-shaped vertebral bodies, avascular necrosis of the humeral heads, cardiomegaly, cholecystectomy clips, absent or calcified spleen, and pulmonary infiltrates.

**HISTORY:** A 12-month-old male with cough

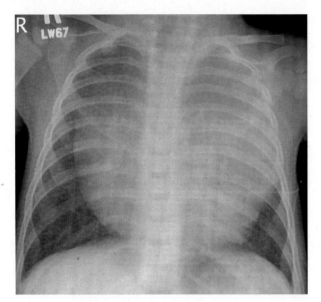

FIGURE 1.24.1

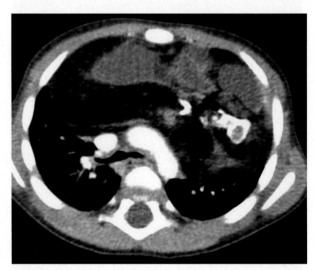

FIGURE 1.24.2

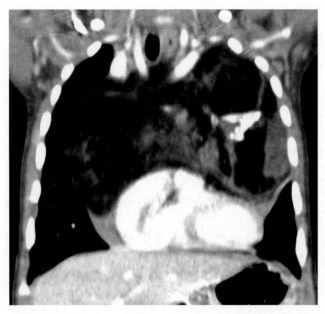

FIGURE 1.24.3

**FINDINGS:** AP chest radiograph (Fig. 1.24.1) demonstrates a large mediastinal mass with well-defined lateral margins and slight lobulations along its left inferolateral aspect. The heart borders are largely obscured. However, the pulmonary vessels and the lateral margins of the vertebral bodies are readily evident consistent with the mass being located in the anterior mediastinum. There are subtle, amorphous areas of calcification within the mass projected over the left midlung. Axial contrast-enhanced chest CT at the level of the aortic arch (Fig. 1.24.2) and coronal reconstruction (Fig. 1.24.3) demonstrate a very large, well-marginated, heterogeneous anterior mediastinal mass. The mass is predominantly of fat attenuation with lobulated areas of soft tissue anteriorly and an irregular soft-tissue attenuation focus posterolaterally. There is faint enhancing septations coursing through the mass and within the soft-tissue components. In addition, large, irregular foci of calcification are present some of which have the appearance of developing teeth.

**DIAGNOSIS:** Mediastinal teratoma

**DISCUSSION:** Mediastinal teratomas comprise approximately 8% of all mediastinal tumors and are benign, slow-growing neoplasms comprising two or more embryonic layers. They typically arise in the anterosuperior mediastinum adjacent to or within the thymus. Most patients are asymptomatic or have symptoms related to some other underlying chest pathology, for example, pneumonia, trauma. However, patients may present with cough, chest pain, and dyspnea. Young patients with large tumors may present in respiratory distress. In rare cases, these tumors can rupture or erode into adjacent mediastinal structures.

Chest radiographs are abnormal in nearly all patients and typically demonstrate a rounded, lobulated, anterior mediastinal mass with sharply delineated margins along the adjacent lung. Associated calcifications may be seen in 20% to 43% of mature teratomas with the visualization of teeth being pathognomic for the diagnosis.

The most common CT findings in a mature teratoma are that of a heterogeneous, well-marginated, partially cystic mass containing fat, soft tissue, fluid, and calcium components. Although less common, fat-fluid levels are nearly diagnostic of a teratoma. Mass effect on the adjacent cardiomediastinal structures, the diaphragm, or the lungs can be seen in nearly three-fourths of patients.

MR imaging, although not as common, may be used to evaluate mature teratomas in young patients in particular with no additional imaging other than a chest radiograph. Here, teratomas, appear as a heterogeneous, anterosuperior mediastinal masses with areas of signal intensity isointense to muscle, areas of fluid intensity signal, and foci of fat intensity signal. Visualization of T1 hyperintensity suggesting fat is helpful in establishing the diagnosis.

In rare cases, sonography may be used in the pediatric patient. Depending on the ratio of cystic to solid components, teratomas can appear as solid, cystic, or complex masses with a complex pattern of hyper- and hypoechogenicity (29–32).

## Aunt Minnie's Pearls

Presence of teeth with an anterosuperior mediastinal mass is pathognomic for a mediastinal teratoma.

Calcifications can be seen on chest radiographs in up to 43% of patients and should suggest the diagnosis of teratoma with CT or MRI recommended for further evaluation.

Fat-fluid levels within an anterior mediastinal mass on CT or MR is nearly diagnostic of a mediastinal teratoma.

HISTORY: A 1-year-old with palpable abdominal mass in the right lower quadrant

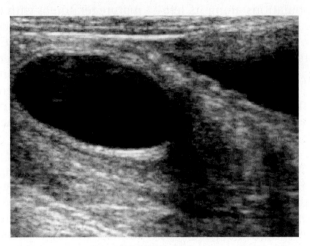

FIGURE 1.25.1

FINDINGS: Sonographic image of the right lower quadrant reveals a cystic mass with an echogenic mucosal lining and hypoechoic rim (Fig. 1.25.1).

DIAGNOSIS: Ileal duplication cyst

DISCUSSION: Duplication cysts by definition are located in or adjacent to the wall of the gastrointestinal mucosa, have smooth muscle in their walls, and are lined by alimentary tract mucosa. The small bowel is the most common location of gastrointestinal duplications, with the ileum being the most common site in the small bowel. Most cases present before the age of 2 years. Several presenting symptoms can occur, including neonatal bowel obstruction, intussusception, palpable mass, vomiting, and abdominal pain. Duplications may contain ectopic gastric or pancreatic mucosa that, when present, can induce intractable abdominal pain, GI bleeding, anemia, and elevated amylase levels. Plain-film findings may include a bowel obstruction or intussusception. Sonographically, a well-defined, spherical or tubular, fluid-filled mass with the characteristic bowel-wall signature of hyperechoic inner lining of mucosa and hypoechoic rim of smooth muscle is specific for duplication. The presence of hemorrhage or proteinaceous debris may produce a complex cystic appearance (33,34).

## Aunt Minnie's Pearl

The presence of a cystic mass with the bowel-wall signature of an inner echogenic mucosal lining and hypoechoic rim of smooth muscle is specific for a gastrointestinal duplication cyst.

**HISTORY:** A 5-year-old with abdominal pain, fever, and vomiting

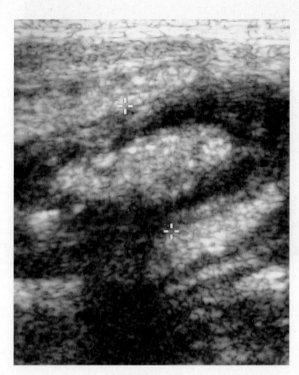

FIGURE 1.26.1

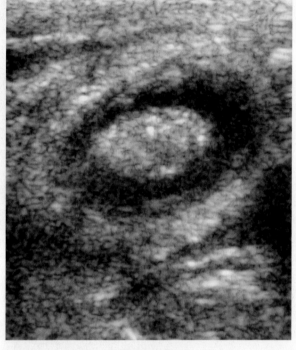

FIGURE 1.26.2

**FINDINGS:** Sagittal (Fig. 1.26.1) and transverse (Fig. 1.26.2) images of the right lower quadrant at the site of maximal pain reveal a non-compressible blind-ending tubular structure, >1 cm in diameter, with a highly echogenic central focus and distal acoustic shadowing.

**DIAGNOSIS:** Acute appendicitis

**DISCUSSION:** Acute appendicitis is the most common surgical emergency in the pediatric population. Typically, the pediatric patient presents with initial history of periumbilical pain that gradually shifts to the right lower quadrant. Abdominal tenderness, fever, anorexia, and/or vomiting and leukocytosis are also present. Sonography is the initial imaging evaluation in children with ambiguous or equivocal clinical findings. Characteristic sonographic features include a non-compressible, blindly ending, tubular structure >6 mm in diameter on longitudinal images. On transverse images, the inflamed appendix has a target appearance consisting of central luminal fluid, a hyperechoic mucosal/submucosal lining, and a hypoechoic muscular wall. When present, as in this case, an associated appendicolith will demonstrate a markedly echogenic focus, with distal acoustic shadowing within the lumen of the appendix (35).

## Aunt Minnie's Pearl

A non-compressible, blindly ending tubular structure in the right lower quadrant >6 mm in diameter in a patient with fever, tenderness, anorexia and leukocytosis = acute appendicitis.

**HISTORY:** Hypotonic short-limbed infant with a rapidly increasing head circumference

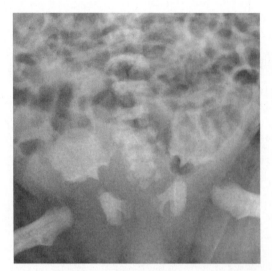

FIGURE 1.27.1

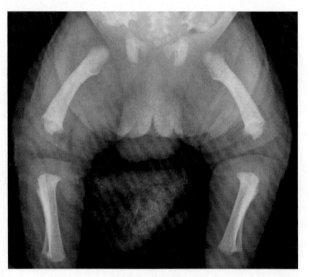

FIGURE 1.27.2

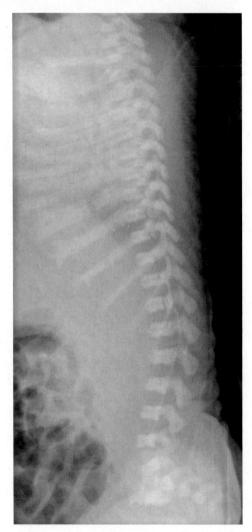

FIGURE 1.27.3

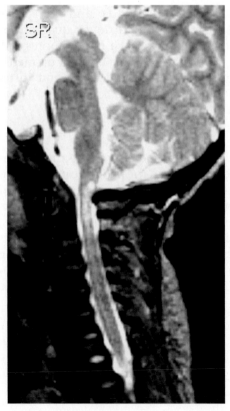

FIGURE 1.27.4

**FINDINGS:** AP film of the pelvis (Fig. 1.27.1) demonstrates progressively decreasing lumbar interpediculate distances, short and squared ilia, narrowed sacrosciatic notches, and horizontal acetabular roofs. AP view of the lower extremities (Fig. 1.27.2) demonstrates short, thick long bones with focal enlargement of the metaphyses. Lateral view of the lumbar spine (Fig. 1.27.3) demonstrates the vertebra to have short pedicles, decreased vertebral body height, and a bullet shape at the thoracolumbar junction. T2-weighted MR image of the cervical spinal cord (Fig. 1.27.4) shows stenosis at the foramen magnum, constricting the spinal canal and focal high signal in the adjacent cervical spinal cord.

**DIAGNOSIS:** Achondroplasia

**DISCUSSION:** Achondroplasia, the most common type of short-limbed dwarfism, results from a defect in endochondral bone formation. Rhizomelia or proximal-limb shortening and craniofacial involvement are the dominant clinical features. Classic plain-film findings of achondroplasia include short and thick tubular bones, which may have a ball-and-socket epiphyseal–metaphyseal configuration reminiscent of telephone receivers. Vertebral changes are characteristic and include decreased vertebral body height, short pedicles, posterior vertebral body scalloping, and progressively decreasing interpediculate distances down the lumbar spine. Because the membranous bone of the calvaria develops normally, these patients have relatively large calvaria. However, the skull base, which is formed from endochondral bone, is underdeveloped. This underdevelopment leads to constriction of the foramen magnum that may result in disabling obstructive hydrocephalus, paraplegia, and infant mortality. Tibial bowing, spinal stenosis with thoracolumbar kyphosis, and hydrocephalus can cause complications later in childhood or adulthood (36,37).

## Aunt Minnie's Pearls

Achondroplasia is the most common rhizomelic dwarfism.

The basic defect is abnormal endochondral bone formation.

One serious complication is narrowing of the foramen magnum, which may cause hydrocephalus and cord compression.

# Case 1.28

**HISTORY:** Term neonate who expired on the first day of life. Provided images are from a postmortem examination.

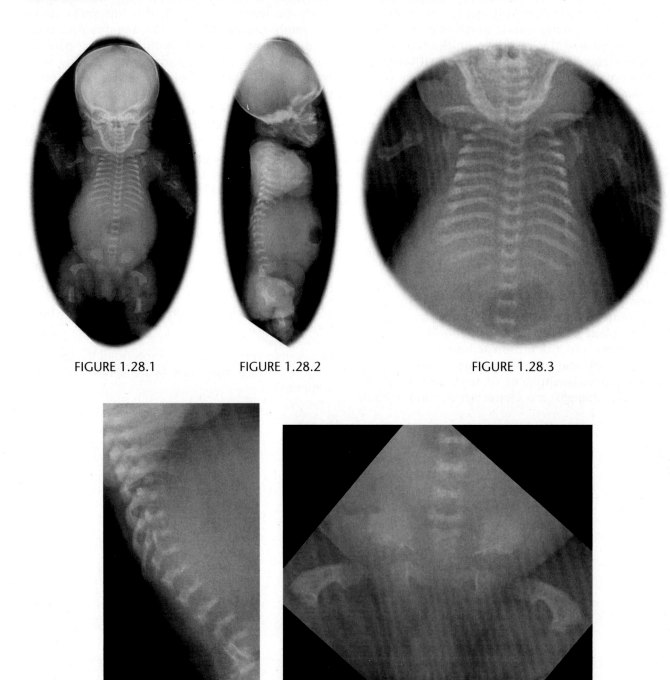

FIGURE 1.28.1

FIGURE 1.28.2

FIGURE 1.28.3

FIGURE 1.28.4

FIGURE 1.28.5

**FINDINGS:** Frontal (Fig. 1.28.1) and lateral (Fig. 1.28.2) whole-body radiographs demonstrate enlargement of the calvarium with relative hypoplasia of the frontal bone and depression of the nasal bridge. There is diffuse spinal platyspondyly seen best on the lateral radiograph (Fig. 1.28.2) with marked rib hypoplasia (Fig. 1.28.3) and associated diminished anteroposterior thoracic dimension. All extremity bones are foreshortened, the pelvis is small with narrowed sacrosciatic notches, and there is bowing of both femora in the classic "French telephone receiver-shaped" pattern. Lateral magnification radiograph of the lumbar spine (Fig. 1.28.4) again demonstrates marked flattening of the vertebral bodies. Lower rib hypoplasia is also partially visualized on this radiograph. Magnification radiograph of the pelvis (Fig. 1.28.5) demonstrates to better advantage hypoplasia of the pelvis with markedly narrowed sacrosciatic notches as well as the classic "French telephone receiver-shaped" deformity of both femora.

**DIAGNOSIS:** Thanatophoric dysplasia (TD)

**DISCUSSION:** Resulting from missense mutations in the gene-encoding fibroblast growth factor receptor 3 (FGFR3), TD is the most common lethal skeletal dysplasia. In fact, the word thanatophoric originates from the Greek word thanatophoros, meaning "bearing death." In general, TD is inherited in an autosomal dominant fashion. The overall incidence is estimated to range from 1/20,000 to 1/50,000. Death generally occurs within the immediate neonatal period secondary to respiratory insufficiency from pulmonary hypoplasia related to diminutive thoracic size or failure of respiratory control resulting from foramen magnum stenosis.

TD can be diagnosed sonographically by prenatal ultrasound or evaluated postnatally by conventional radiographs. Both modalities show similar findings. TD is characterized by markedly foreshortened ribs with associated narrowed thorax, platyspondyly, extremely short (micromelic) extremities that may be either bowed or straight, macrocephaly with frontal bossing, and a diminutive, flared pelvis with narrowed sacrosciatic notches. One classic radiographic feature of TD results from premature closure of the coronal sutures giving the skull a unique clover-like shape, aptly termed the "cloverleaf" skull deformity (German = kleeblattschädel). Another classic radiographic sign associated with TD is the "French telephone receiver-shaped" femora resulting from marked curvature and shortening of both femora (38–42).

## Aunt Minnie's Pearls

TD is the most common lethal skeletal dysplasia

Classic radiographic signs in TD include "cloverleaf-shaped" skull and "French telephone receiver-shaped" femora.

Most die shortly after birth owing to pulmonary hypoplasia resulting from marked rib hypoplasia and subsequent decreased anteroposterior thoracic dimension.

**HISTORY:** Term neonate who subsequently expired 2 days after delivery. Provided images are from a postmortem examination.

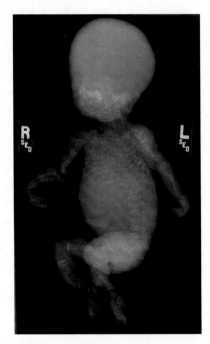

FIGURE 1.29.1

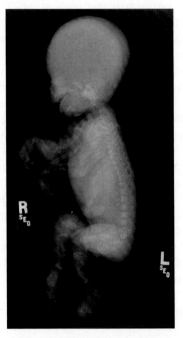

FIGURE 1.29.2

**FINDINGS:** Anteroposterior and lateral postmortem whole-body skeletal radiographs (Figs. 1.29.1 and 1.29.2) demonstrate marked osteopenia of the entire skeleton. The bones are thinned and overtubulated seen best in the humeri and femora. There is extensive fracturing within all of the bones of the appendicular skeleton with multiple bilateral posterior and anterolateral rib fractures. The bilateral tibias, fibulas, radii, and ulni are deformed, fractured and bowed. Macrosomia with frontal bossing and basilar invagination are best demonstrated on the lateral radiograph (Fig. 1.29.2). There is subtle, biconvexity of the vertebral bodies of the cervical spine (Fig. 1.29.2).

**DIAGNOSIS:** Osteogenesis imperfecta

**DISCUSSION:** Osteogenesis imperfect (OI) (aka: van der Hoeve–de Kleyn syndrome) is a heterogeneous group of disorders resulting from gene mutations encoding for type I collagen. OI is inherited almost entirely in an autosomal dominant fashion with only OI type III demonstrating an autosomal recessive pattern. The overall prevalence is 1 in 28,500 live births. There are seven subtypes first proposed by Sillence that range in severity from mild/no deformity (OI type I) to lethal (OI type II). Given the numerous subtypes, there is a wide variety of radiologic presentations, and OI subtyping should

be based on clinical grounds. The major radiologic findings in OI are at least some degree of osteopenia; decreased ossification of calvarial bone with multiple wormian bones (10 or more); wedged or collapsed vertebral bodies; thin, overtubulated bones; and rib fractures. On sonographic evaluation, the weight of the ultrasound probe may compress the skull in severe cases. Death often results from respiratory failure related to thorax deformity, in OI type II in particular. Milder cases, especially in the setting of isolated posterior rib fractures, can be mistaken for NAT and may require genetic testing for its confirmation or exclusion (40,43).

## Aunt Minnie's Pearls

Multiple appendicular skeletal fractures in overtubulated, thinned, and osteopenic bones are the best radiographic clues.

Milder forms of OI can be confused with nonaccidental trauma and should be considered in the appropriate clinical setting.

Dynamic sonographic compression of the cranial vault may be seen in severe form of OI on prenatal ultrasound.

HISTORY: A 2-year-old with bowed lower extremities

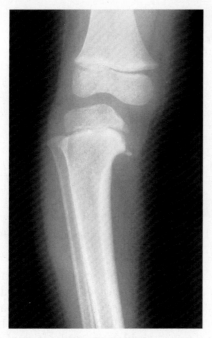

FIGURE 1.30.1

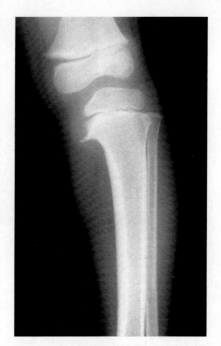

FIGURE 1.30.2

FINDINGS: AP views of the right (Fig. 1.30.1) and left (Fig. 1.30.2) tibias show beaking, fragmentation, and depression of the medial tibial metaphyses. Hypoplasia and medial sloping of the proximal tibial epiphyses are also evident.

DIAGNOSIS: Blount disease (infantile tibia vara)

DISCUSSION: The underlying abnormality in Blount disease is faulty endochondral bone formation in the medial proximal tibia, which results from abnormal mechanical stresses on the physis. Blount disease may present in infants or adolescents. Infantile Blount disease, or tibia vara, represents persistent physiologic bowing or genu varum that fails to regress as the child begins to walk. Radiographs are useful to differentiate the various causes of bowed legs, such as physiologic bowing, rickets, Blount disease, posttraumatic physeal arrest, and focal fibrocartilaginous dysplasia. Infantile Blount disease may be unilateral or bilateral and asymmetric. Adolescent Blount disease occurs in older children who are overweight. This form of the disease is usually milder, often unilateral, and posttraumatic. Either form may resolve spontaneously, but tibial osteotomies are frequently required (44,45).

## Aunt Minnie's Pearls

Blount disease results from abnormal stresses on the medial proximal tibial physis.

Beaking, fragmentation, and sloping characterize the medial proximal tibia.

Infantile and adolescent varieties occur.

**HISTORY:** An 18-month-old female with left hip instability

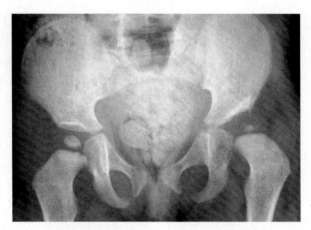

FIGURE 1.31.1

**FINDINGS:** AP radiograph of the pelvis with hips in neutral position (Fig. 1.31.1) reveals lateral and superior displacement of the left femur, increased angulation of the left acetabular roof, and delayed ossification of the left femoral head.

**DIAGNOSIS:** Developmental dysplasia of the hip (DDH)

**DISCUSSION:** DDH has replaced the term *congenital hip dislocation*. It is thought that hip dysplasia results from a combination of joint laxity, acetabular shallowness, and intrauterine position. Females are more commonly affected than males, whites more than blacks, and there is higher incidence among Native Americans. Other risk factors include family history and breech presentation. The left hip (as in this case) is more frequently involved than the right. Sonography is used in the newborn period for infants with abnormal physical exam or risk factors for DDH. Plain-film findings of DDH are late and include persistent increased angulation of the acetabular roof, absence of a central concavity and distinct lateral edge in the acetabulum, lateral and superior displacement of and disparity in size and ossification of the involved femoral head. When instability or dislocation is identified in an infant or young child, the child is placed in a harness or cast in flexion, abduction, and external rotation to obtain satisfactory acetabular–femoral relationships. If this conservative management fails, surgical reduction may be required. Appropriate treatment before the age of 4 will result in reversal of the secondary signs and a normal acetabular–femoral relationship in more than 95% of the cases of DDH (46).

## Aunt Minnie's Pearls

DDH is characterized by femoral head subluxation superiorly, laterally, and posteriorly with respect to the acetabulum, increased angulation of the acetabular roof, and disparity in size and ossification of the involved femoral head.

Risk factors include breech presentation, female gender, and family history.

HISTORY: A 13-year-old boy with T-cell acute lymphoblastic leukemia (ALL) and pain in the left thigh

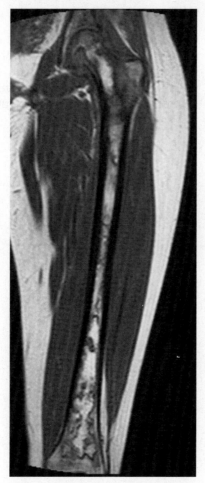

FIGURE 1.32.1

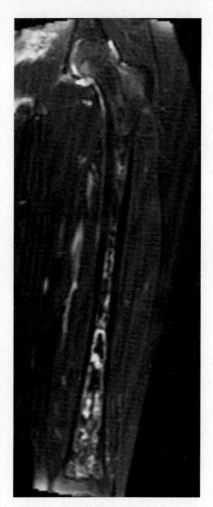

FIGURE 1.32.2

FINDINGS: Coronal T1 (Fig. 1.32.1) and T2 (Fig. 1.32.2) images of the left femur show well-defined geographic areas of heterogeneous signal abnormalities in the proximal and distal marrow of the left femur.

DIAGNOSIS: Medullary osteonecrosis/bone infarcts

DISCUSSION: Osteonecrosis is bone death secondary to ischemic insult. Hemoglobinopathies are a common cause of osteonecrosis in childhood. Other causes include trauma, corticosteroids, irradiation, malignancy (ALL in particular) and its treatment, pancreatitis, Gaucher's disease, Caisson disease, and idiopathic causes, such as Legg–Calve–Perthes disease. The epiphysis and metaphysis of long tubular bones are susceptible because of their limited arterial supply and limited venous drainage. Furthermore, epiphyseal osteonecrosis may be complicated by subchondral collapse and secondary osteoarthritis. Osteonecrosis complicating the treatment of ALL tends to affect white teenage females, 10 to 15 years of age, and is often multifocal. Conventional radiographs are not sensitive in the diagnosis of osteonecrosis or avascular necrosis. MRI has a very high sensitivity and specificity. In the early phase of osteonecrosis, MRI shows nonspecific edema without distinct margins, findings that are indistinguishable from infection or tumor. However, in the subacute or chronic phases after the onset of bony repair, the "double line/double rim sign" is a characteristic MR finding seen on T2-weighted images in up to 80% of patients with osteonecrosis. Around the outer edges of the geographic or serpiginous borders of the infarct there is an inner zone of high signal intensity surrounded by peripheral low signal intensity. The inner hyperintense zone on T2 represents hyperemic granulation tissue and the peripheral low signal intensity, present on all sequences, represents sclerotic bone (47,48).

## Aunt Minnie's Pearls

MRI is very sensitive and specific in the diagnosis of subacute osteonecrosis.

Geographic lesions with sharply defined serpiginous margins and the "double line/double rim sign," consisting of an inner zone of high signal intensity and peripheral zone of low signal intensity on T2-weighted images are characteristic MRI features of osteonecrosis.

**HISTORY:** A 17-year-old with recurrent bouts of epigastric pain

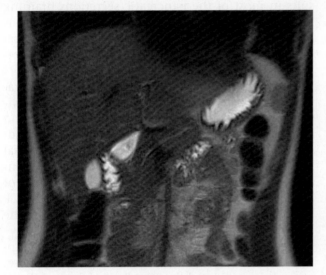

FIGURE 1.33.1

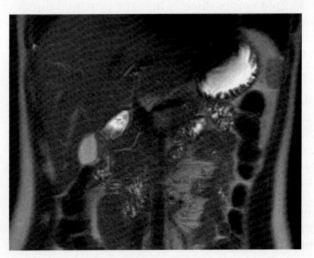

FIGURE 1.33.2

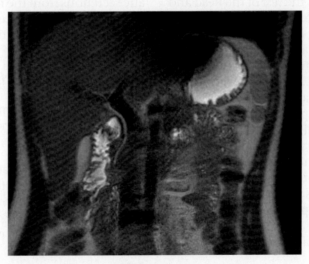

FIGURE 1.33.3

**FINDINGS:** Coronal T2 Haste images from an MR cholangiopancreaticogram (MRCP) reveal the dorsal accessory pancreatic duct (Figs. 1.33.1 and 1.33.2) to empty directly into the proximal duodenum via the minor papilla, separate from the distal common bile duct (Fig. 1.33.3) and ventral pancreatic duct (not well seen on these images) that empty into the ampulla of Vater.

**DIAGNOSIS:** Pancreas divisum

**DISCUSSION:** Pancreas divisum is the most common pancreatic ductal anatomic variation where the main pancreatic duct drains mostly or almost completely through the minor papilla into the duodenum.

The pancreas develops from a dorsal bud and a ventral bud. The dorsal part arises as a diverticulum from the dorsal aspect of the duodenum and forms the entire body and tail as well as portions of pancreatic head and uncinate process of the pancreas. The ventral portion arises as a diverticulum from the primitive bile duct and forms the rest of the head and uncinate process of the pancreas. The duct of the dorsal part (accessory pancreatic duct) therefore empties directly into the duodenum, and the duct of the ventral part joins the distal common bile duct. At about the sixth week of gestation, the dorsal and ventral portions fuse to form the pancreas and their ducts communicate. The terminal portion of the accessory pancreatic duct remains small, whereas the rest of the ducts enlarge resulting in the normal anatomy where the pancreatic duct angles inferiorly to finally drain at the ampulla of Vater. Almost all of the pancreatic secretions drain through this path even if the terminal portion of the accessory pancreatic duct remains open draining at the minor papillae, located more proximally than the major papilla in the duodenum.

Pancreas divisum is caused by nonfusion of the dorsal and ventral pancreatic portions. This results in most of the pancreatic secretions draining through the minor papilla. In most cases there is no communication between the dorsal and ventral pancreatic ducts. In some cases the ventral pancreatic duct may be totally absent.

Endoscopic retrograde cholangiopancreatography was typically used to diagnose pancreas divisum but now MRCP offers a noninvasive method of diagnosing this entity. The characteristic finding of pancreas divisum on MRCP is that the dorsal pancreatic duct extends more horizontally to continue with the accessory pancreatic duct (duct of Santorini) and drains into the minor papilla. MRCP done with secretin helps in better delineation of the pancreatic ductal anatomy.

Most people with pancreas divisum are asymptomatic but this can be a cause for recurrent pancreatitis. It is postulated that the duct of Santorini and the minor papilla are too small to drain the pancreatic secretions from the body and tail of the pancreas adequately thereby causing functional obstruction that predisposes the patient to pancreatitis (49).

## Aunt Minnie's Pearls

Pancreas divisum is the most common pancreatic ductal anatomic variation and can contribute to recurrent pancreatitis.

On MRCP, the major pancreatic duct from the body and tail extends horizontally to continue and drain into the minor papilla which is located cephalad to and separate from the common bile duct that drains normally at the ampulla of Vater.

# Case 1.34

**HISTORY:** A 2-year-old male unrestrained passenger in a motor vehicle accident was unresponsive upon presentation to the trauma center

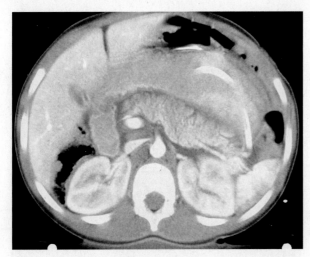

FIGURE 1.34.1

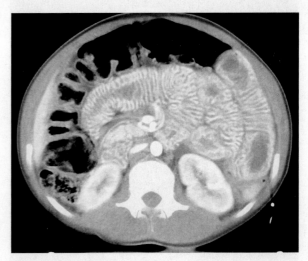

FIGURE 1.34.2

**FINDINGS:** Images from a contrast-enhanced CT of the abdomen reveals (Figs. 1.34.1 and 1.34.2) dilated, fluid-filled bowel with intense enhancement of the bowel wall, aorta, inferior cava, pancreas, and kidneys.

**DIAGNOSIS:** Hypoperfusion complex

**DISCUSSION:** Given recent advances in trauma care, most children with blunt abdominal trauma are treated nonoperatively. CT is the primary method of assessing the presence and severity of intraabdominal injuries in children, and the results will dictate operative versus conservative management. A subgroup of severely injured children has been identified with a constellation of imaging findings characterized by intense enhancement of bowel wall, kidneys, aorta, and IVC. The bowel loops are dilated and fluid-filled,

and the aorta and IVC demonstrate a diminished caliber. This so-called hypoperfusion complex suggests tenuous hemodynamic stability and is associated with a high incidence of mortality (85%). Recognition that the CT findings are owing to hypovolemic shock rather than a visceral injury may enable the surgeon to avoid unnecessary laparotomy (50).

## Aunt Minnie's Pearls

Intense enhancement of dilated and fluid-filled bowel wall, kidneys, aorta, and IVC on contrast-enhanced CT are indicative of the hypoperfusion complex secondary to hypovolemic shock.

The hypoperfusion complex is a poor prognostic indicator, with high associated mortality.

HISTORY: Teenage female with seizure disorder

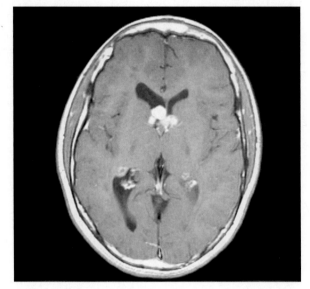

FIGURE 1.35.1

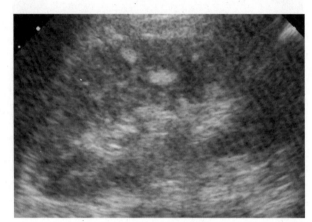

FIGURE 1.35.2

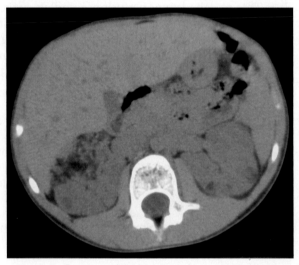

FIGURE 1.35.3

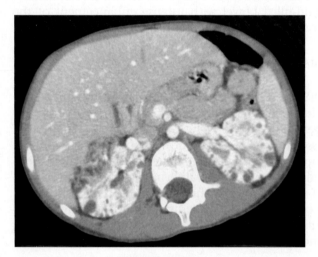

FIGURE 1.35.4

**FINDINGS:** Contrast-enhanced MR of the head reveals (Fig. 1.35.1) enhancing masses in the subependymal regions bilaterally. Sonographic image of the kidney (Fig. 1.35.2) reveals bright echogenic foci in the renal cortex. CT images of the abdomen without (Fig. 1.35.3) and with IV contrast enhancement (Fig. 1.35.4) reveal multiple low-density masses in the kidneys bilaterally and a large soft-tissue mass of heterogenous density in the right kidney.

**DIAGNOSIS:** Tuberous sclerosis (Bourneville's disease)

**DISCUSSION:** Tuberous sclerosis is one of the phakomatoses, a group of disorders characterized by dysplasia and tumors of the embryonic ectoderm, including the skin, nervous system, and eyes. Children with tuberous sclerosis have the classic clinical triad of mental retardation, seizures, and adenoma sebaceum. Typical imaging findings include cysts and hamartomas of the kidneys (angiomyolipomas), hamartomas of the heart (rhabdomyomas), and hamartomas (tubers) of the central nervous system (CNS). Renal angiomyolipomas are characterized in part by their increased echogenicity on ultrasound and low density on CT consistent with fat. The amount of fat within the angiomyolipomas, however, may vary. Characteristic CNS abnormalities are present in 95% of affected patients on neuroimaging examinations. The CNS tubers occur in the subependymal regions, subcortical white matter, and in the cortex. They may calcify. In 5% to 10%, the subependymal tubers may enlarge and enhance, growing into the ventricle and causing hydrocephalus, and are termed *giant-cell tumors*. In rare cases, these tumors may undergo degeneration into a higher grade. Treatment is controversial but may include shunting and/or surgical resection (51).

## Aunt Minnie's Pearls

A fat-containing lesion in the kidney is diagnostic of an angiomyolipoma.

Multiple, bilateral angiomyolipomas of the kidneys are diagnostic of tuberous sclerosis.

Subependymal calcifications are characteristic of tuberous sclerosis.

Contrast enhancement and enlargement of a subependymal intracranial tuber suggest development of giant-cell tumor.

**HISTORY:** A 6-month-old with unusually shaped head

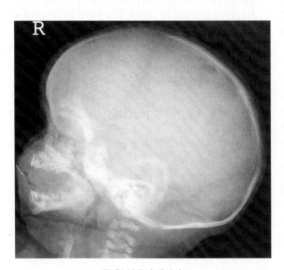

FIGURE 1.36.1

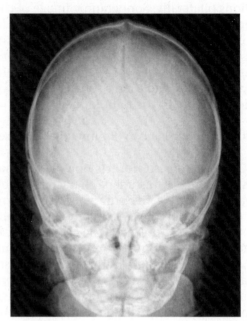

FIGURE 1.36.2

**FINDINGS:** Lateral radiograph of the skull (Fig. 1.36.1) reveals an elongated skull. Frontal radiograph (Fig. 1.36.2) reveals narrowing and sharpening of the sagittal suture and a sclerotic ridge of bone at the expected location of the sagittal suture.

**DIAGNOSIS:** Scaphocephaly or dolichocephaly secondary to premature sagittal craniosynostosis

**DISCUSSION:** Craniosynostosis is the premature closure of a cranial suture, with the sagittal suture being most commonly affected. Growth along the edges of the suture is impaired, producing an extremely long, narrow "boat-like" skull. Plain films are the initial imaging modality of choice, as the sutural abnormality is usually easily seen. In difficult or incomplete cases of synostosis, CT with 3D reconstruction is the best method of identifying the abnormality. Surgical correction is performed to create a more normal appearance and to prevent potential injury to the underlying brain (52).

## Aunt Minnie's Pearls

Plain films characterize most calvarial and sutural changes of premature craniosynostosis.

Three-dimensional CT is accurate in the detection and assessment of craniosynostosis, in particular the subtle or incomplete sutural abnormalities.

**HISTORY:** Newborn with back mass

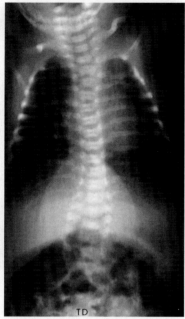

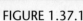

FIGURE 1.37.1

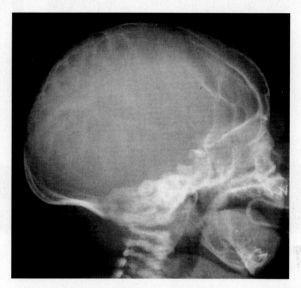

FIGURE 1.37.2

**FINDINGS:** AP radiograph of the spine (Fig. 1.37.1) reveals a splaying of the posterior elements of the lumbar spine consistent with a spinal dysraphism. Lateral view of the skull (Fig. 1.37.2) reveals calvarial fenestrations or lacunae primarily in the parietal bones.

**DIAGNOSIS:** Luckenschadel or lacunar skull

**DISCUSSION:** Lacunar skull is almost invariably associated with dysraphisms, including meningoceles, encephaloceles, and meningomyeloceles. It is a temporary phenomenon that resolves by 4 to 6 months of age. It is probably not based on increased intracranial pressure but because of a defect in membranous bone formation of unknown etiology.

Therefore, the fenestrations are most pronounced in the membranous portions of the skull (parietal and superior portions of the frontal and occipital bones) and spare those portions of the skull formed by endochondral bone formation (skull base and lower half of the frontal and occipital bones) (53).

## Aunt Minnie's Pearls

Luckenschadel is a temporary abnormality in the bony calvaria associated with dysraphic defects.

It is characterized by fenestrations within the parietal bones and superior portions of the frontal and occipital bones.

HISTORY: A 2-year-old with head trauma

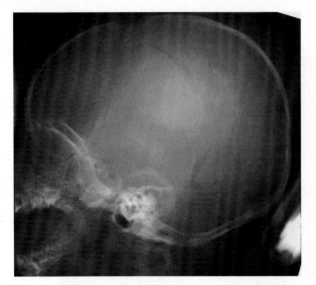

FIGURE 1.38.1

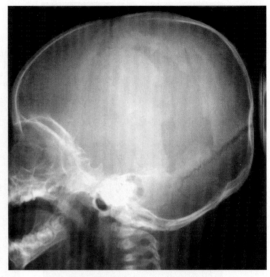

FIGURE 1.38.2

FINDINGS: Lateral view of the skull at the time of the trauma (Fig. 1.38.1) reveals a diastatic linear parietal skull fracture; 2 months later (Fig. 1.38.2), there is a larger radiolucent defect with relatively smooth and sclerotic edges in the parietal bone.

DIAGNOSIS: Leptomeningeal cyst

DISCUSSION: A leptomeningeal cyst or "growing fracture" is an uncommon late complication of a skull fracture. Instead of healing, the fracture "grows." If the underlying dura is torn at the time of the initial injury, subarachnoid membrane may herniate into the fracture site. The persistent pulsations of subarachnoid fluid prevent healing of the fracture fragments and produce a smooth-edged gradually widening fracture line. Clinically, the patient has a pulsatile soft-tissue mass at the site of the defect (54).

## Aunt Minnie's Pearls

Leptomeningeal cyst is characterized by a progressively widening smooth-edged calvarial defect with overlying pulsatile soft-tissue mass in a patient with prior history of skull fracture.

HISTORY: Newborn with congestive failure and bruit over the anterior fontanelle

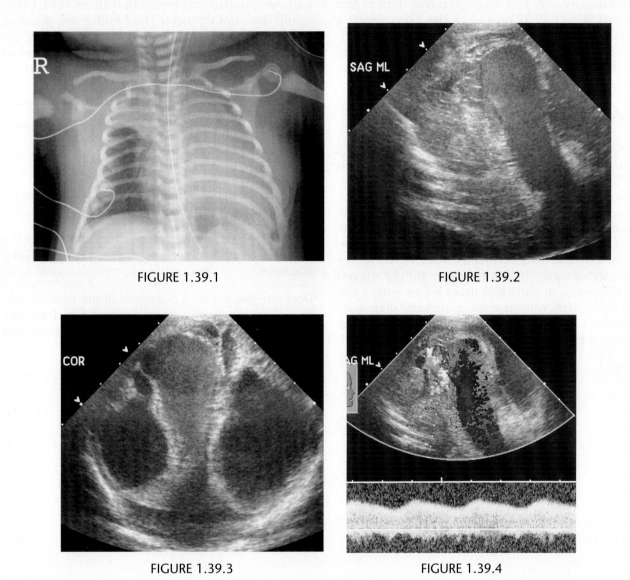

FIGURE 1.39.1

FIGURE 1.39.2

FIGURE 1.39.3

FIGURE 1.39.4

**FINDINGS:** Radiograph of the chest reveals marked cardiomegaly (Fig. 1.39.1). Sagittal (Fig. 1.39.2) and coronal (Fig. 1.39.3) images of the brain reveal a mass in the midline posterior to the third ventricle containing mobile echogenic speckles. Doppler evaluation of the mass demonstrates the lesion to be vascular with arteriovenous shunting (Fig. 1.39.4).

**DIAGNOSIS:** Vein of Galen aneurysm

**DISCUSSION:** The term *vein of Galen aneurysm* is a misnomer because it is actually an arteriovenous malformation, not an aneurysm. The arteriovenous malformation (AVM) is of variable size and may present with high-output congestive failure caused by shunting through the malformation. The AVM may also produce obstruction to the ventricular system and hydrocephalus. Congestive failure and cardiomegaly in the newborn should suggest the diagnosis, in particular in an infant with a cranial bruit. The entity is most commonly diagnosed by cranial ultrasound. Typical ultrasound findings include a hypoechoic mass behind the third ventricle. Color Doppler demonstrates its vascular nature, and pulsed Doppler wave forms demonstrate a pulsatile venous pattern consistent with an AVM. Ultrasound does not delineate the feeding and draining vessels adequately for treatment planning. MR angiography or traditional angiography is therefore required for further workup prior to definitive treatment via endovascular embolization. Doppler sonography may be used to follow the hemodynamic changes after embolization therapy (55,56).

## Aunt Minnie's Pearls

The vein of Galen aneurysm is an arteriovenous malformation, not an aneurysm, involving the vein of Galen.

High-output congestive failure in a newborn with a cranial bruit is highly suggestive of a vein of Galen aneurysm.

Doppler sonography is diagnostic of the vascular malformation, but arteriography is required to determine the precise vascular anatomy prior to endovascular embolization.

# Case 1.40

**HISTORY:** A 32-week-old premature infant at risk for intracranial hemorrhage

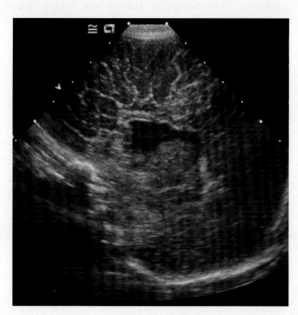

FIGURE 1.40.1

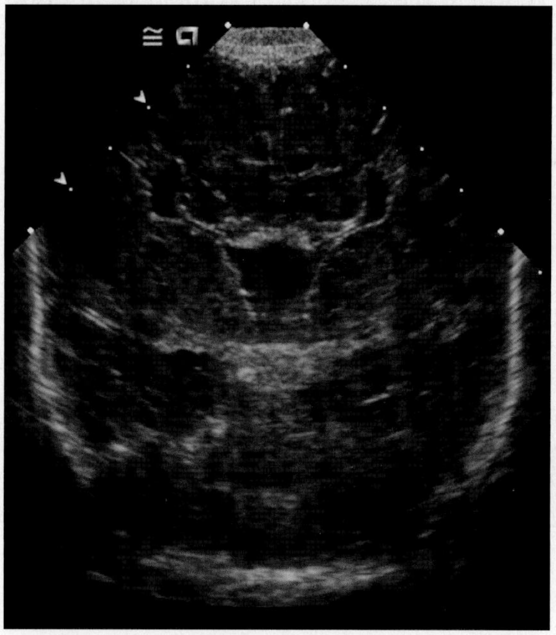

FIGURE 1.40.2

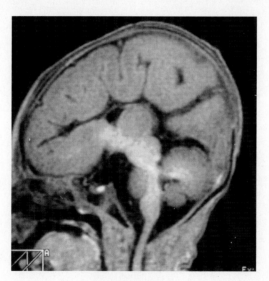

FIGURE 1.40.3

**FINDINGS:** Sagittal midline ultrasound reveals an elevated third ventricle and sulci radiating from the third ventricle (Fig. 1.40.1). A coronal ultrasound image (Fig. 1.40.2) reveals the typical horizontal orientation of the lateral ventricles producing the characteristic "longhorn" appearance. Sagittal midline T1 MR image (Fig. 1.40.3) reveals absence of the corpus callosum, elevation of the third ventricle, and radiating sulci.

**DIAGNOSIS:** Agenesis of the corpus callosum (ACC)

**DISCUSSION:** ACC is frequently an isolated congenital abnormality of the brain but may be associated with various CNS anomalies. The imaging findings are characteristic and consist of absence of the corpus callosum, widely separated lateral ventricles with a "longhorn" configuration, with indentations medially caused by the thickened Probst bundles, a high-riding third ventricle, and a radiating pattern of pericallosal sulci in a sunburst pattern. The occipital horns are larger than the frontal (i.e., colpocephaly), and the bodies of the lateral ventricles have a parallel course. Frequent associations include dorsal midline cysts (30%) and Dandy–Walker malformations (57,58).

## Aunt Minnie's Pearls

Widely separated, angled lateral ventricles with a "longhorn" configuration, high-riding third ventricle, and radiating pattern of pericallosal sulci = ACC.

ACC may occur in isolation or in association with other congenital anomalies of the CNS.

# Case 1.41

**HISTORY:** A 30-week gestational age infant with severe lung disease

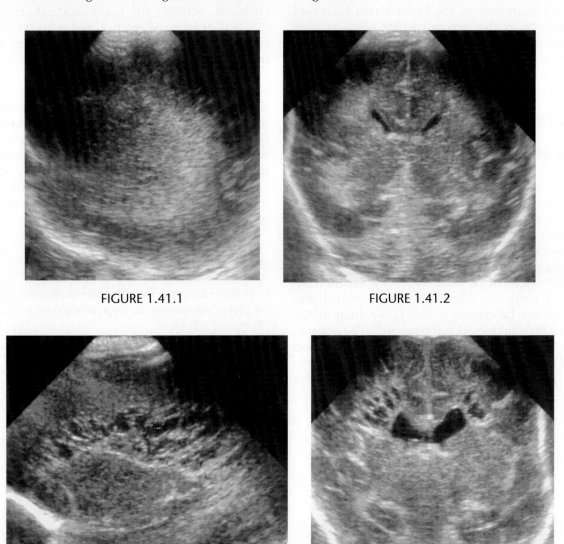

FIGURE 1.41.1

FIGURE 1.41.2

FIGURE 1.41.3

FIGURE 1.41.4

**FINDINGS:** Sagittal (Fig. 1.41.1) and coronal (Fig. 1.41.2) images of the brain reveal increased echogenicity in the periventricular white matter. Sagittal (Fig. 1.41.3) and coronal (Fig. 1.41.4) images 3 weeks later reveal cystic degeneration in the areas of increased echogenicity on the previous scans and slight dilatation of the lateral ventricles.

**DIAGNOSIS:** Periventricular leukomalacia (PVL)

**DISCUSSION:** PVL is a watershed infarction of the periventricular white matter that occurs in premature infants after a hypoxic insult, resulting in the clinical entity of spastic diplegia or cerebral palsy. It may be nonhemorrhagic or hemorrhagic, limited or extensive. Typically, PVL demonstrates increased echogenicity anteriorly and/or posteriorly adjacent to the lateral ventricles on cranial sonography. This echogenicity must be differentiated from the normal periventricular blush of the periventricular white matter. Echogenicity that is less than in the adjacent choroid plexus is considered to be normal. Coarse, echogenic areas equal to or greater than that of the adjacent choroid are suspicious for PVL. When in doubt, scanning through the posterior fontanelle will eliminate the normal periventricular blush, whereas the pathologic echogenicity of PVL will persist. Between 2 and 3 weeks after the ischemic insult, cystic degeneration occurs, and the increased echogenicity is replaced by a number of Swiss cheese–like cysts (i.e., cystic encephalomalcia). Ultimately, the fluid and cysts are resorbed, there is thinning or loss of the periventricular white matter, ventricles dilate in an *ex vacuo* phenomenon, and interhemispheric fissures and sulci become more prominent. Sonography is the initial imaging modality of choice for diagnosis. MR and/or CT are used to evaluate the most severely affected individuals and for follow-up to determine extent of injury (59).

## Aunt Minnie's Pearls

Increased echogenicity in the periventricular white matter that undergoes cystic degeneration with time = PVL.

Imaging through the posterior fontanelle may aid the sonographer in differentiating early periventricular leukomalacia from the normal periventricular blush.

**HISTORY:** A 11-year-old with 3-day history of scrotal pain

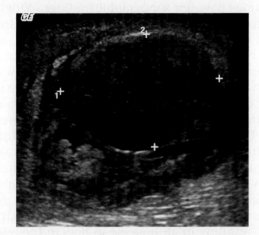

FIGURE 1.42.1

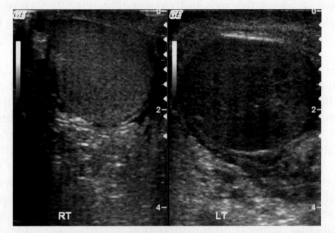

FIGURE 1.42.2

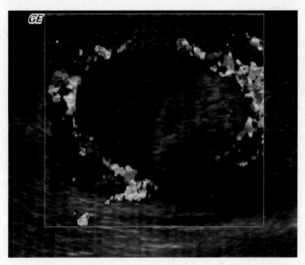

FIGURE 1.42.3

**FINDINGS:** Transverse gray-scale images through the symptomatic testis (Fig. 1.42.1) and comparative transverse views through both testes (Fig. 1.42.2) reveal the left testis to be enlarged, slightly heterogeneous, and diffusely hypoechoic in echotexture compared with the right. There is some thickening of the left epididymis as well. Color Doppler of the left testis (Fig. 1.42.3) reveals absence of intratesticular flow and a ring of increased flow in the capsule around the testicle.

**DIAGNOSIS:** Testicular torsion with infarction

**DISCUSSION:** Testicular torsion results from a twisting of the testis and spermatic cord, obstructing testicular blood flow and causing acute pain secondary to testicular ischemia and/or infarction. Infants and adolescent males are most commonly affected. There are two types of torsion—intravaginal and extravaginal, with intravaginal being the more common. Extravaginal torsion occurs in utero secondary to poor fixation and subsequent twisting of the spermatic cord within the inguinal canal. Therefore, at birth, the neonate has a swollen, discolored scrotum, and the affected testis is frequently already necrotic. Intravaginal torsion, common in adolescents and young adults, is caused by an embryologic failure of fixation of the testicle to the tunica vaginalis the "bell-clapper" deformity), which enables the testicle to rotate freely on the vascular pedicle within the scrotal sac.

The child with acute scrotal pain constitutes a medical emergency, as delay in surgical intervention reduces the likelihood of testicular salvage. If the torsed testicle is detorsed within 6 hours of symptom onset, nearly 100% are viable. However, if torsion persists for more than 24 hours, seldom is a testis salvageable. Doppler sonography is considered the imaging modality of choice when clinical findings are equivocal or presentation is delayed. Early on, the testis may have few sonographic findings. With time and the development of testicular edema, the torsed testis enlarges and becomes hypoechoic. In addition, there may be epididymal swelling and reactive hydrocele formation. A whirlpool sign of the twisted spermatic cord has been described in literature (46). With color Doppler, there is diminished or no flow within the torsed testicle compared with the affected side. Therefore, it is always useful to evaluate the asymptomatic side first as a baseline. As in this case of late torsion, once the testicle has infarcted, there is absence of flow within the testicle and hyperemia in the peritesticular soft tissues, creating the "rim sign." Occasionally, a twisted testis will spontaneously detorse, resulting in an increase in flow in the testicle as well as peritesticular tissues at sonography and clinical resolution of pain (60,61).

## Aunt Minnie's Pearls

Acute scrotal pain constitutes a medical emergency.

Gray-scale ultrasound findings vary with the duration of torsion. Very early on, the testis is normal or near normal in appearance. As time passes, the testis enlarges and becomes hypoechoic.

Color Doppler sonography is the imaging modality of choice to evaluate the acute scrotum.

The color Doppler findings of torsion are diminished or absent testicular flow on the affected side.

In late or missed torsion, there is increased peritesticular flow around the avascular testis producing a rim sign.

**HISTORY:** A 6-year-old with wheezing

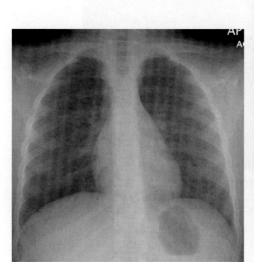

FIGURE 1.43.1

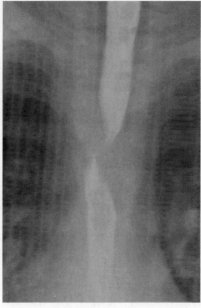

FIGURE 1.43.2

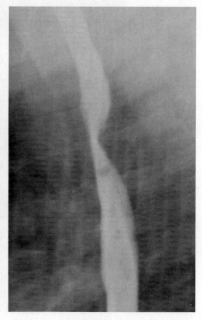

FIGURE 1.43.3

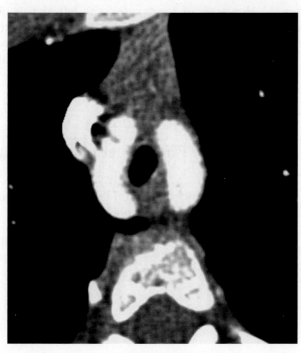

FIGURE 1.43.4

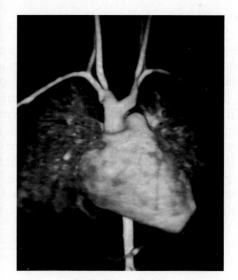

FIGURE 1.43.5A

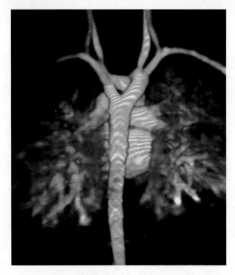

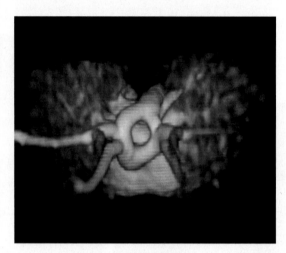

FIGURE 1.43.5B

FIGURE 1.43.5C

**FINDINGS:** Frontal radiograph of the chest (Fig. 1.43.1) reveals loss of the intrathoracic tracheal air column. Frontal (Fig. 1.43.2) and lateral (Fig. 1.43.3) views from a barium swallow reveal bilateral and posterior extrinsic impressions on the thoracic esophagus. An axial CT image of the thorax (Fig. 1.43.4) reveals a vascular ring surrounding and compressing the trachea. AP (Fig. 1.43.5A), PA (Fig. 1.43.5B), and craniocaudal (Fig. 1.43.5C) 3D reconstruction views from a thoracic CT angiogram demonstrate a double aortic arch.

**DIAGNOSIS:** Double aortic arch (DAA)

**DISCUSSION:** The DAA is the most common symptomatic vascular ring. Although esophageal compression may produce symptoms, respiratory findings, including distress, wheezing, or stridor, predominate. On plain films, the DAA will demonstrate a right arch and generalized overaeration. Displacement or indentations on the trachea may be seen, or there may be complete loss of the tracheal air column on frontal projection, as in this case. The esophagram, however, is more valuable as the DAA produces a characteristic reverse S indentation on

the esophagus. The upper indentation is produced by the right-sided arch and the lower indentation by the left-sided arch. A posterior indentation is produced by the encircling posterior arch. In most cases (80%), the right arch is higher, larger, and more posterior than the smaller anterior left arch. However, in some cases, the left arch is dominant, or the arches are symmetric. CT and MRI have replaced aortography, as they noninvasively confirm the diagnosis and clearly delineate the arch anatomy for surgical planning (62,63).

## Aunt Minnie's Pearls

Respiratory symptoms predominate in patients with DAA.

Reverse S indentation on the esophagus in an esophagram is characteristic of DAA.

CT angiography and MRI are the current imaging modalities of choice to confirm the diagnosis and delineate the arch anatomy.

**HISTORY:** Infant with stridor

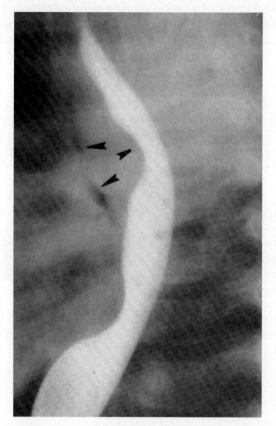

FIGURE 1.44.1

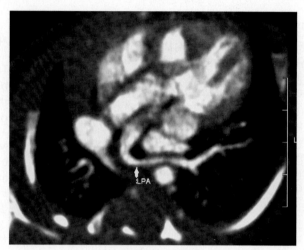

FIGURE 1.44.2

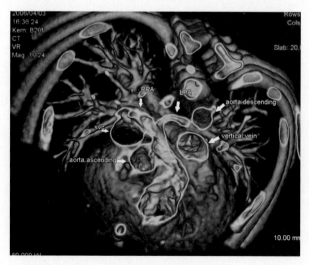

FIGURE 1.44.3

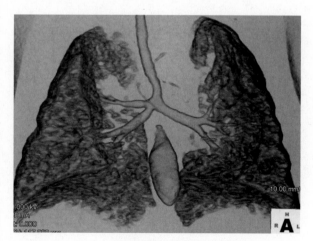

FIGURE 1.44.4

FINDINGS: Lateral view from an esophagram (Fig. 1.44.1) reveals a mass between the trachea and esophagus, compressing the trachea. IV-enhanced CT image of the thorax (Fig. 1.44.2) reveals the left pulmonary artery passing posterior to the trachea. A 3D reconstruction looking down on the heart and great vessels (Fig. 1.44.3) demonstrates the left pulmonary artery arising from the right pulmonary artery, whereas 3D coronal CT reconstruction of the airway (Fig. 1.44.4) reveals rightward displacement and compression of the distal trachea.

DIAGNOSIS: Pulmonary artery sling

DISCUSSION: An anomalous left pulmonary artery arising from the right pulmonary artery, passing around the distal trachea and then between the trachea and esophagus to reach the left lung, has been termed a *pulmonary artery sling*. It typically presents with respiratory distress in the neonatal period. It is the only vascular ring to pass between the trachea and esophagus. As it courses just above and around the distal trachea and right mainstem bronchus, it is frequently accompanied by asymmetric hyperinflation on the right. In 50% of patients, the anomalous left pulmonary artery may be accompanied by a long-segment tracheal stenosis secondary to complete tracheal rings, the so-called ring–sling complex. These patients tend to have severe respiratory distress and bilateral air trapping. In addition to complete tracheal rings, the pulmonary sling is often associated with other congenital anomalies, including congenital heart disease (this patient also had total anomalous pulmonary venous return) and gastrointestinal anomalies, such as tracheoesophageal fistula. Multidetector CT of the thorax is an outstanding modality to identify the pulmonary sling, its effect on the airway, and any associated cardiac anomalies (62–64).

## Aunt Minnie's Pearls

The pulmonary sling is the only vascular ring to pass between the trachea and esophagus, compressing the trachea from behind and producing an anterior impression on the esophagus.

Multidetector CT is the best imaging modality to demonstrate a pulmonary sling and its effect on the airway in a critically ill infant.

**HISTORY:** A 6-week-old male with nonbilious projectile vomiting

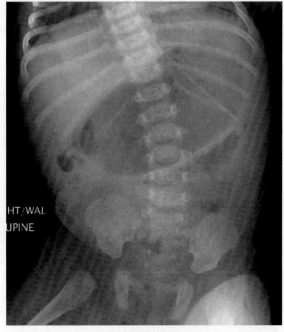

FIGURE 1.45.1

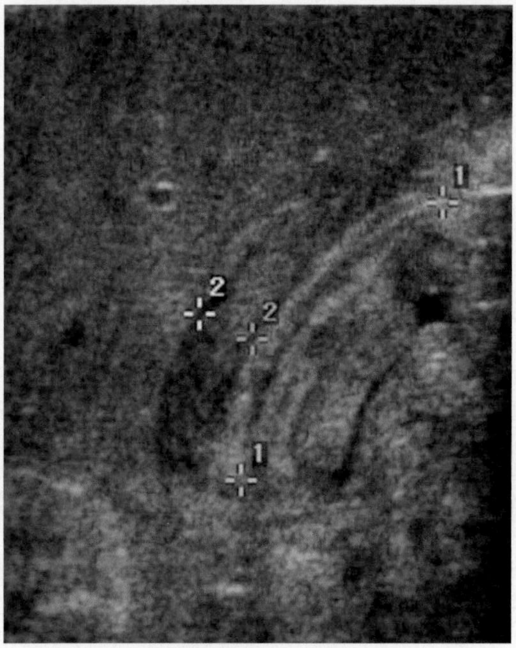

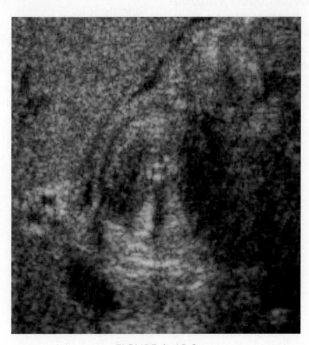

FIGURE 1.45.2

FIGURE 1.45.3

**FINDINGS:** Abdominal radiograph (Fig. 1.45.1) reveals the stomach to be distended with gas. Longitudinal (Fig. 1.45.2) and transverse (Fig. 1.45.3) images through the right epigastrium reveal marked thickening of the pyloric musculature (5 mm) and elongation of the pyloric channel (19 mm). With real-time observation, there was no evidence of passage of gastric contents through the pyloric channel.

**DIAGNOSIS:** Infantile hypertrophic pyloric stenosis (IHPS)

**DISCUSSION:** IHPS, frequently called *pyloric stenosis*, is the most common cause of intestinal obstruction in infancy. It has a 4:1 male predominance as well as a familial predisposition. Hypertrophy and hyperplasia of the circular and longitudinal musculature of the pylorus cause a gastric outlet obstruction resulting in the most common presentation, progressive, nonbilious vomiting in an infant 2 to 8 weeks of age. Without intervention, the repetitive vomiting of gastric contents results in weight loss, despite a voracious appetite, and loss of sodium, potassium, and hydrochloric acid, producing a hypochloremic acidosis. Sonography is the imaging modality of choice, as it provides direct visualization of the anatomy of the pylorus with an accuracy approaching 100%. Pyloric channel thickness >3.0 mm is considered diagnostic, but frequently it is much thicker than that. The lumen is full of redundant, echogenic mucosa. A pyloric channel length >17 mm is also considered abnormal; however, it is often practically difficult to get an accurate length measurement owing to the presence of a distended stomach and the resulting curvature of the pylorus posteriorly. The actual numeric measurements are less important than the overall appearance of the musculature and real-time observation of a persistently thickened and elongated pyloric channel. If the pylorus is difficult to localize, the infant may be rolled into a right anterior or right posterior oblique position to displace gas or fluid and afford better visualization of the pylorus. Using these positional maneuvers usually obviates the need for additional fluid or for placement of a nasogastric tube to decompress the stomach. IHPS is differentiated from pylorospasm by the persistence of the thickened pylorus throughout the examination and lack of normal peristalsis in the thickened pyloric channel. Treatment is surgical with a Ramstedt pyloromyotomy in which the hypertrophied muscle is split longitudinally down to the level of the mucosa. It may be performed via an abdominal incision or laparoscopically (65).

## Aunt Minnie's Pearls

Nonbilious forceful or "projectile" vomiting in an infant of 2 to 8 weeks of age is highly suggestive of pyloric stenosis.

Ultrasound is the imaging modality of choice and, sonographic diagnostic criteria are increased pyloric muscle thickness >3 mm, elongation of the pyloric channel >17 mm, and persistent delay in emptying of gastric contents through the pylorus throughout the course of the examination.

**HISTORY:** A 2-year-old child with 24-hour history of intermittent, crampy abdominal pain and bloody stools

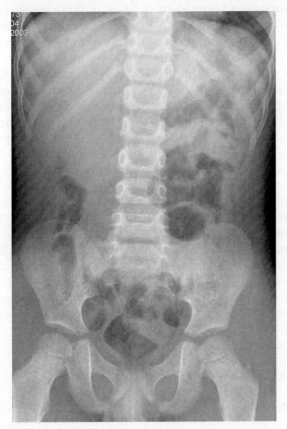

FIGURE 1.46.1

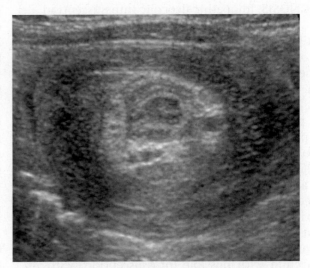

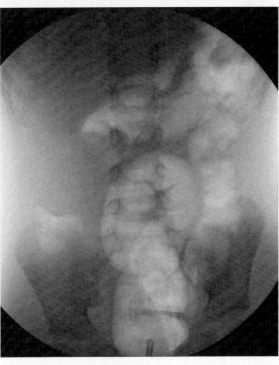

FIGURE 1.46.2

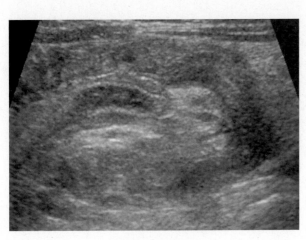

FIGURE 1.46.3

FIGURE 1.46.4

**FINDINGS:** A supine radiograph of the abdomen (Fig. 1.46.1) reveals air scattered in small bowel with a questionable soft-tissue mass in the right upper quadrant. A transverse (Fig. 1.46.2) sonographic image of the right upper quadrant reveals a target sign with multiple concentric rings of bowel within bowel. The longitudinal image (Fig. 1.46.3) reveals the "sandwich" or "pseudokidney" sign. A single image during an air-contrast enema (Fig. 1.46.4) reveals an intraluminal soft-tissue mass in the hepatic flexure.

**DIAGNOSIS:** Idiopathic ileocolic intussusception

**DISCUSSION:** Ileocolic intussusception, a telescoping or invagination of small bowel into the colon, is the most common cause of small-bowel obstruction in childhood. Typically, intussusception occurs between the ages of 5 months and 3 years and presents with irritability, intermittent abdominal pain, vomiting, bloody stools, and/or lethargy. Plain abdominal radiographs have a poor sensitivity (45%) but may demonstrate absence of bowel gas in the ascending colon, a soft-tissue mass within the expected course of the colon, characteristically the proximal transverse colon as in this case, or a small-bowel obstruction with a completely empty colon. Ultrasound is extremely valuable in the evaluation of a child with possible intussusception, with reported accuracies and sensitivities of 98% to 100%. Scanning the abdomen with high-frequency linear transducers is recommended. The identification of a complex, several-centimeter mass with multiple concentric alternating rings, the bowel with bowel, producing a target sign in transverse and a sandwich or pseudokidney sign in longitudinal plane, confirms the diagnosis of intussusception by ultrasound. The presence of flow within the mass on color Doppler suggests that the bowel is viable and therefore, potentially reducible. In addition, ultrasound may identify a lead point or suggest that it is not ileocolic but localized in the small bowel. Common lead points include Meckel's diverticulum, duplication cysts, and lymphoma.

Once the diagnosis of intussusception has been confirmed and the surgical team that the patient is appropriately hydrated and has no signs of peritonitis, sepsis, or perforation, the radiologist typically performs a fluoroscopically guided intussusception reduction. Barium and water-soluble contrast have been used; however, air is the current contrast agent of choice because it is effective, avoids the risk of barium peritonitis or electrolyte disturbances should there be a perforation, and is often faster, thereby reducing irradiation exposure to the patient. Alternatively, in some parts of the world, saline enemas are used under sonographic guidance. Reflux of air or contrast into the small bowel signifies a successful reduction. If there is a question of incomplete reduction after enema, ultrasound again may be useful to verify the persistent intussusception or confirm a successful reduction (66).

## Aunt Minnie's Pearls

Ileocolic intussusception typically presents with colicky abdominal pain ± blood stools in children between the ages of 5 months and 3 years.

Ultrasound is highly sensitive (approaching 100%) in the diagnosis of intussusception.

Air enema (pneumatic reduction) is the procedure of choice in the nonoperative management of intussusception. Resolution of the soft tissue mass and reflux of air into small bowel are the hallmarks of successful reduction.

**HISTORY:** Newborn infant girl with a right renal cyst noted on a prenatal sonogram

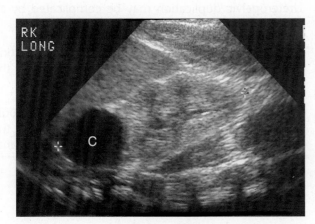

FIGURE 1.47.1

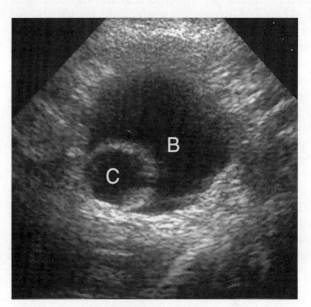

FIGURE 1.47.2

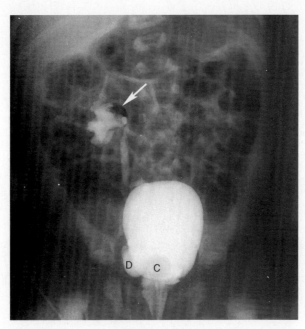

FIGURE 1.47.3

**FINDINGS:** A sagittal ultrasound image of the right kidney (Fig. 1.47.1) demonstrates a right upper pole cyst (*C*). A transverse view (Fig. 1.47.2) of the bladder (*B*) shows a cystic structure (*C*) in the right inferolateral aspect of the right bladder, producing a classic "cyst-within-a-cyst" appearance. The voiding cysto-ureterogram (Fig. 1.47.3) shows a filling defect (*C*) in the bladder, right paraureteral diverticulum (*D*), and right vesicoureteral reflux into the lower moiety of a duplicated right intrarenal collecting system, also known as the famous "drooping-lily" sign (*arrow*).

**DIAGNOSIS:** Ureteropelvic duplication with an ectopic ureterocele

DISCUSSION: Ureteropelvic duplication complicated by an ectopic ureterocele is an important surgical cause of urinary tract infections in infants and young children. The Weigert–Meyer rule dictates that the upper pole ureter inserts into the bladder inferomedially to the lower pole ureter, which inserts in the normal anatomic location. The ectopic ureter may also insert into the urethra, vagina, or vestibule in female patients, leading to continuous urinary incontinence. In the male population, the ectopic ureter may insert into the posterior urethra, seminal vesicles, or prostate, and because these structures are proximal to the urethral sphincter, incontinence does not occur. In general, the upper pole ureter is obstructed by an ectopic ureterocele, and the lower pole ureter refluxes. The ectopic ureterocele may obstruct the ipsilateral lower pole ureter, the contralateral ureter, or even the bladder outlet. The examiner should remember that an ectopic ureterocele is a common cause of bilateral hydronephrosis, especially in infant girls (67).

## Aunt Minnie's Pearls

Ureteropelvic duplication may be complicated by an ectopic ureterocele.

The ureterocele obstructs the upper pole collecting system and may obstruct the lower pole ureter, the opposite ureter, or the bladder outlet.

The Weigert–Meyer rule dictates that the upper pole ureter inserts into the bladder inferomedially to the lower pole ureter, which inserts in the normal anatomic location.

**HISTORY:** Neonate with jaundice, decreased hematocrit, and a right flank mass

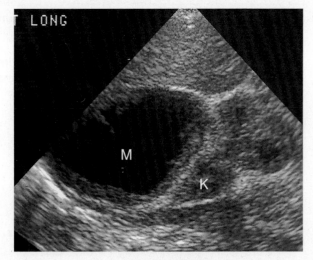

FIGURE 1.48.1

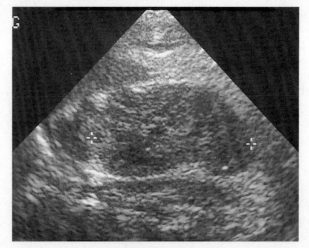

FIGURE 1.48.2

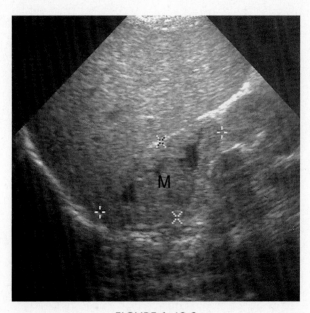

FIGURE 1.48.3

**FINDINGS:** An initial longitudinal image of the right flank (Fig. 1.48.1) reveals a right adrenal mass (*M*) with peripheral solid and central cystic components located superior to the kidney (*K*). Left kidney and adrenal are normal (Fig. 1.48.2); 1 month later, the right adrenal mass (*M*) is smaller (Fig. 1.48.3).

**DIAGNOSIS:** Adrenal hemorrhage

**DISCUSSION:** Adrenal hemorrhage is the most common neonatal adrenal mass. Patients at increased risk include infants of diabetic mothers and babies experiencing perinatal stress from conditions such as sepsis, hypoxia, birth trauma, shock, renal vein thrombosis, and extracorporeal membrane oxygenation (ECMO). Adrenal hemorrhage is more frequently right-sided than left-sided and may be bilateral. Adrenal insufficiency is seldom observed. Significant complications include extracapsular hemorrhage with shock and renal vein thrombosis with diminished renal function. The major differential diagnostic consideration is congenital adrenal neuroblastoma. There are no pathognomonic sonographic features that allow differentiation of the two lesions on the initial examination. Adrenal hemorrhage, however, does decrease in size and becomes more homogeneous on follow-up examinations, whereas neuroblastoma shows interval growth (68).

## Aunt Minnie's Pearls

Risk factors for adrenal hemorrhage include infants of diabetic mothers and babies stressed because of sepsis, hypoxia, birth trauma, shock, renal vein thrombosis, and ECMO.

Think adrenal hemorrhage in a newborn with jaundice, anemia, and an abdominal mass.

Follow-up examinations are critical to differentiate adrenal hemorrhage from congenital adrenal neuroblastoma.

**HISTORY:** Neonate with abnormal prenatal sonography

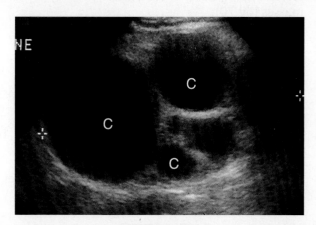

FIGURE 1.49.1

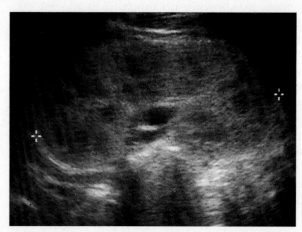

FIGURE 1.49.2

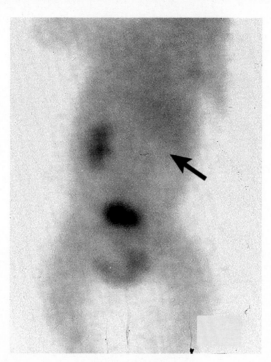

FIGURE 1.49.3

**FINDINGS:** The right kidney (Fig. 1.49.1) is replaced by multiple cysts (*C*) of various sizes that do not intercommunicate and are separated by echogenic parenchyma. The left kidney (Fig. 1.49.2) is sonographically normal. A posterior image from a renogram shows a normally functioning left kidney and absent renal function on the right (Fig. 1.49.3, *arrow*).

**DIAGNOSIS:** Right multicystic dysplastic kidney (MCDK)

**DISCUSSION:** Classic MCDK is thought to result from early in utero atresia of the proximal ureter, renal pelvis, and infundibula. MCDK is the second most common neonatal abdominal mass after congenital ureteropelvic junction obstruction, and most cases present with an abnormal prenatal sonogram. One easy and reliable ultrasonographic sign of MCDK is that the largest cyst is never central, as is the case with congenital ureteropelvic junction obstruction, in which the largest cyst is central and represents the dilated renal pelvis. Nuclear medicine can also assist in differentiating between these two diagnoses by showing no function in the MCDK, and it is also helpful in examining the contralateral kidney, which is abnormal in up to 20% of patients. The most frequent abnormalities observed in the contralateral kidney are vesicoureteral reflux and ureteropelvic junction obstruction. Bilateral MCDK is not compatible with life.

Though MCDKs were traditionally resected because of initial studies suggesting that the masses may be responsible for the development of hypertension, MCDK is now managed nonoperatively because it usually decreases in size, calcifies, and does not produce symptoms. Serial imaging studies are indicated for surveillance of regression or enlargement, and nephrectomy is an option for enlarging, complicated, or atypical cystic renal masses (69,70).

## Aunt Minnie's Pearls

MCDK causes numerous cysts that are not connected on ultrasound images.

Nuclear medicine studies confirm the diagnosis by showing no function on the affected side.

Look for anomalies involving the contralateral kidney.

**HISTORY:** A 10-week-old infant with jaundice and acholic stools

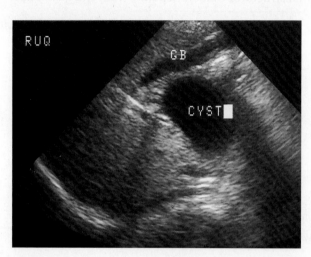

FIGURE 1.50.1

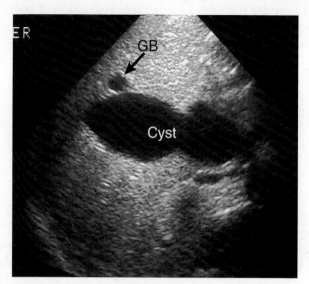

FIGURE 1.50.2

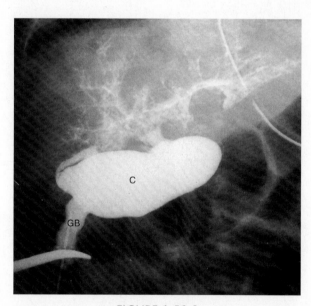

FIGURE 1.50.3

**FINDINGS:** Longitudinal (Fig. 1.50.1) and transverse (Fig. 1.50.2) images through the porta hepatis reveal a bilobed cystic mass (*CYST*) located in the porta hepatis and separate from the gallbladder (*GB*). An operative cholangiogram (Fig. 1.50.3) obtained by injection of the gallbladder shows the large bilobed cyst (*C*) communicating with the gallbladder and an attenuated intrahepatic biliary tree. Notice the absence of contrast distally in the gastrointestinal tract.

**DIAGNOSIS:** Choledochal cyst associated with distal extrahepatic biliary atresia

**DISCUSSION:** The neonatal choledochal cyst is congenital in origin and is often associated with extrahepatic biliary atresia. The clinical presentation is indistinguishable from that of neonatal hepatitis and biliary atresia. Children with choledochal cysts not associated with biliary atresia present later in life with an abdominal mass, pain, or jaundice. Sonography, hepatobiliary scintigraphy, and operative cholangiography are required for complete evaluation of the neonate. Nuclear scintigraphy may reveal only the lack of excretion of radionuclide into the gastrointestinal tract, consistent with biliary atresia, but may fail to visualize the choledochal cyst. Early diagnosis of biliary atresia is crucial because performance of a Kasai procedure (i.e., portoenterostomy) before 12 weeks of age improves the prognosis (71).

## Aunt Minnie's Pearls

Choledochal cysts are seen on sonograms as cystic portal structures that are separate from the gallbladder.

In neonates, this disorder may be associated with extrahepatic biliary atresia.

HISTORY: Infant born prematurely

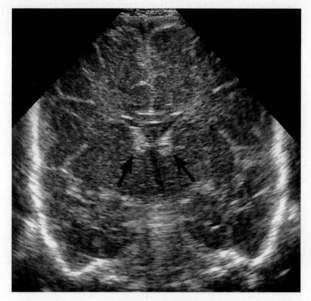

FIGURE 1.51.1

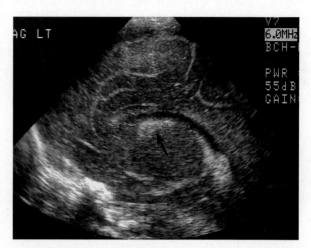

FIGURE 1.51.2

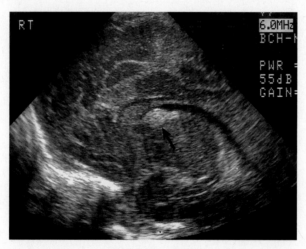

FIGURE 1.51.3

FINDINGS: A coronal image of the neonatal brain (Fig. 1.51.1) shows bilateral hyperechoic masses (*arrows*) that are inferolateral to the floors of the frontal horns and medial to the caudate. On the sagittal images (Figs. 1.51.2 and 1.51.3), the hyperechoic masses appear as a bulge anterior to the caudothalamic groove (*arrows*).

DIAGNOSIS: Bilateral germinal matrix or subependymal hemorrhages

DISCUSSION: The germinal matrix is a bed of highly vascular subependymal tissue that is located adjacent to the lateral ventricles in the caudothalamic groove. In premature infants, the stresses of delivery and extrauterine life can lead to thrombosis, bleeding, and infarction in the delicate tissues of the germinal matrix. Intracranial hemorrhage occurs in 25% to 40% of premature infants born at <32 weeks gestation and weighing <1,500 g. Hyperechoic masses that are centered on the caudothalamic groove are characteristic of germinal matrix hemorrhages. Look for ventricular and parenchymal extension of the hemorrhage and hydrocephalus because prognosis is affected by the presence of these complicating features. As the hemorrhagic areas evolve, they become less echogenic and may even result in cystic encephalomalacia.

Screening sonography of the head is usually performed in this population at days 7 and 14 of life because approximately 90% of intracranial hemorrhages occur by day 6 of life, and most cases of posthemorrhagic hydrocephalus present by day 14. A discharge study is also performed for prognostic assessment, and neurodevelopmental outcome is generally proportional to the severity of the intracranial hemorrhage and degree of ventricular dilatation (72).

## Aunt Minnie's Pearls

Hyperechoic masses in the caudothalamic groove in a premature infant (<32 weeks or <1,500 g) are germinal matrix hemorrhages.

Check for ventricular and parenchymal extension and for the development of hydrocephalus.

HISTORY: Term infant with low Apgar scores, hypotonia, seizures, and metabolic acidosis

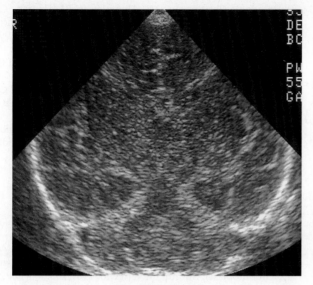

FIGURE 1.52.1

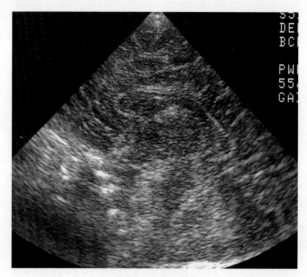

FIGURE 1.52.2

FINDINGS: Coronal (Fig. 1.52.1) and sagittal (Fig. 1.52.2) images of the neonatal brain demonstrate diffusely increased brain echogenicity, poor sulcal–gyral differentiation, and small ventricles.

DIAGNOSIS: Perinatal asphyxia or diffuse hypoxic–ischemic injury

DISCUSSION: Perinatal asphyxia is a common cause of diffuse hypoxic–ischemic injury in the term infant. Neurologic outcome correlates with the sonographic appearance because 90% of patients with abnormal brain echogenicity progress to death or neurologic sequelae. The sonographic findings of diffuse echogenicity and sulcal effacement reflect neuronal necrosis and mass effect from cerebral edema. Focal areas of infarction may be seen as increased echogenicity in the basal ganglia, middle cerebral artery territories, and watershed areas. Late findings of diffuse injury include cystic encephalomalacia, parenchymal calcifications, and atrophy with ventriculomegaly (73).

## Aunt Minnie's Pearls

Diffuse increased echogenicity and sulcal effacement are diagnostic of hypoxic-ischemic injury.

Focal areas of infarction may be seen in the basal ganglia, middle cerebral artery territory, or watershed areas.

# REFERENCES

1. Pracos JP, Sann L, Genin G, et al. Ultrasound diagnosis of midgut volvulus: The "whirlpool" sign. Pediatr Radiol 1992; 22(1):18–20.

2. Stringer DA, Babyn PS. Pediatric gastrointestinal imaging and intervention. Hamilton, ON: BC Decker, 2000:311–332.

3. Stringer DA, Babyn PS. Pediatric gastrointestinal imaging and intervention. Hamilton, ON: BC Decker, 2000:332–336.

4. Lonergan GJ, Baker AM, Morey MK, et al. Child abuse: Radiologic–pathologic correlation. Radiographics 2003;23: 811–845.

5. Kleinman PK. Diagnostic imaging of child abuse. St Louis, MO: Mosby, 1998:8–25, 110–148, 285–342.

6. Slovis TL, Sty JR, Haller JO. Imaging of the pediatric urinary tract. Philadelphia, PA: Saunders, 1989:87–89.

7. Lonergan GJ, Schwab CM, Suarez ES, et al. Neuroblastoma, ganglioneuroblastoma, and ganglioneuroma: Radiologic–pathologic correlation. Radiographics 2002;22:911–934.

8. Stringer DA, Babyn PS. Pediatric gastrointestinal imaging and intervention. Hamilton, ON: BC Decker, 2000:174–190.

9. Taylor GA, Eggli KD. Lap belt injuries of the lumbar spine in children: A pitfall in CT diagnosis. AJR Am J Roentgenol 1988;150:1355–1358.

10. Rampton J. Signs in radiology: The football sign. Radiology 2004;231:81–82.

11. Siegal MJ, Coley BD. Pediatric imaging. Philadelphia, PA: Lippincott Williams & Wilkins, 2006:13–15.

12. Stringer DA. Pediatric gastrointestinal imaging. Hamilton, ON: BC Decker, 2000:496–499.

13. Epelman M, Daneman A, Navarro OM, et al. Necrotizing enterocolitis: Review of state-of-the-art imaging findings with pathologic correlation. Radiographics 2007;27:285–305.

14. Ryan S. Postnatal imaging of chest malformations. In: Donoghue V (ed.). Radiological imaging of the neonatal chest. Berlin, Germany: Springer-Verlag, 2002:98.

15. Gudjonsson U, Brown J. Scimitar syndrome. Semin Thorac Cardiovasc Surg Pediatr Card Surg Ann 2006;9:56–62.

16. Midyat L, Demir E, Aşkin M, et al. Eponym: Scimitar syndrome. Eur J Pediatr 2010;169:1171–1177. doi:10.1007/s00431-010-1152-4.

17. Stringer DA, Babyn PS. Pediatric gastrointestinal imaging and intervention. Hamilton, ON: BC Decker, 2000:342–348.

18. Stringer DA, Babyn PS. Pediatric gastrointestinal imaging and intervention. Hamilton, ON: BC Decker, 2000:363–365.

19. Swischuk L. Imaging of the newborn, infant, and young child. Baltimore, MD: Lippincott Williams & Wilkins, 1997:775–777.

20. Ozonoff MB. Pediatric orthopedic radiology. Philadelphia, PA: Saunders, 1992:293–300.

21. Bar-Ziv J, Koplowitz BZ, Agid R. Imaging of foreign body aspiration in the respiratory tract. In: Lucaya J, Strife J (eds.). Pediatric chest imaging: Chest imaging in infants and children. Berlin, Germany: Springer, 2002:171–183.

22. Stringer DA, Babyn PS. Pediatric gastrointestinal imaging and intervention. Hamilton, ON: BC Decker, 2000:238–246.

23. Christison-Lagay E, Kelleher CM, Langer JC. Neonatal abdominal wall defects. Semin Fetal Neonatal Med 2011;16(3): 164–172.

24. Ledbetter DJ. Congenital abdominal wall defects and reconstruction in pediatric surgery: Gastroschisis and omphalocele. Surg Clin North Am. 2012;92(3):713–727.

25. Stringer DA, Babyn PS. Pediatric gastrointestinal imaging and intervention. Hamilton, ON: BC Decker, 2000:486–490.

26. Stringer DA, Babyn PS. Pediatric gastrointestinal imaging and intervention. Hamilton, ON: BC Decker, 2000:440–442.

27. Lonergan GJ, Cline DB, Abbondanzo SL. Sickle cell anemia. Radiographics 2001;21:971–994.

28. Ejindu VC, Hine AL, Mashayekhi M, et al. Musculoskeletal manifestations of sickle cell disease. Radiographics 2007;27:1005–1021.

29. Moeller KH, Rosado-de-Christenson ML, Templeton PA. Mediastinal mature teratoma: Imaging features. AJR Am J Roentgenol 1997;169(4):985–990.

30. Rosado-de-Christenson ML, Templeton PA, Moran CA. From the archives of the AFIP. Mediastinal germ cell tumors: Radiologic and pathologic correlation. Radiographics 1992; 12(5):1013–1030.

31. Lewis BD, Hurt RD, Payne WS, et al. Benign teratomas of the mediastinum. J Thorac Cardiovasc Surg 1983;86(5):727–731.

32. Ikezoe J, Morimoto S, Arisawa J, et al. (1986). Ultrasonography of mediastinal teratoma. J Clin Ultrasound 1986;14(7): 513–520.

33. MacPherson RI. Gastrointestinal tract duplications: Clinical, pathologic, etiologic, and radiologic considerations. Radiographics 1993;13:1063–1080.

34. Seigel MJ. Pediatric sonography. Philadelphia, PA: Lippincott Williams & Wilkins, 2011:364–365.

35. Seigel MJ, Coley BD. Pediatric imaging. Philadelphia, PA: Lippincott Williams & Wilkins, 2006:245–249.

36. Taybi LR. Radiology of syndromes, metabolic disorders, and skeletal dysplasias. St Louis, MO: Mosby, 1996:643–646.

37. Kao SC, Waziri MH, Smith WL, et al. MR imaging of the craniovertebral junction, cranium, and brain in children with achondroplasia. AJR Am J Roentgenol 1989;153:565–569.

38. Tavormina PL, Shiang R, Thompson LM, et al. Thanatophoric dysplasia (types I and II) caused by distinct mutations in fibroblast growth factor receptor 3. Nat Genet 1995;9(3):321–328.

39. Sahinoglu Z, Uludogan M, Gurbuz A, et al. Prenatal diagnosis of thanatophoric dysplasia in the second trimester: Ultrasonography and other diagnostic modalities. Arch Gynecol Obstet 2003;269(1):57–61.

40. Dighe M, Fligner C, Cheng E, et al. Fetal skeletal dysplasia: An approach to diagnosis with illustrative cases. Radiographics 2008;28(4):1061–1077.

41. Orioli IM, Castilla EE, Barbosa-Neto JG. The birth prevalence rates for the skeletal dysplasias. J Med Genet 1986; 23(4):328–332.

42. Baker KM, Olson DS, Harding CO, et al. Long-term survival in typical thanatophoric dysplasia type 1. Am J Med Genet 1997;70(4):427–436.

43. Sillence DO, Senn A, Danks DM. Genetic heterogeneity in osteogenesis imperfecta. J Med Genet 1979;16(2):101–116.

44. Langenskiold A. Tibia vara: A critical review. Clin Orthop Relat Res 1989;246:195–207.

45. Ozonoff MB. Pediatric orthopedic radiology. Philadelphia, PA: Saunders, 1992:324–331.

46. Ozonoff MB. Pediatric orthopedic radiology. Philadelphia, PA: Saunders, 1992:190–209.

47. Kan JH, Kleinman PK. Pediatric and adolescent musculoskeletal MRI: A case-based approach. New York, NY: Springer, 2007:166–173.

48. Mattano LA Jr, Sather HN, Trigg ME, et al. Osteonecrosis as a complication of treating acute lymphoblastic leukemia in children: A report from the Children's Cancer Group. J Clin Oncol 2000;18(18):3262–3272.

49. Yu J, Turner MS, Fulcher AS, et al. Congenital anomalies and normal variants of the pancreaticobiliary tract and the pancreas in adults: Part 2, pancreatic duct and pancreas. AJR Am J Roentgenol 2006;187(6):1544–1553. doi:10.2214/AJR.05.0774.

50. Sivit CJ, Taylor GA, Bulas DI, et al. Posttraumatic shock in children: CT findings associated with hemodynamic instability. Radiology 1992;182:723–726.

51. Altman NR, Purser RK, Post MJ. Tuberous sclerosis: Characteristics at CT and MR imaging. Radiology 1988;167(2):527–532.

52. Swischuk LE. Imaging of the newborn, infant, and young child. Baltimore, MD: Lippincott Williams & Wilkins, 1997:904–913.
53. Swischuk LE. Imaging of the newborn, infant, and young child. Baltimore, MD: Lippincott Williams & Wilkins, 1997:933–935.
54. Swischuk LE. Imaging of the newborn, infant, and young child. Baltimore, MD: Lippincott Williams & Wilkins, 1997:949.
55. Siegel MJ. Pediatric sonography. Philadelphia, PA: Lippincott Williams & Wilkins, 2011:81–83.
56. Brunelle F. Arteriovenous malformation of the vein of Galen in children. Pediatr Radiol 1997;27:501–513.
57. Sztriha L. Spectrum of corpus callosum agenesis. Pediatr Neurol 2005;32(2):94–101.
58. Siegel MJ. Pediatric sonography. Philadelphia, PA: Lippincott Williams & Wilkins, 2011:90–92.
59. Siegel MJ. Pediatric sonography. Philadelphia, PA: Lippincott Williams & Wilkins, 2011:72–75.
60. Vijayaraghavan SB. Sonographic differential diagnosis of acute scrotum: Real-time whirlpool sign, a key sign of torsion. J Ultrasound Med 2006;25:563–574.
61. Siegel MJ. The acute scrotum. Radiol Clin North Am 1997; 35:959–976.
62. Schulman M. Vascular rings: A practical approach to imaging and diagnosis. Pediatr Radiol 2005;35(10):961–979.
63. Backer CL. Vascular rings and pulmonary artery sling. In: Mavroudis C, Backer CL (eds.). Pediatric cardiac surgery, 3rd ed. Philadelphia, PA: Mosby, 2003:234–250.
64. Berdon WE. Rings, slings, and other things: Vascular compression of the infant trachea updated from the midcentury to the millennium—the legacy of Robert E. Gross, MD, and Edward B. D. Neuhauser, MD. Radiology 2000;216(3):624–632.
65. Hernanz-Schulman M. Infantile hypertrophic pyloric stenosis. Radiology 2003;227:319–331.
66. Applegate KE. Clinically suspected intussusception in children: Evidence-based review and self-assessment module. AJR Am J Roentgenol 2005;185:S175–S183.
67. Nussbaum AR, Dorst JP, Jeffs RD, et al. Ectopic ureter and ureterocele: Their varied sonographic manifestations. Radiology 1986;159:227–235.
68. Shackelford GD. Adrenal glands, pancreas, and other retroperitoneal structures. In: Siegel MJ (ed.). Pediatric sonography, 2nd ed. New York, NY: Raven, 1995:306–310.
69. Strife JL, Souza AS, Marks DR, et al. Multicystic dysplastic kidney in children: US follow-up. Radiology 1993;186: 785–788.
70. Atiyeh B, Husmann D, Baum M. Contralateral renal abnormalities in multicystic dysplastic kidney disease. J Pediatr 1992;121:65–67.
71. Torrisi JM, Haller JO, Velcek FT. Choledochal cyst and biliary atresia in the neonate: Imaging findings in five cases. AJR Am J Roentgenol 1990;155:1273–1276.
72. Siegel MJ. Brain. In: Siegel MJ (ed.). Pediatric sonography, 2nd ed. New York, NY: Raven, 1995:40–49.
73. Siegel MJ, Shackelford GD, Perlman JM, et al. Hypoxic–ischemic encephalopathy in term infants: Diagnosis and prognosis evaluated by ultrasound. Radiology 1984;152: 395–399.

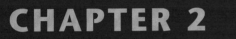

# CHAPTER 2

# MUSCULOSKELETAL SYSTEM

**Catherine C. Roberts / Laura W. Bancroft / Thomas L. Pope Jr.**

*The authors and editors acknowledge the contribution of the Chapter 2 author from the second edition: Riyadh Al-Okaii, MD*

**HISTORY:** A 39-year-old man fell

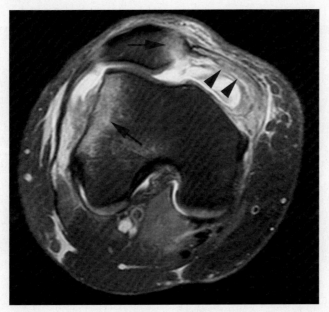

FIGURE 2.1.1

**FINDINGS:** Axial, T2-weighted fat-suppressed MR image (Fig. 2.1.1) shows bone contusions in the medial patella and the lateral femoral condyle (*arrows*) with an associated tear of the medial retinaculum (*arrowheads*).

**DIAGNOSIS:** Acute patellar dislocation-relocation (PDR)

**DISCUSSION:** Acute PDR is a common injury that occurs with a variety of activities and accounts for 2% to 3% of knee injuries overall, but has a higher incidence in active populations (1). It characteristically occurs with internal rotation of the femur on a fixed and externally rotated tibia or a direct blow to the medial side of the knee. In PDR, the patella dislocates laterally, and the medial patellar facet impinges on the lateral femoral condyle, producing bone contusions at both sites. Because the bone contusions result from direct impaction as they are in the transient dislocation of the knee associated with ACL tears, the contusions may also be called "kissing contusions." Clinical evaluation of the patient with PDR is often difficult because of the large knee joint effusion and because the patella is usually relocated to its near anatomic position at the time of presentation. The patient may not realize that patellar dislocation has occurred.

Radiographs may show a lipohemarthrosis or a chip fracture adjacent to the donor site of the medial facet of the patella. MR findings associated with PDR include any or all of the following: disruption or sprain of the medial retinaculum, lateral patellar tilt or subluxation, lateral femoral condylar and medial patellar osseous contusions, osteochondral injury to the medial patella or lateral femur, intraarticular sliver-like osseus fragment, damage to Hoffa's fat pad, and joint effusion or lipohemarthrosis (2–6). MR imaging is recommended for all patients with PDR since they often have concomitant injury to the major ligaments of the knee or the menisci (7). Redislocation occurs in up to 63% of patients, and more than one-half of these untreated patients will have fair to poor outcomes. Surgical repair versus closed management is tailored to the patient's clinical situation (8).

## Aunt Minnie's Pearls

Bone contusions of the medial patellar facet and lateral femoral condyle (i.e., "kissing contusions") are seen with PDR.

Meniscal or ligamentous injuries are often associated findings in PDR.

Aggressive surgical repair is indicated to avoid chronic, repetitive dislocation and morbidity.

## Case 2.2

**HISTORY:** A 61-year-old woman with shoulder pain (Figs. 2.2.1 and 2.2.2). (Fig. 2.2.3 is described under **Discussion.**)

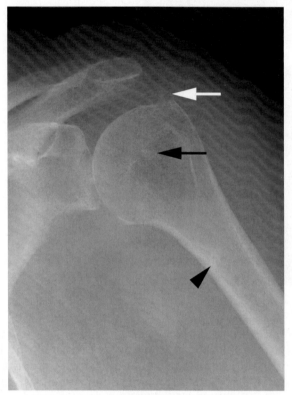

FIGURE 2.2.1

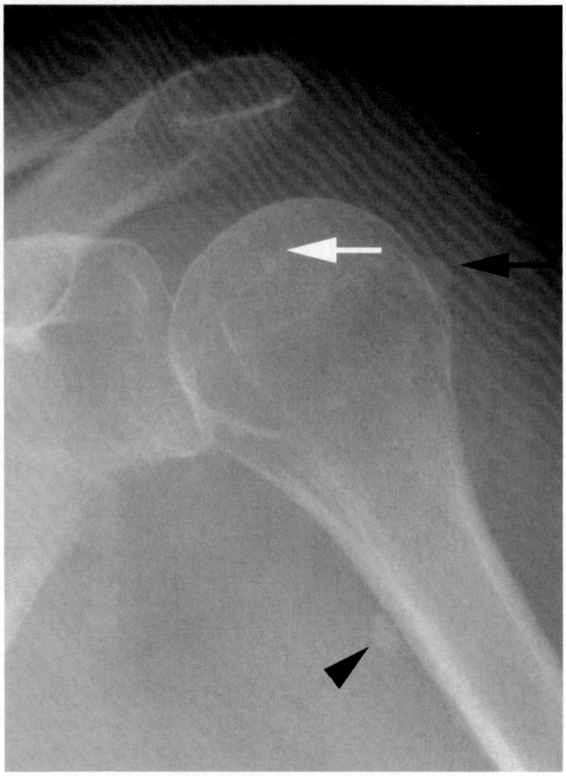

FIGURE 2.2.2

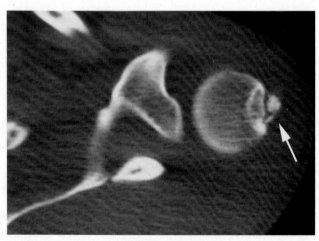

FIGURE 2.2.3

**FINDINGS:** AP radiographs of the left shoulder in external (Fig. 2.2.1) and internal (Fig. 2.2.2) rotation demonstrate globular foci of calcification in the expected location of the supraspinatus (*white arrow*), infraspinatus (*black arrow*), and pectoralis major (*arrowheads*) tendons.

**DIAGNOSIS:** Hydroxyapatite deposition disease (HADD)

**DISCUSSION:** HADD consists of crystal deposition in and around joints, without a known cause (9). Two-thirds of patients are asymptomatic (10). HADD can be the cause of acute pain and be associated with fever, increased erythrocyte sedimentation rate, and C-reactive protein. Other terms used to describe this entity include calcific tendonitis, hydroxyapatite rheumatism, calcific periarthritis, and peritendinitis calcarea.

On radiographs, the calcium deposits appear cloud-like and amorphous and can involve the tendon, ligament, bursa, or joint capsule. Intraarticular crystal deposition can destroy the joint space, resulting in a condition referred to as "Milwaukee shoulder." The shoulder is most commonly involved. On CT, accompanying erosion of the underlying bone can be seen (Fig. 2.2.3). If the interpreting radiologist is not familiar with this entity, bone erosion from HADD can be misinterpreted as reflecting an aggressive malignant process. Biopsy of these areas in equivocal cases can exclude malignancy, but the hydroxyapatite crystals are beyond the resolution of light microscopy, so a specific pathologic diagnosis of HADD will not result unless electron microscopy or electron diffraction studies are utilized. Alizarin S stain can screen for crystals but identifies other calcium crystals as well. The CT appearance has been described as commonly having a flame-shaped or comet-tail configuration of the calcifications (11,12). If calcification and erosion occur in a region not typical for HADD, additional workup to exclude malignancy is necessary.

## Aunt Minnie's Pearls

HADD is commonly referred to as calcific tendinosis and usually has an innocuous appearance on radiographs consisting of cloud-like calcification.

HADD typically is asymptomatic until migration of the calcification can be the cause of acute pain.

HADD can have an aggressive, erosive appearance on CT, especially when involving the pectoralis major origin, which can be misinterpreted as malignancy.

**HISTORY:** Three individuals with foot pain

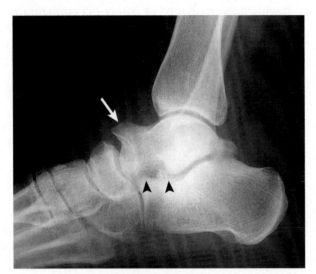

FIGURE 2.3.1

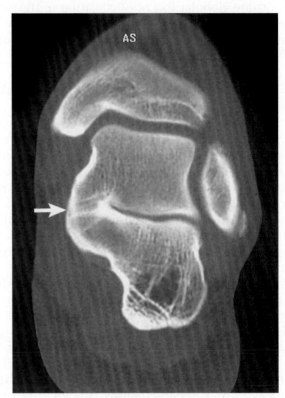

FIGURE 2.3.2

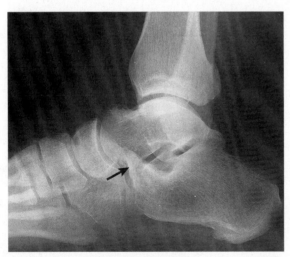

FIGURE 2.3.3

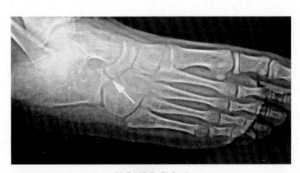

FIGURE 2.3.4

**FINDINGS:** A lateral radiograph of the left foot (Fig. 2.3.1) demonstrates a prominent talar beak (*arrow*) and bony sclerosis overlying the middle facet (*arrowheads*). Coronal CT through the middle facet shows talocalcaneal fusion, with bony bridging between the talus and the sustentaculum tali of the calcaneus (Fig. 2.3.2, *arrow*). Figures 2.3.3 to 2.3.6 are explained under **Discussion.**

**DIAGNOSIS:** Tarsal coalition

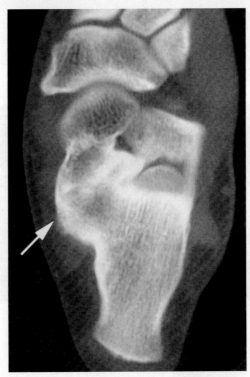

FIGURE 2.3.5

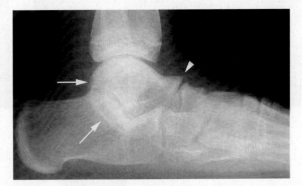

FIGURE 2.3.6

**DISCUSSION:** Tarsal coalition, an abnormal fusion of one or more of the tarsal bones, may be fibrous, cartilaginous, or osseous and may be posttraumatic or result from articular disease, infection, or surgery. It may be congenital, usually a consequence of autosomal dominant inheritance, and it has been linked to several syndromes. Research on defining the exact DNA point mutations is ongoing (13–15). The most common tarsal coalitions are calcaneonavicular and talocalcaneal (16). Almost all talocalcaneal coalitions occur between the sustentaculum tali of the calcaneus and the middle facet of the talus. The incidence of tarsal coalition is <1% (17,18). The disorder is more common in male patients, may be bilateral in up to 50% of patients, and is most commonly discovered during the second and third decades of life (14,19). Multiple ipsilateral coalitions have been described (14). The peroneal spastic flatfoot deformity may be the initial clinical manifestation in many of these patients because of decreased subtalar motion (20).

Radiographically, calcaneonavicular coalition may be suspected because of elongation of the anterior facet of the calcaneus on radiographs (i.e., anteater sign; Fig. 2.3.3, *arrow*). The 45-degree medial oblique view is the best diagnostic radiographic projection to demonstrate this type of coalition (Fig. 2.3.4). CT can also be used to confirm coalition and shows sclerosis at the articulation (Fig. 2.3.5). Congenital coalition usually evolves from fibrous to osseous coalition and may not be apparent on the initial evaluation.

Talocalcaneal coalition can result in dorsal beaking of the talar head (Fig. 2.3.6, *arrowhead*), the so-called C-sign (Fig. 2.3.6, *arrows*), a ball-and-socket ankle mortise, asymmetry of the inferior talar necks, widening of the lateral talar process, nonvisualization of the subtalar joint medial facet (21), and close approximation between the talus and calcaneus. For definitive diagnosis of either type of coalition, CT is the preferred investigation in most cases (22).

## Aunt Minnie's Pearls

The most common types of tarsal coalition are talocalcaneal and calcaneonavicular.

Talocalcaneal coalition is bilateral in approximately 25% to 50% of patients.

CT is the investigation of choice for the diagnosis of tarsal coalition.

The anteater sign is seen in calcaneonavicular coalition.

A talar beak, obscured middle facet, and C-sign are seen in talocalcaneal coalition.

**HISTORY:** A 23-year-old man with pain in the right hip

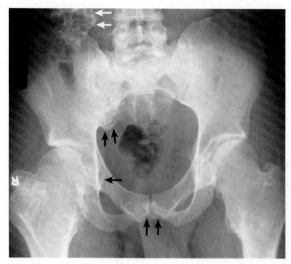

FIGURE 2.4.1

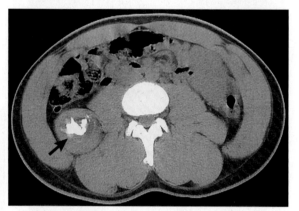

FIGURE 2.4.2

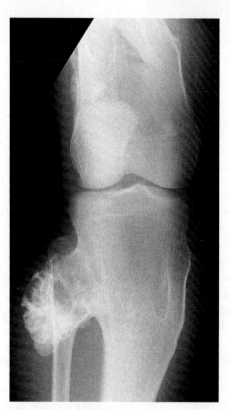

FIGURE 2.4.3

**FINDINGS:** An anteroposterior view of the pelvis (Fig. 2.4.1) shows flaring of the metaphyseal regions of the proximal femurs and numerous osteochondromas arising from the right iliac crest, pubic bones, and proximal right femur (*arrows*). An axial CT image through the upper pelvis demonstrates a large, right exostosis with an associated soft-tissue mass (Fig. 2.4.2, *arrow*). An anteroposterior radiograph of the knee shows multiple osteochondromas arising from the femur and the fibula (Fig. 2.4.3). Figures 2.4.4 and 2.4.5 show the classic radiographic findings in the distal femur and forearm in other patients with this same disorder.

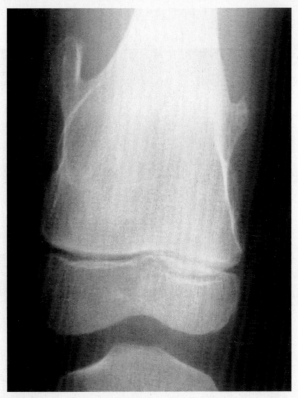

FIGURE 2.4.4

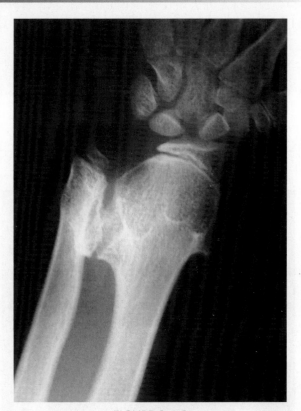

FIGURE 2.4.5

**DIAGNOSIS:** Multiple hereditary exostosis (i.e., diaphyseal aclasia)

**DISCUSSION:** Multiple hereditary exostosis is an autosomal dominant disorder that usually manifests in the first or second decades of life. Pain may be the presenting symptom because of compression of neurovascular structures by the osteochondromas. Initial signs of the disorder may include decreased range of motion, deformities caused by bowing or shortening of the involved bones, and palpable masses adjacent to joints. The osteochondromas are generally bilateral and most commonly involve the femur, tibia, fibula, and humerus. The scapula, innominate bone, ribs, radius, and ulna may also be affected.

Complications occurring in multiple hereditary exostosis are the same as those associated with solitary exostosis: fracture, vascular injury, bursal formation, neurologic compromise, osseous deformity, and malignant transformation. The risk of malignant transformation is 5% in the patient with multiple hereditary exostoses and <1% in those with solitary exostosis. Clinical features of pain, swelling, palpable mass, and imaging findings showing growth of a previously stable exostosis, new bony erosion, or development of new or increasing calcifications are signs of potential malignant transformation. The definitive diagnosis of a developing malignancy is determined by open biopsy and pathologic examination. The most frequently associated malignant tumor is chondrosarcoma, usually developing in the femur, tibia, humerus, or innominate bone (Fig. 2.4.2, *arrow*) (23,24).

## Aunt Minnie's Pearls

Abnormal modeling of bone and osseous deformity are characteristic of multiple hereditary exostosis.

New pain, mass, bony erosion, or calcifications may indicate malignant transformation.

Definitive diagnosis of malignant degeneration requires open biopsy and pathologic examination.

HISTORY: Three patients with the same diagnosis

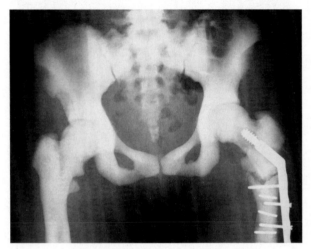

FIGURE 2.5.1

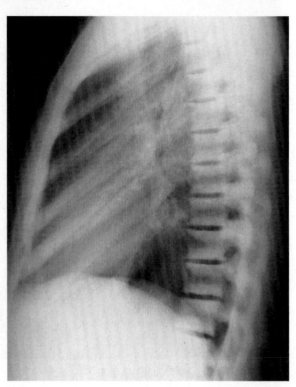

FIGURE 2.5.2

**FINDINGS:** Anteroposterior view of the pelvis (Fig. 2.5.1) in a 22-year-old woman shows diffuse, uniform, bony sclerosis and a subtrochanteric fracture of the proximal left femur. A lateral chest radiograph of another patient (Fig. 2.5.2) shows the sandwich appearance of the vertebral bodies caused by increased sclerosis of the superior and inferior end plates. Radiographs of the knees in a younger patient (Fig. 2.5.3) show splaying of the metaphyses and alternating radiolucent bands in the distal femurs and proximal tibias and fibulas bilaterally.

**DIAGNOSIS:** Osteopetrosis

**DISCUSSION:** Osteopetrosis is a complex hereditary disorder characterized by a defect in osteoclastic resorption. Four subtypes are described with distinct clinical and radiographic features. The two most common subtypes are the precocious and delayed types. The autosomal recessive, precocious form is lethal, and the patients usually die shortly after birth or survive for only a few years. Clinically, they are characterized by hepatosplenomegaly, failure to thrive, and blindness. Patients with the autosomal dominant, delayed form are generally asymptomatic but may have mild anemia, cranial nerve deficits, pathologic fracture, or bleeding problems after tooth extraction (25).

The imaging features of osteopetrosis consist of generalized osteosclerosis and diffuse cortical thickening with narrowing of the medullary cavity. Typical radiographic features include the bone-within-bone appearance, metaphyseal undermodeling and widening (i.e., Erlenmeyer flask deformity), radiolucent

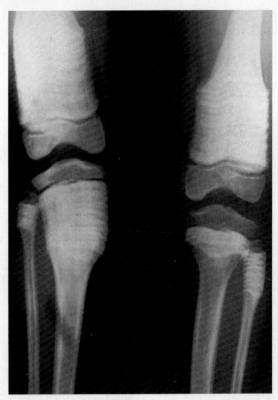

FIGURE 2.5.3

and radiodense bands near the ends of long bones, and obliteration of mastoid air cells and paranasal sinuses. Potential complications of osteopetrosis include fractures (i.e., bones are weaker than normal), crowding of normal bone marrow spaces resulting in pancytopenia and extramedullary hematopoiesis, and osteosclerosis of the basal foramina of the skull with resultant cranial nerve deficits (26).

## Aunt Minnie's Pearls

Osteosclerosis + alternating radiolucent bands + metaphyseal widening = osteopetrosis.

The major complications are pathologic fractures, pancytopenia, and cranial nerve defects.

# Case 2.6

HISTORY: A 11-year-old boy with right arm pain after a fall (Figs. 2.6.1 and 2.6.2). Figure 2.6.3 shows the same lesion in the femur of a different patient.

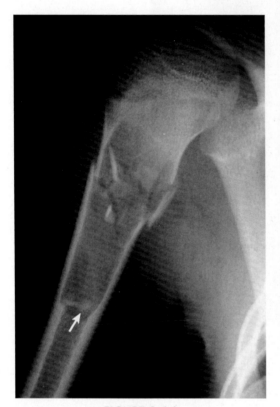

FIGURE 2.6.1

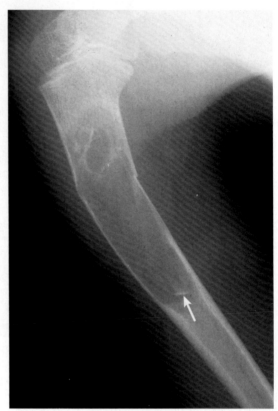

FIGURE 2.6.2

FINDINGS: Anteroposterior and lateral views of the proximal right humerus (Figs. 2.6.1 and 2.6.2) demonstrate a well-circumscribed, geographic, lytic metaphyseal lesion with cortical thinning. The lesion has well-defined margins and no demonstrable matrix. A comminuted fracture has occurred, and fragments of the cortex have fallen to the dependent portion of the lesion (arrows). Figure 2.6.3 exhibits the same lesion in the femur of a 7-year-old boy.

DIAGNOSIS: Unicameral bone cyst

DISCUSSION: Unicameral or simple bone cysts are benign lesions of unknown origin that are often initially discovered because of pathologic fracture. The "fallen-fragment sign" is the distinguishing feature in these lesions because the fragments can reach this position only in purely cystic lesions (27). These tumors are uncommon, comprising only 5%

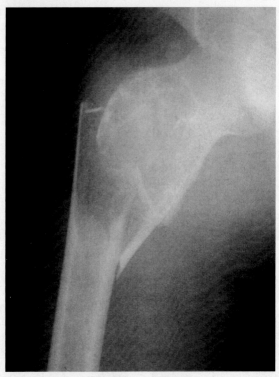

FIGURE 2.6.3

of all primary bone tumors. The most common sites of involvement are the proximal humerus, femur, tibia, or fibula. Most lesions are identified in the second decade, and there is a 2:1 male predominance. Lesions near the metaphysis are active, but as the patient grows, the lesion migrates to the diaphysis of the bone and becomes inactive. Treatment includes curettage and packing with bone chips or steroid injection. Lesions have been reported to resolve spontaneously (28).

## Aunt Minnie's Pearls

Unicameral bone cysts are most common in the proximal humerus and femur.

The fallen-fragment sign confirms the cystic nature of this lesion.

**HISTORY:** A 55-year-old woman (Fig. 2.7.1) and 47-year-old man (Figs. 2.7.2 to 2.7.5), both with foot pain

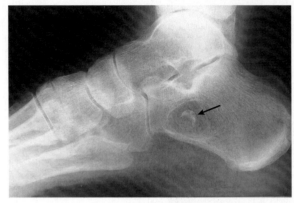

FIGURE 2.7.1

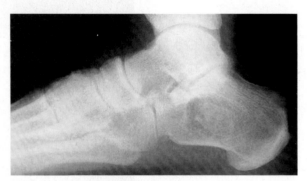

FIGURE 2.7.2

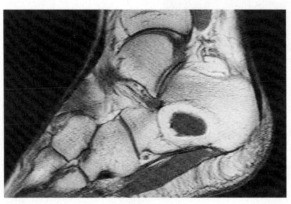

FIGURE 2.7.3

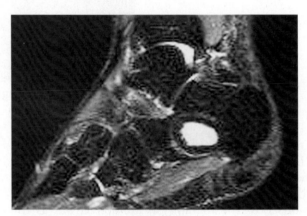

FIGURE 2.7.4

**FINDINGS:** A lateral radiograph of the left foot (Fig. 2.7.1) shows a nonaggressive, well-defined lytic lesion in the anterior aspect of the calcaneus with a thin sclerotic border and central calcification. A lateral radiograph of the foot (Fig. 2.7.2) shows a lytic lesion in the calcaneus with central calcification. Sagittal T1-weighted (Fig. 2.7.3) and short tau inversion recovery (STIR) (Fig. 2.7.4) MR images demonstrate a lesion with signal characteristics of peripheral fat and a cystic center. No soft-tissue mass is present. Figure 2.7.5 is explained under **Discussion**.

**DIAGNOSIS:** Intraosseous lipoma

**DISCUSSION:** Intraosseous lipomas, comprising <1% of all primary bone tumors, are most commonly diagnosed in the fourth to sixth decades of

life. However, the lesions have been reported in patients up to 75 years of age. Male and female patients are equally affected. The lesion averages 4 cm in diameter and is usually found within the metaphyses of the long tubular bones of the femur, tibia, and fibula or within the calcaneus (29,30). Multiple intraosseous lipomas are rare.

The intraosseous lipoma is characterized radiographically by radiolucency; a thin, sclerotic margin; and occasionally by lobulation or intraosseous ridges. Bony expansion, when it occurs, is usually within the small tubular bones. In the calcaneus, this lesion typically resides in a relatively lucent triangle anteriorly and may, as in this case, show a central area of calcification or ossification. Lipomas arising in the proximal femur may be associated with ossification along the margin of the intertrochanteric line. Histologically, intraosseous and extraosseous lipomas are

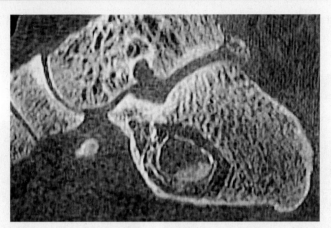

FIGURE 2.7.5

identical (31). CT or MRI can be used as adjunct imaging tests to confirm the diagnosis of intraosseous lipoma. On MRI, the lesion has signal characteristics identical to fat, and CT demonstrates the fat within the lesion (Fig. 2.7.5). Treatment is usually unnecessary when characteristic lesions are seen in asymptomatic patients. If the patient complains of pain, a biopsy followed by bone grafting may be required.

## Aunt Minnie's Pearls

A lytic lesion with a thin, sclerotic border and central calcification (especially within the calcaneus) represents an intraosseous lipoma until proven otherwise.

The average size of intraosseous lipoma is 4 cm.

**HISTORY:** Adolescent child with pain in the leg (Figs. 2.8.1 and 2.8.2). Figure 2.8.3 is the same lesion in the humerus of a different patient.

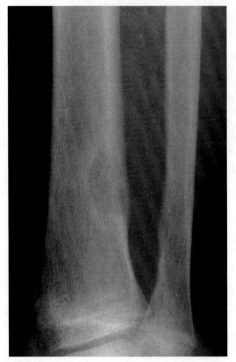

FIGURE 2.8.1                    FIGURE 2.8.2

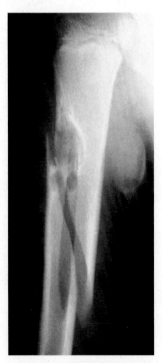

FIGURE 2.8.3

FINDINGS: There is a well-defined, eccentric, radiolucent lesion with a thin, sclerotic border adjacent to the cortex of the distal tibia (Fig. 2.8.1). A repeat study 7 years later shows a well-defined sclerotic lesion in the same location (Fig. 2.8.2). Figure 2.8.3 shows an identical lesion in a different patient with a pathologic fracture, an uncommon complication of this lesion.

DIAGNOSIS: Fibrous cortical defect (FCD) or nonossifying fibroma (NOF)

DISCUSSION: FCD, the common designation for this entity, is often used synonymously with NOF. Although the lesions are identical histologically, some authorities call lesions 2 cm and larger NOF, whereas those <2 cm are called FCD. These lesions are usually discovered as an incidental finding on imaging done for other reasons and rarely cause symptoms (32).

FCD or NOF occurs in up to 40% of children older than 2 years; 95% of the lesions occur in patients younger than 20 years. Eighty percent of the lesions occur in the lower extremity, and about 25% of lesions are polyostotic. Polyostotic forms are often associated with neurofibromatosis, fibrous dysplasia, and Jaffe-Campanacci syndrome. Lesions originally arise adjacent to the physis, and as limb lengthening occurs, they migrate away from the joint. The typical FCD or NOF is radiolucent; has a thin, sclerotic margin; and shows no periosteal reaction. Rarely, it may be expansile or undergo pathologic fracture, as the lesion in Figure 2.8.3. The natural history of FCD or NOF is to involute during adolescence and to become sclerotic, as in the patient of Figures 2.8.1 and 2.8.2. When the characteristic imaging features are encountered on radiography, no further imaging or treatment is necessary. The only indication for treatment is if there has been a pathologic fracture through the lesion and fracture fixation is needed (33).

## Aunt Minnie's Pearls

Eccentric, well-defined, lucent lesion in a young asymptomatic patient is most likely an FCD or NOF.

When classic, uncomplicated radiographic findings are present, no treatment or further imaging is necessary.

**HISTORY:** A 12-year-old boy with pain in the lower leg (Figs. 2.9.1 and 2.9.2) and 10-year-old boy with pain in the foot (Figs. 2.9.3 and 2.9.4). Figure 2.9.5 is the same lesion in a different patient.

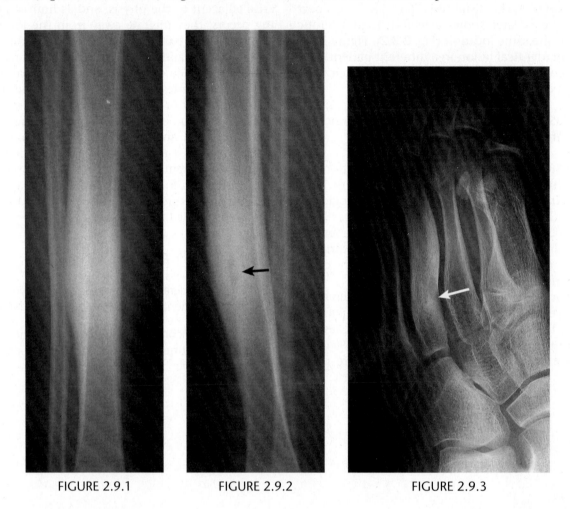

FIGURE 2.9.1    FIGURE 2.9.2    FIGURE 2.9.3

**FINDINGS:** Anteroposterior (Fig. 2.9.1) and lateral (Fig. 2.9.2) radiographs of the lower leg in the first patient show a focal area of sclerosis in the midshaft of the tibia with a central area of radiolucency (*arrow*). In the second patient, an oblique view of the left foot (Fig. 2.9.3) shows sclerosis of the shaft of the fourth metatarsal with an associated central radiolucency (*arrow*). A corresponding axial CT image (Fig. 2.9.4) demonstrates the region of sclerosis and confirms the central radiolucency (*arrow*). An axial, gadolinium-enhanced, fast spoiled-gradient echo image (Fig. 2.9.5) from another patient demonstrates the intensely enhancing nidus (*arrow*) in the anterior aspect of the distal femur.

**DIAGNOSIS:** Osteoid osteoma

**DISCUSSION:** Osteoid osteoma is a benign osteoblastic neoplasm composed of a central core of vascular osteoid tissue and a peripheral zone of sclerotic bone. The cause is unknown. Most osteoid osteomas occur in patients between the ages of 5 and 25 years, and there is a 3:1 male predominance. With rare exceptions, pain is a hallmark of osteoid osteoma, and without this symptom, the diagnosis should be questioned. The characteristic history of pain, which is worse at night and relieved by small doses of aspirin (salicylates), can be elicited from about 50% of patients. Symptoms and signs of a systemic illness are generally absent, and results of laboratory tests are usually normal (34).

Osteoid osteoma has a predilection for the diaphysis of the long bones of the lower extremity, and about 60% of the lesions occur in the femur and tibia. Other common sites are the humerus, bones of the hands and feet, and posterior elements of the spine, where the lesions are usually located

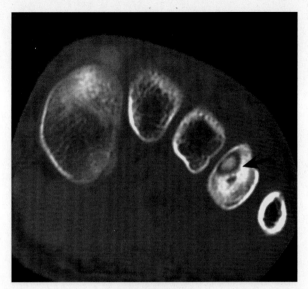

FIGURE 2.9.4

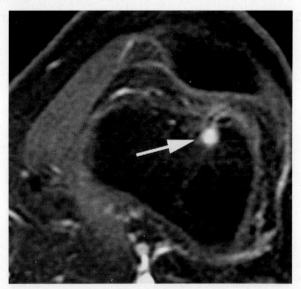

FIGURE 2.9.5

at the base of the transverse process, pedicle, or lamina (35). Multifocal lesions are rare (36,37).

The classic radiographic appearance, virtually diagnostic of osteoid osteoma, is demonstrated in these two examples: a centrally located ovoid radiolucent area (nidus), measuring <1 cm in diameter and surrounded by a zone of uniform bony sclerosis. There may also be a focus of calcification within the radiolucent nidus. Additional modalities helpful in diagnosing osteoid osteoma are bone scintigraphy, CT, and MRI. On the radionuclide bone scan, the double-density sign with intense accumulation centrally and less marked uptake in the periphery is characteristic of osteoid osteoma. Bone-seeking radiopharmaceuticals may be used for intraoperative or percutaneous therapeutic guidance (38). CT is particularly useful for evaluating lesions in the spine, pelvis, or femoral neck.

Prompt arterial enhancement on dynamic MR can help differentiate osteoid osteoma from Brodie abscess and stress injuries in equivocal cases (39). Conventional therapy includes open or percutaneous excision of the entire nidus (34). Radiofrequency ablation is an excellent minimally invasive option for treatment (40).

## Aunt Minnie's Pearls

Pain that is worse at night and relieved by salicylates is characteristic of osteoid osteoma.

The nidus is the radiolucent area on radiographs and the enhancing region on MRI.

Ablation or excision of the entire nidus is usually curative; recurrence is rare.

**HISTORY:** A 35-year-old woman with pain in the right knee

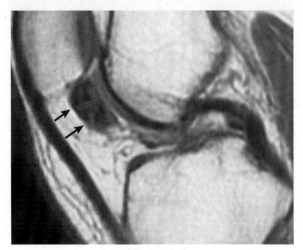

FIGURE 2.10.1

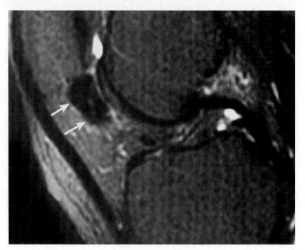

FIGURE 2.10.2

**FINDINGS:** Sagittal proton-density (Fig. 2.10.1) and fast spin-echo, T2-weighted fat-suppressed (Fig. 2.10.2) MR images of the right knee joint demonstrate a low-signal-intensity mass in the upper aspect of the infrapatellar fat pad (i.e., Hoffa's fat pad) on both imaging sequences (*arrows*).

**DIAGNOSIS:** Pigmented villonodular synovitis (PVNS)

**DISCUSSION:** PVNS is a proliferative disorder of the synovium that usually affects adults in the third and fourth decades of life. The exact cause is unknown, but it is likely related to inflammatory or posttraumatic processes. The knee is the most commonly involved joint, followed in descending frequency by the hip, elbow, and ankle, although any joint may be affected. Generally, the disorder is monarticular but multicentric involvement may be encountered (41). The disease affects the sexes equally, with some series showing predominance of disease in either gender (42–44). A history of trauma can be elicited in about 50% of cases.

Symptoms depend on whether the disease is focal or diffuse and include pain, swelling, and diminished range of motion. Aspiration of the joint may show the hemorrhagic and characteristic "chocolate" effusion.

Classic radiographic features of PVNS include soft-tissue swelling, joint effusion, preservation of articular space, absence of osteoporosis, and bony erosions or cysts. Although there are rare reports of atypical cases that contain calcium (45,46), evidence of calcification or metaplastic cartilage in essence excludes the diagnosis of PVNS. The MR features of low signal intensity on T1-weighted, T2-weighted, or gradient-echo sequences result from the hemosiderin deposition in PVNS. However, hemosiderin deposition within hemophilia, synovial hemangioma, or neuropathic osteoarthropathy, all of which are associated with a chronic hemarthrosis, may also result in low signal intensity on these MR sequences (47–49). Treatment of PVNS is arthroscopic or surgical excision of the lesions with synovectomy.

## Aunt Minnie's Pearls

Lesions of PVNS, because of the hemosiderin deposits, generally have low signal intensity on T1- and T2-weighted MR images.

Hemosiderin deposits (low T1- and T2-weighted signal) may also be seen in hemophilia, synovial hemangioma, and neuropathic osteoarthropathy.

Aspiration of the hemorrhagic or "chocolate" effusion is typical of PVNS.

**HISTORY:** A 52-year-old man with a prior shoulder injury (Figs. 2.11.1 to 2.11.4)

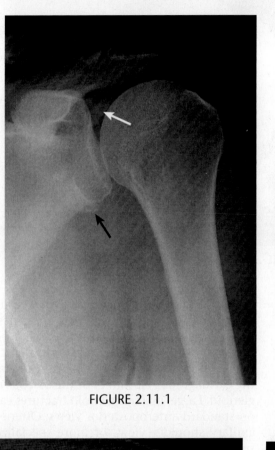

FIGURE 2.11.1

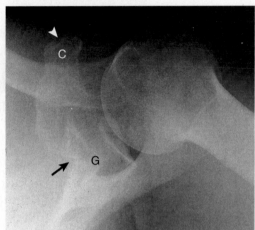

FIGURE 2.11.2

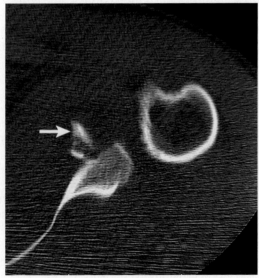

FIGURE 2.11.3

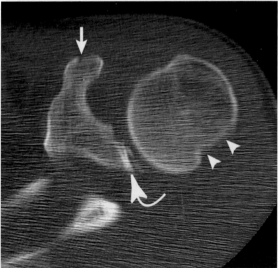

FIGURE 2.11.4

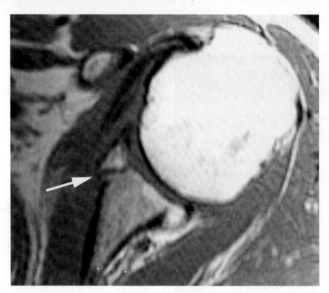

FIGURE 2.11.5

**FINDINGS:** Anteroposterior (Fig. 2.11.1) and axillary (Fig. 2.11.2) views of the left shoulder show small fragments of bone (*arrows*) adjacent to the superior and inferior aspect of the glenoid (*G*) and a nondisplaced coracoid (*C*) fracture (*arrowhead*). Axial CT images through the shoulder joint show a fracture of the anteroinferior aspect of the glenoid (i.e., Bankart lesion) (Fig. 2.11.3, *arrow*). Another CT image (Fig. 2.11.4) reveals fractures of the superior glenoid (*curved arrow*), coracoid process (*arrow*), and a compression fracture of the posterolateral aspect of the humeral head (i.e., Hill–Sachs lesion; *arrowheads*). Figure 2.11.5 is explained under **Discussion.**

**DIAGNOSIS:** Bony Bankart lesion of the shoulder with an associated Hill–Sachs deformity of the humeral head caused by anterior glenohumeral dislocation

**DISCUSSION:** The classic Bankart lesion is an avulsion of the anterior labroligamentous structures from the anterior glenoid rim. A bony Bankart consists of injury to the glenoid labrum and the anterior and inferior rim of the glenoid. Figure 2.11.5 of another patient shows the bony Bankart lesion with a fracture of the anterior and inferior aspect of the glenoid (*arrow*).

With anterior glenohumeral dislocation, the humeral head dislocates anteriorly and inferiorly in relation to the glenoid and may result in any or all of the following lesions: compression fracture of the superior and posterolateral aspect of the humeral head (i.e., Hill–Sachs lesion), stripping of the anterior capsule of the joint, and fractures of the cartilaginous labrum or of the osseous rim of the glenoid. Large, osseous glenoid fractures can be seen on standard anteroposterior views. Often, however, axillary shoulder views or more specialized views, such as the West Point view, are necessary to visualize more subtle bony injuries (50). Demonstration of the fibrocartilaginous Bankart lesion requires CT arthrography or MRI (51–53).

## Aunt Minnie's Pearls

The Bankart lesion of the anterior inferior glenoid labrum is caused by traumatic anterior dislocation of the shoulder.

A compression fracture of the posterolateral humeral head (i.e., Hill–Sachs deformity) is often an associated finding.

MRI or CT arthrography is required to diagnose the purely fibrocartilaginous Bankart lesion.

HISTORY: A 16-year-old basketball player with pain in his left knee (Figs. 2.12.1 to 2.12.3). Figures 2.12.4 to 2.12.6 are from a different patient and are explained under **Discussion.**

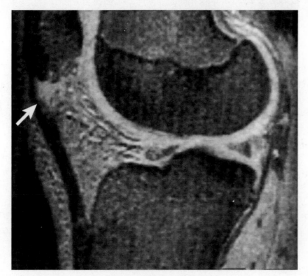

FIGURE 2.12.1

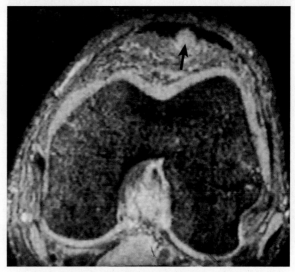

FIGURE 2.12.2

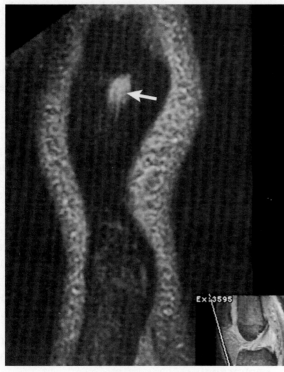

FIGURE 2.12.3

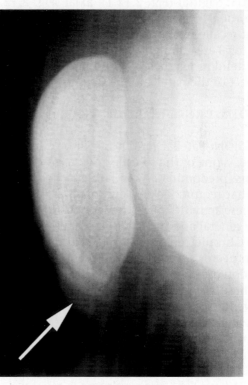

FIGURE 2.12.4

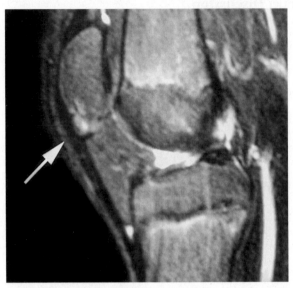

FIGURE 2.12.5

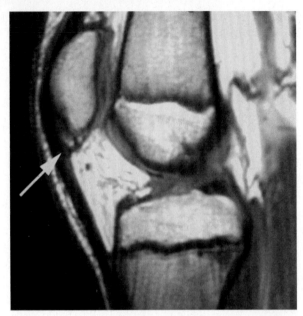

FIGURE 2.12.6

**FINDINGS:** Sagittal (Fig. 2.12.1), axial (Fig. 2.12.2), and coronal (Fig. 2.12.3) three-dimensional, gradient-recalled echo MR images of the left knee show a focal area of high signal intensity within the patellar tendon just below its origin from the inferior aspect of the patella (*arrows*).

**DIAGNOSIS:** Patellar tendinosis (i.e., jumper's knee)

**DISCUSSION:** Patellar tendinosis, also called jumper's knee, is one of the so-called overuse syndromes. It occurs predominately in athletes involved in sports that require kicking, jumping, and running. All of these activities place tremendous stress on the knee in general and the patellofemoral joint in particular. Chronic repetitive stress without rest may result in necrosis, fibrosis, and degeneration within the tendon and may over time lead to tendon rupture. These changes result in anterior knee pain with swelling and tenderness in the anterior aspect of the patella, the patella-patellar tendon junction, or the proximal patellar tendon.

A similar clinical scenario can occur in adolescents with an associated bony fragmentation of the lower pole of the patella. This syndrome is referred to as Sinding-Larsen-Johansson disease, one of the osteochondroses (54,55). Figure 2.12.4 is a coned-down, lateral knee radiograph of a 13-year-old athlete with anterior knee pain and shows fragmentation of the inferior pole of the patella (*arrow*). The sagittal T2-weighted MR image (Fig. 2.12.5) confirms the fragmentation of the patella and shows prepatellar edema and edema within the proximal patellar tendon (*arrow*). The sagittal T1-weighted MR image (Fig. 2.12.6) shows the fragmentation of the patella that is characteristic of this disorder (*arrow*).

MRI is the diagnostic investigation of choice to confirm the clinical suspicion of patellar tendinosis. The MR features, as shown in this example, are an enlarged proximal patellar tendon with areas of increased signal intensity on any imaging sequence. The areas of abnormal, increased signal intensity may be more evident on inversion-recovery or fat-suppressed sequences that are more sensitive to edema or fluid. If a patellar tendon disruption is encountered, axial images should be obtained so that the degree of tendon injury can be estimated (56). Ultrasound is another alternative test for identifying abnormalities of tendons in general and the patellar tendon in particular (57).

## Aunt Minnie's Pearls

Patellar tendinosis (i.e., jumper's knee) is common in sports requiring jumping and abrupt quadriceps contraction.

Inversion-recovery or fat-suppressed MR sequences are preferred to identify the extent of the tendon injury.

Ultrasound is an alternative test to make the diagnosis of jumper's knee.

**HISTORY:** A 21-year-old man with worsening pain in the left wrist after an injury 6 months earlier (Fig. 2.13.1). Figures 2.13.2 and 2.13.3 are of a 46-year-old man with wrist pain and are explained under **Discussion.**

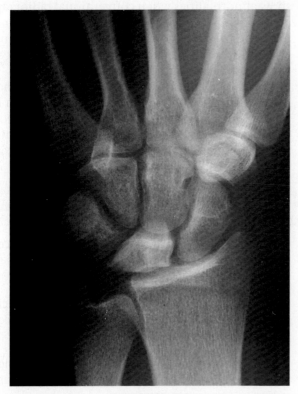

FIGURE 2.13.1

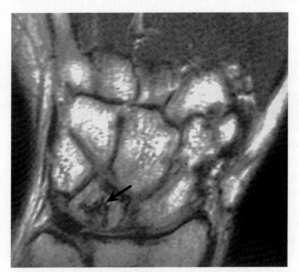

FIGURE 2.13.2

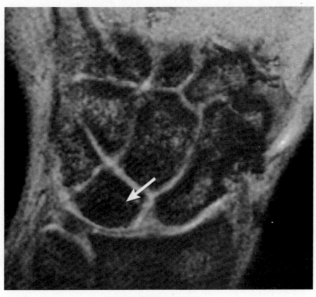

FIGURE 2.13.3

**FINDINGS:** Anteroposterior view of the left wrist (Fig. 2.13.1) shows an ulna that is shorter than the radius (i.e., negative ulnar variance or ulnar minus variance) and a lunate that is sclerotic and somewhat irregular in shape.

**DIAGNOSIS:** Kienböck disease (i.e., lunatomalacia)

**DISCUSSION:** Kienböck disease, or lunatomalacia, is osteonecrosis of the lunate. It is most common in patients 20 to 40 years old and has a predilection for the dominant hand in individuals involved in manual labor. The exact cause of this disorder is unknown. However, single or repetitive trauma is thought to be the primary cause in most cases. The lunate is considered vulnerable to injury from trauma because of its precarious blood supply and its fixed position in the wrist (58,59). A shortened ulna in relation to the radius (i.e., negative ulnar variance or ulnar minus variance) is seen in up to 75% of patients with lunatomalacia and is considered a major cause of the disorder. It is thought that this variation redistributes the compressive forces from the distal ulna to the lunate, thereby increasing the likelihood that the lunate will undergo osteonecrosis (60,61).

The imaging findings, which do not always correlate with the patient's symptoms, include increased density or sclerosis of the lunate and, eventually, alteration in the normal bony shape with collapse on radiographs. MRI allows diagnosis of the early, reversible stage of bone marrow edema and may show abnormalities when conventional radiographs are normal (61). For example, in a 46-year-old man with wrist pain, a coronal T1-weighted image (Fig. 2.13.2) demonstrates low signal intensity in the lunate (*arrow*) and negative ulnar variance. The gradient-recalled echo MR image (Fig. 2.13.3) shows the signal intensity within the lunate to remain low (*arrow*). These features are diagnostic of osteonecrosis (i.e., Kienböck disease). Surgical intervention includes lunate replacement, radial shortening, and ulnar lengthening.

## Aunt Minnie's Pearls

Negative ulnar variance (i.e., ulnar minus variance) is seen in about 75% of patients with lunatomalacia, or Kienböck disease.

On radiographs, sclerosis of the lunate, especially when associated with negative ulnar variance, is highly suggestive of Kienböck disease.

MRI is indicated for symptomatic patients with negative ulnar variance and a normal lunate on radiographs.

HISTORY: An 18-year-old man with acute injury of the right knee (Figs. 2.14.1 to 2.14.3). Figures 2.14.4 and 2.14.5 are explained under **Discussion.**

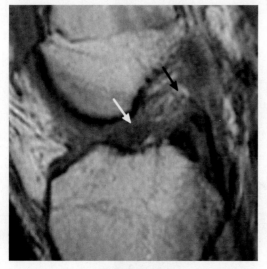

FIGURE 2.14.1

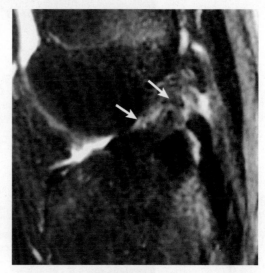

FIGURE 2.14.2

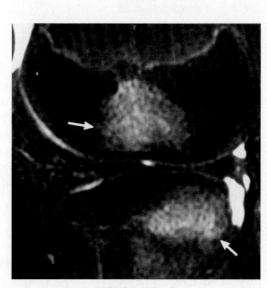

FIGURE 2.14.3

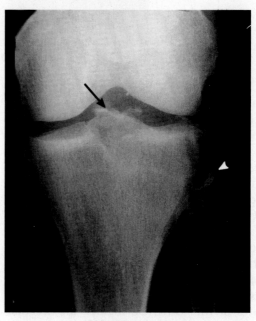

FIGURE 2.14.4

FINDINGS: Sagittal proton-density (Fig. 2.14.1) and fast spin-echo, T2-weighted fat-suppressed (Fig. 2.14.2) MR images show an area of increased signal intensity within the anterior cruciate ligament (ACL), the so-called pseudo-mass (*arrows*); nonvisualization of the normal ACL fibers; and a joint effusion. A sagittal fast spin-echo, T2-weighted fat-suppressed MR image through the lateral joint compartment (Fig. 2.14.3) shows high-signal-intensity areas in the subchondral regions of the midportion of the lateral

femoral condyle and the posterolateral tibial plateau, the so-called "kissing contusions" (*arrows*).

DIAGNOSIS: Full-thickness tear of the ACL

DISCUSSION: ACL injury is a frequent sequela of knee trauma, occurring in up to 70% of patients with hemarthroses in the acute setting. The classic mechanisms of injury include indirect trauma from deceleration, hyperextension, or twisting forces

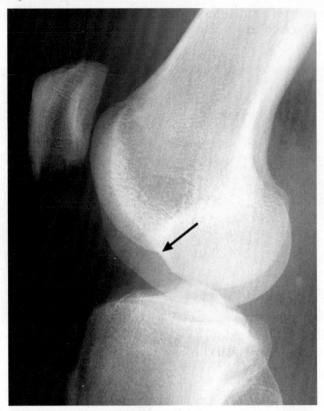

FIGURE 2.14.5

(e.g., "clipping"), often accompanied by an audible pop and the rapid onset of pain, swelling, and disability. About one-third of patients with an ACL injury have other associated ligamentous disruptions or meniscal tears.

Conventional radiographic findings of an ACL tear include avulsion fractures from the femoral or tibial attachment of the ACL (Fig. 2.14.4, *arrow*), the Segond fracture (Fig. 2.14.4, *arrowhead*), or a deep lateral sulcus sign (Fig. 2.14.5, *arrow*). On the lateral radiograph, anterior translation of the tibia may also be seen, and a lateral femoral sulcus deeper than 1.5 mm is highly associated with ACL injury (62). MRI features of the torn ACL include an irregular or wavy contour with decreased angulation on the sagittal images (i.e., "lying down" or vertically oriented ACL), increased signal intensity on all MRI sequences in the region of the ACL (i.e., so-called "pseudo-mass"), posterior displacement of the lateral meniscus (i.e., "uncovered lateral meniscus" sign), loss of the normal obtuse curvature with increased angulation of the posterior cruciate ligament, undulation of the patellar tendon, and the "empty notch" sign, which is also seen on arthroscopy (63). Bone impaction from transient subluxation results in the characteristic osseous contusions involving the posterolateral tibial plateau and midportion of the lateral femoral condyle (i.e., "kissing contusions"). These contusions are found in about 70% to 80% of patients and may remain up to 9 weeks after injury (3,64,65). Long-term sequelae of an ACL tear include premature osteoarthrosis and anterior cruciate ligament ganglion formation. Various ACL reconstruction procedures are available, and most operations can be performed arthroscopically.

## Aunt Minnie's Pearls

Approximately 70% of acute traumatic knee hemarthroses have ACL injuries.

On radiographs, a lateral femoral condylar sulcus of >1.5 mm (i.e., deep sulcus sign) strongly suggests an ACL tear.

Increased signal within the ligament, loss of slope of the ligament, and associated bone contusions are important features of ACL tears on MRI.

"Kissing contusions" of the posterolateral tibia and the anterolateral femoral condyle are commonly associated with an ACL tear.

**HISTORY:** A 19-year-old man with worsening pain in the right knee after a recent injury (Figs. 2.15.1 to 2.15.3). Figures 2.15.4 and 2.15.5 are explained under **Discussion.**

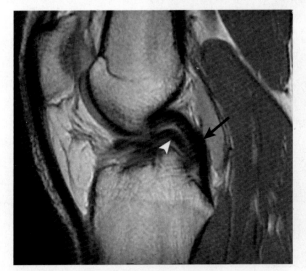

FIGURE 2.15.1

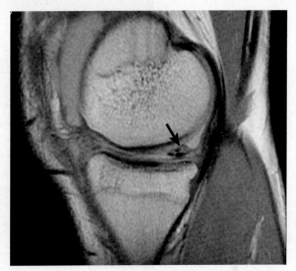

FIGURE 2.15.2

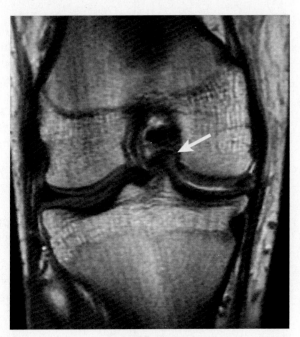

FIGURE 2.15.3

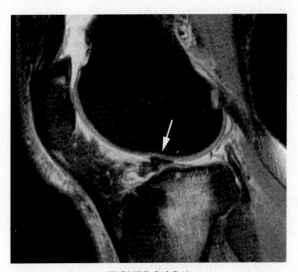

FIGURE 2.15.4

**FINDINGS:** A sagittal proton-density MR image of the right knee (Fig. 2.15.1) shows a normal posterior cruciate ligament (PCL, *arrow*) with an apparent second PCL underneath (i.e., "double-PCL" sign; *arrowhead*). A sagittal proton-density image through the edge of the medial meniscus (Fig. 2.15.2) shows increased signal intensity in the posterior horn of the medial meniscus (*arrow*), diminished visualization of the anterior horn, and lack of the characteristic bow-tie appearance of the

meniscus at this site. A corresponding coronal proton-density image reveals the displaced meniscal fragment in the intercondylar notch (Fig. 2.15.3, *arrow*).

**DIAGNOSIS:** Displaced bucket-handle tear of the medial meniscus

**DISCUSSION:** The bucket-handle tear, usually caused by acute trauma, is a longitudinal meniscal tear in

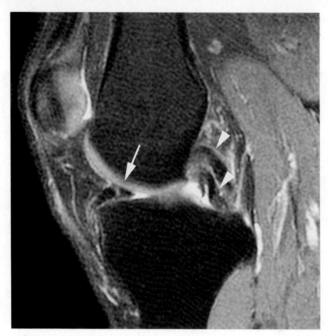

FIGURE 2.15.5

which the central, unstable fragment migrates into the intercondylar notch. As seen arthroscopically, the migrated fragment represents the handle of the bucket, and the portion of the meniscus remaining in situ represents the bucket (66).

Many MRI features suggest a bucket-handle tear. On 4-mm sagittal images, the medial meniscus should have a bow-tie appearance on at least three consecutive MR slices. If the meniscus is not seen on all these slices, then the coronal images must be scrutinized to confirm that the meniscus is intact.

The double-PCL sign is produced by displacement of the meniscal handle fragment into the intercondylar notch, where it comes to rest anterior and inferior to the PCL. Another associated morphologic sign of a bucket-handle tear of the meniscus is the so-called "flipped meniscus" sign. This sign consists of a shortened posterior horn with an abnormally tall anterior horn (>6 mm) on sagittal images (Fig. 2.15.4) or an additional triangular meniscal fragment located just posterior to the

normally shaped anterior horn (67,68). The differential diagnosis for the double-PCL sign includes a full-thickness tear of the ACL, which can coexist with a meniscal tear. Both of these diagnoses are demonstrated in Figure 2.15.5, in which there is a full-thickness ACL tear causing a double-PCL sign (*arrowheads*) and a bucket-handle tear of the meniscus that is flipped anteriorly, causing an abnormally tall meniscal anterior horn (*arrow*).

## Aunt Minnie's Pearls

On sagittal MR images, the double-PCL and flipped meniscus signs are highly characteristic of a bucket-handle tear.

The separated handle of the bucket-handle meniscal tear lying within the intercondylar notch on coronal MR images is also typical of a bucket-handle tear.

The major differential diagnosis for the double-PCL sign is a full-thickness tear of the ACL.

HISTORY: A 19-year-old man with pain in the left knee (Figs. 2.16.1 to 2.16.3). Figure 2.16.4 is explained under **Discussion.**

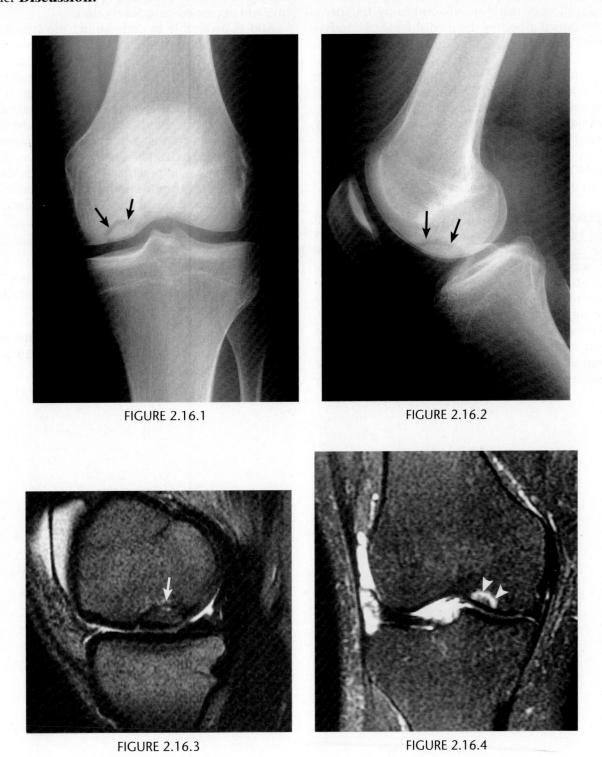

FIGURE 2.16.1

FIGURE 2.16.2

FIGURE 2.16.3

FIGURE 2.16.4

**FINDINGS:** Anteroposterior (Fig. 2.16.1) and lateral (Fig. 2.16.2) radiographs of the left knee show a semicircular lucency, with an adjacent bony fragment, on the lateral aspect of the medial femoral condyle (*arrows*). An accompanying sagittal T2-weighted MR image in the same patient demonstrates minimal linear increased signal intensity in the same region as the lucency, located between the subchondral bone and the fragment (Fig. 2.16.3, *arrow*). The fragment has low signal intensity and is not completely covered by cartilage.

**DIAGNOSIS:** Osteochondritis dissecans (osteochondrosis) of the medial femoral condyle

**DISCUSSION:** Osteochondritis dissecans is most frequently encountered during adolescence and is believed to result from an osteochondral fracture that was initially caused by shearing, rotatory, or tangentially aligned impaction forces. Common locations for osteochondritis dissecans include the knee (involvement of the lateral aspect of the medial femoral condyle is 10 times more common than lateral condylar involvement), humeral head, capitellum of the elbow, and dome of the talus (69). Bilateral involvement has been described in as many as one-third of cases involving the femur (70). Clinically, patients may complain of pain, swelling, locking, and decreased range of motion.

MRI is invaluable in determining the stability of these lesions. The presence of linear high T2-weighted signal intensity between the fragment and donor site indicates fluid or granulation tissue and strongly suggests instability of the fragment (i.e., loose *in situ* fragment) (Fig. 2.16.4, *arrowheads*). Focal cystic areas beneath the fragment or denudation of articular cartilage are also MR signs suggesting an unstable fragment. All patients with radiographic evidence of osteochondritis dissecans could potentially benefit from MRI to assess the integrity of the donor fragments before any surgical or arthroscopic intervention or therapy (71).

## Aunt Minnie's Pearls

The medial femoral condyle, dome of the talus, and capitellum are the most common sites of osteochondritis dissecans.

Encircling fluid or focal cystic areas between the medullary canal and the fragment on MRI suggests a potentially loose or unstable fragment.

HISTORY: A 34-year-old man with an acute knee injury (Figs. 2.17.1 and 2.17.2). Figures 2.17.3 and 2.17.4 are explained under **Discussion.**

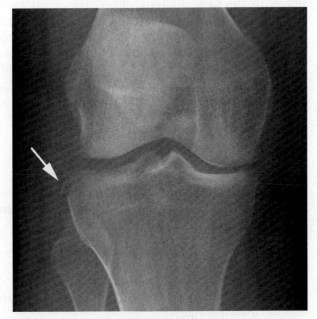

FIGURE 2.17.1

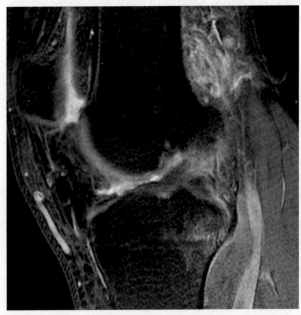

FIGURE 2.17.2

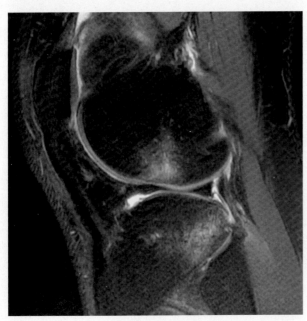

FIGURE 2.17.3

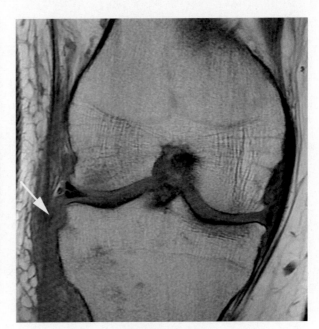

FIGURE 2.17.4

FINDINGS: Anteroposterior view of the right knee shows a linear sliver of bone adjacent to the lateral aspect of the lateral tibial plateau (Fig. 2.17.1, *arrow*). A sagittal proton-density MR image of the knee in the same patient shows an ACL tear and a tibial plateau contusion (Fig. 2.17.2).

DIAGNOSIS: Segond fracture

DISCUSSION: The Segond fracture is usually caused by internal rotatory and varus forces. The avulsion occurs posteriorly and proximal to Gerdy's tubercle, the insertion site of the iliotibial band, and is therefore classically thought to represent an avulsion fracture of the lateral capsular ligament from its insertion site on the lateral tibial plateau; however, the actual structure avulsed has been challenged in the literature (72). The presence of a Segond fracture fragment should alert the interpreting imager to underlying anteroposterior instability of the knee, because nearly 90% of these patients have ACL tears, and of these, up to 60% have associated meniscal tears (73).

On MRI, the Segond fracture fragment can be a subtle finding because of its small size. Figure 2.17.3, a sagittal proton-density, fat-suppressed MR image, shows "kissing contusions" typical for an ACL tear. Figure 2.17.4, the coronal T1-weighted MR image in the same patient, shows the small avulsion fracture fragment characteristic of the Segond fracture. In most cases, however, trabecular microfracture or bone marrow edema is seen adjacent to the avulsion fracture (74). A medial Segond-type fracture, a similar avulsion fracture affecting the medial tibial plateau, has been described and is associated with injury to the posterior cruciate ligament (75).

## Aunt Minnie's Pearls

An avulsion fracture involving the lateral aspect of the lateral tibial plateau = Segond fracture.

A Segond fracture is associated with an ACL tear in up to 90% of patients.

A high percentage of patients with the Segond fracture also has meniscal injuries.

HISTORY: A 54-year-old man with pain in the left shoulder (Figs. 2.18.1 and 2.18.2). Figures 2.18.3 and 2.18.4 are from different patients and are explained under **Discussion.**

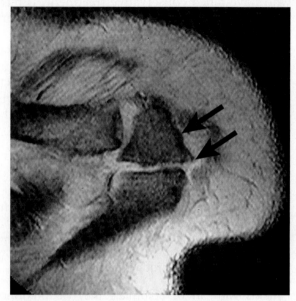

FIGURE 2.18.1

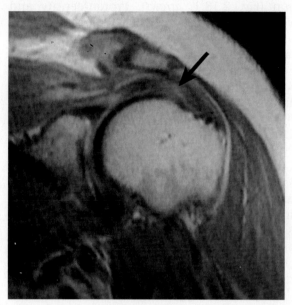

FIGURE 2.18.2

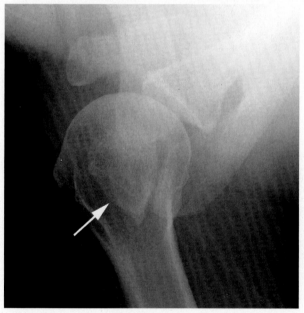

FIGURE 2.18.3

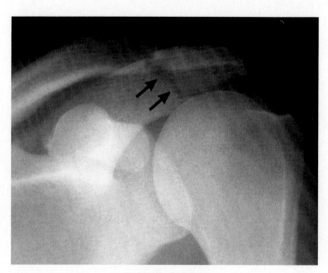

FIGURE 2.18.4

**FINDINGS:** An axial gradient-recalled echo image of the left shoulder shows a well-corticated triangular bony structure in the region of the acromion (Fig. 2.18.1, *arrows*). Proton-density and T2-weighted, coronal, oblique MR images of the shoulder show hypertrophic changes that involve the acromioclavicular joint, causing impingement and increased signal intensity within the distal aspect of the supraspinatus tendon, indicative of tendinosis (Fig. 2.18.2, *arrow*).

**DIAGNOSIS:** Os acromiale

**DISCUSSION:** An os acromiale is a persistent separate ossification center for the acromion that is associated with rotator cuff tendon impingement and tearing. The ossification center for the acromion fuses in normal individuals before 25 years of age. Lack of fusion of this ossification site may normally occur in up to 15% of individuals and is often bilateral (76). The os acromiale, triangular and variable in size, generally forms a synchondrosis with the acromion and also articulates with the clavicle. This variation is important clinically because it can be symptomatic due to rotator cuff impingement and tear, especially when associated with a step-off deformity (77). Open reduction and internal fixation in symptomatic patients with this anomaly, who have failed conservative treatment, is recommended to treat symptoms and prevent further rotator cuff injury (78,79).

The os acromiale (Fig. 2.18.3, axillary radiograph, *arrow*), with its smooth sclerotic margins, can be easily distinguished from an acute acromial fracture (Fig. 2.18.4, anteroposterior radiograph, *arrows*) since an acute fracture has no sclerosis around the fragment.

## Aunt Minnie's Pearls

The normal ossification center of the acromion fuses before 25 years of age.

A persistent ossification center, the os acromiale, can occur in up to 15% of individuals.

Patients with an os acromiale may be predisposed to impingement and rotator cuff tear, and therapy is often recommended.

HISTORY: An anteroposterior radiograph was obtained for an 81-year-old man who fell. He entered the emergency room with his arm locked in an abducted position high above his head.

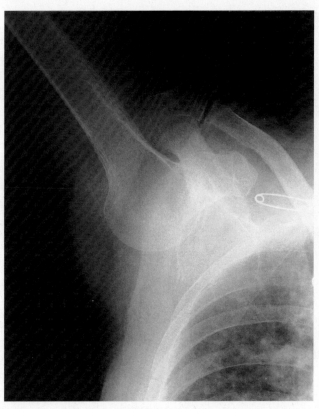

FIGURE 2.19.1

FINDINGS: The right humeral head is dislocated inferiorly at the glenohumeral joint. The superior aspect of the humeral head does not contact the inferior aspect of the glenoid rim, and the arm is held over the patient's head in a fixed position (Fig. 2.19.1).

DIAGNOSIS: Luxatio erecta

DISCUSSION: Luxatio erecta is an uncommonly encountered clinical scenario and comprises <1% of all shoulder dislocations (80,81). Bilateral cases of luxatio erecta have been reported in the literature (82,83). It usually occurs when a direct, axial force is applied to a fully abducted arm or when a hyperabduction force leads to leverage of the humeral head across the acromion, resulting in inferior dislocation of the humerus. Clinically, the patient holds the arm in an elevated, immobile position over the head because the humeral head is fixed below the inferior aspect of the glenoid.

With luxatio erecta, the inferior joint capsule is almost always torn. There may also be associated fractures of the greater tuberosity, acromion, clavicle, coracoid process, and glenoid. The most serious complications are injuries to the brachial plexus and axillary artery. Long-term sequelae of luxatio erecta include adhesive capsulitis and recurrent subluxations or dislocations (80,81). The treatment of luxatio erecta is closed reduction (usually under general anesthesia) and imaging evaluation for associated injuries.

Luxatio erecta is a term also rarely used for inferior dislocation of the hip with inversion of the femoral shaft (84).

## Aunt Minnie's Pearls

The patient who holds an arm in a fixed, elevated position over the head probably has an inferior shoulder dislocation, aka luxatio erecta.

Serious potential complications of luxatio erecta include injuries to the brachial plexus and axillary artery.

**HISTORY:** A 65-year-old woman with insulin-dependent diabetes and recent swelling of the left foot (Fig. 2.20.1). Figure 2.20.2 is explained under **Discussion.**

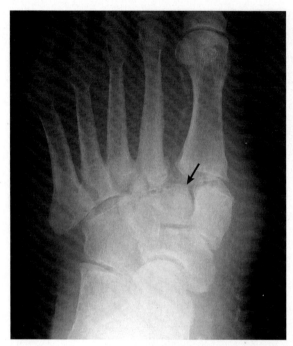

FIGURE 2.20.1

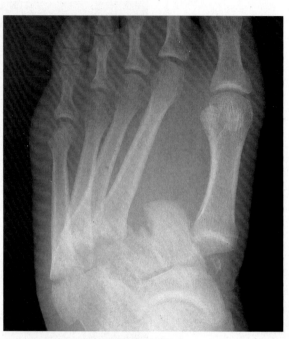

FIGURE 2.20.2

**FINDINGS:** Anteroposterior view of the left foot (Fig. 2.20.1) demonstrates vascular calcification, soft-tissue swelling, lateral subluxation of the second through the fifth metatarsals in relation to the cuneiforms, and early destructive changes at the tarsal-metatarsal joints. Notice the disruption of the normal parallel alignment of the medial aspect of the second cuneiform with the medial aspect of the second metatarsal base (*arrow*).

**DIAGNOSIS:** Lisfranc fracture-dislocation, homolateral type

**DISCUSSION:** The Lisfranc fracture-dislocation was named for Napoleon's surgeon, Lisfranc, who described an amputation procedure through the tarsometatarsal joints. On imaging, the Lisfranc fracture-dislocation is seen as dorsal and lateral dislocation of the metatarsal bases in relation to the cuneiforms. It is the most common dislocation in the foot. The injury may result from various acute traumatic mechanisms but most commonly develops as a result of neuropathic changes, often from diabetes mellitus. There are two distinct forms of the Lisfranc fracture-dislocation: homolateral and divergent. In the homolateral type, all metatarsals are dislocated laterally in relation to the cuneiforms (Fig. 2.20.1).

In the divergent type, there is lateral displacement of the second through the fifth metatarsals and medial or dorsal shift of the first metatarsal (Fig. 2.20.2).

Diabetics develop neuropathic changes because of the peripheral loss of pain and proprioceptive sensations. The neuropathic changes primarily involve the tarsometatarsal (Lisfranc), intertarsal, and metatarsal-phalangeal joints of the foot. The characteristic radiographic changes include soft-tissue swelling, vascular calcification, bone destruction and fragmentation, multiple fractures, and soft-tissue ossific debris from the destructive changes (85,86). Soft-tissue infection also occurs in this setting, and distinguishing noninfected neuropathic changes from osteomyelitis may be problematic by imaging preoperatively, but enhanced MR imaging can be useful in detecting bone marrow edema, subcutaneous abscess, and sinus tracts (87).

## Aunt Minnie's Pearls

Lisfranc fracture-dislocation is common in the setting of diabetic neuropathy.

Lack of parallel alignment of the medial aspects of the second cuneiform and the second metatarsal is the most important finding in making the diagnosis of a Lisfranc injury in the midfoot.

**HISTORY:** A 21-year-old man with a prior puncture wound to the leg

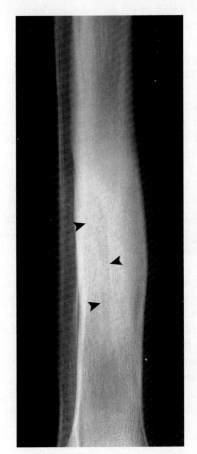

FIGURE 2.21.1

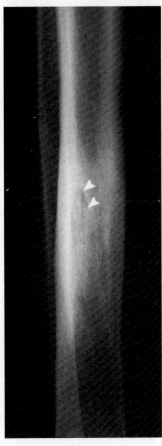

FIGURE 2.21.2

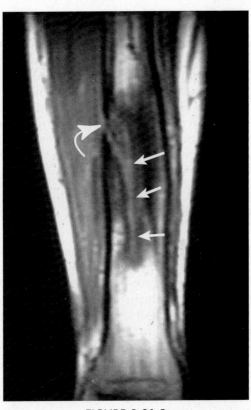

FIGURE 2.21.3

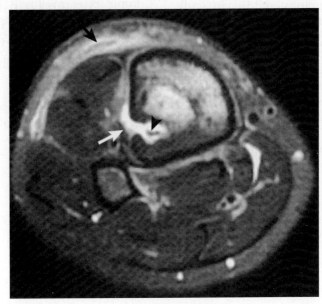

FIGURE 2.21.4

**FINDINGS:** Radiographs of the right tibia and fibula (Figs. 2.21.1 and 2.21.2) show a vague, irregular linear radiolucency within an area of sclerosis in the distal third of the tibia (*arrowheads*). Coronal T1-weighted MRI of the tibia reveals a serpiginous region of decreased marrow signal extending over several centimeters (Fig. 2.21.3, *arrows*) and a defect in the lateral tibial cortex (*curved arrow*). Axial T2-weighted MRI through the same region demonstrates a bony sequestrum (Fig. 2.21.4, *arrowhead*) and increased signal intensity (i.e., marrow edema) within the tibia. A sinus tract extends through the lateral aspect of the posterior tibia (*white arrow*) to the skin surface anteriorly (*black arrow*), with edematous changes in the subcutaneous tissues.

**DIAGNOSIS:** Chronic osteomyelitis with a draining sinus tract

**DISCUSSION:** Osteomyelitis may be classified as acute, subacute, or chronic. The three basic mechanisms responsible for dissemination of osteomyelitis and septic arthritis are hematogenous seeding, contiguous spread of infection from adjacent structures, and penetrating injury or surgery. Most cases of osteomyelitis are caused by *Staphylococcus aureus*. However, in patients with sickle cell anemia, *Salmonella* is common, and in intravenous drug abusers and compromised hosts, the *Serratia* and *Pseudomonas* species often prevail.

The imaging workup of the patient with suspected osteomyelitis should include radiographs, nuclear imaging, ultrasonography, or MRI. In acute osteomyelitis, the earliest radiographic sign is obscuration of the normal fat planes as a result of soft-tissue swelling. Bony changes usually do not appear until 1 to 2 weeks after the onset of the infection. Osteomyelitis typically affects the epiphysis in infants and adults and the metaphysis in children and is multifocal in neonates. The MRI features of acute osteomyelitis include areas of diminished signal intensity on short TE images within the normally high signal intensity of the fatty bone marrow. Long TE images with fat-suppression or inversion-recovery images usually show areas of increased signal intensity in muscle, cortical bone, and periosteum that are not well demonstrated on short TE sequences. T1-weighted fat-suppressed, gadolinium-enhanced images increase sensitivity and specificity in the diagnosis of infection (88).

Chronic osteomyelitis results from inadequately treated or untreated acute osteomyelitis. The radiographic findings of chronic osteomyelitis include prominent cortical thickening and a mixed pattern of osteosclerosis and osteolysis. Signs suggesting reactivation of infection include the development of new, ill-defined areas of osteolysis; thin, linear periostitis; or the presence of a sequestrum and draining sinus tract (89).

Radionuclide scanning with technetium methylene diphosphonate, gallium, and indium may be used in the investigation of chronic osteomyelitis. Positron-emission tomography (PET), when negative, makes the presence of osteomyelitis highly unlikely (90). Overall, MRI is the best imaging study to define the extent of the process (87).

An unusual complication of a long-standing draining sinus tract in chronic osteomyelitis is squamous cell carcinoma. Clinical clues to this complication are changes in the amount, composition, or color of the chronic drainage.

## Aunt Minnie's Pearls

Chronic osteomyelitis is characterized by sequestra formation, a draining sinus tract, and mixed areas of osteosclerosis and osteolysis.

*Staphylococcus aureus* is the most common organism in this disease.

Squamous cell carcinoma is an unusual complication of long-standing draining sinus tract in chronic osteomyelitis.

HISTORY: Two 50-year-old patients who complained of joint pain

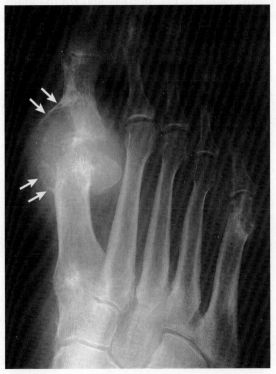

FIGURE 2.22.1

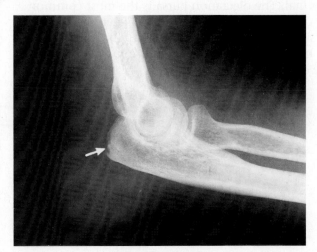

FIGURE 2.22.2

FINDINGS: Anteroposterior view of the right foot of the first patient shows soft-tissue swelling, extensive periarticular erosions with sclerotic borders, overhanging edges in the first metatarsophalangeal joint, and preservation of the articular space (Fig. 2.22.1, *arrows*). A lateral view of the right elbow in a different patient reveals marked soft-tissue swelling and a faint radiopacity in the region of the olecranon bursa. Minimal erosive changes are present in the posterior surface of the olecranon (Fig. 2.22.2, *arrow*).

DIAGNOSIS: Gout

DISCUSSION: Gout is seen in patients with elevated uric acid levels and results from deposition of negatively birefringent monosodium urate crystals in synovial fluid. The disease has a male-to-female ratio of 20:1, is usually first discovered in middle-aged or elderly males, and occurs mainly in the joints of the lower extremities, particularly the first metatarsophalangeal joint, the intertarsal joints, the ankle, and the knee. The first metatarsophalangeal joint is a frequent site of the initial attack and becomes involved in up to 75% to 90% of patients, a condition called *podagra*. The radiographic changes of gout occur in about 50% of patients with elevated uric acid levels, and the changes require 6 to 12 years to develop. The most common findings are punched-out erosions with sclerotic borders and overhanging cortical margins, referred to as overhanging edges or margins. The erosions may be intraarticular, periarticular, or located some distance from the joint. Soft-tissue tophi, producing masses adjacent to the areas of bony erosion, may occasionally contain faint calcification within them. Generally, the articular space is preserved, and periarticular osteopenia is minimal. The olecranon bursa is the most common site of gouty bursal involvement. Bilateral olecranon bursitis strongly suggests gout (91,92). Dual-energy CT has shown significant promise in the noninvasive diagnosis of gout (93).

## Aunt Minnie's Pearls

Erosions with sclerotic borders and overhanging margins with preservation of the articular space are typical of gout.

The olecranon bursa is the most commonly involved bursa in patients with gout.

Bilateral olecranon bursitis usually indicates gout as the cause.

HISTORY: A 23-year-old patient with a chronic disease

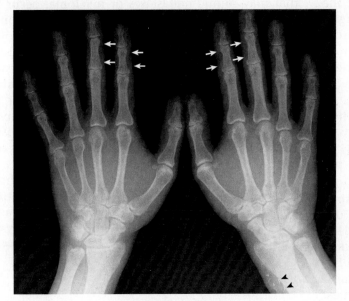

FIGURE 2.23.1

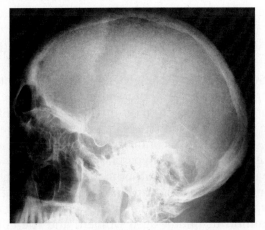

FIGURE 2.23.2

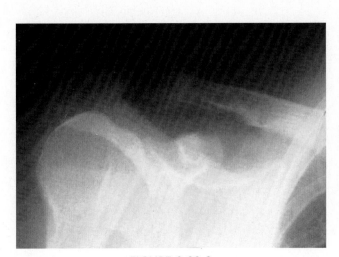

FIGURE 2.23.3

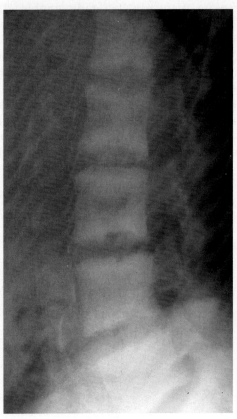

FIGURE 2.23.4

**FINDINGS:** Anteroposterior view of the hands of a patient with chronic renal failure shows subperiosteal resorption along the radial aspect of the middle phalanges of the index and middle fingers (Fig. 2.23.1, *arrows*). There are vascular clips from a graft at the radial aspect of the right wrist (*arrowheads*). A lateral view of the skull in the same patient (Fig. 2.23.2) shows a salt-and-pepper appearance.

**DIAGNOSIS:** Secondary hyperparathyroidism (HPT)

**DISCUSSION:** HPT is a general term referring to an increased serum level of parathyroid hormone. Primary HPT results from an intrinsic abnormality in the parathyroid gland (e.g., an adenoma, hyperplasia, carcinoma). Secondary HPT is caused by a diffuse, adenomatous hyperplasia, and tertiary HPT develops from an autonomous parathyroid adenoma caused by the chronic overstimulation of hyperplastic glands in renal insufficiency. HPT is most common in middle-aged women, and the clinical findings are generally attributable to renal, skeletal, and gastrointestinal changes (94).

There are many distinct radiographic changes of HPT. Bone resorption along the radial aspect of the middle phalanges of the hand (especially of the second and third digits) is considered diagnostic of this disorder. Bone resorption at other sites, including the sacroiliac joints, symphysis pubis, and distal end of the clavicle, occur in HPT but are less specific signs of the disease (e.g., distal clavicular resorption; Fig. 2.23.3). Bone softening may lead to basilar invagination, wedged vertebrae, bowing of long bones, and slipped capital femoral epiphyses. Brown tumors, which are lytic, expansile lesions that may mimic metastases or myeloma, occur in the jaw, rib, and pelvis and are more commonly seen in primary HPT. Osteosclerosis, more commonly seen in secondary HPT, is characterized by bandlike sclerosis on the superior and inferior surfaces of the vertebral body (i.e., rugger-jersey spine; Fig. 2.23.4). Soft-tissue calcifications can occur in the viscera, cornea, periarticular regions, and hyaline or fibrocartilage, causing chondrocalcinosis. Erosive arthritis-simulating rheumatoid arthritis occurs but is a rare complication of this disorder.

The major complications of HPT include nephrocalcinosis, fractures, peptic ulcers, and pancreatitis (95–98). Imaging is important in the diagnosis and plays a role in preoperative planning, especially in complicated cases (99,100).

## Aunt Minnie's Pearls

Subperiosteal resorption along the radial aspects of the second and third middle phalanges of the hand is diagnostic of hyperparathyroidism.

Resorption occurs at other sites, including the sacroiliac joints, symphysis pubis, and distal clavicle.

Chondrocalcinosis and brown tumors are more commonly seen in primary hyperparathyroidism.

Soft-tissue calcifications and osteosclerosis are more commonly seen in secondary hyperparathyroidism.

**HISTORY:** Four elderly patients with pain

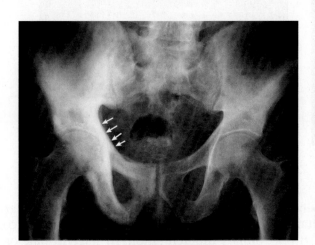

FIGURE 2.24.1

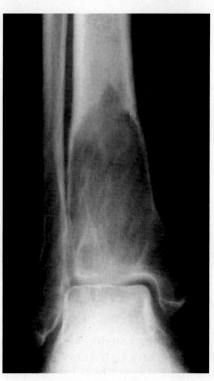

FIGURE 2.24.2

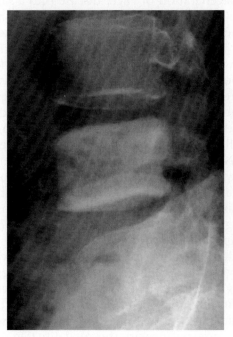

FIGURE 2.24.3

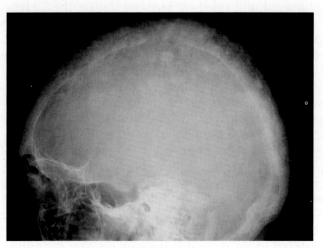

FIGURE 2.24.4

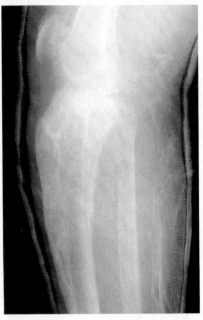

FIGURE 2.24.5

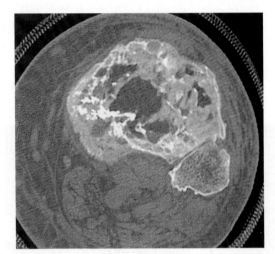

FIGURE 2.24.6

**FINDINGS:** An anteroposterior view of the pelvis (Fig. 2.24.1) in an elderly man shows extensive thickening of the right iliopectineal line (*arrows*) with coarsening of the trabecular pattern and increased sclerosis throughout the entire right hemipelvis.

**DIAGNOSIS:** Paget disease (i.e., osteitis deformans)

**DISCUSSION:** The exact cause of Paget disease is unknown, though it is suspected to be caused by a slow virus. Its highest incidence is in the countries that were conquered and ruled by England during the height of the British Empire. Paget disease is most common in men older than 40 years of age and has a higher incidence in temperate climates. The essential pathologic abnormality is disordered bone remodeling affecting osteoblastic and osteoclastic activity. Osseous involvement may be monostotic or polyostotic, and 80% of the patients are asymptomatic at the time of the discovery of the disease, usually as an incidental finding on radiography or because of elevated serum alkaline phosphatase and elevated serum and urinary hydroxyproline.

Paget disease may be divided into four stages. In stage I (acute phase), active and unbalanced osteoclastic bone resorption usually causes areas of lytic bone destruction. In stage II (intermediate phase), increased osteoblastic activity results in thickening of the cortex, coarsening of the trabecular pattern, generalized bone overgrowth, and loss of corticomedullary differentiation. In stage III (late or inactive phase), there is a diffuse increase in the density of involved bone. Stage IV is the superimposed malignant degeneration of Paget disease into a sarcoma. The major cause of the second peak of osteosarcoma in the elderly patient is underlying Paget disease.

The characteristic, but not entirely pathognomonic, radiographic findings in the acute phase are osteoporosis circumscripta, in which an advancing lytic area is seen in the frontal or occipital regions of the skull, and subarticular osteolysis in the diaphyses of the tubular bones, especially the tibia, yielding a flame-shaped or "blade-of-grass" appearance (Fig. 2.24.2). In the intermediate stage, there may be bowing of the long bones, an "ivory" or "picture frame" vertebral body (Fig. 2.24.3), and more extensive calvarial osteosclerosis superimposed on a background of osteolysis, resulting in the cotton-wool appearance of the skull (Fig. 2.24.4).

In the long bones of the lower extremity, cortical thickening, increased trabecular coarseness, and bowing can be seen (Fig. 2.24.5), and CT can confirm these findings (Fig. 2.24.6). MRI also shows the classic characteristics of Paget disease, but these findings are nonspecific with this modality (Fig. 2.24.7). The most important role for MRI in the patient with

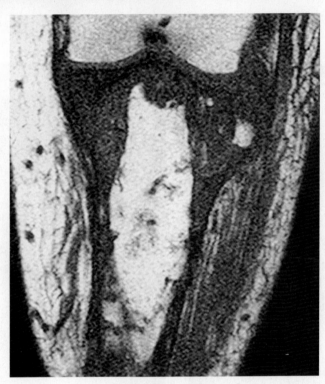

FIGURE 2.24.7

Paget disease is to detect malignant sarcomatous degeneration by showing new bone destruction, soft-tissue masses, and bone and soft-tissue edema.

Potential complications of Paget disease include spinal cord compression from basilar invagination or compression fracture, cranial nerve involvement, high-output cardiac failure caused by arteriovenous shunting within pagetoid bone, protrusio acetabuli from bone-softening, pathologic fractures of tubular bones, and premature degenerative arthritis. The most serious complication, however, is sarcomatous degeneration, most often to an osteosarcoma, which occurs in about 10% of the patients. Giant-cell tumor is also a well-recognized secondary lesion that has a predilection for the skull and facial bones (101,102).

## Aunt Minnie's Pearls

Elevated serum alkaline phosphatase and serum and urine hydroxyproline levels are characteristic of Paget disease.

Characteristic, but not entirely pathognomonic, patterns of Paget disease include the flame-shaped lucency within the long bones, the "ivory" and "picture frame" vertebral body, and osteoporosis circumscripta or cotton-wool appearance of the skull.

Sarcomatous degeneration, usually to an osteosarcoma, can occur in up to 10% of patients.

HISTORY: A 20-year-old woman with generalized bone pain

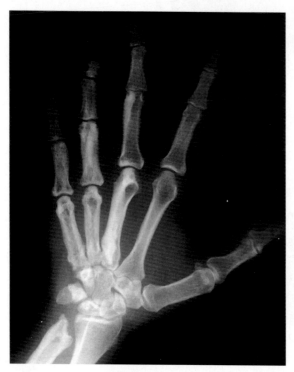

FIGURE 2.25.1

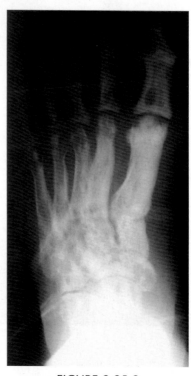

FIGURE 2.25.2

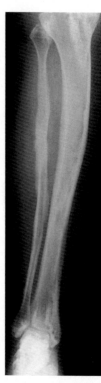

FIGURE 2.25.3

FINDINGS: An anteroposterior view of the left hand demonstrates wavy hyperostosis involving the periosteal and endosteal surfaces of the middle-, ring-, and little-finger metacarpals and the phalanges in each finger. These are distributed along the sensory distribution of the ulnar nerve. Shortening of the ulna is also seen in this view (Fig. 2.25.1). Anteroposterior views of the left foot and of the right tibia and fibula demonstrate similar involvement of the bony structures of the lower extremity. Hyperostosis, deformity, and enlargement of the tarsal and metatarsal bones are most marked in the medial ray (Figs. 2.25.2 and 2.25.3).

DIAGNOSIS: Melorheostosis

DISCUSSION: Patients with melorheostosis, a rare disorder of unknown origin that affects men and women equally, usually present in early childhood with pain, swelling, decreased range of motion, stiffness, and soft-tissue contractures. These symptoms and signs may become quite profound as the disease progresses. The bones of the lower extremities are most commonly involved, and the condition usually involves multiple bones in the same extremity or ray. Patterns of involvement may be monostotic, monomelic, or polyostotic, and the distribution usually corresponds to dermal sclerotomes (103).

A highly characteristic radiographic finding in melorheostosis is areas of undulating hyperostosis adjacent to the intramedullary cortical regions that extend along the length of a bone. This appearance has been likened to candle wax dripping down the side of a candle (Fig. 2.25.1). These undulating areas of subcortical marrow excrescence may involve only one side of the tubular bones in the upper or lower extremity or may extend distally to involve the carpal and tarsal bones or the metacarpals, metatarsals, and phalanges. Rarely, this process may cross a joint, with resultant fusion. Endosteal hyperostosis may be so extensive that it obliterates the medullary cavity. Soft-tissue ossification and calcification may also be seen in the periarticular regions (103,104).

## Aunt Minnie's Pearls

Intramedullary subcortical wavy hyperostosis resembling candle wax drippings is highly characteristic of melorheostosis.

The bony and soft-tissue involvement typically conforms to spinal sensory nerve dermatomal distribution.

# Case 2.26

**HISTORY:** A 41-year-old man with knee pain (Fig. 2.26.1). Figures 2.26.2 and 2.26.3 are different patients and are explained under **Discussion.**

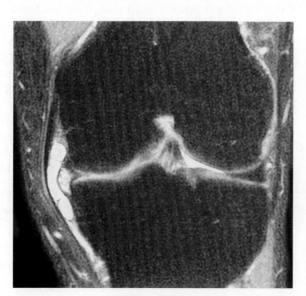

FIGURE 2.26.1

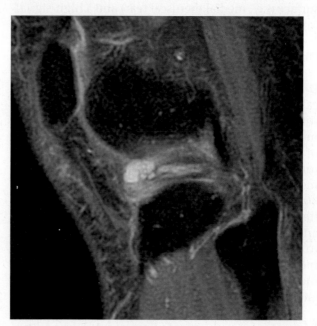

FIGURE 2.26.2

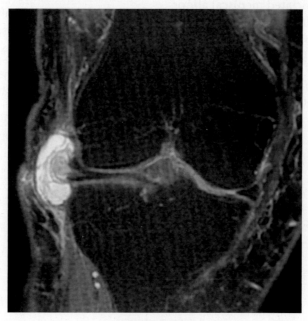

FIGURE 2.26.3

**FINDINGS:** Coronal, proton-density, fat-suppressed MRI (Fig. 2.26.1) shows high signal intensity in the medial meniscus communicating with an articular surface (i.e., medial meniscal tear) and a high-signal-intensity mass adjacent to the medial meniscus.

**DIAGNOSIS:** Medial meniscal cyst

**DISCUSSION:** Most authorities believe that meniscal cysts are formed by passage of synovial fluid through a meniscal tear into adjacent tissue after meniscal trauma or degeneration. As many as 8% of meniscal specimens obtained from meniscectomy contain cysts. Meniscal cysts are more commonly seen in men and occur at an average age of 30 to 40 years (105). Cysts of the lateral meniscus historically (on the basis of physical examination and arthroscopy data) have been estimated to be 3 to 10 times more common than cysts of the medial meniscus. MR imaging data, however, suggest that medial meniscal cysts may be more common than lateral cysts (105).

Radiographs may demonstrate smooth extrinsic bony erosion in the tibial plateau without periosteal reaction or a focal noncalcified soft-tissue mass at or adjacent to the joint line (106). MRI most clearly defines the cysts and any associated meniscal abnormalities. Classic MR findings include a nonaggressive, high-signal-intensity, unilocular, or multilocular mass of variable size in the parameniscal tissues. Lateral meniscal cysts are often confined by soft-tissue planes and are therefore usually small, close to the joint line, and more often symptomatic (Fig. 2.26.2)

although they can become large (Fig. 2.26.3). Medial meniscal cysts are less confined by the soft tissues and capsule and are usually larger and extend farther away from the joint, remaining attached to the meniscus by a stalk. These medial meniscal cysts can extend posteriorly into the popliteal fossa and mimic a popliteal cyst clinically and radiographically. Meniscal cysts generally follow fluid signal on all MR sequences. However, there have been reports of meniscal cysts with components that are seen as high signal intensity on T1-weighted MRI, possibly owing to hemorrhage.

The most common therapy is total excision of the cyst and treatment of any associated meniscal abnormality by arthroscopy or surgery (107). Rarely, conservative measures may result in more than temporary relief of symptoms (108).

## Aunt Minnie's Pearls

Meniscal pathology (usually a meniscal tear) almost always coexists with a meniscal cyst.

A meniscal cyst is likely to recur if the underlying meniscal pathology is not repaired.

Conventional radiographs are typically normal but rarely show a soft-tissue mass or nonaggressive extrinsic bony erosion.

Lateral meniscal cysts tend to be smaller but often more symptomatic than the larger medial meniscal cysts.

HISTORY: Withheld

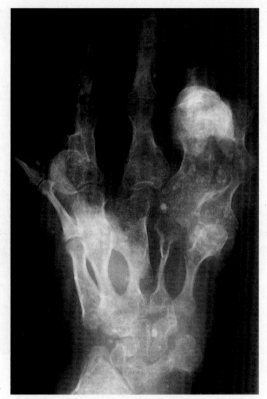

FIGURE 2.27.1

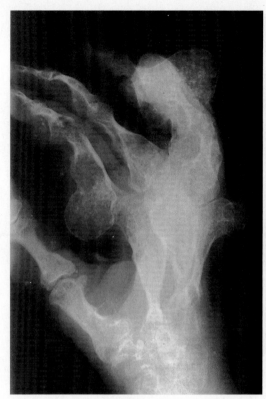

FIGURE 2.27.2

FINDINGS: Anteroposterior and oblique views of the right hand (Figs. 2.27.1 and 2.27.2) show multiple metacarpal and phalangeal lesions with chondroid matrix, representing enchondromas and numerous hand and finger soft-tissue masses containing phleboliths.

DIAGNOSIS: Maffucci syndrome (i.e., multiple enchondromatosis with soft-tissue hemangiomas)

DISCUSSION: The diagnosis of Maffucci syndrome is made on the basis of a combination of multiple nonhereditary enchondromatosis and soft-tissue hemangiomas. The hemangiomas, usually detected at birth or shortly thereafter, are variable in size and number and can become quite large, resulting in growth disturbance. Their distribution does not correlate with that of the enchondromas. Hemangiomas that occur in the head, neck, or gastrointestinal tract can lead to stridor, epistaxis, and dysphagia (109). There is also a higher rate of malignant transformation of enchondromas into chondrosarcoma in patients with Maffucci syndrome (as high as 27% in some series). Other malignancies, including hemangiosarcomas, lymphangiosarcomas, and fibrosarcomas, have also been described (109).

The imaging appearance of Maffucci syndrome is similar to that of Ollier disease, except that patients with Maffucci syndrome also have soft-tissue masses and phleboliths. Involvement of the hands and feet is usually severe, and CT or MRI is useful to evaluate the extent of the soft-tissue and bony lesions.

## Aunt Minnie's Pearls

Multiple enchondromas + soft tissue hemangiomas = Maffucci syndrome.

Involvement of the hands and feet is frequent and severe.

**HISTORY:** A 76-year-old woman with hand pain

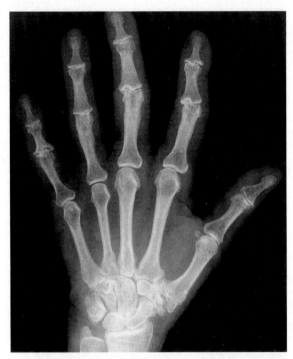

FIGURE 2.28.1

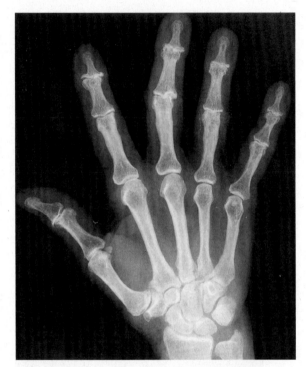

FIGURE 2.28.2

**FINDINGS:** Radiographs show the left (Fig. 2.28.1) and right (Fig. 2.28.2) hands of an elderly woman with intermittent bilateral hand pain.

**DIAGNOSIS:** Erosive osteoarthritis (EOA), also called erosive osteoarthrosis or Kellgren arthritis

**DISCUSSION:** EOA is an inflammatory form of osteoarthritis that occurs in postmenopausal women and is usually limited to the hands. Most patients have a history of chronic, intermittent hand pain that may, by its presentation and symptoms, mimic rheumatoid arthritis clinically. The most characteristic radiographic finding is central articular erosions, which are most prominent at the proximal interphalangeal joints, the so-called "gull wing" or "seagull" erosions. These erosive changes, most remarkably narrowing of the first carpometacarpal joints, are often superimposed on the standard radiographic features of osteoarthritis seen in patients of this age. The radiographic appearance may also resemble rheumatoid involvement. However, the distal interphalangeal and the first carpometacarpal joint involvement seen in EOA is uncommon in rheumatoid arthritis and usually allows differentiation of the two processes. The joints involved by EOA may eventually undergo bony ankylosis, which rarely occurs in the more common form of primary osteoarthritis. When ankylosis occurs, the findings must then be distinguished from the ankylosis occurring in the interphalangeal joints in patients with psoriasis or, less commonly, with Reiter syndrome. Involvement of the carpometacarpal joint helps make this distinction in most cases (92,110,111).

## Aunt Minnie's Pearls

The symptoms of patients with EOA may mimic rheumatoid arthritis.

Central articular erosions (i.e., "gull wing" or "seagull" erosions), ankylosis, and osteoporosis are typical for EOA and uncommon in primary osteoarthritis.

First carpometacarpal narrowing is a feature commonly associated with EOA but is an unusual feature of the arthritis associated with psoriasis or Reiter syndrome.

**HISTORY:** A 34-year-old man with sudden onset of calf pain during a tennis match

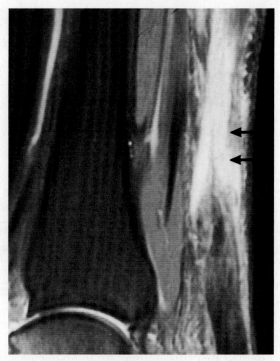

FIGURE 2.29.1

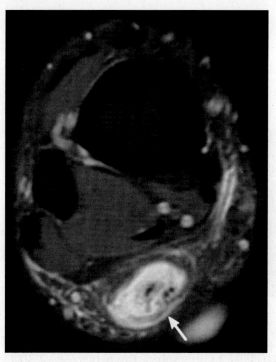

FIGURE 2.29.2

**FINDINGS:** Sagittal fat-suppressed proton-density MRI of the lower calf (Fig. 2.29.1) demonstrates increased signal intensity at the musculotendinous junction of the Achilles tendon (*arrows*). An axial fat-suppressed proton-density image through this area reveals a mass of increased signal intensity in the expected location of the Achilles tendon (Fig. 2.29.2, *arrow*).

**DIAGNOSIS:** Achilles tendon tear, full thickness

**DISCUSSION:** The Achilles tendon, formed by the confluence of the gastrocnemius and soleus tendons, is the strongest and longest tendon of the lower leg. The critical zone, the site of most acute tears, is 2 to 6 cm proximal to the insertion site at the posterior aspect of the calcaneus and is an area of relative hypovascularity. The typical patient who develops acute Achilles tendon tears is the middle-aged man who is sedentary during the week and then participates in sports on the weekends (i.e., a "weekend warrior"). Most of these individuals tear their Achilles when they engage in strenuous activities requiring sudden or forceful dorsiflexion or push-off of the foot (e.g., tennis, racquetball, squash).

Radiographs may support the clinical diagnosis by showing marked soft-tissue swelling behind the distal tibia and ankle and obliteration of the pre-Achilles fat pad. Ultrasonography can reliably show the degree of tendon injury and has the advantage of enabling the evaluation of the patient in a real-time format (112); however, the technique is operator dependent. MRI features of a partial tear of the Achilles tendon include tendon enlargement, discontinuity of some of the tendon fibers, intratendinous areas of increased signal intensity on T2-weighted or inversion-recovery sequences, and surrounding soft-tissue edema. Axial MR images are important for estimating the degree of tendon disruption. In the complete Achilles tendon rupture, an intratendinous gap is present and is generally filled with high-signal-intensity blood and edema (as shown in this case) (113).

## Aunt Minnie's Pearls

Most Achilles tendon tears occur 2 to 6 cm proximal to the calcaneal insertion site in a region of relative hypovascularity.

Achilles tendon tears are most common in the "weekend warrior."

MRI and ultrasonography help assess severity of the tear.

**HISTORY:** A 75-year-old man with history of bilateral total hip replacement and worsening hip pain

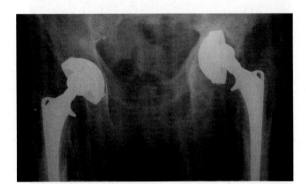

FIGURE 2.30.1

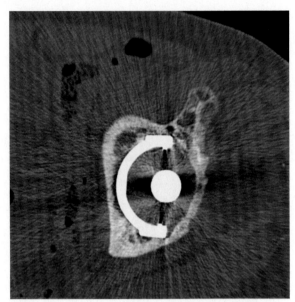

FIGURE 2.30.2

**FINDINGS:** AP radiograph of the pelvis (Fig. 2.30.1) demonstrates an unusually vertical orientation of the acetabular component on the left. Additionally, the bones of the left hemipelvis are enlarged and have coarsened trabeculae. An axial CT through the left hip (Fig. 2.30.2) confirms rotation of the acetabular component and the coarsened bone trabeculae.

**DIAGNOSIS:** Loose total hip replacement, Paget disease

**DISCUSSION:** Hip replacement is the most common orthopedic operation performed. There are numerous styles of prostheses and several types of materials used in hip replacements. This variability in appearance can make it challenging to evaluate for complication, especially when there is no prior study from which to evaluate interval change. Complications such as periprosthetic fracture and dislocation are relatively straightforward to detect. Signs of prosthesis loosening can be more subtle. Loosening is most commonly caused by the body's inflammatory reaction to particles from wear of the polyethylene liner. Infection also causes prosthesis loosening.

When evaluating hip replacements, there are several areas that should be assessed (114). First, the entire prosthesis should be imaged. The location and orientation of each component should be evaluated. In this case, the left acetabular opening is more vertically

oriented than the normal 30- to 50-degree angle relative to a horizontal line drawn through the ischial tuberosities. The location of the femoral head component within the acetabular component should be confirmed. An eccentric location of the femoral head can reflect wear of the polyethylene liner, though there are some styles of liner that are asymmetrically manufactured to cause an eccentric location of the femoral component head. Images should be scrutinized for signs of loosening, which include widening of the lucent zone at the cement-bone or prosthesis-bone interface >2 mm (present surrounding the inferomedial aspect of the acetabular component in this case), migration of the components (present in this case), cement fracture, periosteal new bone formation, and gross osteolysis involving the surrounding bone. Loosening in this case was due to poor structural integrity of the pagetoid bone, as opposed to polyethylene wear.

## Aunt Minnie's Pearls

Lucency measuring >2 mm at the cement-bone or prosthesis-bone interface suggests loosening.

Pagetoid bone is softer than normal bone and more prone to complication.

The most common causes of joint prosthesis loosening are polyethylene wear and infection.

# REFERENCES

1. Hsiao M, Owens BD, Burks R, et al. Incidence of acute traumatic patellar dislocation among active-duty United States military service members. Am J Sports Med 2010;38:1997–2004.
2. Haas JP, Collins MS, Stuart MJ. The "sliver sign": A specific radiographic sign of acute lateral patellar dislocation. Skeletal Radiol 2012;41:595–601.
3. Davis KW. Imaging pediatric sports injuries: Lower extremity. Radiol Clin North Am 2010;48:1213–1235.
4. Pope TL Jr. MR imaging of patellar dislocation and relocation. Semin Ultrasound CT MR 2001;22:371–382.
5. Quinn SF, Brown TR, Demlow TA. MR imaging of patellar retinacular ligament injuries. J Magn Reson Imaging 1993;3:843–847.
6. Spritzer CE, Courneya DL, Burk DL Jr, et al. Medial retinacular complex injury in acute patellar dislocation: MR findings and surgical implications. AJR Am J Roentgenol 1997;168:117–122.
7. Tuite MJ, Daffner RH, Weissman BN, et al. ACR appropriateness criteria® acute trauma to the knee. J Am Coll Radiol 2012;9:96–103.
8. Stefancin JJ, Parker RD. First-time traumatic patellar dislocation: A systematic review. Clin Orthop Relat Res 2007;455:93–101.
9. Garcia GM, McCord GC, Kumar R. Hydroxyapatite crystal deposition disease. Semin Musculoskelet Radiol 2003;7:187–193.
10. Bosworth B. Calcium deposits in the shoulder and subacromial bursitis: A survey of 12,122 shoulders. JAMA 1941;116:2477–2482.
11. Hayes CW, Rosenthal DI, Plata MJ, et al. Calcific tendinitis in unusual sites associated with cortical bone erosion. AJR Am J Roentgenol 1987;149:967–970.
12. Cahir J, Saifuddin A. Calcific tendonitis of pectoralis major: CT and MRI findings. Skeletal Radiol 2005;34:234–238.
13. Settle SH Jr, Rountree RB, Sinha A, et al. Multiple joint and skeletal patterning defects caused by single and double mutations in the mouse Gdf6 and Gdf5 genes. Dev Biol 2003;254:116–130.
14. Clarke DM. Multiple tarsal coalitions in the same foot. J Pediatr Orthop 1997;17:777–780.
15. Graham JM Jr, Braddock SR, Mortier GR, et al. Syndrome of coronal craniosynostosis with brachydactyly and carpal/tarsal coalition due to Pro250Arg mutation in FGFR3 gene. Am J Med Genet 1998;77:322–329.
16. Cass AD, Camasta CA. A review of tarsal coalition and pes planovalgus: Clinical examination, diagnostic imaging, and surgical planning. J Foot Ankle Surg 2010;49:274–293.
17. Zaw H, Calder JD. Tarsal coalitions. Foot Ankle Clin 2010;15:349–364.
18. Varich L, Bancroft L. Radiologic case study. Talocalcaneal coalition. Orthopedics 2010;33:374–452.
19. Lemley F, Berlet G, Hill K, et al. Current concepts review: Tarsal coalition. Foot Ankle Int 2006;27:1163–1169.
20. Rodriguez N, Choung DJ, Dobbs MB. Rigid pediatric pes planovalgus: Conservative and surgical treatment options. Clin Podiatr Med Surg 2010;27:79–92.
21. Liu PT, Roberts CC, Chivers FS, et al. Absent middle facet: A sign on unenhanced radiography of subtalar joint coalition. AJR Am J Roentgenol 2003;181:1565–1572.
22. Crim J. Imaging of tarsal coalition. Radiol Clin North Am 2008;46:1017–1026.
23. Richardson RR. Variants of exostosis of the bone in children. Semin Roentgenol 2005;40:380–390.
24. Stieber JR, Dormans JP. Manifestations of hereditary multiple exostoses. J Am Acad Orthop Surg 2005;13:110–120.
25. McAlister W, Herman T. Osteochondrodysplasias, dysostoses, chromosomal aberrations, mucopolysaccharidoses, and mucolipidoses. In: Resnick D (ed.). Diagnosis of bone and joint disorders. Philadelphia, PA: WB Saunders, 2002:4449–4533.
26. Stoker DJ. Osteopetrosis. Semin Musculoskelet Radiol 2002;6:299–305.
27. Motamedi K, Seeger LL. Benign bone tumors. Radiol Clin North Am 2011;49:1115–1134.
28. Damante JH, Da SGEN, Ferreira O Jr. Spontaneous resolution of simple bone cysts. Dentomaxillofac Radiol 2002;31:182–186.
29. Campbell RS, Grainger AJ, Mangham DC, et al. Intraosseous lipoma: Report of 35 new cases and a review of the literature. Skeletal Radiol 2003;32(4):209–222.
30. Murphey MD, Carroll JF, Flemming DJ, et al. From the archives of the AFIP: Benign musculoskeletal lipomatous lesions. Radiographics 2004;24:1433–1466.
31. Resnick D. Tumors and tumor-like lesions of bone: Radiographic principles. In: Resnick D (ed.). Diagnosis of bone and joint disorders. Philadelphia, PA: WB Saunders, 2002:3745–3762.
32. Smith SE, Kransdorf MJ. Primary musculoskeletal tumors of fibrous origin. Semin Musculoskelet Radiol 2000;4:73–88.
33. Iagaru A, Henderson R. PET/CT follow-up in nonossifying fibroma. AJR Am J Roentgenol 2006;187:830–832.
34. Kransdorf MJ, Stull MA, Gilkey FW, et al. Osteoid osteoma. Radiographics 1991;11:671–696.
35. Atesok KI, Alman BA, Schemitsch EH, et al. Osteoid osteoma and osteoblastoma. J Am Acad Orthop Surg 2011;19:678–689.
36. Schai P, Friederich N, Kruger A, et al. Discrete synchronous multifocal osteoid osteoma of the humerus. Skeletal Radiol 1996;25:667–670.
37. Gonzalez G, Abril JC, Mediero IG, et al. Osteoid osteoma with a multicentric nidus. Int Orthop 1996;20:61–63.
38. Tse WL, Hung LK, Law B, et al. Enhanced localization of osteoid osteoma with radiolabeling and intraoperative gamma counter guidance: A case report. J Hand Surg Am 2003;28:699–703.
39. Liu PT, Chivers FS, Roberts CC, et al. Imaging of osteoid osteoma with dynamic gadolinium-enhanced MR imaging. Radiology 2003;227:691–700.
40. Motamedi D, Learch TJ, Ishimitsu DN, et al. Thermal ablation of osteoid osteoma: Overview and step-by-step guide. Radiographics 2009;29:2127–2141.
41. Mukhopadhyay K, Smith M, Hughes PM. Multifocal PVNS in a child—followed over 25 years. Skeletal Radiol 2006;35:539–542.
42. Ottaviani S, Ayral X, Dougados M, et al. Pigmented villonodular synovitis: A retrospective single-center study of 122 cases and review of the literature. Semin Arthritis Rheum 2011;40:539–546.
43. Adelani MA, Wupperman RM, Holt GE. Benign synovial disorders. J Am Acad Orthop Surg 2008;16:268–275.
44. Mendenhall WM, Mendenhall CM, Reith JD, et al. Pigmented villonodular synovitis. Am J Clin Oncol 2006;29:548–550.
45. Farrokh D. Atypical form of pigmented villonodular synovitis of the knee containing calcifications. J Belge Radiol 1996;79:203–205.
46. Oda Y, Izumi T, Harimaya K, et al. Pigmented villonodular synovitis with chondroid metaplasia, resembling chondroblastoma of the bone: A report of three cases. Mod Pathol 2007;20:545–551.
47. Kim HK, Zbojniewicz AM, Merrow AC, et al. MR findings of synovial disease in children and young adults: Part 1. Pediatr Radiol 2011;41:495–511.
48. Walker EA, Fenton ME, Salesky JS, et al. Magnetic resonance imaging of benign soft tissue neoplasms in adults. Radiol Clin North Am 2011;49:1197–1217.
49. Frick MA, Wenger DE, Adkins M. MR imaging of synovial disorders of the knee: An update. Radiol Clin North Am 2007;45:1017–1031.
50. Roberts CC. Shoulder overview. In: Manaster BJ (ed.). Diagnostic and surgical imaging anatomy: Musculoskeletal. Philadelphia, PA: Lippincott Williams & Wilkins, 2006:2–75.

51. Omoumi P, Teixeira P, Lecouvet F, et al. Glenohumeral joint instability. J Magn Reson Imaging 2011;33:2–16.

52. Davis KW. Imaging pediatric sports injuries: Upper extremity. Radiol Clin North Am 2010;48:1199–1211.

53. Sanders TG, Zlatkin M, Montgomery J. Imaging of glenohumeral instability. Semin Roentgenol 2010;45:160–179.

54. Iwamoto J, Takeda T, Sato Y, et al. Radiographic abnormalities of the inferior pole of the patella in juvenile athletes. Keio J Med 2009;58:50–53.

55. Peace KA, Lee JC, Healy J. Imaging the infrapatellar tendon in the elite athlete. Clin Radiol 2006;61:570–578.

56. El-Khoury GY, Wira RL, Berbaum KS, et al. MR imaging of patellar tendinitis. Radiology 1992;184:849–854.

57. Weinberg EP, Adams MJ, Hollenberg GM. Color Doppler sonography of patellar tendinosis. AJR Am J Roentgenol 1998;171:743–744.

58. Paksima N, Canedo A. Kienböck's disease. J Hand Surg Am 2009;34:1886–1889.

59. Schuind F, Eslami S, Ledoux P. Kienbock's disease. J Bone Joint Surg Br 2008;90:133–139.

60. Chung KC, Spilson MS, Kim MH. Is negative ulnar variance a risk factor for Kienböck's disease? A meta-analysis. Ann Plast Surg 2001;47:494–499.

61. Lisle DA, Shepherd GJ, Cowderoy GA, et al. MR imaging of traumatic and overuse injuries of the wrist and hand in athletes. Magn Reson Imaging Clin N Am 2009;17:639–654.

62. Cobby MJ, Schweitzer ME, Resnick D. The deep lateral femoral notch: An indirect sign of a torn anterior cruciate ligament. Radiology 1992;184:855–858.

63. Roberts CC, Towers JD, Spangehl MJ, et al. Advanced MR imaging of the cruciate ligaments. Magn Reson Imaging Clin N Am 2007;15:73–86.

64. Miller TT. MR imaging of the knee. Sports Med Arthrosc 2009;17:56–67.

65. White LM, Miniaci A. Cruciate and posterolateral corner injuries in the athlete: Clinical and magnetic resonance imaging features. Semin Musculoskelet Radiol 2004;8:111–131.

66. Fox MG. MR imaging of the meniscus: Review, current trends, and clinical implications. Radiol Clin North Am 2007;45:1033–1053.

67. Wright DH, De Smet AA, Norris M. Bucket-handle tears of the medial and lateral menisci of the knee: Value of MR imaging in detecting displaced fragments. AJR Am J Roentgenol 1995;165:621–625.

68. Dorsay TA, Helms CA. Bucket-handle meniscal tears of the knee: Sensitivity and specificity of MRI signs. Skeletal Radiol 2003;32:266–272.

69. Sanders RK, Crim JR. Osteochondral injuries. Semin Ultrasound CT MR 2001;22:352–370.

70. Connolly SA, Connolly LP, Jaramillo D. Imaging of sports injuries in children and adolescents. Radiol Clin North Am 2001;39:773–790.

71. Moktassi A, Popkin CA, White LM, et al. Imaging of osteochondritis dissecans. Orthop Clin North Am 2012;43:201–211.

72. Campos JC, Chung CB, Lektrakul N, et al. Pathogenesis of the Segond fracture: Anatomic and MR imaging evidence of an iliotibial tract or anterior oblique band avulsion. Radiology 2001;219:381–386.

73. Resnick D. Internal derangements of joints. In: Resnick D (ed.). Diagnosis of bone and joint disorders. Philadelphia, PA: WB Saunders, 2002:3019–3376.

74. Gottsegen CJ, Eyer BA, White EA, et al. Avulsion fractures of the knee: Imaging findings and clinical significance. Radiographics 2008;28:1755–1770.

75. Hall FM, Hochman MG. Medial Segond-type fracture: Cortical avulsion off the medial tibial plateau associated with tears of the posterior cruciate ligament and medial meniscus. Skeletal Radiol 1997;26:553–555.

76. Sammarco VJ. Os acromiale: Frequency, anatomy, and clinical implications. J Bone Joint Surg Am 2000;82:394–400.

77. Ouellette H, Thomas BJ, Kassarjian A, et al. Re-examining the association of os acromiale with supraspinatus and infraspinatus tears. Skeletal Radiol 2007;36:835–839.

78. Harris JD, Griesser MJ, Jones GL. Systematic review of the surgical treatment for symptomatic os acromiale. Int J Shoulder Surg 2011;5:9–16.

79. Kurtz CA, Humble BJ, Rodosky MW, et al. Symptomatic os acromiale. J Am Acad Orthop Surg 2006;1:12–19.

80. Krug DK, Vinson EN, Helms CA. MRI findings associated with luxatio erecta humeri. Skeletal Radiol 2010;39:27–33.

81. Yamamoto T, Yoshiya S, Kurosaka M, et al. Luxatio erecta (inferior dislocation of the shoulder): A report of 5 cases and a review of the literature. Am J Orthop 2003;32:601–603.

82. Marks TO, Kelsall NK, Southgate JJ. Bilateral luxatio erecta: Recognition and reduction. Emerg Med Australas 2011;23:510–511.

83. Camarda L, Martorana U, D'Arienzo M. A case of bilateral luxatio erecta. J Orthop Traumatol 2009;10:97–99.

84. Brogdon BG, Woolridge DA. Luxatio erecta of the hip: A critical retrospective. Skeletal Radiol 1997;26:548–552.

85. Morrison WB, Ledermann HP. Work-up of the diabetic foot. Radiol Clin North Am 2002;40:1171–1192.

86. Schweitzer ME, Morrison WB. MR imaging of the diabetic foot. Radiol Clin North Am 2004;42:61–71.

87. Russell JM, Peterson JJ, Bancroft LW. MR imaging of the diabetic foot. Magn Reson Imaging Clin N Am 2008;16:59–70.

88. Resnick D. Osteomyelitis, septic arthritis and soft tissue infection: Mechanisms and situations. In: Resnick D (ed.). Diagnosis of bone and joint disorders. Philadelphia, PA: WB Saunders, 2002:2377–2480.

89. Tehranzadeh J, Wong E, Wang F, et al. Imaging of osteomyelitis in the mature skeleton. Radiol Clin North Am 2001;39:223–250.

90. van der Bruggen W, Bleeker-Rovers CP, Boerman OC, et al. PET and SPECT in osteomyelitis and prosthetic bone and joint infections: A systematic review. Semin Nucl Med 2010;40:3–15.

91. Dhanda S, Jagmohan P, Quek ST. A re-look at an old disease: A multimodality review on gout. Clin Radiol 2011;66:984–992.

92. Monu JU, Pope TL Jr. Gout: A clinical and radiologic review. Radiol Clin North Am 2004;42:169–184.

93. Desai MA, Peterson JJ, Garner HW, et al. Clinical utility of dual-energy CT for evaluation of tophaceous gout. Radiographics 2011;31:1365–1375.

94. Gleason DC, Potchen EJ. The diagnosis of hyperparathyroidism. Radiol Clin North Am 1967;5:277–287.

95. Resnick DL. Erosive arthritis of the hand and wrist in hyperparathyroidism. Radiology 1974;110:263–269.

96. Marcocci C, Cetani F. Clinical practice. Primary hyperparathyroidism. N Engl J Med 2011;365:2389–2397.

97. Murphey MD, Sartoris DJ, Quale JL, et al. Musculoskeletal manifestations of chronic renal insufficiency. Radiographics 1993;13:357–379.

98. Fraser WD. Hyperparathyroidism. Lancet 2009;374:145–158.

99. Buckley O, Halpenny D, Torreggiani WC. Role of the radiologist in the preoperative evaluation of primary hyperparathyroidism. AJR Am J Roentgenol 2008;190:W82.

100. Johnson NA, Carty SE, Tublin ME. Parathyroid imaging. Radiol Clin North Am 2011;49:489–509.

101. Theodorou DJ, Theodorou SJ, Kakitsubata Y. Imaging of Paget disease of bone and its musculoskeletal complications: Review. AJR Am J Roentgenol 2011;196:S64–S75.

102. Resnick D. Paget's disease. In: Resnick D (ed.). Diagnosis of bone and joint disorders. Philadelphia, PA: WB Saunders, 2002:1947–2000.

103. Suresh S, Muthukumar T, Saifuddin A. Classical and unusual imaging appearances of melorheostosis. Clin Radiol 2010;65:593–600.

104. Ihde LL, Forrester DM, Gottsegen CJ, et al. Sclerosing bone dysplasias: Review and differentiation from other causes of osteosclerosis. Radiographics 2011;31:1865–1882.

105. Campbell SE, Sanders TG, Morrison WB. MR imaging of meniscal cysts: Incidence, location, and clinical significance. AJR Am J Roentgenol 2001;177:409–413.

106. Blair TR, Schweitzer M, Resnick D. Meniscal cysts causing bone erosion: Retrospective analysis of seven cases. Clin Imaging 1999;23:134–138.

107. Ryu RK, Ting AJ. Arthroscopic treatment of meniscal cysts. Arthroscopy 1993;9:591–595.

108. Chang A. Imaging-guided treatment of meniscal cysts. HSS J 2009;5:58–60.

109. McDermott AL, Dutt SN, Chavda SV, et al. Maffucci's syndrome: Clinical and radiological features of a rare condition. J Laryngol Otol 2001;115:845–847.

110. Brower A, Flemming D. Arthritis in black and white, 2nd ed. Philadelphia, PA: WB Saunders, 1997:273–292.

111. Greenspan A. Erosive osteoarthritis. Semin Musculoskelet Radiol 2003;7:155–159.

112. Fessell DP, Jacobson JA. Ultrasound of the hindfoot and midfoot. Radiol Clin North Am 2008;46:1027–1043.

113. Tuite MJ. MR imaging of the tendons of the foot and ankle. Semin Musculoskelet Radiol 2002;6:119–131.

114. Roberts CC, Chew FS. Radiographic imaging of hip replacement hardware. Semin Roentgenol 2005;40:320–332.

# CHAPTER 3

# CARDIOVASCULAR AND INTERVENTIONAL RADIOLOGY

Stephen P. Loehr

*The authors and editors acknowledge the contribution of the Chapter 3 author from the second edition: Adam Henn, MD.*

HISTORY: Two patients with sudden onset of pain radiating to the back. Figures 3.1.1 and 3.1.2 are of the first patient; Figure 3.1.3 is of the second patient.

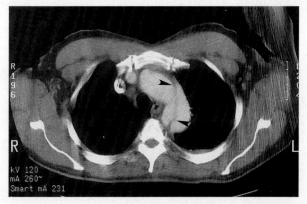

FIGURE 3.1.1

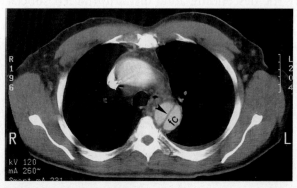

FIGURE 3.1.2

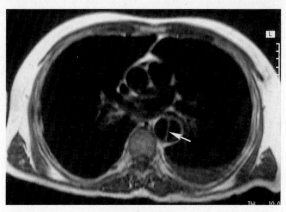

FIGURE 3.1.3

FINDINGS: Axial contrast-enhanced CT images through the chest reveal an intimal flap within the aortic lumen that originates near the left subclavian artery (Fig. 3.1.1, *arrowheads*) and extends inferiorly down the thoracic aorta (Fig. 3.1.2, *arrowhead*). The larger, false channel (*fc*) is located in the posterolateral descending aorta. The ascending aorta is normal. No active extravasation of contrast material from the aorta is identified. In a different patient with the same abnormality, an axial echocardiography (ECG)-gated, T1-weighted magnetic resonance imaging (MRI) also demonstrates an intimal flap (Fig. 3.1.3, *arrow*).

DIAGNOSIS: Aortic dissection (i.e., DeBakey type III or Stanford type B)

DISCUSSION: Dissection of the aorta occurs when a pathologic communication develops between the true aortic lumen and the aortic wall. The most common predisposing factor to the development of aortic dissection is hypertension (1). Other predisposing factors include Marfan and Ehlers–Danlos syndromes, pregnancy, trauma, aortic valve disease, and coronary artery bypass surgery (2). Dissections that involve the ascending aorta (i.e., DeBakey types I and II and Stanford type A) can lead to rapid death because of rupture into the pericardium, acute valvular insufficiency, or coronary artery occlusion (3). These types of dissections are managed with emergent surgery (4). Dissections that involve only the descending aorta distal to the left subclavian artery (i.e., DeBakey type III or Stanford type B) are usually managed medically by control of the patient's hypertension. Aortic dissections in selected patients have been successfully treated using endovascular methods (i.e., stent-grafts) (5,6).

## Aunt Minnie's Pearls

Emergent surgery is required for Stanford type A dissections.

Always check for aortic rupture and branch vessel involvement.

If dissection involves the ascending aorta, look for pericardial hematoma.

**HISTORY:** Cyanosis

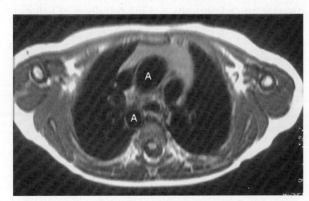

FIGURE 3.2.1

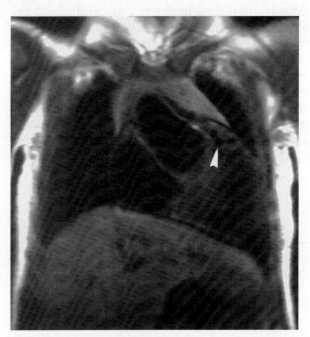

FIGURE 3.2.2

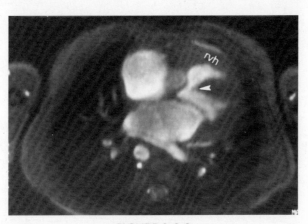

FIGURE 3.2.3

**FINDINGS:** The axial ECG-gated, T1-weighted MR image (Fig. 3.2.1) at the level of the great vessels demonstrates a right aortic arch (*A*). The coronal T1-weighted MR image demonstrates hypoplasia of the pulmonary infundibulum (Fig. 3.2.2, *arrowhead*). Axial gradient-recalled-echo MR images through the heart (Fig. 3.2.3) reveal right ventricular hypertrophy (*rvh*) and a high membranous ventricular septal defect (VSD) (*arrowhead*).

**DIAGNOSIS:** Tetralogy of Fallot

**DISCUSSION:** Tetralogy of Fallot is characterized by a combination of infundibular pulmonic hypoplasia, VSD, right ventricular hypertrophy, and overriding of the aortic root above the VSD (7). The pulmonic infundibular stenosis and overriding of the aorta facilitate shunting of deoxygenated blood from the right ventricle to the aorta, thereby producing cyanosis. Approximately one-fourth of patients with tetralogy of Fallot also have a right aortic arch, usually with mirror-image branching. The plain-film findings of right aortic arch with decreased pulmonary vasculature should strongly suggest this diagnosis. These patients usually do not have cardiomegaly.

MRI is often used to detect intracardiac and extracardiac abnormalities (8). In planning surgery for tetralogy of Fallot, it is important to assess the degree of hypoplasia of the pulmonary arteries and the development of collateral vessels from the systemic to pulmonary arteries. MRI analysis of measurements of the pulmonary artery and aortic root diameters has led to several methods for assisting in planning surgical repair and for predicting postoperative heart failure (9–11). Surgical correction varies from palliative shunt procedures (e.g., Blalock–Taussig) to complete repair of the infundibular outflow obstruction and patching of the VSD (i.e., Lillehei procedure).

## Aunt Minnie's Pearls

Infundibular stenosis + VSD + overriding aorta + right ventricular hypertrophy = tetralogy of Fallot.

Right arch + decreased pulmonary flow + no cardiomegaly on radiographs = think tetralogy of Fallot.

# Case 3.3

HISTORY: Two newborns with cyanosis

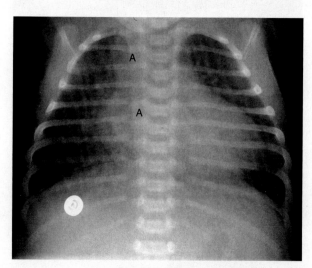

FIGURE 3.3.1

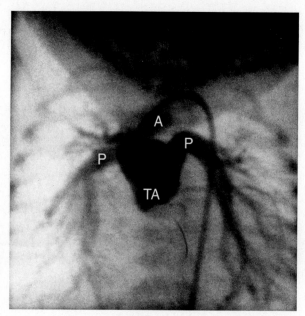

FIGURE 3.3.2

FINDINGS: A frontal chest radiograph demonstrates a right-sided aortic arch (A), cardiomegaly, and increased pulmonary blood flow (Fig. 3.3.1). An angiogram on another patient obtained by injection of contrast material into the aortic root (Fig. 3.3.2) reveals a single vascular trunk (TA), which gives rise to the aorta (A) and the pulmonary arteries (P).

DIAGNOSIS: Persistent truncus arteriosus

DISCUSSION: Between the fifth and seventh weeks of embryologic development, the aorta, pulmonary artery, and high ventricular septum are formed by fusion of the truncoconal ridges, which divide the truncus arteriosus into the aorta and pulmonary artery (12). Failure of the ridges to fuse causes a persistent truncus arteriosus and a defect in the ventricular septum. Radiographically, this diagnosis is strongly suggested when a right aortic arch (35% of cases), cardiomegaly, and increased pulmonary vascularity are present. Angiography or MRI can confirm the diagnosis by visualization of the persistent truncus. The truncal valve has two to five leaflets

but is most commonly tricuspid (13). The most familiar classification scheme for persistent truncus arteriosus is the Collett and Edward's system (14) that is based on the variable origin of the pulmonary arteries from the truncus. A main pulmonary artery arising from the left posterolateral aspect of the truncus (type 1) is the most common type. Surgical correction involves creating a new pulmonary outflow tract with synthetic graft material, although the truncal vessel becomes the aortic root. Before surgery, it is important to assess the position and origins of the coronary arteries on the imaging studies so that they are not inadvertently injured during the surgical procedure.

## Aunt Minnie's Pearls

Embryologic separation of the aorta from the pulmonary artery fails to occur in persistent truncus arteriosus.

Right arch + increased pulmonary flow + cyanosis = think persistent truncus arteriosus.

**HISTORY:** An 18-year-old woman with cyanosis as a newborn (Figs. 3.4.1 and 3.4.2). Figure 3.4.3 is of a different patient.

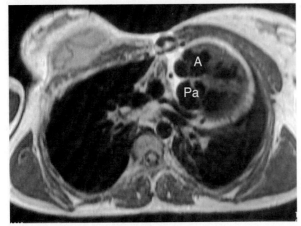

FIGURE 3.4.1

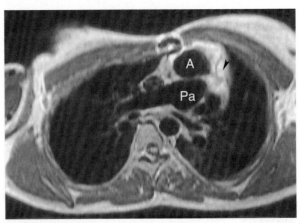

FIGURE 3.4.2

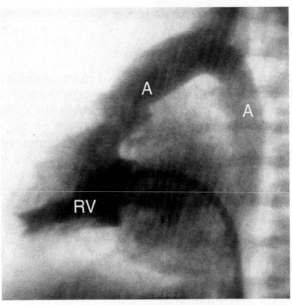

FIGURE 3.4.3

**FINDINGS:** Axial ECG-gated, spin-echo, T1-weighted MR images of the heart were obtained. The abnormal position of the aortic valve and aorta (A) anterior to the pulmonic valve and pulmonary artery (Pa) (Figs. 3.4.1 and 3.4.2) defines d-transposition. A coronary artery is seen originating from the aortic root (Fig. 3.4.2, *arrowhead*). In a different patient, a lateral view from an angiogram obtained with injection of contrast material into the right ventricle (RV) (Fig. 3.4.3) shows contrast opacifying the anteriorly displaced aorta (A).

**DIAGNOSIS:** d-transposition of the great vessels

**DISCUSSION:** Transposition of the great arteries is the most common congenital cyanotic heart lesion in the newborn. MRI allows a specific diagnosis of this lesion if the segmental method of cardiac analysis described by Van Praagh (15) is followed. In normal cardiac development, the inferior vena cava empties into a right-sided atrium, and the aortic valve is located posterior to and to the right of the pulmonic valve. This arrangement describes situs solitus, normal aortic position, and a normal d-bulboventricular loop, respectively. The aorticopulmonary septum, which is responsible for dividing the truncus arteriosus into the two great vessels, normally undergoes a clockwise spiral. If this fails to occur, the aortic valve will lie anteriorly to the pulmonic valve, thereby defining transposition (16).

A VSD is present in 40% of these patients, and valvular or subvalvular stenosis may occur in 30% of patients. Aortic transposition results in ventriculoarterial discordance (i.e., the right ventricle empties into the aorta). Atrioventricular concordance still exists in d-transposition; the venous blood travels from the right atrium to the right ventricle and out the aorta. An atrial septal defect (ASD), VSD, or patent ductus arteriosus is necessary to allow blood to mix between the systemic and pulmonary circulations.

## Aunt Minnie's Pearls

If the aortic valve is anterior to the pulmonic valve, transposition is present.

The dextro designation (d) indicates that the aortic valve is to the right of the pulmonic valve.

Surgical repair is necessary within 6 months to 1 year for optimal survival.

HISTORY: Young woman with severe cyanosis as a newborn

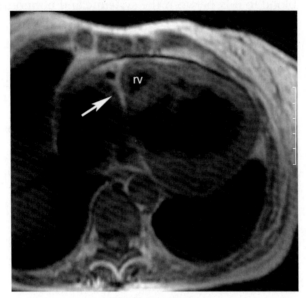

FIGURE 3.5.1

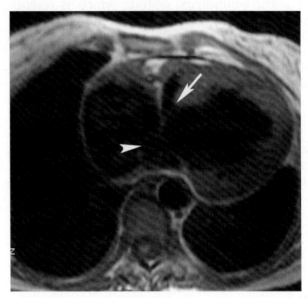

FIGURE 3.5.2

FINDINGS: ECG-gated, T1-weighted, spin-echo MR image reveals a linear bar of high signal intensity in the expected location of the tricuspid valve (Fig. 3.5.1, *arrow*). A large atrial septal artery on chest film = valvular pulmonic stenosis. An ASD (Fig. 3.5.2, *arrowhead*) and a large VSD (*arrow*) are present, as is an extremely hypoplastic right ventricle (*rv*) (Fig. 3.5.1).

DIAGNOSIS: Tricuspid atresia

DISCUSSION: When the tricuspid atrioventricular valve fails to develop normally, tricuspid atresia is present. The newborn presents with cyanosis, and radiographs classically demonstrate decreased pulmonary vascularity. MRI reveals a muscular and fatty ridge of tissue that separates a large right atrium from the hypoplastic right ventricle. A patent foramen ovale or ASD is necessary for blood to bypass the atretic valve and flow into the left atrium. The patient's VSD allows a small amount of blood to pass into the pulmonary circulation through the hypoplastic right ventricle. Approximately 30% of patients with tricuspid atresia also have transposition of the great vessels (17), and pulmonic stenosis is also a common coexistent lesion. The presence of these associated lesions can have a great impact on the associated radiographic findings. Surgical correction involves palliative shunts to the pulmonary artery from the superior vena cava (Glenn) or right atrium (Fontan) and correction of the accompanying intracardiac shunts or transposition.

## Aunt Minnie's Pearls

Chest radiograph in tricuspic atresia shows decreased pulmonary vascularity.

MRI demonstrates a muscular and fatty ridge in the location of tricuspid valve and a hypoplastic right ventricle.

Tricuspid atresia is associated with an ASD and a VSD in all cases and transposition of the great vessels in 30% of patients.

HISTORY: Mild cyanosis and a long systolic murmur identified on physical examination

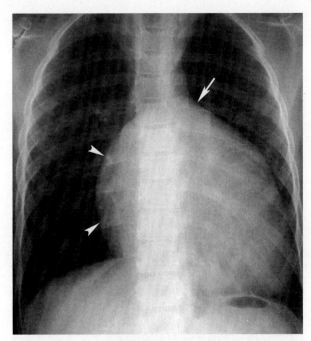

FIGURE 3.6.1

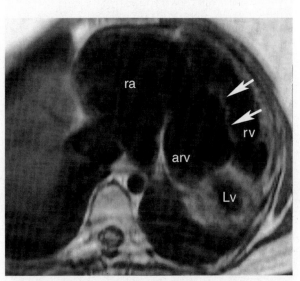

FIGURE 3.6.2

FINDINGS: Frontal view of the chest demonstrates an elongated and enlarged right atrium, which results in a box-shaped contour (Fig. 3.6.1, *arrowheads*). The pulmonary vascularity is decreased, and the area of the main pulmonary artery is concave on the frontal view (Fig. 3.6.1, *arrow*). In a different patient, an axial, ECG-gated, T1-weighted MR image of the heart reveals downward displacement and tethering of the tricuspid valve into the right ventricle (Fig. 3.6.2, *arrows*). This image also shows that a portion (*arv*) of the right ventricle (*rv*) is incorporated into the right atrium (*ra*). The left ventricle is also seen (*Lv*).

DIAGNOSIS: Ebstein anomaly

DISCUSSION: The Ebstein anomaly is abnormal downward displacement of the septal and posterior leaflets of the tricuspid valve into the right ventricle. As a result of this displacement, much of the right ventricle is anatomically incorporated into the right atrium, or "atrialized" (Fig. 3.6.2, *arv*). This portion of the ventricle has an abnormally thin wall, and

tricuspid regurgitation occurs. An associated patent foramen ovale or secundum ASD is present in most cases. Radiographs may demonstrate a nearly pathognomonic appearance of an elongated and enlarged right atrium with a box-shaped contour, as seen in this case. Echocardiography, MRI, or angiography can confirm the diagnosis by demonstrating the displaced tricuspid leaflets and associated abnormalities. ECG abnormalities are frequently found and include right bundle branch block, prolonged PR intervals, and Wolff–Parkinson–White syndrome (18). An association has been described between this anomaly and the use of lithium in early pregnancy (19).

## Aunt Minnie's Pearls

Downward displacement of the septal and posterior leaflets of the tricuspid valve into the right ventricle indicates the Ebstein anomaly.

The Ebstein anomaly is associated with ECG conduction abnormalities and in utero lithium exposure.

HISTORY: Acyanotic 11-year-old girl with upper-extremity hypertension

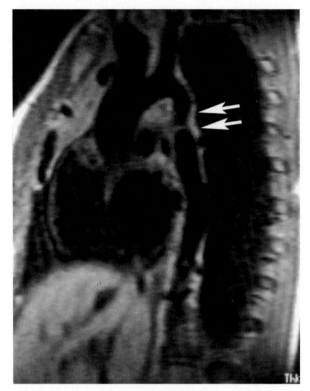

FIGURE 3.7.1

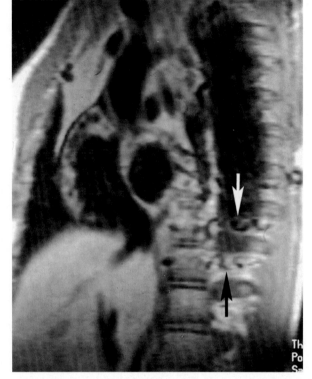

FIGURE 3.7.2

FINDINGS: Oblique sagittal, ECG-gated, T1-weighted MR image of the aorta demonstrates an area of abnormal narrowing in the region of the aortic isthmus (Fig. 3.7.1, *arrows*). Another image obtained off the midline reveals dilated, tortuous intercostal arterial collaterals (Fig. 3.7.2, *arrows*).

DIAGNOSIS: Coarctation of the aorta

DISCUSSION: The juxtaductal portion of the aorta is congenitally narrowed in coarctation of the aorta. If the narrowing occurs proximal to the ductus, blood is shunted to the descending thoracic aorta through the patent ductus. After the ductus closes, clinical symptoms may quickly develop with congestive heart failure and left-to-right shunting across a VSD. Postductal coarctations produce the more familiar presentation in which the radiographs demonstrate left ventricular hypertrophy, an indistinct aortic knob with a "three" contour, and bilateral rib notching. Coarctation of the aorta is associated with bicuspid aortic valve, VSD, patent ductus

arteriosus, berry aneurysms, and Turner syndrome. Pseudo-coarctation refers to elongation of the thoracic aorta with kinking in the juxtaductal region, but no significant pressure gradient exists across the narrowing and no collateral vessels are present (20).

Surgical correction in patients younger than 10 years usually involves placement of a patch across the posterior aorta. Older patients, who are less subject to physical growth, are treated with a subclavian artery patch. Postsurgical restenosis is often treated with balloon dilatation.

MRI permits accurate follow-up evaluation after balloon angioplasty or surgical repair (21).

### Aunt Minnie's Pearls

Coarctation = juxtaductal narrowing of aortic arch with pressure gradient across the lesion (pseudo-coarctation = no pressure gradient).

This anomaly is frequently associated with bicuspid aortic valve, VSD, and patent ductus arteriosus.

HISTORY: A 24-year-old woman with rapidly worsening ascites

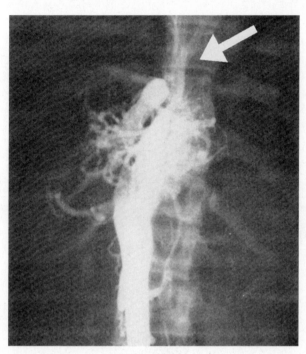

FIGURE 3.8.1

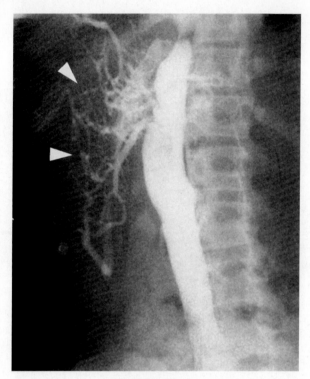

FIGURE 3.8.2

FINDINGS: Anteroposterior (AP; Fig. 3.8.1) and oblique lateral (Fig. 3.8.2) inferior vena cava (IVC) cavagrams demonstrate stenosis of the suprahepatic IVC (*arrow*) and a spider-web appearance (*arrowhead*) of the hepatic vein elements.

DIAGNOSIS: Budd–Chiari syndrome

DISCUSSION: Hepatic venous obstruction (i.e., Budd–Chiari syndrome) is an uncommon cause of portal hypertension. Patients usually present with hepatosplenomegaly and rapid onset of ascites. Hepatic vein occlusion in adults can be the result of various hypercoagulable states (e.g., polycythemia vera or oral contraceptive use) or tumor invasion, as is seen in cases of hepatocellular or renal cell carcinoma. Often, a specific cause is not determined.

Hemodynamic evaluation shows evidence of postsinusoidal venous obstruction, with elevated free and wedged hepatic vein pressures. The spider-web appearance of the wedged hepatic venogram is characteristic (22).

## Aunt Minnie's Pearls

A spider-web appearance of intrahepatic venous collaterals is characteristic of Budd–Chiari syndrome.

Hypercoagulable states and tumor invasion of the cava are common causes in adults.

Associated portal vein thrombosis may occur in 20% of patients with Budd–Chiari.

HISTORY: An 8-year-old girl with hypertension and postprandial abdominal pain

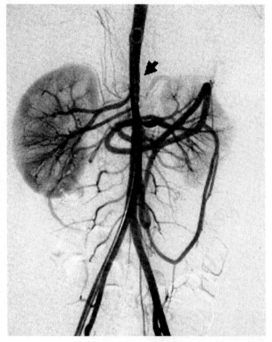

FIGURE 3.9.1

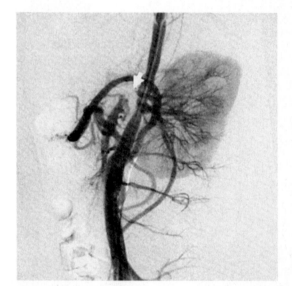

FIGURE 3.9.2

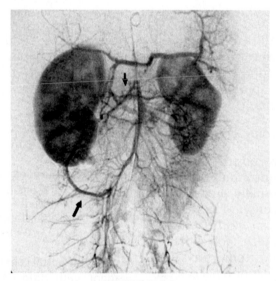

FIGURE 3.9.3

**FINDINGS:** Anteroposterior and lateral abdominal aortograms (Figs. 3.9.1 and 3.9.2) demonstrate occlusion of the celiac axis and superior mesenteric artery (*arrows*) and severe tapering of middle aorta. Late-phase image (Fig. 3.9.3) reveals reconstitution of these vessels through mesenteric collaterals (*arrows*).

**DIAGNOSIS:** Midaortic syndrome (MAS)

**DISCUSSION:** MAS is a rare vascular abnormality manifested by narrowing of the abdominal aorta and including the renal and visceral branches. This condition accounts for 0.5% to 2.0% of aortic coarctations and has also been referred to as coarctation of the abdominal aorta and subisthmic coarctation (23–25). This is a potential cause of renovascular hypertension in children and adolescents, typically manifesting after the age of 5 years (26). MAS is a noninflammatory, nonatheromatous condition of unknown origin. The diagnosis is made with angiography. Angiography demonstrates smooth, segmental stenosis of the abdominal aorta, primarily involving the infrarenal aorta and bilateral proximal renal arteries. The disease may extend cephalad over time to involve the suprarenal aorta and the origin of the superior mesenteric artery. The inferior mesenteric artery is often spared (26).

Differential diagnosis considerations include Takayasu's arteritis and neurofibromatosis. In Takayasu's arteritis, the patients are older and present with systemic inflammatory signs and symptoms. Neurofibromatosis can have midabdominal aortic stenosis, but the diagnosis is usually known from other manifestations of the disease. Arterial bypass surgery is a highly successful treatment that can be curative. Balloon angioplasty can be used, but the results are often short term because of the progressive intimal and medial hyperplasia associated with the condition. Angioplasty may be useful for temporary relief of hypertension and as a bridge to surgery.

## Aunt Minnie's Pearls

MAS is a rare noninflammatory nonatheromatous vascular abnormality that accounts for 0.5% to 2% of aortic coarctations.

The cause is unknown.

Typical presentation is after the age of 5 years.

# Case 3.10

**HISTORY:** A 28-year-old trauma patient with absent right lower-extremity pulses

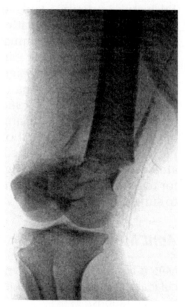

FIGURE 3.10.1

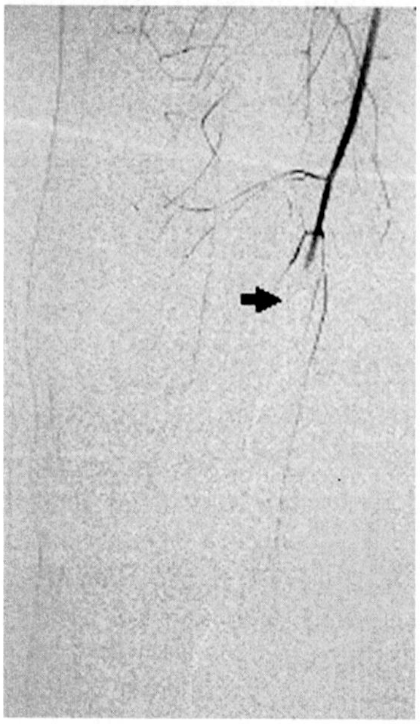

FIGURE 3.10.2

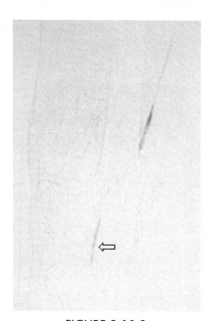

FIGURE 3.10.3

**FINDINGS:** Select right lower-extremity arteriogram shows a comminuted fracture of the distal femur (Fig. 3.10.1) with occlusion of the popliteal artery (Fig. 3.10.2, *arrow*). There is a trace amount of blood flow below the knee (Fig. 3.10.3, *open arrow*).

**DIAGNOSIS:** Popliteal artery occlusion (traumatic)

**DISCUSSION:** Injury to the popliteal artery accounts for 5% to 19% of civilian arterial injuries and results in more amputations than any other vascular injury (27,28). Intimal injury, associated with thrombosis and transection, occurs more often with blunt than penetrating trauma. Knee dislocations are the most common type of associated musculoskeletal injury (29). Because of its course, the popliteal artery is anatomically vulnerable to trauma. The artery is tethered between the tendinous arch of adductor magnus and soleus muscle, rendering it susceptible to stretch injuries and unprotected from direct trauma. Popliteal artery thrombosis can also be complicated by venous injury and compartment syndrome.

Early recognition and treatment is crucial for limb salvage. Emergent arteriography can make the diagnosis and provide a road map for vascular reconstruction (30). However, arteriography should not delay revascularization if severe ischemia is clinically apparent. Physical findings include transient or permanent loss or decrease in distal pulses, gross instability of the knee owing to dislocation or fracture, skin pallor, and motor or sensory changes in the affected limb.

## Aunt Minnie's Pearls

Early recognition and treatment of popliteal artery occlusion is crucial for limb salvage.

Of nonfracture injuries, posterior knee dislocations are commonly associated with acute vascular injury.

HISTORY: A 23-year-old woman with left arm weakness and fever

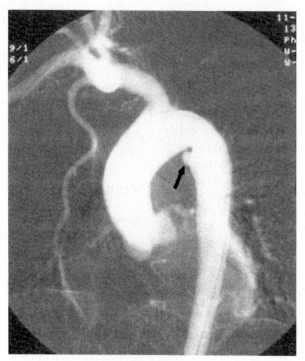

FIGURE 3.11.1

FINDINGS: Thoracic left anterior oblique arteriogram demonstrates large innominate artery and right internal mammary artery with proximal occlusions of the left common carotid artery and left subclavian artery (Fig. 3.11.1). A saccular pseudoaneurysm (*arrow*) is identified near the isthmus.

DIAGNOSIS: Takayasu's arteritis type 1

DISCUSSION: Takayasu's arteritis is a large-vessel vasculitis characterized by inflammation and fibrosis of the aorta and its major branches. Dr. Takayasu, a Japanese ophthalmologist, described the first case in 1908, when he reported vascular malformations in the retina (31). It was later discovered that these retinal vascular structures are a response to narrowing of the neck arteries. Takayasu's arteritis is pathologically similar to giant-cell arteritis. The cause remains unknown, but there may be a relationship to tuberculosis, genetic influences, or immunologic factors. Takayasu's arteritis is most common in female patients (>80%) of Asian descent and typically manifests before 30 years (32,33).

Clinical presentation is divided into two stages. Stage I is the systemic phase characterized by fever, arthralgias, and weight loss. Stage II consists of the fibrotic changes that lead to vessel stenosis and aneurysmal formation. These findings have led to use of the term *pulseless disease*. The spectrum of disease is variable, ranging from asymptomatic individuals to those with hypertension, stroke, or myocardial infarctions. Approximately 50% of patients have pulmonary artery involvement.

The diagnosis is typically made with angiography showing characteristic occlusions, stenoses, and aneurysms. Multiple sites of involvement are typical. Elevated erythrocyte sedimentation rate and thrombocytosis are typical laboratory findings. Antiinflammatory medications (i.e., corticosteroids) are the mainstay of medical therapy. Surgical and angioplastic revascularization is often necessary, but an optimal approach has not been determined. Deaths are most often the result of congestive heart failure, arrhythmias, and stroke.

## Aunt Minnie's Pearls

Takayasu's arteritis is a large-vessel vasculitis most commonly affecting female patients (>50%).

The disease affects all racial and ethnic categories but has an Asian predominance.

Typical presentation occurs before 30 years.

**HISTORY:** A 35-year-old woman with refractory hypertension

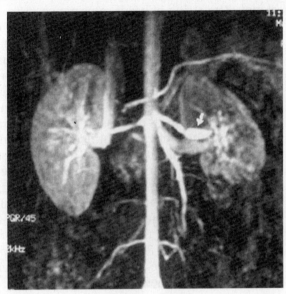

FIGURE 3.12.1

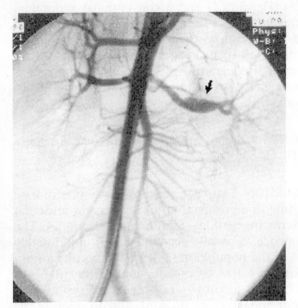

FIGURE 3.12.2

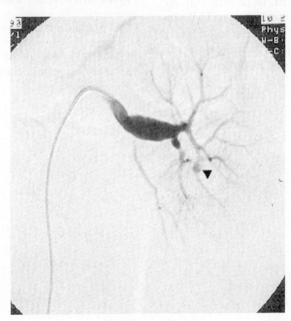

FIGURE 3.12.3

**FINDINGS:** A coronal, three-dimensional, gadolinium-enhanced, abdominal magnetic resonance angiogram (MRA) (Fig. 3.12.1) and a conventional abdominal arteriogram (Fig. 3.12.2) demonstrate a normal right renal artery and poststenotic fusiform dilatation of the distal left main renal artery (*arrow*). A selective left renal arteriogram (Fig. 3.12.3) also demonstrates a small branch vessel aneurysm not seen on MRA (*arrowhead*).

**DIAGNOSIS:** Renal artery fibromuscular dysplasia (FMD)

**DISCUSSION:** FMD is a composite vascular disease resulting in a proliferation of fibrous and muscular elements in medium- and large-sized arteries. The prevalence is small, accounting for proximately 0.5% of the population (34). FMD accounts for approximately 10% of cases of renal artery stenosis. The cause is unknown, but theory suggests genetics, hormonal factors, smoking, and disorders of the vasa vasorum. FMD may affect any element of the vessel wall (i.e., intima, medium, or adventitia). Almost 90% of renal artery stenosis owing to FMD involves the media (i.e., medial hyperplasia). FMD is more common in the female population and tends to occur between 15 and 50 years. In children, FMD is largely of the intimal type (35).

The renal arteries are the most common site (60%–75%), although disease can be seen in any vascular bed, including the craniocervical, visceral, and iliac arteries. The string-of-beads appearance (associated with medial fibrodysplasia) results from multiple, small aneurysms found in the middle and distal arteries. FMD can be associated with spontaneous dissection and thrombosis of the renal artery, which leads to impaired renal function and infarction. This is more common with the intimal and adventitial forms. The diagnosis is made with renal angiography or MRA, and the preferred treatment is percutaneous transluminal renal angioplasty (36). Intravascular stents are not the treatment of choice in this setting but are used in cases that fail standard treatment, including significant stenosis despite adequate balloon angioplasty, focal vessel perforation, or a large flow-limiting intimal dissection. Surgical revascularization is generally reserved for cases of failed angioplasty that are not amenable to percutaneous treatment or lesions in need of emergent surgical repair (37).

### Aunt Minnie's Pearls

FMD in children is most often the intimal type.

Renal artery FMD is the most common cause of renovascular hypertension in the adolescent population.

HISTORY: A 40-year-old male trauma patient

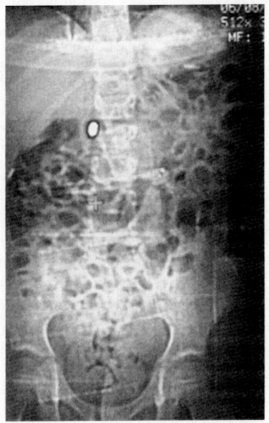

FIGURE 3.13.1

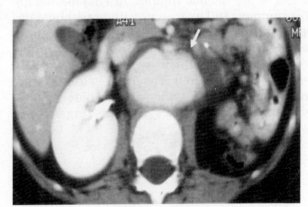

FIGURE 3.13.2

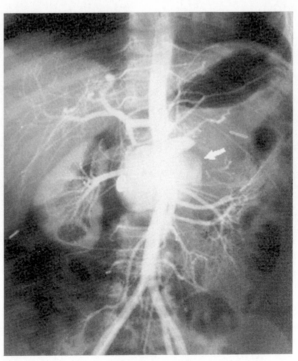

FIGURE 3.13.3

FINDINGS: The anteroposterior scout radiograph (Fig. 3.13.1) depicts multiple distended bowel loops and radiopaque foreign body. Axial computed tomography (CT) with contrast (Fig. 3.13.2) and abdominal arteriogram (Fig. 3.13.3) demonstrate large aortic pseudoaneurysm (*arrows*) resulting from a gunshot wound.

DIAGNOSIS: Traumatic aortic pseudoaneurysm

DISCUSSION: Vascular injuries can result from blunt or penetrating traumatic injuries. Blunt injuries cause approximately 10% to 15% of traumatic vascular injuries, most often from motor vehicle accidents (38). Penetrating injuries from gunshots and sharp objects (including fractures) account for the rest of the vascular injuries. Arterial injuries are most common and may occur with or without concomitant venous injury. Isolated venous injuries are rare. The extremities are the most susceptible location for vascular injuries, accounting for 75% to 80% of the cases (39). The lower extremities are more often involved. Other sites include cervical, visceral, and aortic injuries (in decreasing order of frequency). Most vascular trauma patients are men between 20 and 40 years.

Vascular injuries can result in the formation of pseudoaneurysms. Pseudoaneurysms differ from a true aneurysm in that there is not dilatation of all vessel layers (i.e., intima, media, and adventitia). Rather, there is contained disruption of the artery by surrounding soft tissues or an intact adventitia. However, some arterial injuries can lead to weakening of the arterial walls and result in a true aneurysm. Possible complications include rupture, neurovascular compression, thrombosis, and infection (40). Mycotic pseudoaneurysms are classically seen in drug abusers. The diagnostic evaluation includes angiography, CT, ultrasound, and arteriography.

## Aunt Minnie's Pearls

Most cases of pseudoaneurysms involve penetrating trauma.

The lower extremities are the most common site of involvement.

## Case 3.14

**HISTORY:** A 23-year-old man with chronic, dull pelvic pain

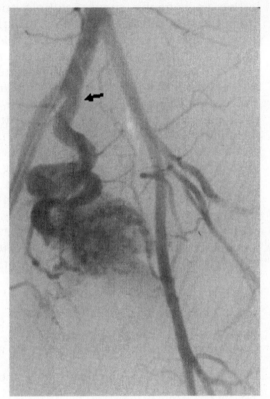

FIGURE 3.14.1

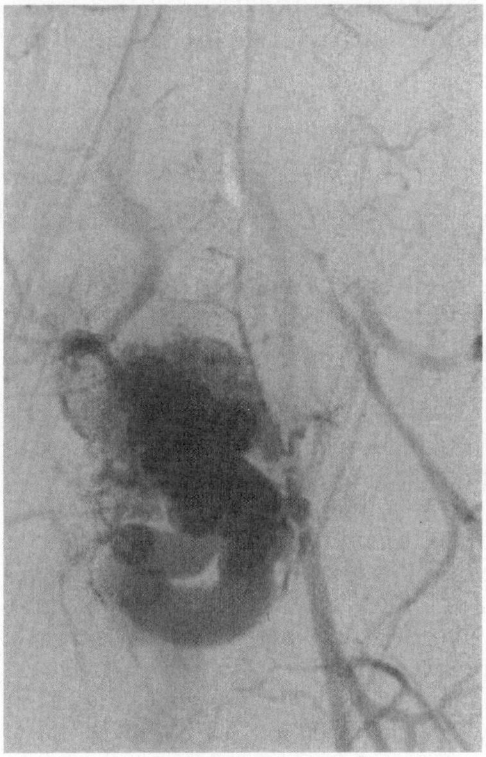

FIGURE 3.14.2

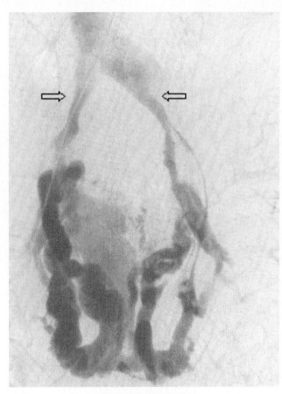

FIGURE 3.14.3

**FINDINGS:** The pelvic arteriogram (Fig. 3.14.1) demonstrates a large arteriovenous malformation (AVM) originating from the right hypogastric artery (*arrow*). Late-phase images (Figs. 3.14.2 and 3.14.3) show drainage into the hypogastric veins and IVC (*open arrows*).

**DIAGNOSIS:** Congenital pelvic arteriovenous malformation

**DISCUSSION:** AVM is an abnormal connection between the arterial and venous systems without an intervening capillary bed and can result in mass formation. AVMs can be congenital or acquired. Acquired lesions are usually caused by penetrating injuries, fractures, and surgical procedures or result from vascular diseases, such as atherosclerosis and mycotic aneurysms. Congenital AVMs can manifest at different ages and typically grow with the patient. AVMs can occur in any organ, but 50% occur in the head and neck (41). Other locations include the CNS, heart, liver, lung, kidney, and gastric mucosa (i.e., Dieulafoy's disease). Small malformations may be asymptomatic. Typical physical findings are swelling, pain, and hemorrhage. A pulsatile mass or bruit can be present if the lesion is relatively superficial. Blood preferentially flows through the low-resistance fistula and results in cyanosis distal to the lesion. Angiography is crucial for diagnostic and therapeutic evaluation. Selective angiography shows multiple anomalous arterial vessels and anastomoses with early filling of veins. Blood vessels are dilated, tortuous, and elongated. Structure of the vascular walls is abnormal, with thinning or hypertrophy of arteries and thickening (or arterialization) of veins. Many AVMs are considered unstable because of their capacity to progressively enlarge. Indications for treatment include congestive heart failure, hemorrhage, cosmetic deformity, and ulcerations. Treatment is tailored to the individual lesion, including surgical resection, embolization, and irradiation. Various materials have been used for embolization therapy, and the diameter of the shunt determines the size of the embolization particles so as to prevent systematic spread. A combination of therapeutic techniques is often used to prevent complications and recurrences (42).

## Aunt Minnie's Pearls

Fifty percent of AVMs occur in the head and neck.

Treatment of giant AVMs includes staged embolization and surgery.

HISTORY: A 25-year-old patient with right leg injury

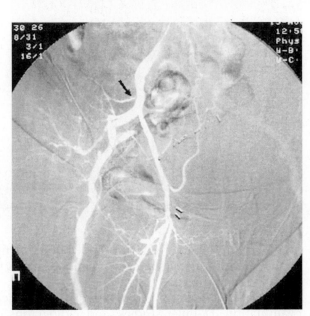

FIGURE 3.15.1

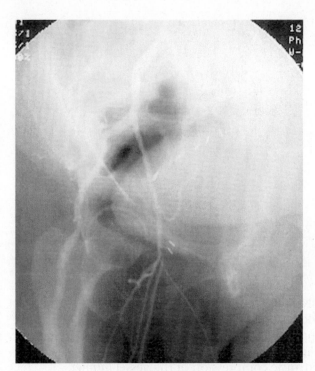

FIGURE 3.15.2

FINDINGS: Right lower-extremity arteriograms (Figs. 3.15.1 and 3.15.2) demonstrate continuation of the right internal iliac artery (*arrow*) below the inguinal ligament.

DIAGNOSIS: Persistent sciatic artery (PSA)

DISCUSSION: PSA is a rare anatomic vascular anomaly. The sciatic artery arises from the umbilical artery to supply the developing embryonic limb, but this vessel is normally replaced by the femoral artery by the third month of gestation. If the sciatic artery persists, it may become the main blood supply to the lower extremity. PSA originates from the hypogastric artery and gives off the superior gluteal and internal pudendal arteries before passing through the greater sciatic notch. The sciatic artery runs down the posterior thigh with the sciatic nerve. PSA is considered complete if it continues down the thigh as the popliteal artery. If PSA is incomplete, the sciatic artery terminates in the posterior thigh without direct communication with the popliteal artery (43).

This vascular anomaly is rare and reportable in most cases. There is a slight male predominance,

without a preference for either side. Approximately 25% of the cases are bilateral (44). Patients present with symptoms of a mass, ischemia, and gluteal pain. PSA is prone to atherosclerosis and aneurysm formation. One-half of patients develop aneurysms that are generally distal to the sciatic notch. Aneurysmal treatments are primarily surgical and include resection of the aneurysm with direct anastomosis, ligation with a bypass, and embolization with a bypass. Few cases have been treated without surgical intervention and involve embolization of an incomplete PSA with a dual vascular supply (45).

## Aunt Minnie's Pearls

The sciatic artery runs down the posterior thigh with the sciatic nerve. The PSA is considered complete if it continues down the thigh as the popliteal artery.

Approximately 25% of cases are bilateral.

PSA is prone to early atherosclerosis and aneurysm formation.

# Case 3.16

HISTORY: A 35-year-old woman with left arm weakness while raising her arm

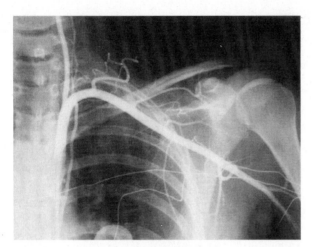

FIGURE 3.16.1

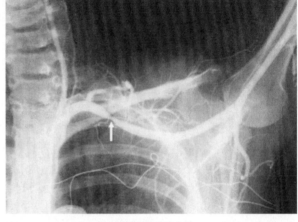

FIGURE 3.16.2

FINDINGS: A left upper-extremity arteriogram in adduction (Fig. 3.16.1) demonstrates the normal appearance of left subclavian artery. In abduction (Fig. 3.16.2), there is a distinct narrowing caused by extrinsic compression of the vessel (*arrow*).

DIAGNOSIS: Thoracic outlet syndrome (TOS)

DISCUSSION: TOS refers to compression of the neurovascular structures passing through the thoracic outlet. The neurovascular structures involved are the brachial plexus, subclavian vein, and subclavian artery. Neurologic compression is most common (95%), followed by venous (4%) and arterial compression (1%). Neurologic compression is more common in women (3:1), and the isolated venous type is more prevalent in men (46).

Arterial complications are the least common but can be the most serious because of the ischemia of the upper extremity. Symptoms usually occur between the third and sixth decades without gender bias. These patients typically have a bony anomaly, such as a cervical rib, that is present in 50% of cases. The most common compression site is the interscalene triangle (47). Extrinsic compression may cause thickening and inflammation of the arterial wall. Poststenotic dilation and aneurysmal formation develop from the flow disturbance and patients may become symptomatic from thromboembolic events in the proximal arteries and microembolizations to the hands and digits.

Arterial compression is diagnosed with physical examination, Doppler studies, and radiographs of the upper thorax and confirmed with arteriography. In suspected cases, arteriography should include the entire upper extremity from the aortic arch to the digits. Findings include poststenotic dilatation, aneurysm, thrombus formation, and intimal changes. Surgery is the primary treatment, involving decompression of the thoracic outlet, arterial reconstruction, and reperfusion. Catheter-directed thrombolytic therapy can be used as a bridge to definitive surgical treatment (48).

## Aunt Minnie's Pearls

Review the chest radiograph to rule out an obvious anatomic cause of TOS (e.g., cervical rib).

TOS may occur in up to 1% of the population.

Provocative maneuvers during arteriography are essential to reveal the abnormality.

Definitive treatment of TOS is surgery.

**HISTORY:** A 55-year-old man with a history of left femoral–to–popliteal artery bypass has fever and left knee pain

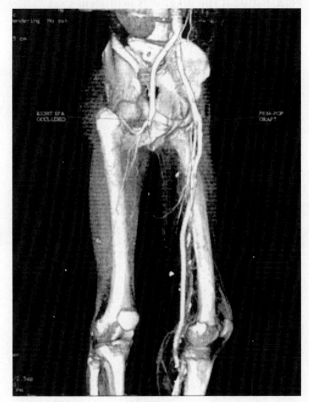

FIGURE 3.17.1

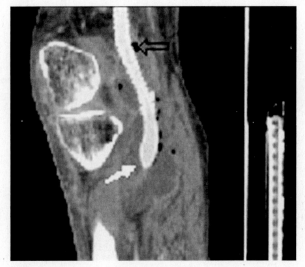

FIGURE 3.17.2

**FINDINGS:** CT angiogram depicts patency of the left femoral–to–popliteal bypass graft (Fig. 3.17.1). There is fluid density surrounding the distal anastomosis (Fig. 3.17.2, *white arrow*). Air pockets are also seen within the fluid density (Fig. 3.17.2, *open arrows*).

**DIAGNOSIS:** Peripheral bypass graft infection (i.e., perigraft abscess)

**DISCUSSION:** Infection of vascular grafts can be a life- or limb-threatening complication. Vascular grafts typically become infected by one of three ways: perioperative contamination, hematogenous spread, and enteric erosion or fistula. Synthetic grafts generally have an increased risk of infection compared with autogenous grafts. Graft infections can occur at any time, but the mean interval after surgery is approximately 2 years. There is increased incidence of graft infections involving groin anastomoses, contaminated wounds, prolonged procedures, and emergent cases. Complications of infection include thrombosis, rupture, enteric fistulas, and pseudoaneurysm formation.

CT is the preferred imaging modality for vascular graft infections because of its high sensitivity and specificity, speed, and availability. Signs of graft infection include perigraft air, fluid, soft-tissue attenuation, and pseudoaneurysm formation (49). Postoperative air is rare after 1 week but does not suggest infection until 1 or 2 months postoperatively. Similarly, perigraft fluid is not considered suspicious until about 3 months postoperatively.

Nuclear medicine studies (e.g., indium-111–labeled leukocytes) can be complementary tests to cross-sectional imaging and may be more sensitive than CT in cases of early graft infection (50,51). However, nuclear medicine studies can also provide false-positive results owing to postoperative inflammation. Interventional procedures with CT can be useful in the diagnosis and management of patients. CT-guided aspiration of perigraft fluid collections can be performed preoperatively to establish antimicrobial therapy and to bridge patients for definitive surgical treatment. CT-guided injection of contrast into perigraft collections can also be diagnostic of enteric fistula if the diagnosis is unclear (52).

### Aunt Minnie's Pearl

CT is the initial imaging modality of choice to diagnose perigraft abscess.

HISTORY: A 50-year-old man with chronic right leg pain and absent right femoral pulses

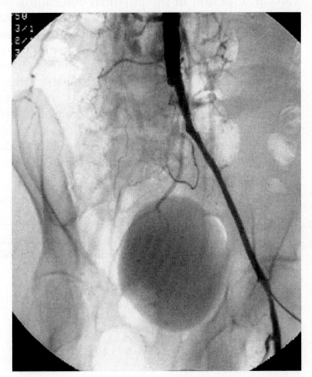

FIGURE 3.18.1

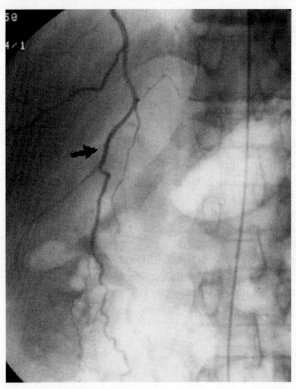

FIGURE 3.18.2

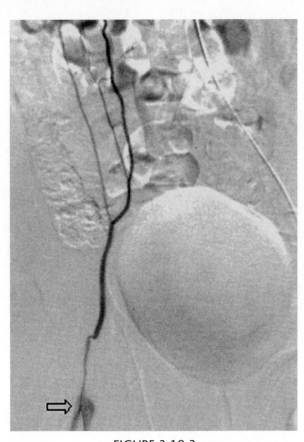

FIGURE 3.18.3

**FINDINGS:** An abdominal angiogram reveals occlusion of the entire right iliac artery (Fig. 3.18.1). Selective right internal mammary artery injection (Fig. 3.18.2) reveals collateral flow from the superior to inferior epigastric artery (*arrow*) and then reconstitution of the right common femoral artery (Fig. 3.18.3, *open arrow*).

**DIAGNOSIS:** Winslow's collateral pathway (i.e., chronic right iliac artery occlusive disease)

**DISCUSSION:** Winslow's collateral pathway applies to a collateral pathway involving the lower extremities in aortoiliac occlusive disease. The pathway is as follows: subclavian artery, internal mammary, superior epigastric, inferior epigastric, and external iliac artery. More common collateral pathways involve the inferior mesenteric artery and the intercostals arteries. Winslow's pathway is more common in congenital coarctations of the aorta and less common in adult-onset vaso-occlusive disease (53).

Selective internal mammary artery arteriography has been suggested in patients with aortoiliac occlusion. Injection in the proximal descending thoracic aorta may also suffice because the intercostal arteries normally connect with the internal mammary arteries. This collateral pathway may present a problem for patients with lower-extremity ischemia and coronary artery disease. Selecting the internal mammary artery as a coronary bypass conduit can cause vascular insufficiency to the associated lower extremity, and selective internal mammary arteriography therefore may be useful during a cardiac catheterization in patients with aortoiliac occlusive disease (54).

## Aunt Minnie's Pearl

Winslow's pathway is more common in congenital coarctation of the aorta.

# Case 3.19

HISTORY: A 20-year-old male pitcher with right arm pain and swelling for 2 weeks

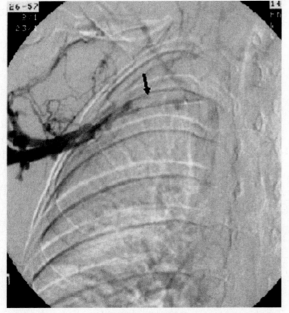

FIGURE 3.19.1

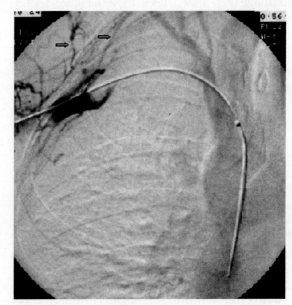

FIGURE 3.19.2

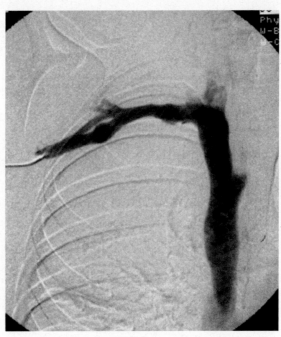

FIGURE 3.19.3

**FINDINGS:** A right upper-arm venogram reveals thrombosis of the right subclavian vein (Fig. 3.19.1, *arrow*). Collateral veins reconstitute the central venous drainage (Fig. 3.19.2, *open arrows*). Figure 3.19.3 demonstrates clearance of the clot after pharmacomechanical thrombolysis.

**DIAGNOSIS:** Paget–Schroetter syndrome (i.e., effort thrombosis)

**DISCUSSION:** The eponym is named after Sir James Paget and Leopold von Schroetter, who described symptoms of thrombosis in the upper extremities during the 19th century (55). The term *effort thrombosis* is widely used for the same entity that describes venous thrombosis of the upper extremities associated with strenuous exercise of the upper extremities and shoulders. Thromboses of the upper extremities account for 2% to 4% of all deep venous thromboses (56). Upper-extremity thrombophlebitis can lead to pulmonary embolism in 1% to 10% of cases. Paget–Schroetter syndrome is most commonly associated with young men and affects the dominant arm. Pathologically, thrombosis is caused by strain on the vein in different positions and results in injury to the intima. Underlying anatomic anomalies, such as a cervical rib or hypertrophied muscles, can cause venous compression and propagate the thrombosis (57). Paget–Schroetter syndrome often manifests as pain, swelling, and discoloration of the involved upper extremity. Diagnosis is usually made with duplex ultrasound and confirmed with venography. The treatment for effort thrombosis is still evolving, and long-term results have shown a poor prognosis with conservative therapy (i.e., anticoagulation and immobilization). Patients with subclavian effort thrombosis undergo catheter-mediated thrombolysis followed by thoracic decompression. Some studies advocate angioplasty and stent placement after thoracic decompression (57).

## Aunt Minnie's Pearls

Effort thrombosis is more common in men and usually affects the dominant arm.

Treatment is catheter-directed thrombolysis and surgery.

HISTORY: A 60-year-old man with an irregular heart rate and syncope

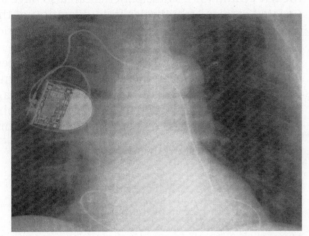

FIGURE 3.20.1

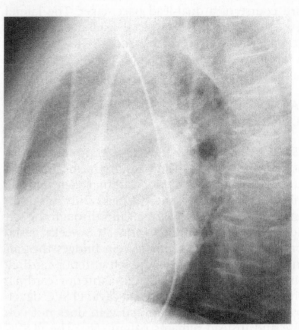

FIGURE 3.20.2

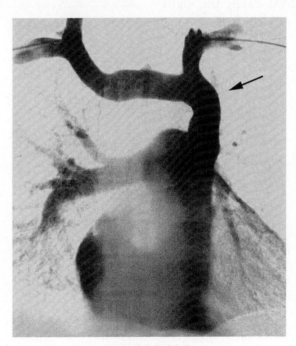

FIGURE 3.20.3

FINDINGS: Posteroanterior and lateral chest radiographs (Figs. 3.20.1 and 3.20.2) demonstrate a leftward course of a dual-lead pacemaker. The lateral view shows the tip of a distal lead overlying expected location of coronary sinus. The venogram reveals persistent left superior vena cava (*arrow*) draining into the coronary sinus (Fig. 3.20.3).

DIAGNOSIS: Persistent left superior vena cava (PLSVC)

DISCUSSION: PLSVC is the most common venous anomaly in the chest and results from abnormal patency of the left anterior cardinal vein. During embryologic development, the head and arms drain venous blood into the right atrium through the left and right anterior cardinal veins. At 8 weeks' gestation, the left brachiocephalic vein bridges the cardinal veins. Subsequently, the left anterior cardinal vein degenerates, and the right anterior cardinal vein becomes the superior vena cava. PLSVC develops if the left anterior cardinal vein does not collapse and instead remains patent (58). The PLSVC typically drains into the right atrium through the coronary sinus. In most PLSVC cases, the right anterior cardinal vein remains patent, resulting in bilateral or double superior vena cavae.

Approximately 0.3% to 0.5% of the population has PLSVC. These patients are usually hemodynamically stable, but they are at increased risk for paradoxical embolism from accompanying lesions, such as ASDs, unroofed coronary sinus, or drainage into the left atrium (59). These patients can also have associated cardiac arrhythmias from dilatation of the coronary sinus that causes stretching of the atrioventricular node and His bundles.

PLSVC is often an incidental finding on a chest radiograph after central line placement, and definitive diagnosis can be made with a variety of imaging modalities. Transesophageal echocardiography is particularly accurate in detecting PLSVC and concomitant cardiac anomalies.

## Aunt Minnie's Pearls

PLSVC occurs in <0.5% of the general population.

Most cases also have a simultaneous patent right superior vena cava.

**HISTORY:** A 20-year-old woman with cough

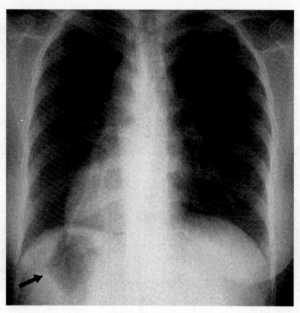

FIGURE 3.21.1

**FINDINGS:** A posteroanterior chest radiograph reveals a cardiac silhouette in right side of chest. A right-sided stomach bubble is present (Fig. 3.21.1, *arrow*).

**DIAGNOSIS:** Situs inversus totalis

**DISCUSSION:** Total situs inversus refers to a reversal of the normal location of the atria and visceral structures. The term *situs solitus* is used for normal positioning. Situs inversus is independent of the cardiac apex position, and situs inversus can be classified with dextrocardia or levocardia. Situs ambiguous or heterotaxy is the term used when the relationship between the atria and viscera are inconsistent.

Situs inversus is found in 0.01% of the population and has no gender or racial predilection (60). Situs inversus with dextrocardia is more common and usually associated with a right aortic arch. These patients have a 3.5% incidence of congenital heart disease (usually transposition of the great vessels) (61).

Situs inversus with levocardia is rare and is highly associated with congenital heart disease. Kartagener syndrome affects 20% of patients with situs inversus (62). These patients have primary ciliary dysfunction and suffer from repeated sinus and pulmonary infections, often resulting in bronchiectasis.

The diagnosis can be made with various imaging modalities. CT, MR, and sonography can accurately demonstrate the location of the abdominal visceral structures. MR and sonography are often helpful in assessing the cardiac atrial locations. Fetal sonography or chest radiography may be the initial imaging studies to suggest the diagnosis of situs inversus.

## Aunt Minnie's Pearls

Situs inversus with dextrocardia = usual variant, with a 4% chance of congenital heart disease.

Situs inversus with levocardia has >95% association with congenital heart disease.

HISTORY: A 74-year-old male having undergone endovascular repair of abdominal aortic aneurysm (EVAR) 12 months earlier

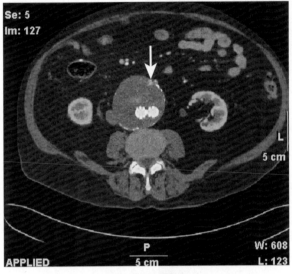

FIGURE 3.22.1

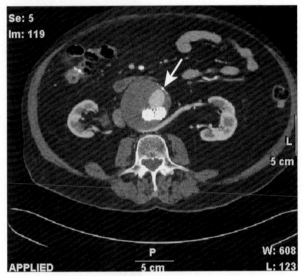

FIGURE 3.22.2

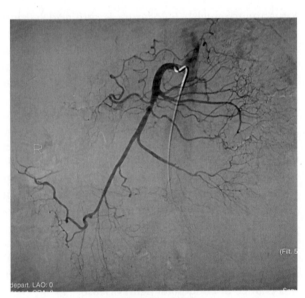

FIGURE 3.22.3

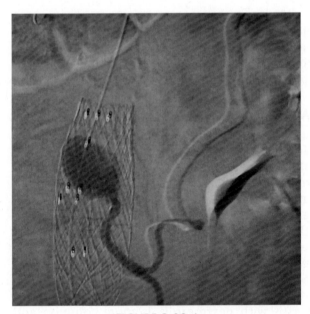

FIGURE 3.22.4

**FINDINGS:** Computed tomography angiogram (CTA) demonstrates an endoleak that appears to arise at the origin of the inferior mesenteric artery (IMA; Figs. 3.22.1 and 3.22.2, *arrows*). Initial flush aortogram with the catheter cephalad to the visceral vessels demonstrates an endoleak. Selective superior mesenteric artery angiogram demonstrates the endoleak resulting from retrograde filling of the IMA (Figs. 3.22.3 and 3.22.4, *arrow*).

**DIAGNOSIS:** Endoleak, Type II, following EVAR.

**DISCUSSION:** EVAR has evolved into a major treatment modality for abdominal aortic aneurysms (AAAs). As many as 70% of AAAs are now treated with endovascular minimally invasive therapy (63). This treatment has spawned a new type of post-procedure issue, the endoleak. An endoleak is persistent flow of systemic arterial blood into the aneurysm sac. Endoleaks result from several factors, and are categorized as types I to V. Type I results from an inadequate anastomotic seal. Type II endoleak occurs when there is retrograde flow from aortic branch vessels (usually lumbar arteries or the IMA). Type III endoleaks are the consequence of device failure, such as separation of modular components or a tear in the fabric of the endograft. Type IV endoleak is typically a transient phenomena occurring with initial endograft placement and relating to graft material porosity. Type V endoleak is a complex phenomena referred to as endotension. There is no demonstrable extravasation of blood from the graft into the aneurysm sac, but the aneurysm does not decrease in size, and often increases. The salient point with respect to endoleaks is the persistence of arterial pressurization of the aneurysm sac, and continued high risk of aneurysm rupture, despite the EVAR. Management is determined by the source. This may include vessel embolization, placement of extension graft or new graft or surgical repair (conversion) (64,65).

## Aunt Minnie's Pearls

Aneurysms that undergo EVAR require lifelong CTA follow-up.

The critical imaging findings are evidence of endoleak and increase in aneurysm sac diameter, which usually require angiographic evaluation.

Angiographic embolization may be appropriate treatment, particularly for Type II endoleaks.

HISTORY: A 32-year-old male who fell on an overturned bar stool, sustaining a straddle injury to his perineum

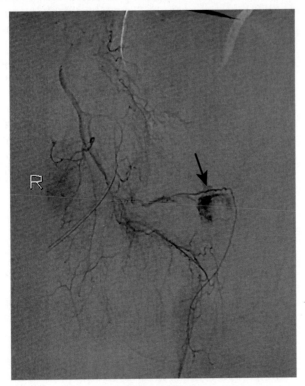

FIGURE 3.23.1

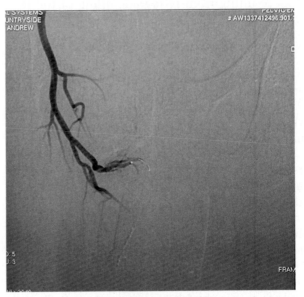

FIGURE 3.23.2

FINDINGS: Initial angiographic evaluation demonstrates unilateral right-sided cavernosal arterial extravasation (Fig. 3.23.1, *arrow*). The following images demonstrate embolization with a single microcoil of the terminal cavernosal branch with resolution of cavernosal leak (Fig. 3.23.2).

DIAGNOSIS: Priapism, high flow, with resolution following superselective embolization

DISCUSSION: Priapism is defined as persistent erection lasting longer than 4 hours. This condition is associated with a number of predisposing factors, including hematologic (sickle cell disease), iatrogenic (erectile dysfunction medications), and trauma. Priapism is clinically divided into low-flow and high-flow states. Low-flow states denote issues with outflow obstruction and represent true emergencies, as tissue ischemia is present, and the therapeutic window for amelioration is short. High-flow states typically indicate increased arterial inflow and are often characterized by a cavernosal leak or acquired arteriovenous fistula, resultant from various traumatic injuries (skateboarding, bicycling, direct blunt trauma to the perineum). Therapy varies for the low-flow versus the high-flow states,

arteriography often being the gold standard for diagnostic differentiation and least invasive treatment for high-flow conditions. Traditional therapy for high-flow priapism required urologic surgical procedures, such as exploration and ligation of the responsible vessel or the creation of a shunt. Successful transarterial embolization was first described in 1977 and has become increasingly the therapy of choice (66,67). A review of 202 reported cases in the literature reports success rate of 89% with transarterial embolization as against 22% with surgical procedures (68).

## Aunt Minnie's Pearls

Priapism is categorized into low-flow and high-flow types, often distinguishable by clinical history.

Pelvic angiography with bilateral selective catheterization of the pudendal arteries is the appropriate diagnostic modality for high-flow priapism; definitive treatment may be rendered transarterially.

Pelvic angiography and embolization are associated with very high success rates and very low incidence of complications, especially erectile dysfunction.

HISTORY: A 38-year-old male carpenter with right-hand pain

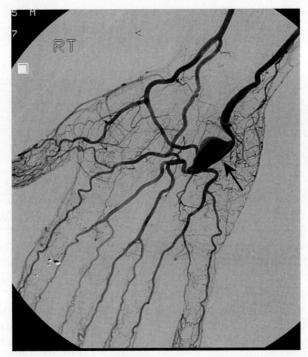

FIGURE 3.24.1

FINDINGS: Digital subtraction angiogram of the right hand shows large saccular aneurysm of the superficial division of the distal ulnar artery (Fig. 3.24.1). No occlusions are identified in the digital arteries or superficial palmar arch.

DIAGNOSIS: Hypothenar hammer syndrome (HHS)

DISCUSSION: HHS is a form of occupation-induced hand ischemia that may manifest as Raynaud's phenomenon (69,70). The etiology is usually from repetitive traumatic hand use during occupational or recreational activities. Patients with HHS often present with hand parathesias, numbness and pain, or coolness and pallor in the hand and fingers.

Angiographic findings of HHS may include occlusion of the distal ulnar artery at the level of the hamate, aneurysm formation of the distal ulnar artery and superficial palmar arch (Fig. 3.24.1, *arrow*), and possible distal embolization to the digital arteries of the affected hand. Oftentimes features of both acute and chronic vascular injury are demonstrated.

Treatment options include conservative and reconstructive approaches. Surgical excision of ulnar aneurysms with vascular interposition grafting results in high patency rates if the condition is diagnosed early. Medical strategies include heparinization and prostaglandin $E_1$ therapy, smoking cessation and lipid control, and avoidance of further repetitive hand trauma. Regional intra-arterial thrombolysis has been utilized successfully in cases of ulnar and digital artery occlusions (71,72).

Color Doppler ultrasound and gadolinium-enhanced MRA are increasingly popular means of noninvasively evaluating suspected HHS. However, digital subtraction angiography (DSA) remains the gold standard. The chief advantages of DSA include providing real-time flow data and improved spatial resolution and offers the ability to perform endovascular treatment.

### Aunt Minnie's Pearls

Distal ulnar artery aneurysm and/or arterial occlusions with history of occupational/recreation hand/wrist trauma = HHS.

More common in the dominant hand and in males.

**HISTORY:** A 35-year-old male with chronic history of tobacco abuse and right-hand pain, coolness, and skin discoloration.

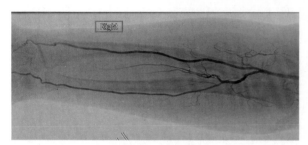

FIGURE 3.25.1

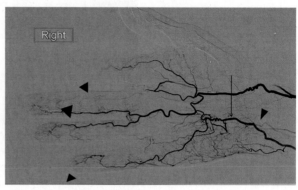

FIGURE 3.25.2

**FINDINGS:** Right forearm arteriogram demonstrates normal brachial artery bifurcation and normal proximal radial, ulnar, and interosseous arteries (Fig 3.25.1). Right-hand selective arteriogram demonstrates abnormal "corkscrew collaterals" (Fig. 3.25.2, *thin arrow*) and multiple segmental occlusions in the digital branches and thenar eminence (Fig. 3.25.2, *arrowheads*).

**DIAGNOSIS:** Buerger's disease

**DISCUSSION:** Buerger's disease, also known has thromboangiitis obliterans (TAO), is a vasoocclusive disorder characterized by non-atheromatous segmental vascular inflammation involving the small and medium-sized arteries and veins of the upper and lower extremities. Buerger's disease is estimated to affect approximately 12 to 20 people per 100,000 in the United States and is more common in males 20 to 40 years of Asian or Eastern European ethnicity (73).

The disease is strongly associated with heavy tobacco use, and progression of the disease is correlated with continued tobacco abuse.

Patients typically present with pain, coolness, or color disturbance in the hands or feet. The patient may also complain of skin changes, painful sores, or ulcers on the hands or feet (74).

Angiographic findings on upper- or lower-extremity arteriography demonstrate classic occlusions with "corkscrew" collateral vessels bridging areas of blockage in the small to medium arteries. Buerger's disease seldom involves the visceral arteries, and it is sometimes necessary to perform angiography of the visceral arterial circulation to exclude other forms of vasculitis (75).

There is no definite cure for Buerger's disease, and the goal of treatment is to control symptoms. It is essential that patients refrain from tobacco use immediately and completely. Other recommended treatments include measures to increase blood flow including applying warmth and exercise and avoidance of cold temperatures. Surgical sympathectomy may control pain in addition to administration of vasodilators and aspirin.

## Aunt Minnie's Pearls

Buerger's disease is associated with heavy or prolonged tobacco abuse and mostly affects males of 20 to 40 years.

Vessels in hands and feet are especially affected.

**HISTORY:** A 56-year-old dialysis patient with right upper-arm arteriovenous fistula (AVF) and right-hand pain and coolness.

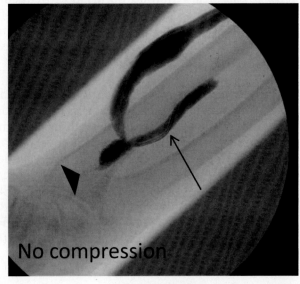

FIGURE 3.26.1

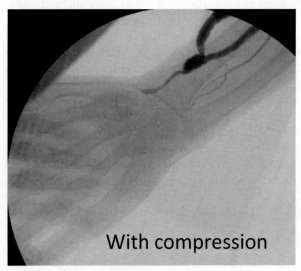

FIGURE 3.26.2

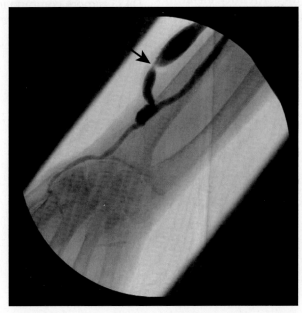

FIGURE 3.26.3

FINDINGS: Right forearm fistulogram with catheter position in afferent radial artery (Fig. 3.26.1, *arrow*) was performed without compression of the fistula. This demonstrates opacification of the fistula with no significant arterial flow distal to the arterial anastomosis (*arrowhead*). Fistulogram with compression of the outflow fistula demonstrates opacification of the afferent radial artery, fistula proximal to compression, and radial artery distal to arterial anastomosis (Fig. 3.26.2).

Radiocephalic fistulogram following minimally invasive limited ligation endoluminal assisted revision (MILLER) banding (Fig. 3.26.3, *arrow*) at the perianastomotic segment of the fistula demonstrates balanced arterial flow proximal and distal to arterial anastomosis and adequate flow in fistula.

DIAGNOSIS: Dialysis access steal syndrome (DASS)

DISCUSSION: DASS is caused by an arterial insufficiency state distal to the dialysis access (AVF or dialysis graft). This usually occurs owing to diversion of flow into the dialysis access with reversal or severe reduction in arterial flow to the extremity distal to the dialysis access. There are five recognized stages of severity of steal syndrome ranging from altered sensation to irreversible neuropathy, gangrene, or limb loss. The overall incidence of DASS is estimated at 3% to 5%. Steal syndrome occurs more frequently in larger brachial–cephalic and brachial–basilic fistulas and least often in snuffbox AVF. The estimated incidence in polytetrafluroethylene or PTFE grafts is 2.2% (76).

Steal syndrome is characterized by hand pain or coolness, altered sensation, absent pulses, poor capillary refill, or severe atrophy, weakness or tissue loss.

Treatment is directed at reversal of ischemia while preserving the dialysis access. Surgical options include distal revascularization–interval ligation (DRIL/DRAL), flow reduction or banding, proximalization of AV anastomosis (PAVA), revision of distal inflow (RUDI), and the MILLER (77,78). The latter procedure is a fluoroscopically guided modified banding technique, which can be performed in the angiography suite.

## Aunt Minnie's Pearls

DASS is more common in larger proximal fistulas.

# REFERENCES

1. Higgins CB. Essentials of cardiac radiology and imaging. Philadelphia, PA: Lippincott-Raven, 1992:184.
2. Williams JE, Honick AB. The great vessels. In: Brant WE, Helms CA (eds.). Fundamentals of diagnostic radiology. Baltimore, MD: Williams & Wilkins, 1994:614–617.
3. DeBakey ME, Henley WS, Cooley DA, et al. Surgical management of dissecting aneurysms of the aorta. J Thorac Cardiovasc Surg 1965;49:130–149.
4. Petasnick JP. Radiologic evaluation of aortic dissection. Radiology 1991;180:297–305.
5. Quinn SF, Duke DJ, Baldwin SS, et al. Percutaneous placement of a low-profile stent-graft device for aortic dissections. J Vasc Interv Radiol 2002;13:791–798.
6. Kato N, Hirano T, Shimono T, et al. Treatment of chronic aortic dissection by transluminal endovascular stent-graft placement: Preliminary results. J Vasc Interv Radiol 2001;12:835–840.
7. Van Praagh R, Van Praagh S, Nebesar RA, et al. Tetralogy of Fallot: Underdevelopment of the pulmonary infundibulum and its sequelae. Am J Cardiol 1970;26:25–33.
8. Mirowitz SA, Gutierrez FR, Canter CE, et al. Tetralogy of Fallot: MR findings. Radiology 1989;171:207–212.
9. McGoon DC, Baird DK, Davis GD. Surgical management of large bronchial collateral arteries with pulmonary stenosis of atresia. Circulation 1975;52:109.
10. Nakata S, Imai Y, Takanashi Y, et al. A new method for the quantitative standardization of cross-sectional areas of the pulmonary arteries in congenital heart disease with decreased pulmonary blood flow. J Thorac Cardiovasc Surg 1984;88:610.
11. Sanchez HE, Cornish EM, Shih FC, et al. The surgical treatment of tetralogy of Fallot. Ann Thorac Surg 1984;37:431.
12. Sadler TW. Langman's medical embryology, 5th ed. Baltimore, MD: Williams & Wilkins, 1985:188.
13. Higgins CB. Essentials of cardiac radiology and imaging. Philadelphia, PA: Lippincott-Raven, 1992:80.
14. Collett RW, Edward JE. Persistent truncus arteriosus: A classification according to anatomic types. Surg Clin North Am 1949;29:1245–1270.
15. Van Praagh R. Diagnosis of complex congenital heart disease: Morphologic–anatomic method and terminology. Cardiovasc Intervent Radiol 1984;7:115–120.
16. Sadler TW. Langman's medical embryology, 5th ed. Baltimore, MD: Williams & Wilkins, 1985:185.
17. Higgins CB. Essentials of cardiac radiology and imaging. Philadelphia, PA: Lippincott-Raven, 1992:77.
18. Behrman RE, Vaughan VC III. The cardiovascular system. In: Nelson textbook of pediatrics, 13th ed. Philadelphia, PA: WB Saunders, 1987:976.
19. Goldberg HL, DiMascio A. Psychotropic drugs in pregnancy. In: Lipton MA, DiMascio A, Killam KF (eds.). Psychopharmacology: A generation of progress. New York, NY: Raven, 1978:1047–1055.
20. Miller SW. Aortic arch stenoses: Coarctation, aortitis, and variants. Appl Radiol 1995;24:15–19.
21. Gomes AS, Lois JF, George B, et al. Congenital abnormalities of the aortic arch: MRI. Radiology 1987;165:691–695.
22. Reuter SR, Redman HC, Cho KJ. Gastrointestinal angiography, 3rd ed. Philadelphia, PA: WB Saunders, 1986;1:286–292.
23. Lewis VD, Meranze SG, Mclean GK. The midaortic syndrome: Diagnosis and treatment. Radiology 1988;167:111–113.
24. O'Neill JA, Berkowitz H, Fellows KJ. Midaortic syndrome and hypertension in childhood. J Pediatr Surg 1995;30:164–171.
25. Bleacher J, Turner ME. Renal autotransplantation for renovascular hypertension caused by midaortic syndrome. J Pediatr Surg 1997;32:248–250.
26. Adams WM, John PR. US demonstration and diagnosis of the midaortic syndrome. Pediatr Radiol 1998;28:461–463.
27. Seybold EA, Busconi BD. Traumatic popliteal artery thrombosis and compartment syndrome of the leg following blunt trauma to the knee: A discussion of treatment and complications. J Orthop Trauma 1996;10:138–141.
28. Peck JJ, Eastman AB. Popliteal vascular trauma. Arch Surg 1990;125:1339–1344.
29. Synder WH. Popliteal and shank arterial injury. Surg Clin North Am 1988;68:787–807.
30. Dhiray SM. Advances in the management of acute popliteal vascular blunt injuries. J Trauma 1985;25:793–797.
31. Loscalzo J, Creager MA, Dzau VJ. Vascular medicine: A textbook of vascular biology and diseases, 2nd ed. Boston, MA: Little, Brown, 1996:1016–1019.
32. Yalcindag A, Sundel R. Vasculitis in childhood. Curr Opin Rheumatol 2001;13:422–427.
33. Gravanis MB. Giant cell arteritis and Takayasu aortitis: Morphologic, pathogenetic and etiologic factors. Int J Cardiol 2000;75:S21–S33.
34. Begelman S, Olin JW. Fibromuscular dysplasia. Curr Opin Rheumatol 2000;12:41–47.
35. Van Bockel JH, Weibull H. Fibrodysplastic disease of the renal arteries. Eur J Vasc Surg 1994;8:655–657.
36. Safian RD, Textor SC. Renal artery stenosis. N Engl J Med 2001;344:431–442.
37. Anderson C, Hansen K. Renal artery fibromuscular dysplasia: Results of current surgical therapy. J Vasc Surg 1995;22:207–216.
38. Chaikof E, Shamberger R, Brewster D. Traumatic pseudoaneurysms of the abdominal aorta. J Trauma 1985;25:169–173.
39. Miller J, Wall M, Mattox K. Ruptured aortic pseudoaneurysm 28 years after gunshot wound: Case report and review of literature. J Trauma 1998;44:214–218.
40. Rathlev N. Peripheral vascular injuries. eMed J 2001;2(6). www.medwebplus.com. Accessed January 2, 2007.
41. Loscalzo J, Creager MA, Dzau VJ. Vascular medicine: A textbook of vascular biology and diseases, 2nd ed. Boston, MA: Little, Brown, 1996:1242–1243.
42. Young JR, Olin JW, Bartholomew JR. Peripheral vascular diseases, 2nd ed. St Louis, MO: Mosby, 1996:591–595.
43. Kubota Y, Kichikawa K. Coil embolization of a persistent sciatic artery aneurysm. Cardiovasc Intervent Radiol 2000;23:245–247.
44. Neiman H, Yao J. Angiography of vascular disease. New York, NY: Churchill Livingstone, 1985:59–61.
45. Shultze WP, Garrett WV. Persistent sciatic artery: Collective review and management. Ann Vasc Surg 1993;7:303–310.
46. Urschel H, Razzuk M. Neurovascular compression in the thoracic outlet. Changing management over 50 years. Ann Surg 1998;4:609–617.
47. Parziale J, Akelman E, Arnold-Peter C. Thoracic outlet syndrome. Am J Orthop 2000;29:353–360.
48. Wilbourn A. Thoracic outlet syndromes. Neurol Clin 1999;17:477–497.
49. Lee JKT. Retroperitoneum: Postoperative complications. In: Lee JKT, Sagel SS, Stanley RJ (eds.). Computed body tomography with MRI correlation. New York, NY: Raven, 1989:707–753.
50. Orton DF, LeVeen RF. Aortic prosthetic graft infections: Radiologic manifestations and implications for management. Radiographics 2000;20:977–993.
51. Rossi P, Arata F. Prosthetic graft infection: Diagnostic and therapeutic role of interventional radiology. J Vasc Interv Radiol 1997;8:271–277.
52. Blunt TJ. Vascular graft infections: An update. Cardiovasc Surg 2001;9:225–233.
53. Grollman JH. Winslow's pathway—It's not the only way. Catheter Cardiovasc Interv 2000;49:445–446.

54. Prager RJ, Akin JR. Winslow's pathway: A rare collateral channel in intrarenal aortic occlusion. AJR Am J Roentgenol 1997;128:485–487.

55. Zell L, Kindermann W. Paget–Schroetter syndrome in sports activities: Case study and literature review. Angiology 2001;52:337–342.

56. Feurgier P, Aleksic I. Long-term results of venous revascularization for Paget–Schroetter syndrome in athletes. Ann Vasc Surg 2001;15:212–218.

57. Kreinberg P, Chang B. Long-term results in patients treated with thrombolysis, thoracic inlet decompression, and subclavian vein stenting for Paget–Schroetter syndrome. J Vasc Surg 2001;33:S100–S105.

58. Sarodia BD, Stoller JK. Persistent left superior vena cava: Case report and literature review. Respir Care 2000;45:411–416.

59. Tak T, Crouch E, Drake GB. Persistent let superior vena cava: Incidence, significance and clinical correlates. Int J Cardiol 2002;82:91–93.

60. Wilhelm A. Situs inversus. eMed J 2002;3(2). www.med webplus.com. Accessed December 5, 2007.

61. Tonkin I, Tonkin A. Visceroatrial situs abnormalities: Sonographic and computed tomographic appearance. AJR Am J Roentgenol 1982;138:509–515.

62. Kinney T, Deluca S. Kartagener's syndrome. Am Fam Physician 1991;44:133–134.

63. Kaufman JA, Lee MJ. Vascular and interventional radiology: The requisites. Philadelphia, PA: Mosby, 2004:252–260.

64. Steinmetz E, Rubin BG. Type II endoleak after endovascular abdominal aortic aneurysm repair: A conservative approach with selective intervention is safe and cost-effective. J Vasc Surg 2004;39:306–313.

65. Jones JE, Atkins MD, Brewster DC, et al. Persistent type II endoleak after endovascular repair of abdominal aortic aneurysm is associated with adverse late outcomes. J Vasc Surg 2007;46:1–8.

66. Wear JR, Crummy AB, Munson BO. A new approach to the treatment of priapism. J Urol 1977;177:252–254.

67. O'Sullivan P, Browne R, McEniff N, et al. Treatment of "high-flow" priapism with superselective transcatheter embolization: A useful alternative to surgery. Cardiovasc Intervent Radiol 2006;29:196–201.

68. Kuefer R, Bartsch G Jr, Herkommer K, et al. Changing diagnostic and therapeutic concepts in high-flow priapism. Int J Impot Res 2005;17:109–113.

69. Conn J Jr, Bergan JJ, Bell JL. Hand ischemia: Hypothenar hammer syndrome. Proc Inst Med Chicago 1970;28:83.

70. Sharma R, Ladd W, Chaisson G, et al. Hypothenar hammer syndrome. Circulation 2002;105:1615.

71. Yakubov SJ, Nappi JF, Candela RJ, et al. Successful prolonged local infusion of urokinase for the hypothenar hammer syndrome. Cathet Cardiovasc Diagn 2003;29(4):301–303.

72. Vayssairat M. Hypothenar hammer syndrome: Seventeen cases with long-term follow-up. J Vasc Surg 1987;5:838–843.

73. Espinoza LR. Buerger's disease: Thromboangiitis obliterans 100 years after the initial description. Am J Med Sci 2009; 337(4):285–286.

74. Olin JW. Thromboangiitis obliterans (Buerger's disease). In: Rutherford RB (ed.). Vascular surgery, 5th ed. Philadelphia, PA: WB Saunders Co, 2000:350–364.

75. Olin JW, Young JR, Graor RA, et al. The changing clinical spectrum of thromboangiitis obliterans (Buerger's disease). Circulation 1990;82(5 suppl):IV3–IV8.

76. Berman SS, Gentile AT, Glickman MH, et al. Distal revascularization–interval ligation for limb salvage and maintenance of dialysis access in ischemic steal syndrome. J Vasc Surg 1997;26:393–402.

77. Tordoir JH, Dammers R, van der Sande FM. Upper extremity ischemia and hemodialysis vascular access. Eur J Vasc Endovasc Surg 2004;27:1–5.

78. Goel N, Miller GA, Jotwani MC, et al. Minimally invasive limited ligation endoluminal-assisted revision (MILLER) for the treatment of dialysis access-associated steal syndrome. Kidney Int 2006;70:765–770.

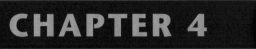

# CHAPTER 4

# ULTRASOUND

**Susan J. Ackerman  /  Abid Irshad  /  Amy S. Campbell  /
Abbie Cluver**

*The authors and editors acknowledge the contribution of the Chapter 4 author
from the second edition: Sunil Kini, MD and from the 3rd edition: Angelle
Harper, MD.*

HISTORY: New kidney transplantation with pain and anuria

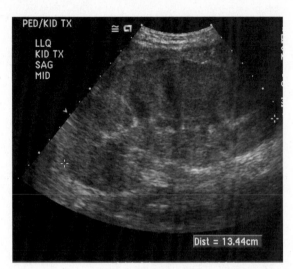

FIGURE 4.1.1

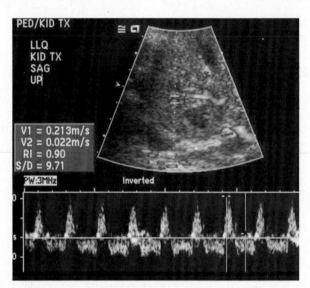

FIGURE 4.1.2

FIGURE 4.1.3

FINDINGS: Echogenic thrombus is noted in the main renal vein (Fig. 4.1.1). In addition, there is no flow on color and spectral Doppler waveforms (Fig. 4.1.2). Reversal of flow is noted in the intrarenal artery (Fig. 4.1.3).

DIAGNOSIS: Renal vein thrombosis in kidney transplantation

DISCUSSION: Renal vein thrombosis usually occurs in the acute postoperative period. It causes acute pain and swelling, in addition to anuria. The diagnostic criteria include gray-scale findings of thrombus within the main renal vein and absence of flow noted in the transplant vein with color Doppler (1). In addition, there is reversal of diastolic flow within the main renal artery and the intrarenal arteries. Rapid diagnosis and intervention such as thrombectomy are important to salvage the kidney. A nephrectomy may be the end point.

## Aunt Minnie's Pearls

The predominant symptom is anuria with pain.

Color Doppler ultrasound shows absence of flow in the main renal vein and reversal of diastolic flow in the main renal artery.

# Case 4.2

HISTORY: Palpable thyroid nodule

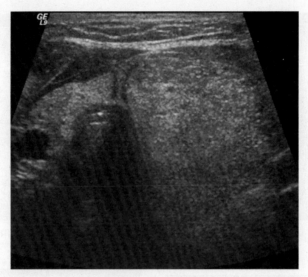

FIGURE 4.2.1

FINDINGS: A well-defined hypoechoic solid mass with diffuse microcalcifications is noted (Fig. 4.2.1).

DIAGNOSIS: Papillary thyroid cancer

DISCUSSION: Papillary thyroid cancer is an epithelial cell cancer that accounts for approximately 80% of all thyroid cancers.

It is most prevalent in young females. The sonographic characteristics include hypoechogeniticity, microcalcifications, and hypervascularity.

The "snowstorm" appearance or diffuse microcalcifications in a hypoechoic nodule has been specifically described with papillary thyroid cancer.

It commonly spreads to the cervical lymph nodes. The cervical lymph node metastasis may contain echogenic foci representing microcalcifications or cystic degeneration.

The mortality rate from papillary thyroid cancer after 20 years is approximately 6%.

## Aunt Minnie's Pearls

Papillary thyroid carcinoma is the most common type of thyroid cancer.

The classic appearance is a hypoechoic nodule with diffuse microcalcifications or "snowstorm" appearance.

HISTORY: A 16-week pregnancy with hyperemesis and vaginal bleeding

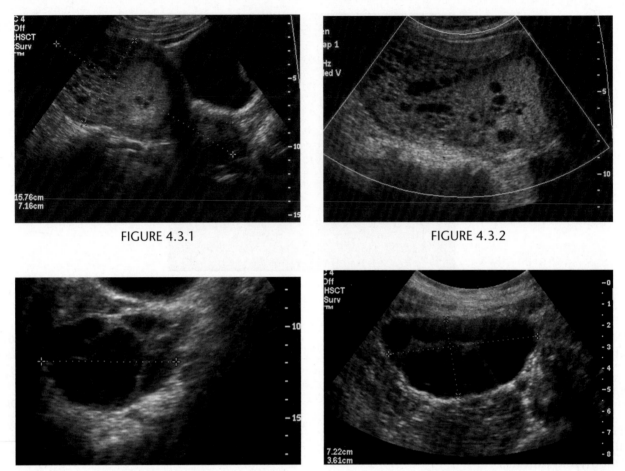

FIGURE 4.3.1

FIGURE 4.3.2

FIGURE 4.3.3

FIGURE 4.3.4

FINDINGS: Transabdominal evaluation of the gravid uterus reveals an echogenic, heterogeneous mass with multifocal small cystic spaces filling the endometrial canal (Figs. 4.3.1 and 4.3.2). In conjunction with this, the ovaries demonstrate frank enlargement with essential replacement by multiple, large cysts (Figs. 4.3.3 and 4.3.4).

DIAGNOSIS: Complete molar pregnancy with bilateral theca lutein cysts

DISCUSSION: Complete molar pregnancy is most often associated with a 46,XX karyotype supplied by all paternal chromosomes. At pathological evaluation, there is no associated fetal development, with only abnormal villi seen. Markedly elevated hCG resulting from excessive trophoblastic proliferation causes characteristic symptoms, including hyperemesis gravidarum. The most frequent presenting symptom is vaginal bleeding, seen in >90% of cases.

Characteristic imaging features of complete molar pregnancy are as above with an echogenic mass containing multiple tiny cystic spaces representing hydropic villi within the abnormal tissue. Theca lutein cysts are an associated finding in 15% to 30% of complete moles as a result of hyperstimulation of the ovaries owing to excessive amounts of circulating serum hCG.

## Aunt Minnie's Pearls

Twenty percent of complete molar pregnancies will develop persistent gestational trophoblastic disease. This includes invasive mole, choriocarcinoma, and placental site trophoblastic tumor.

Theca lutein cysts are a result of hyperstimulation and are seen in the setting of molar pregnancy and assisted fertility. These can undergo hemorrhage, rupture, and torsion.

HISTORY: A 30-week pregnancy with suspected twin gestation and no prior prenatal care

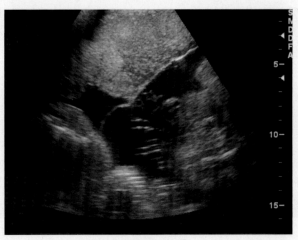

FIGURE 4.4.1

FINDINGS: Sonographic evaluation of the gravid uterus demonstrates two fused anteriorly located placentas with a thick intertwin membrane. A triangular piece of placental tissue can be seen to extend into this membrane where it tapers sharply (Fig. 4.4.1).

DIAGNOSIS: Dichorionic twin pregnancy (the twin peak sign)

DISCUSSION: Determination of chorionicity and amnionicity is a primary goal of obstetric ultrasound in multiple gestations as this dramatically effects prognosis (2). Best seen at approximately 10 to 14 weeks' gestational age, the "twin peak" or "lambda" sign is an extremely specific sign of dichorionicity, regardless of the stage at which it is detected (3). However, as the pregnancy progresses, the interdigitating placental villi will regress, and this becomes progressively less evident, with variable persistence and visibility into the later stages of pregnancy (4).

## Aunt Minnie's Pearls

An easily seen intertwin membrane with extension of chorion/placenta into it = dichorionic pregnancy.

Absence of twin peak sign is not helpful in late second and third trimester as it is inconsistently seen later in pregnancy.

HISTORY: A 45-year-old male presents with history of chronic scrotal discomfort

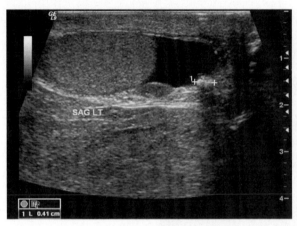

FIGURE 4.5.1

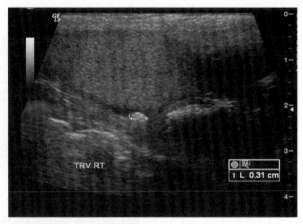

FIGURE 4.5.2

FINDINGS: A transverse image through the left scrotum (Fig. 4.5.1) and a longitudinal image through the right scrotum (Fig. 4.5.2) show normal appearance to the testicles. Both sides show an echogenic focus in the tunica vaginalis cavity outside the testicle that demonstrates posterior acoustic shadow suggesting a calcified lesion. Presence of fluid makes it easily visible.

DIAGNOSIS: Scrotoliths or scrotal pearls

DISCUSSION: Scrotoliths occur as calcifications within the layers of tunica vaginalis that are usually seen as an incidental finding. This is a benign entity and has no association with testicular cancer as opposed to testicular microlithiasis, which has been associated with testicular malignancy. The scrotoliths may be associated with previous trauma or inflammation and have been more commonly seen in mountain bikers, likely from repetitive scrotal trauma. There are various theories regarding their formation. These may form by deposition of calcium on a nidus that may result either from inflammation or torsion of the appendix testis or epididymal appendage (5,6). Macroscopically, these masses are usually seen as rubbery, white, rounded loose bodies. Microscopically, these are a mixture of fibrinoid material and calcium and usually contain a central nidus.

Clinically, these patients are usually asymptomatic; however, they may occasionally feel these as palpable nodules. These are usually seen as an incidental finding on ultrasound. Ultrasound usually demonstrates single or multiple extra-testicular stones within the layers of the tunica vaginalis that may be freely mobile, especially in the presence of hydrocele. These are frequently seen in association with hydrocele, and presence of fluid also makes it easy to identify these stones. The diagnosis is usually straightforward as these usually have a typical appearance. Other causes of extra-testicular calcifications include epididymal calcification seen in chronic epididymitis, tuberculosis, and schistosomiasis.

### Aunt Minnie's Pearls

Single or multiple extra-testicular, usually mobile, calcified masses (scrotoliths) occur between the layers of tunica vaginalis.

These are not associated with testicular neoplasms and are usually of no clinical significance.

**HISTORY:** A 34-year-old gravid woman (estimated gestational age of 22.5 weeks) with maternal serum alpha-fetoprotein level of 5.3 multiples of the median

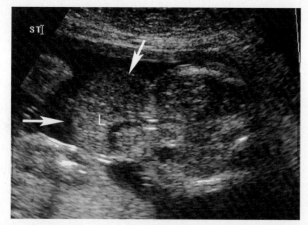

FIGURE 4.6.1

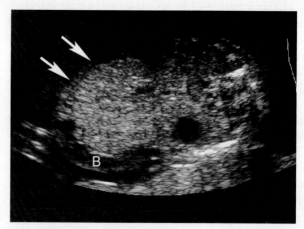

FIGURE 4.6.2

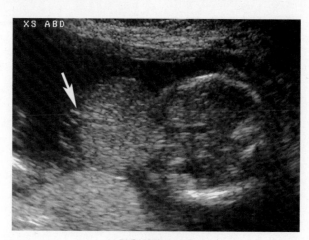

FIGURE 4.6.3

**FINDINGS:** A 3.5-cm defect of the ventral aspect of the fetal anterior abdominal wall can be seen on these transverse views of the fetal abdomen. Through this defect protrudes a solid mass of approximately 4 cm in diameter (Fig. 4.6.1, *arrows*). This mass contains liver (*L*) and bowel (*B*) and is covered by a thin membrane (Fig. 4.6.2, *arrows*). Figure 4.6.3 reveals that the umbilical cord inserts into the mass (*arrow*).

**DIAGNOSIS:** Omphalocele

**DISCUSSION:** Omphaloceles (exomphalos) occur in 1 of 4,000 live births and are usually detected during routine sonographic examination of the fetal abdomen or in the workup for elevated alpha-fetoprotein levels. The defect consists of herniation of abdominal contents into the base of the umbilical cord. The cord inserts into the apical–caudal aspect of the mass, unlike gastroschisis, in which the cord inserts normally into the abdominal wall. Although the delineating peritoneal--amniotic membrane is not always easily visible, its presence can be inferred from the smooth surface of the herniated mass. This should be contrasted to gastroschisis, in which there is no delineating membrane and the loops of bowel float freely within the amniotic cavity. The presence of liver within an omphalocele can be inferred by the homogeneous appearance of the herniated mass, the presence of intrahepatic vessels, and the large size of the defect (7–9).

Associated anomalies have been reported in 67% to 88% of fetuses with omphalocele identified prenatally. These anomalies include karyotype abnormalities and nonchromosomal structural anomalies. Chromosome abnormalities have been more strongly associated with small omphalocele sacs that do not contain liver.

## Aunt Minnie's Pearls

Herniation of abdominal contents into the base of the umbilical cord = omphalocele.

Small omphaloceles that do not contain liver have a stronger association with chromosomal abnormalities than larger omphaloceles.

Associated anomalies have been reported in up to 88% of fetuses with omphalocele.

# Case 4.7

HISTORY: A 32-year-old gravid woman with maternal serum alpha-fetoprotein of 2.6 multiples of the median

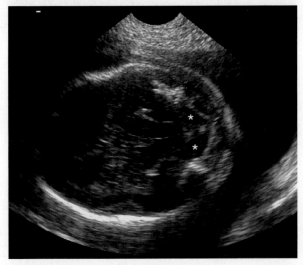

FIGURE 4.7.1

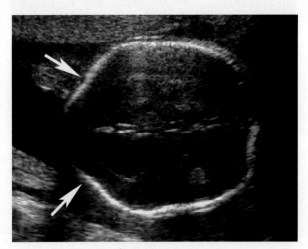

FIGURE 4.7.2

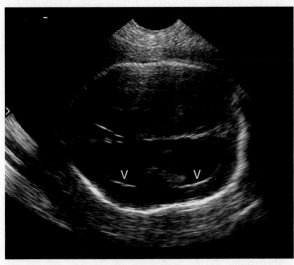

FIGURE 4.7.3

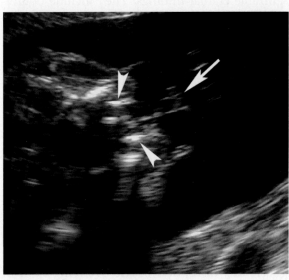

FIGURE 4.7.4

FINDINGS: Classic "banana sign" (i.e., obliteration of posterior fossa and curved appearance of the herniated cerebellum; Fig. 4.7.1, *asterisks*) and "lemon sign" (i.e., abnormal bifrontal concavity; Fig. 4.7.2, *arrows*) are seen in the cranium of this fetus of 20 weeks' gestation. Mild ventriculomegaly (*V*) is present (Fig. 4.7.3), and the lateral ventricles measure 13 mm (up to 10 mm is normal). Axial (Fig. 4.7.4) and sagittal (Fig. 4.7.5) views of the spine demonstrate the flared laminae (Fig. 4.7.4, *arrowheads*), which are diagnostic of spina bifida and the associated meningomyelocele (Figs. 4.7.4 and 4.7.5, *arrows*) extending from approximately

L3 through S3. Bilateral clubfeet were also present (only the right foot is shown; Fig. 4.7.6).

DIAGNOSIS: Chiari II (Arnold–Chiari) malformation and associated meningomyelocele

DISCUSSION: Open neural tube defects are the most common central nervous system malformations (10,11). Direct visualization of a meningomyelocele may be difficult, however, and even the most skilled examiner may worry about false-negative results. Fortunately for the sonographer, meningomyeloceles are almost always accompanied by the

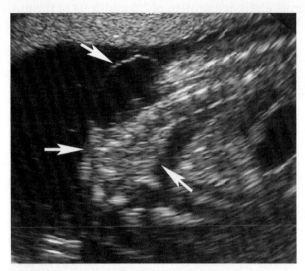

FIGURE 4.7.5

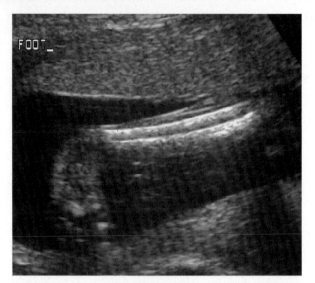

FIGURE 4.7.6

Arnold–Chiari malformation, which has more easily recognizable cranial findings. They include obliteration of the cisterna magna, the lemon sign, ventricular dilatation, and a disproportionately small biparietal diameter.

Posterior fossa abnormalities, including obliteration of the cisterna magna and banana-shaped cerebellum are almost diagnostic of associated open meningomyelocele. Conversely, a normal cisterna magna virtually eliminates the possibility of spina bifida. The "lemon sign," although quite useful, is not specific for meningomyelocele (12,13). Resolution of the lemon sign in fetuses with meningomyelocele invariably occurs by the 34th week of gestation.

The presence of these characteristic cranial findings serves as a marker for a meningomyelocele. The bony spinal defect should be imaged as should the associated soft-tissue findings (i.e., myelomeningocele sac, disruption of the overlying skin, or both). The level and extent of the defect should be reported.

As with all detected prenatal abnormalities, the remainder of the fetus should be carefully examined for associated abnormalities. The neuromuscular anomalies, in particular, caused by the spinal defect lead to the development of clubfoot. Meningomyelocele also may be associated with an increased risk of karyotype abnormality (14).

Neural tube defects are usually accompanied by abnormally high levels of maternal serum alpha-fetoprotein. The rate of neural tube defects and the risk of recurrence can be decreased by maternal folate supplementation around the time of conception (15).

## Aunt Minnie's Pearls

"Lemon" and "banana" signs imply meningomyelocele.

Neural tube defects are commonly associated with abnormally high levels of maternal serum alpha-fetoprotein.

**HISTORY:** A 30-year-old woman had a fetus imaging at 21 weeks' gestation. Prior sonography was performed in Australia at 8 weeks' gestation (a routine study was requested as part of initial patient evaluation in the United States)

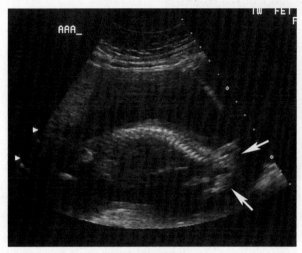

FIGURE 4.8.1

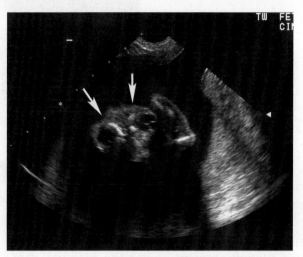

FIGURE 4.8.2

**FINDINGS:** Transabdominal sagittal view of the fetal spine does not demonstrate a normal head (Fig. 4.8.1, *arrows*). Transvaginal coronal view of the face confirms absence of the calvarium and brain cephalad to the orbits (Fig. 4.8.2, *arrows*).

**DIAGNOSIS:** Anencephaly

**DISCUSSION:** Anencephaly, which results from failure of the rostral neuropore to close by the 24th day of fetal life, is the most common type of neural tube defect; it is reported in 1 of 1,000 births (10,11). A distinct female predominance is seen in anencephaly; the female-to-male ratio is 4:1. Elevated alpha-fetoprotein levels can be detected early in pregnancy, and polyhydramnios is seen in up to one-half of cases after 26 weeks' gestation. Symmetric loss of both brain tissue and calvarium cephalad to the bony orbits is the most reliable feature of this anomaly and is best demonstrated on a coronal image of the fetal face.

Angiomatous stroma may be seen above the fetal orbits (i.e., area cerebrovasculosa); in such cases, it may be difficult to distinguish this disorder from congenital absence of the calvarium (i.e., exencephaly), in which some brain tissue is present above the orbits. Because the bony calvarium cannot be identified with transvaginal sonography before 11.5 weeks' gestation, anencephaly should not be diagnosed before this time.

Up to one-third of cases of anencephaly may have additional anomalies, most commonly spina bifida. If identified, the spinal dysraphism can help to distinguish anencephaly from exencephaly in difficult cases (16). This distinction is important, because the risk of neural tube defects in future pregnancies is greater in mothers of anencephalic children. Periconceptional folate acid supplementation decreases the risk of anencephaly.

## Aunt Minnie's Pearls

Anencephaly = loss of brain tissue and calvarium in a fetus older than 11.5 weeks' gestation.

Elevated alpha-fetoprotein levels and polyhydramnios are associated findings in anencephaly.

Up to one-third of anencephalic babies have additional anomalies; the most common is spina bifida.

**HISTORY:** A 33-year-old woman with a history of polysubstance abuse at 33 weeks' gestation underwent cesarean section for persistent vaginal bleeding

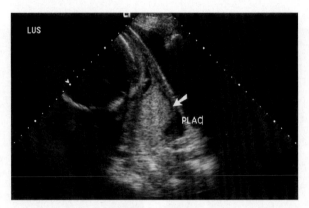

FIGURE 4.9.1

**FINDINGS:** A sagittal image (Fig. 4.9.1, *arrow*) of the lower uterine segment shows the placenta completely covering the cervical os.

**DIAGNOSIS:** Complete placenta previa

**DISCUSSION:** Placenta previa is defined as the implantation of the placenta over the cervical os. There are three recognized variations of placenta previa: complete, partial, and marginal.

In complete placenta previa, the placenta is implanted on both sides of the internal cervical os, bridging the os. This type presents the most serious maternal risk because it is associated with greater blood loss than with marginal or partial previa. The frequency of total placenta previa has been reported as low as 20% and as high as 43%. As a leading cause of third-trimester hemorrhage, patients with placenta previa classically present with painless bleeding. Massive vaginal bleeding can result in fetal and maternal death if vaginal delivery is attempted.

Complete placenta previa always requires cesarean section (17). Potential sources of false-positive diagnosis include an overdistended urinary bladder, contraction in the lower uterine segment, and subchorionic hematoma (18).

Significant risk factors are maternal age older than 35 years and African American or other minority race.

## Aunt Minnie's Pearls

In complete placenta previa, the placenta covers the entire cervix.

Placenta previa is a major cause of third-trimester bleeding.

Complete placenta previa always requires cesarean section.

Significant risk factors are maternal age older than 35 years and African American or other minority race.

HISTORY: A 27-year-old gravid woman with a history of a second-trimester spontaneous abortion

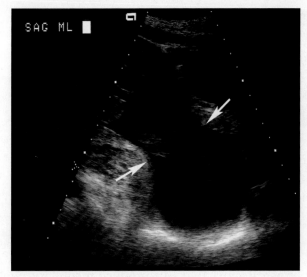

FIGURE 4.10.1

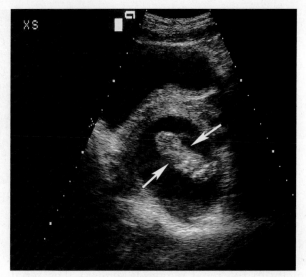

FIGURE 4.10.2

FINDINGS: A sagittal image reveals that the cervix is dilated to 3 cm, and the classic hourglass, bulging membranes protrude into the vagina (Fig. 4.10.1, *arrows*). The fetal foot is seen on a transverse image of the cervix (Fig. 4.10.2, *arrows*).

DIAGNOSIS: Cervical incompetence

DISCUSSION: Cervical incompetence is a functional condition in patients who often present with a history of recurrent, usually painless second-trimester spontaneous abortions. Sonographic findings of a cervix <3 cm long, a gaping internal os, and funneling or tunneling of the patient's membranes into the endocervical canal can be associated with preterm delivery (19). The shorter the cervix, the more likely the patient will deliver prematurely. Cervical cerclage is the treatment of choice.

The cervix can change, often dramatically, during the sonographic examination. The cervix may appear completely normal at one point in the examination and grossly abnormal at another. For high-risk patients, the cervix should be imaged more than once and observed continuously for several minutes (20).

## Aunt Minnie's Pearls

Hourglass membranes gaping through cervical os = severe cervical incompetence.

In high-risk patients, the cervix should be imaged more than once and continuously for several minutes.

HISTORY: Repeated bouts of urinary colic

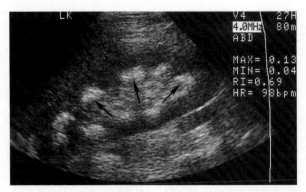

FIGURE 4.11.1

FINDINGS: A longitudinal view of the kidney (Fig. 4.11.1) demonstrates markedly increased echogenicity in the renal pyramids (*arrows*). The renal cortex is normal in echogenicity, and no hydronephrosis is identified. The kidneys are normally shaped and are otherwise unremarkable.

DIAGNOSIS: Medullary nephrocalcinosis

DISCUSSION: Nephrocalcinosis is defined as abnormal deposition of calcium salts in the renal cortex (i.e., cortical nephrocalcinosis) or pyramids (i.e., medullary nephrocalcinosis). This should be distinguished from urinary stone formation, which is called *urolithiasis*. Medullary nephrocalcinosis can be recognized on ultrasonography as markedly hyperechoic renal pyramids, which may produce distal acoustic shadowing. Early medullary nephrocalcinosis may appear as hyperechoic rings around the pyramids. Sonography is more sensitive than radiographs for the diagnosis of nephrocalcinosis; therefore, correlation with a supine abdomen film is not always helpful (21).

The three leading causes of medullary nephrocalcinosis include hyperparathyroidism (40%), medullary sponge kidney (20%), and distal type I renal tubular acidosis (20%) (22). Other causes of hypercalcemia that can produce medullary nephrocalcinosis include drugs (i.e., steroids and furosemide), sarcoidosis, immobilization, milk-alkali syndrome, paraneoplastic syndromes, hypervitaminosis D, and hyperthyroidism. If the calcification is noticeably segmental, medullary sponge kidney is the primary consideration because other leading causes of medullary nephrocalcinosis typically produce diffuse and bilateral renal involvement. The combination of cortical and medullary nephrocalcinosis strongly suggests primary oxaluria.

## Aunt Minnie's Pearls

Hyperechoic renal pyramids with or without distal acoustic shadowing = medullary nephrocalcinosis.

Hyperparathyroidism, medullary sponge kidney, and distal renal tubular acidosis are the leading causes of medullary nephrocalcinosis.

**HISTORY:** A 58-year-old woman with cryptogenic cirrhosis

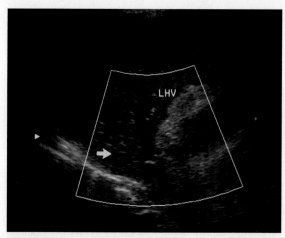

FIGURE 4.12.1

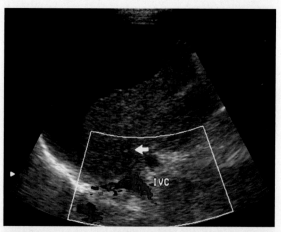

FIGURE 4.12.2

**FINDINGS:** Doppler images (Figs. 4.12.1 and 4.12.2, *arrows*) show absence of flow in the right and middle hepatic veins as they drain into the inferior vena cava. Other findings include a small nodular liver and perihepatic free fluid, representing ascites.

**DIAGNOSIS:** Budd–Chiari syndrome

**DISCUSSION:** Budd–Chiari is a rare syndrome caused by partial or complete obstruction of one or more hepatic veins or the inferior vena cava. If the hepatic veins are visualized on gray scale and there is no detectable flow or reversed flow on color Doppler, the sensitivity for diagnosing Budd–Chiari syndrome is very high (23). There are numerous causes of Budd–Chiari, the most common being idiopathic. Other causes include tumor thrombus, pregnancy, hypercoagulable states, trauma, sepsis, dehydration, and some medications (24). The predominant

presenting features are hepatomegaly and ascites. It is more common in women, and patients may present acutely with abdominal pain or have an insidious onset. Overall, mortality is high in early acute disease, but once an acute episode is terminated, the prognosis is good. Treatment options include anticoagulation, measures to control ascites and gastrointestinal bleeding, and procedures such as shunts to restore hepatic blood outflow (25).

## Aunt Minnie's Pearls

The predominant presenting symptoms of Budd–Chiari syndrome are hepatomegaly and ascites.

Doppler ultrasound images will show absence of flow of one or more hepatic veins in patients with Budd–Chiari syndrome.

HISTORY: Mentally challenged patient who gives a history of a left nephrectomy

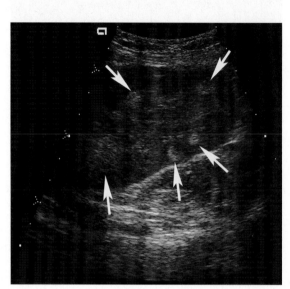

FIGURE 4.13.1

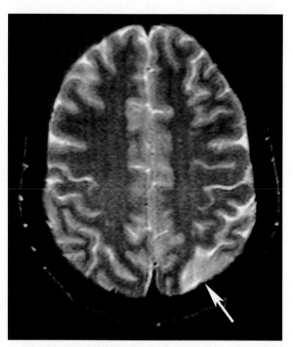

FIGURE 4.13.2

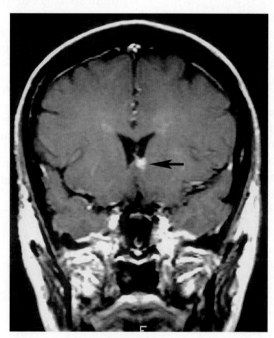

FIGURE 4.13.3

**FINDINGS:** A longitudinal ultrasound image of the right kidney (Fig. 4.13.1) demonstrates numerous homogeneously hyperechoic masses originating in the renal cortex (*arrows*). A previously acquired MRI of the brain reveals findings of cortical tubers (Fig. 4.13.2, *arrow*) and a giant-cell astrocytoma near the foramen of Monro (Fig. 4.13.3, *black arrow*).

**DIAGNOSIS:** Renal angiomyolipomas in a patient with tuberous sclerosis

**DISCUSSION:** A solitary hyperechoic mass in the kidney can be caused by several benign and malignant processes. When innumerable, well-defined, hyperechoic masses are seen, however, the differential diagnosis is more limited; most of these cases represent angiomyolipomas in patients with tuberous sclerosis. However, approximately 5% of patients with innumerable renal angiomyolipomas do not have stigmata of tuberous sclerosis (26). To make a confident imaging-specific diagnosis, correlation with other imaging modalities is necessary, such as CT of the fatty renal lesions or MRI for the characteristic brain findings in tuberous sclerosis. In rare cases, multiple fatty renal lesions are lipomas or teratomas, but in such cases, the characteristic imaging features of tuberous sclerosis would be absent elsewhere in the body.

Tuberous sclerosis, or Bourneville disease (27), is an autosomal dominant, neurocutaneous disorder that leads to renal anomalies in most patients. Angiomyolipomas are seen in approximately 80% and renal cysts in 20% to 40% of patients. Larger angiomyolipomas (>4 cm) have a tendency to bleed and therefore may require urgent nephrectomy, as in this patient, or embolization (28). Renal masses are the most common cause of spontaneous perinephric hemorrhage, and renal cell carcinoma and angiomyolipoma lead the list. Angiography of angiomyolipomas reveals characteristic microaneurysms in the mass.

## Aunt Minnie's Pearls

Multiple, bilateral, hyperechoic renal masses in a patient with tuberous sclerosis are almost certainly angiomyolipomas.

Angiomyolipomas are seen in up to 80% of patients with tuberous sclerosis (i.e., Bourneville disease).

HISTORY: Patient with history of gallstones and recent weight loss

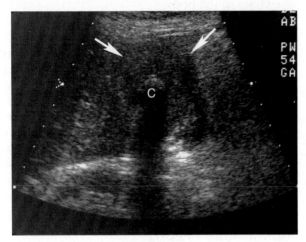

FIGURE 4.14.1

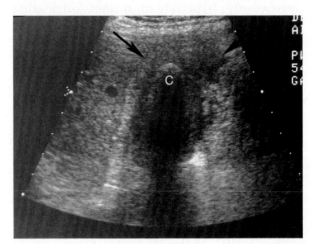

FIGURE 4.14.2

FINDINGS: Transverse (Fig. 4.14.1) and longitudinal (Fig. 4.14.2) images through the gallbladder show a soft-tissue mass in the expected location of the gallbladder (*arrows*). A dense, round structure in the center of the soft-tissue mass casts a clean acoustic shadow and therefore is most likely a gallbladder calculus (*C*). The patient had no tenderness over the gallbladder (i.e., negative Murphy's sign) and no history suggestive of cholecystitis.

DIAGNOSIS: Cholelithiasis and gallbladder carcinoma

DISCUSSION: Approximately 75% of patients with gallbladder carcinoma have gallstones. Although poorly understood, the chronic inflammation associated with gallstones is believed to result in epithelial dysplasia and the development of adenocarcinoma. One of the most common imaging presentations of gallbladder carcinoma is that of a soft-tissue mass in the gallbladder surrounding a gallstone. Other presentations include a polypoid intraluminal mass or focal wall thickening. Calcification of the gallbladder wall (i.e., "porcelain" gallbladder) also predisposes

to carcinoma (29). Although the quoted risk for developing carcinoma ranges from 16% to 60%, most agree that a porcelain gallbladder is an indication for cholecystectomy.

As a result of early spread of tumor to the liver or regional lymph nodes, gallbladder carcinoma carries a dismal 20% 5-year survival rate.

Hematogenous dissemination to distal organs is unusual. Invasion of the tumor into the hepatoduodenal ligament may result in obstruction of the common bile duct, and the hepatic flexure of the colon is sometimes involved.

## Aunt Minnie's Pearls

A soft-tissue mass that replaces the gallbladder lumen and is associated with a gallstone = gallbladder carcinoma in most cases.

Look for liver invasion or metastases and regional lymph node enlargement.

The 5-year survival rate for gallbladder carcinoma is about 20%.

HISTORY: A 55-year-old woman with diabetes

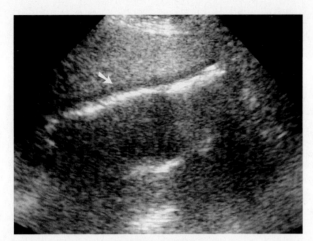

FIGURE 4.15.1

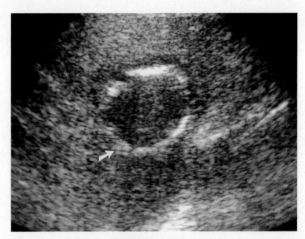

FIGURE 4.15.2

FINDINGS: Sagittal (Fig. 4.15.1, *arrow*) and transverse (Fig. 4.15.2, *arrow*) images of the gallbladder demonstrate a highly reflective outline of the entire gallbladder wall with a dirty acoustic shadow.

DIAGNOSIS: Emphysematous cholecystitis

DISCUSSION: Emphysematous cholecystitis is a severe variant of acute cholecystitis, characterized by the presence of gas in the gallbladder wall, lumen, or pericholecystic tissues in the absence of an abnormal communication between the biliary system and the gastrointestinal tract. It occurs most often in men, and associated factors include diabetes and cholelithiasis. The initial insult is ischemia with developing infection from a gas-forming organism, most commonly *Clostridia perfringens*, *Escherichia coli*, and *Bacteroides fragilis*. Mortality and morbidity rates are high, and emergency surgery is needed to reduce the high incidence of perforation and gangrene (30).

## Aunt Minnie's Pearls

Acute emphysematous cholecystitis primarily affects elderly diabetic men.

Bright reflections with "dirty" acoustic shadowing from a nondependent portion of the gallbladder wall suggest the diagnosis.

The most common infecting organisms are *C. perfringens*, *E. coli*, and *B. fragilis*.

Emergency surgery is indicated in emphysematous cholecystitis.

HISTORY: Patient with intermittent pelvic pain

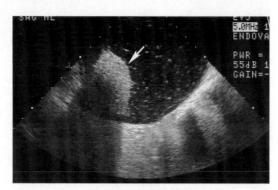

FIGURE 4.16.1

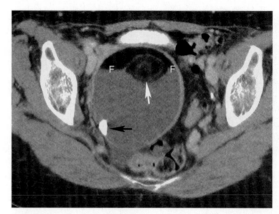

FIGURE 4.16.2

FINDINGS: A transverse ultrasound image in the region of the right adnexa (Fig. 4.16.1) reveals a cystic mass that contains diffuse, low-level internal echogenicity. A hyperechoic nodule inside the mass (*arrow*) produces marked posterior acoustic shadowing. A contrast-enhanced CT scan at the same level (Fig. 4.16.2) shows the soft-tissue nodule floating inside the lesion (*white arrow*) and an internal calcification (*black arrow*) and fat-fluid level (*F*).

DIAGNOSIS: Ovarian dermoid

DISCUSSION: This benign germ cell tumor of the ovary is named *dermoid* because the internal lining of the cystic mass contains skin and dermal appendages. *Ovarian teratoma* may be a more appropriate name because these masses contain elements from all three primitive germ cell lines. Although ovarian dermoids are histologically benign, their clinical behavior is not always benign. These neoplasms can cause ovarian torsion, and malignant degeneration (usually into squamous cell carcinoma) occurs rarely in older individuals. These masses are usually removed at the time of diagnosis.

Dermoids may be diagnosed with various imaging modalities by identifying the characteristic ectodermal elements of hair, teeth, and bone. A specific sonographic diagnosis can be made by identifying plugs of hair, fat, and calcium floating within the cystic mass. These Rokitansky plugs are hyperechoic on sonograms and often produce prominent posterior acoustic shadowing. Identification of a sebum-fluid level and calcification is also diagnostic of this tumor (31).

## Aunt Minnie's Pearls

A cystic adnexal mass with fat-fluid level and Rokitansky plug = ovarian dermoid.

These masses are removed because they predispose to ovarian torsion and may undergo malignant degeneration.

**HISTORY:** Two patients with vague scrotal discomfort

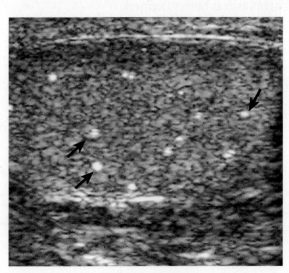

FIGURE 4.17.1

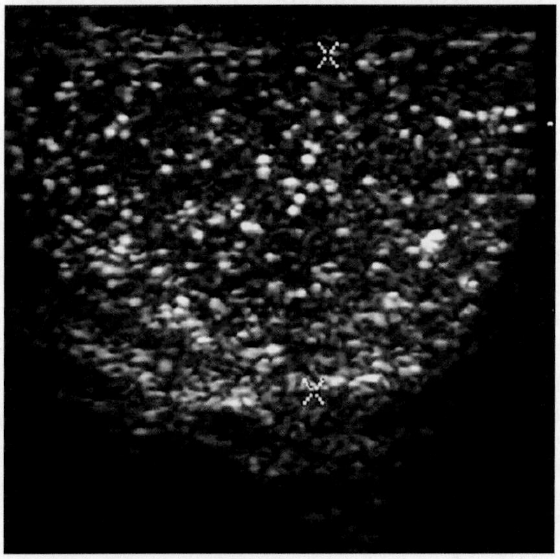

FIGURE 4.17.2

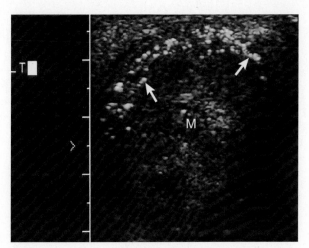

FIGURE 4.17.3

**FINDINGS:** A single longitudinal view of the left testicle in patient A (Fig. 4.17.1) reveals numerous tiny hyperechoic, non-shadowing foci (*black arrows*). The other testicle had the same appearance. The testicles are otherwise normal in echogenicity and size. A longitudinal view of the right testicle in patient B (Fig. 4.17.2) demonstrates tiny hyperechoic foci. However, in this patient, a transverse view of the left testicle (Fig. 4.17.3) reveals numerous, tiny, hyperechoic foci displaced to the periphery of the testicle (*arrows*) by a large heterogeneous mass (*M*).

**DIAGNOSIS:** Testicular microlithiasis (patient A) and testicular microlithiasis with seminoma (patient B)

**DISCUSSION:** Testicular microlithiasis occurs when degenerated tubular epithelium sloughs into the lumen of the seminiferous tubule and calcifies. These tiny (<2 mm) hyperechoic foci produce no acoustic shadowing and are almost always bilateral. Testicular microlithiasis can be differentiated from other causes of testicular calcification by its characteristic appearance and distribution. Associated conditions include cryptorchidism, the Klinefelter and Down syndromes, male pseudohermaphroditism, and pulmonary alveolar microlithiasis (32).

Testicular microlithiasis may coexist with an overt testicular neoplasm, as in patient B, or with the premalignant condition of intratubular germ cell neoplasia. Although various malignant germ cell tumors have been found in patients with testicular microlithiasis, the degree of increased risk for the development of neoplasm is unknown (32,33). When testicular microlithiasis is discovered with ultrasonography, the testicles should be carefully surveyed for neoplasm in all patients, and ultrasonographic follow-up in 6 months to 1 year should be performed until the degree of increased risk for neoplasm is better defined.

## Aunt Minnie's Pearls

Numerous tiny foci of calcium in both testicles = testicular microlithiasis.

Be aware of the association of testicular microlithiasis with testicular neoplasms.

When a testicular mass is discovered, always survey the retroperitoneum for metastatic adenopathy.

# Case 4.18

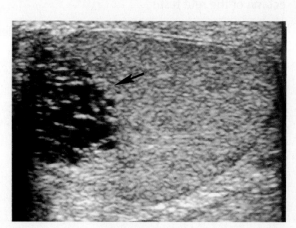

FIGURE 4.18.1

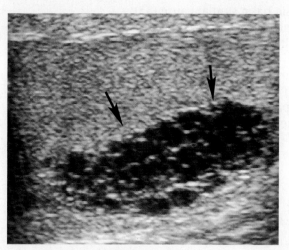

FIGURE 4.18.2

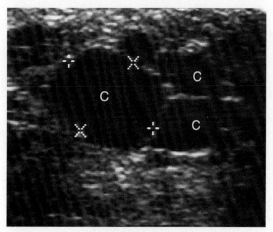

FIGURE 4.18.3

**FINDINGS:** Transverse (Fig. 4.18.1) and longitudinal (Fig. 4.18.2) views of the left testicle reveal numerous small cystic structures adjacent to the mediastinum testis (*black arrows*). Figure 4.18.3 shows bilateral cysts originating in the epididymis (*C*), which probably account for the patient's palpable mass. The testes are otherwise normal.

**DIAGNOSIS:** Tubular ectasia of the rete testis and spermatoceles

**DISCUSSION:** The rete testis is a latticework of tubules that are located in the mediastinum testes and connect the seminiferous tubules to the efferent ductules. If the rete testis becomes abnormally dilated, a unique appearance of dilated, serpiginous tubules near the mediastinum is seen on sonograms. In most cases, this tubular ectasia of the rete testis is associated with spermatoceles, intratesticular cysts, or both. The process is usually bilateral but may be asymmetric (34). Although the cause is obscure, the association of testicular cysts with previous trauma or infection has led to the assumption that tubular ectasia has a similar cause (35).

The sonographic appearance of tubular ectasia parallels a spectrum of severity from mild serpiginous dilatation of the tubules to cysts in the region of the mediastinum. The condition is usually identified in middle-aged men, and the lesion itself is nonpalpable and usually asymptomatic. No serious sequelae of the abnormality are known.

## Aunt Minnie's Pearls

Small, cystic spaces in the mediastinum testis = tubular ectasia of the rete testis.

Most cases are associated with spermatoceles or testicular cysts.

**HISTORY:** A 54-year-old man with elevated liver function test results, hepatomegaly, and chronic hepatitis who recently underwent endoscopic retrograde cholangiopancreatography (ERCP) and liver biopsy

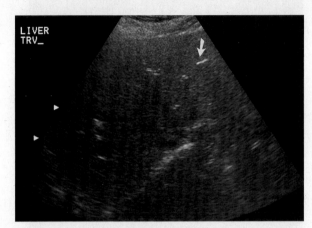

FIGURE 4.19.1

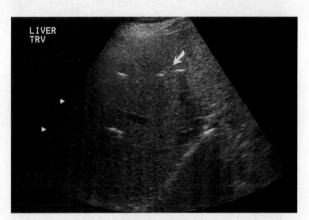

FIGURE 4.19.2

**FINDINGS:** Multiple linear echogenic foci within the bile ducts with distal acoustic shadowing are demonstrated on these sonographic images (Figs. 4.19.1 and 4.19.2, *arrows*).

**DIAGNOSIS:** Pneumobilia

**DISCUSSION:** Pneumobilia can be caused by any process that results in biliary–enteric or biliary–cutaneous communication. There are several causes, including diverting surgeries that result in choledochojejunostomy or choledochoduodenostomy. Any condition that results in distortion or incompetence of the sphincter of Oddi can also cause air to reflux into the biliary tree. This may be the result of sphincterotomy at ERCP or inflammatory processes affecting the duodenum, such as peptic ulcer disease or Crohn's disease. Biliary–enteric fistulas can result from cholecystitis with erosion of a stone through the gallbladder wall creating a fistulous tract between the gallbladder and the adjacent bowel. If the passed stone causes downstream obstruction or ileus, this combination of findings is referred to as *gallstone ileus*. Pneumobilia appears on radiographs and CT as linear branching lucencies within the

liver. Gas is bright on ultrasound, and pneumobilia appears sonographically as intrahepatic hyperechogenic foci that often produce distal acoustic shadowing. The air collections are generally centralized as a result of hepatofugal flow of bile. This distinguishes pneumobilia from air in the portal system that is carried peripherally with portal blood flow. A common false-positive diagnosis of pneumobilia is intrabiliary stones. In most cases, gas produces a brighter reflection and a "dirtier" shadow than stones. Ringdown artifact is seen only behind gas and, when seen, is useful in making the diagnosis (36).

## Aunt Minnie's Pearls

Pneumobilia or air in the biliary tree results when there is abnormal communication between the biliary system and bowel.

Sonographically, pneumobilia is demonstrated as linear hyperechogenic foci within the biliary system.

A common false-positive sign of pneumobilia is intrabiliary stones.

**HISTORY:** Patient who underwent a cardiac catheterization 1 day earlier

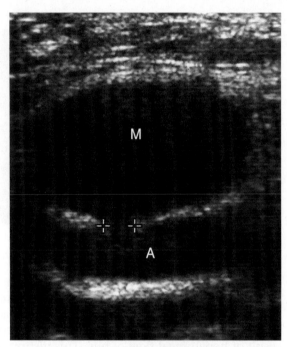

FIGURE 4.20.1

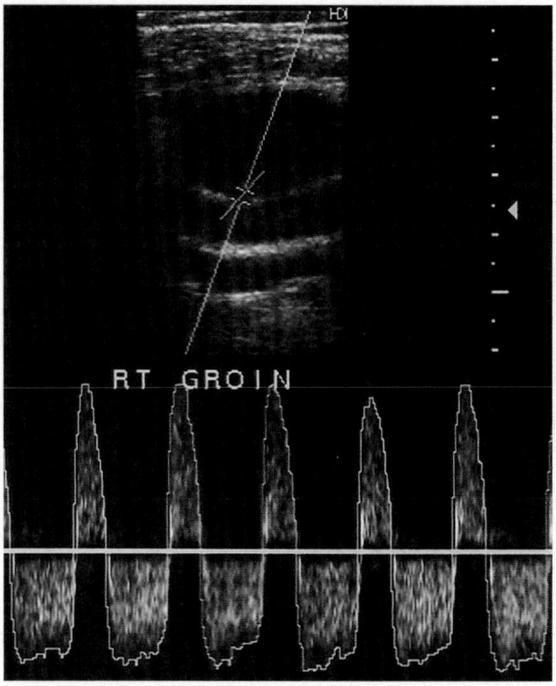

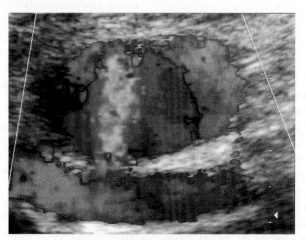

FIGURE 4.20.2

FIGURE 4.20.3

**FINDINGS:** On this single, longitudinal, gray-scale image of the right common femoral artery (Fig. 4.20.1), a round, anechoic mass (*M*) is present anterior to the artery (*A*). A Doppler waveform (Fig. 4.20.2) obtained in an area of communication between the artery and the anechoic mass demonstrates flow both toward (above baseline) and then away from (below baseline) the transducer, or a to-and-fro appearance. A corresponding color Doppler image (Fig. 4.20.3) reveals a swirling color-flow pattern in the cystic mass.

**DIAGNOSIS:** Postcatheterization femoral artery pseudoaneurysm

**DISCUSSION:** A pseudoaneurysm is a localized rupture of an artery contained by the surrounding soft tissues. The wall of the aneurysm does not contain intima, media, and adventitia and is therefore called a *pseudoaneurysm*. Femoral artery pseudoaneurysm is a well-known complication of percutaneous angiography that occurs when arterial blood communicates with an extravascular collection of blood through the puncture site. Ultrasonography is used to differentiate between a pseudoaneurysm and a periarterial hematoma. The pseudoaneurysm can sometimes be treated with ultrasound by compressing the area until complete thrombosis of the pseudoaneurysm occurs.

A characteristic Doppler finding is the to-and-fro waveform obtained at the neck of the pseudoaneurysm. Blood entering the pseudoaneurysm during systole produces flow above the baseline, and blood exiting during diastole produces flow below the baseline (37). The normal transient diastolic flow reversal seen from small arterial branches of the femoral artery should not be confused with the pandiastolic flow reversal seen at pseudoaneurysm necks.

Color Doppler examination of the area reveals the swirling color pattern similar to the yin–yang symbol in Chinese dualistic philosophy.

### Aunt Minnie's Pearls

A pseudoaneurysm has a characteristic to-and-fro waveform at its neck.

A characteristic yin–yang swirling color Doppler flow pattern is seen within the pseudoaneurysm.

# Case 4.21

**HISTORY:** A 71-year-old female with hyperparathyroidism

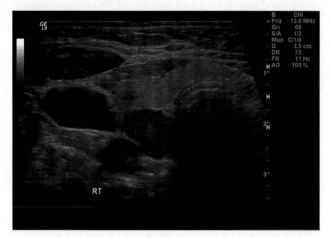

FIGURE 4.21.1

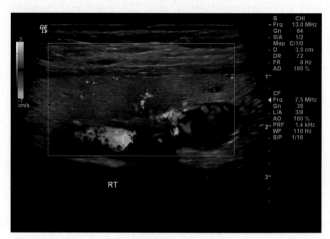

FIGURE 4.21.2

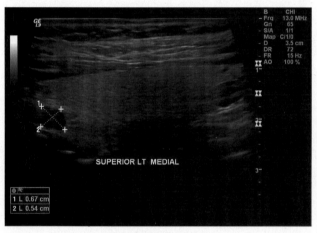

FIGURE 4.21.3

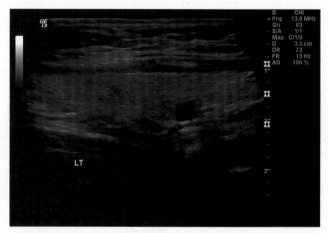

FIGURE 4.21.4

**DIAGNOSIS:** Multiple parathyroid adenomas

**FINDINGS:** A well-defined, hypoechoic, reniform mass is noted posterior to the right lobe (Fig. 4.21.1). Internal vascularity is noted (Fig. 4.21.2). Evaluation of the left thyroid lobe reveals smaller but similar appearing lesions superior and inferior to the gland (Figs. 4.21.3 and 4.21.4).

**DISCUSSION:** Parathyroid adenomas may be oval or flat as the glands develop longitudinal in fascial planes (38). Most have a thin echogenic capsule and are hypoechoic to thyroid. Some adenomas may have cystic changes (Fig. 4.21.2). Color Doppler demonstrates flow within the parenchyma.

## Aunt Minnie's Pearls

Parathyroid adenomas are the most common cause of primary hyperparathyroidism.

Ultrasound is the primary initial imaging modality to diagnose parathyroid adenomas around the thyroid gland.

HISTORY: A 21-year-old female with hirsutism, obesity, and amenorrhea

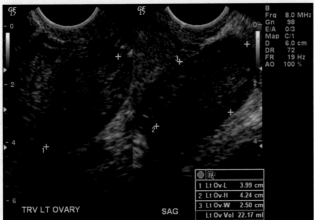

FIGURE 4.22.1

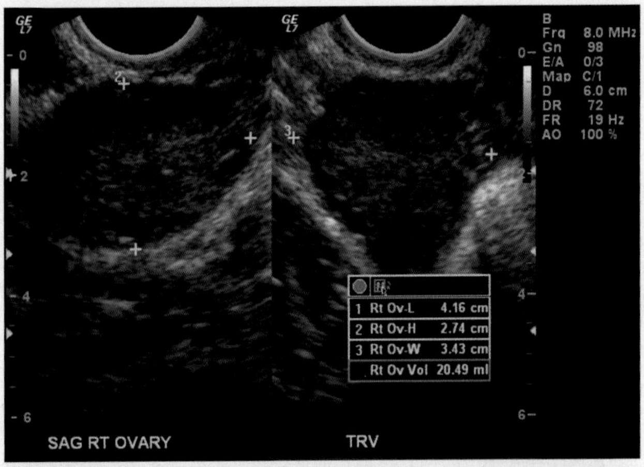

FIGURE 4.22.2

FINDINGS: Figures 4.22.1 and 4.22.2 demonstrate that both ovaries are enlarged. Furthermore, noted are >10 follicles per ovary, all of which measure <10 mm.

DIAGNOSIS: Polycystic ovarian syndrome

DISCUSSION: To diagnose polycystic ovarian syndrome, two of three criteria must be present:

Polycystic ovaries
Anovulation
Hyperandrogenism (39)

Imaging findings include enlarged ovaries with volume >10 cc and >12 follicles per ovary measuring <10 mm in diameter (39).

## Aunt Minnie's Pearls

Polycystic ovarian syndrome is the most common cause of anovulatory infertility.

Imaging findings in one ovary are sufficient to diagnose polycystic ovarian syndrome.

HISTORY: A 65-year-old female with history of myelodysplastic syndrome presents with increasing right upper quadrant pain.

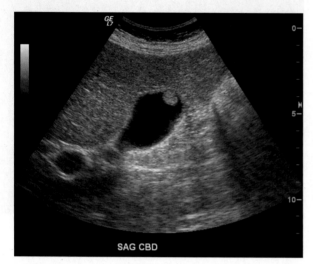

FIGURE 4.23.1

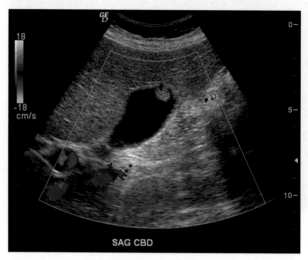

FIGURE 4.23.2

FINDINGS: Rounded echogenic mass is seen within the nondependent portion of the gallbladder fundus (Fig. 4.23.1). There is a feeding vessel identified at the junction with the gallbladder wall (Fig. 4.23.2).

DIAGNOSIS: Biliary papillary adenoma

DISCUSSION: Gallbladder adenomas comprise <5% of benign gallbladder lesions. They typically present as homogeneously echogenic, solitary lesions (40). These polyps are frequently pedunculated and sonographic interrogation with Doppler imaging can demonstrate blood flow in the pedicle, as seen in this case.

The differential for benign masses of the gallbladder also includes cholesterol polyps and inflammatory polyps, with cholesterol polyps comprising over half of all benign lesions of the gallbladder (40,41). Multiplicity and lesion size <10 mm are often a good predictors of benignity. Gallbladder malignancies are much less common and include primary gallbladder adenocarcinomas, melanoma metastatic to the gallbladder, and secondary invasion from adjacent hepatocellular carcinoma (40).

### Aunt Minnie's Pearl

The presence of pedicle flow and size >10 mm in a solitary polyp are concerning imaging features. These lesions are typically excised for pathologic examination.

# Case 4.24

**HISTORY:** A 30-year-old female presents with an enlarging palpable breast mass

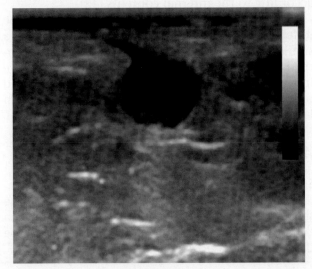

FIGURE 4.24.1

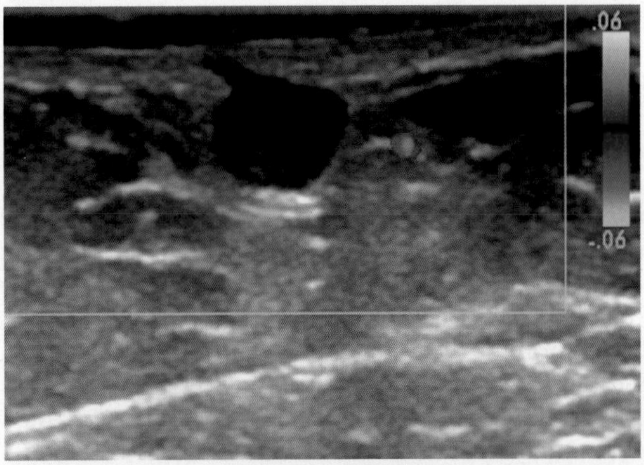

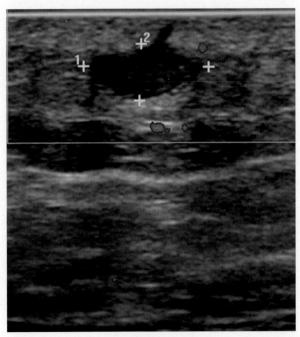

FIGURE 4.24.2

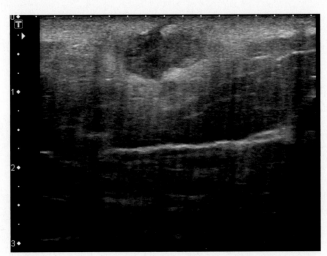

FIGURE 4.24.3

FIGURE 4.24.4

**FINDINGS:** Predominately anechoic structure originating within the subcutaneous fat. Standoff technique allows for clear visibility of a neck extending through the dermis to an opening in the skin (Fig. 4.24.1). There is no identifiable flow within the lesion (Fig. 4.24.2). Similar additional lesions demonstrating varying degrees of internal debris (Figs. 4.24.3 and 4.24.4).

**DIAGNOSIS:** Sebaceous cyst

**DISCUSSION:** Sebaceous cysts are of skin origin and arise predominately in the hair-bearing areas of the body. They frequently present in breast imaging as a palpable mass in the axillary regions. Classically these lesions are considered to lie entirely within the skin (Fig. 4.24.3), but can also lie within the subcutaneous fat (Figs. 4.24.1 and 4.24.4). Lesions in the subcutaneous fat often demonstrate a gland-shaped neck coursing through the skin, as in this case. The internal echogenicity of a sebaceous cyst will vary according to the internal contents (42).

Epidermal inclusion cysts are considered in the differential for cysts of skin origin and occur in a similar anatomic distribution (43). What differentiates an epidermal inclusion cyst is its distinctive internal echogenicity with the classically described onion-skin arising from the sloughing of keratin layers into the cyst lumen (42).

## Aunt Minnie's Pearl

Sebaceous cyst is classically described as arising entirely within the skin. However, it can also arise in the subcutaneous tissues. In these cases the presence of a demonstrable neck coursing through the skin can be diagnostic.

HISTORY: A 22-year-old female presented with severe right lower quadrant pain, nausea, and vomiting

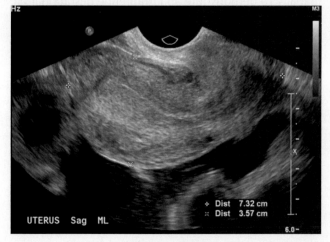

FIGURE 4.25.1

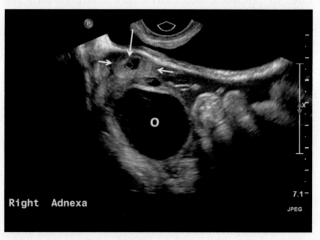

FIGURE 4.25.2

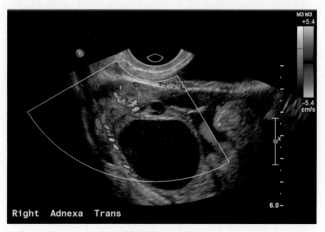

FIGURE 4.25.3

FINDINGS: Transvaginal scan, sagittal image through the uterus (Fig. 4.25.1) shows normal endometrial stripe without any intrauterine gestational sac. There is significant amount of free fluid noted posterior to the uterus. Figure 4.25.2 through the right adnexa shows a large anechoic cystic mass (O), which represents right ovary with corpus luteal cyst. Anterior to that, there is an echogenic ring-like structure (*short arrows*) that represents an extrauterine gestational sac. A small yolk sac (*long arrow*) is also present within the gestation sac. Figure 4.25.3 is a color Doppler US image through the right adnexal region showing increased vascularity around the gestational sac.

DIAGNOSIS: Right ectopic pregnancy

DISCUSSION: The incidence of ectopic pregnancy has increased in recent years and is seen in 1% to 2% of all pregnancies in United States (44–46). It most commonly occurs in fallopian tubes (97%) but can occur in cervix, ovary, cornua of the uterus or even intra-abdominally. Among the tubal pregnancies, ampulla is the most common site of implantation. If the patient's beta-hCG is more than 1,500 to 2,000 mIU/mL and an intrauterine pregnancy is not seen on a transvaginal scan, an ectopic pregnancy should be suspected (New9). Patients usually present with lower abdominal pain. The risk factors include previous tubal surgery, previous ectopic pregnancy, infertility treatment, and intrauterine contraceptive device. On ultrasound, tubal pregnancy usually presents as a complex adnexal mass, which may show increased peripheral vascularity frequently termed as ring of fire appearance. Presence of complex free fluid and a complex adnexal mass suggests ruptured ectopic pregnancy in the appropriate setting. Uterine endometrium may show thickening owing to decidual reaction but without a gestational sac. Occurrence of concomitant intrauterine and ectopic pregnancy is extremely rare (1:30,000). Ovaries may show cystic changes from corpus luteum formation and increased peripheral vascularity, which in many cases may be mistaken for an ectopic pregnancy.

## Aunt Minnie's Pearls

Inability to demonstrate an intrauterine gestational sac with transvaginal scan in a patient with beta-hCG levels of >2,000 mIU/mL should always raise suspicion for an ectopic pregnancy.

Endometrial (decidual) cysts may be seen even with ectopic pregnancy (pseudosac) and should not be mistaken for a true sac. Demonstration of a yolk sac within an intrauterine gestational sac more accurately confirms an intrauterine pregnancy.

HISTORY: A 58-year-old male presented with vague testicular pain bilaterally

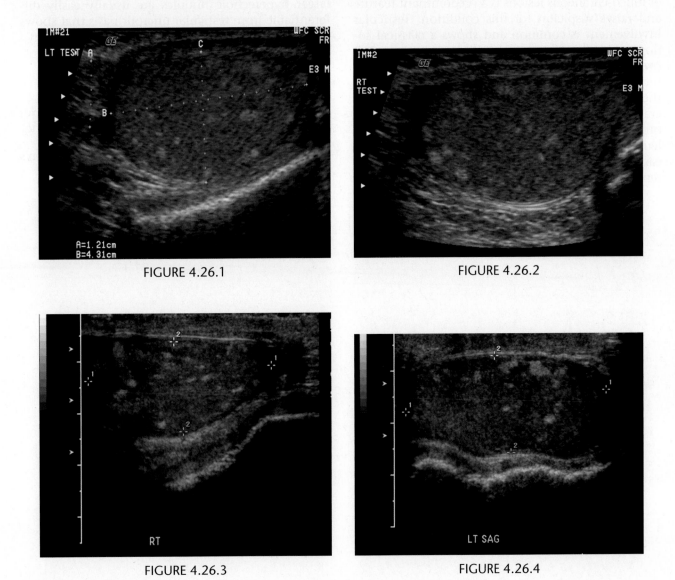

FIGURE 4.26.1

FIGURE 4.26.2

FIGURE 4.26.3

FIGURE 4.26.4

FINDINGS: Figures 4.26.1 and 4.26.2 are gray-scale US images of the right and left testicles. Both testicles show multiple echogenic foci scattered throughout the testicles. These foci are larger than typical micro-lithiasis, are homogeneous, circumscribed, and do not show any posterior shadowing. Figures 4.26.3 and 4.26.4 are of the same patient seen 3 years later. No significant interval change in the appearance of these nodules is seen.

DIAGNOSIS: Lipohamartomas of testicles

DISCUSSION: Testicular lipohamartomas are almost always associated with Cowden disease. Isolated lipomas are rare. Cowden disease is also known as multiple hamartoma syndrome. This is a rare condition with prevalence of about 1:250,000 (47). Patients can have multiple benign or malignant neoplasms and hamartomas in various organ systems such as breast, thyroid, endometrium, and skin. Presence of muco-cutaneous lesions is a predominant feature and raises suspicion for this condition. Testicular involvement is common and shows a classical sonographic appearance of multiple echogenic foci owing to the fat content. These show typical findings of fat-containing lesions on MRI and on biopsy, the lesions show interstitial lipomatosis (48). Bilateral multiple testicular lesions can be seen in many other conditions such as malignancy, lymphoma, leukemia, metastatic disease, granulomatous disease, and adrenal rests. Most of these conditions tend to have hypoechoic lesions or heterogeneous, mixed echogenicity lesions. Lipohamartomas with larger hyperechoic nodules are usually easily differentiable from testicular microlithiasis that shows multiple tiny punctate hyperechoic foci bilaterally.

## Aunt Minnie's Pearls

Appearance of homogeneous hyperechoic bilateral lesions in the testicles without any posterior shadowing.

Presence of other stigmata associated with Cowden's disease is clue for diagnosis.

**HISTORY:** A 42-year-old male with tense left scrotal mass

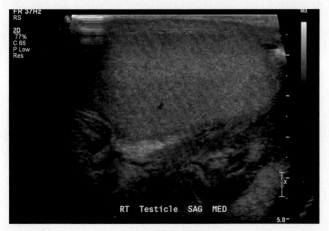

FIGURE 4.27.1

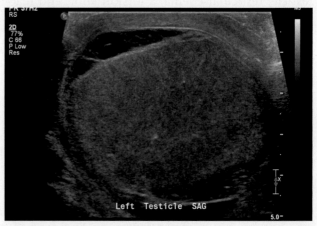

FIGURE 4.27.2

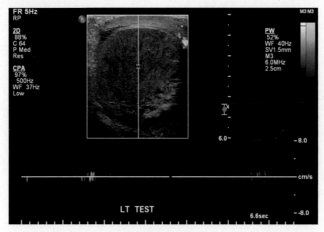

FIGURE 4.27.3

**FINDINGS:** Sagittal images through the right testicle (Fig. 4.27.1) and left testicle (Fig. 4.27.2) show heterogeneous and decreased echogenicity throughout the left testicle with normal echogenicity in the right testicle. Pulse wave Doppler image of the left testicle (Fig 4.27.3) shows no detectable flow in the left testicle with flow in the scrotal wall.

**DIAGNOSIS:** Left testicular torsion

**DISCUSSION:** Testicular torsion occurs as a result of the faulty attachment of the testis to the scrotal wall. The most common anatomic anomaly producing this faulty attachment is the bell-clapper deformity. It consists of a tunica vaginalis that completely surrounds the testis, causing the testis to be attached only to the spermatic cord and the testis is freely suspended in the scrotum, like the clapper in a bell. The first hemodynamic consequence is venous obstruction. This is followed by arterial inflow obstruction and testicular ischemia. Testicle viability depends on duration of the torsion and number of twists of the spermatic cord. Infarction can occur in 4 hours after the onset of symptoms. The goal is for urologists to operate within 6 hours after the onset of symptoms (49,50).

Gray-scale sonography may show nonspecific abnormalities such as decreased echogenicity of testicle, testicular edema, a torsion knot, and reactive hydroceles. A torsed testicle may also appear normal on gray-scale imaging. If the testis is hypoechoic or inhomogeneous, it may be infarcted and possibly nonviable. Color Doppler imaging can show absent or asymmetrically decreased testicular vascularity in the torsed testis. In prolonged torsion there may be reactive edema of the scrotal wall. Color Doppler analysis can also document detorsion by showing return of vascular flow to the testis (49,50).

Color Doppler imaging is the preferred method of evaluating patients with suspected testicular torsion.

## Aunt Minnie's Pearls

Gray-scale imaging of a torsed testicle may be normal or it may show enlarged hypoechoic testis, a torsion knot, a reactive hydrocele, and scrotal edema.

The diagnosis is made by color Doppler imaging, which can show decreased or absent vascular flow to the testis.

**HISTORY:** A 64-year-old female with elevated liver function tests, abdominal pain, and dilated common bile duct

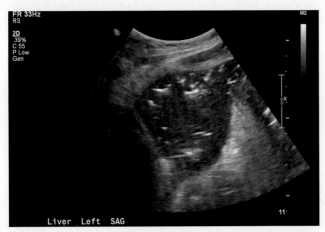

FIGURE 4.28.1

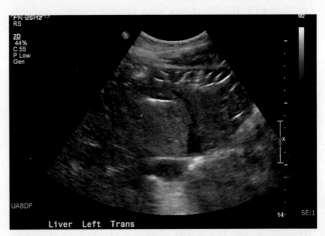

FIGURE 4.28.2

**FINDINGS:** Sagittal (Fig. 4.28.1) and transverse (Fig. 4.28.2) gray-scale sonographic images of the left lobe of the liver show multiple echogenic foci predominantly in the periphery of the liver.

**DIAGNOSIS:** Hepatic portal venous gas

**DISCUSSION:** Hepatic portal venous gas is characteristically described as peripheral and branching gas lucencies within the liver noted to extend to within 2 cm of the liver capsule. The peripheral location is owing to the centrifugal flow of the blood in the portal vein. On ultrasound the gas will appear as peripheral echogenic foci and on CT or radiographs as lucencies that approach the liver capsule. Portal venous gas should be distinguished from centrally located pneumobilia related to gas within the biliary system. Distinguishing between these clinical entities is important as the predisposing factors and pathophysiological processes have very different modes of therapy. With hepatic portal venous gas, more air typically accumulates in the left portal venous system as it is more anterior on ultrasound or CT imaging. However, on plain radiographs linear lucencies will accumulate in the right portal venous system (51,52).

Initially associated with bowel necrosis and a very high mortality rate, portal venous gas is now being imaged in many benign conditions. Portal venous gas has many possible causes including ischemic bowel, necrotic/ulcerated colorectal carcinoma, inflammatory bowel disease, and perforated peptic ulcer (51,52). Other causes include pancreatitis, abdominal abscess, diverticulitis, trauma, and bowel obstruction. Upper and lower endoscopies can cause iatrogenic portal venous gas.

## Aunt Minnie's Pearls

Portal venous gas appears on ultrasound as echogenic foci in periphery of the liver.

Distinguishing from pneumobilia and finding the cause of the portal venous gas is important owing to high mortality rate associated with many causes of hepatic portal venous gas.

# REFERENCES

1. Sidhu P, Baxter G. Ultrasound of abdominal transplantation. Leipzig, Germany: Thieme, 2002.

2. Sherer DM. Adverse perinatal outcome of twin pregnancies according to chorionicity: Review of the literature. Am J Perinatol 2001;18(1):23–27.

3. Finberg HJ. The "twin peak" sign: Reliable evidence of dichorionic twinning. J Ultrasound Med 1992;11:571–577.

4. Sepulveda W, Sebire NJ, Hughes J, et al. Evolution of the lambda or twin/chorionic peak sign in dichorionic twin pregnancies. Obstet Gynecol 1997;89:439–441.

5. Dewbury KC. Scrotal ultrasonography: An update. BJU Int 2000;86(suppl 1):143–152.

6. Horstman WG. Scrotal imaging. Urol Clin North Am 1997; 24:653–671.

7. Goncalves LF, Jeanty P. Ultrasound evaluation of fetal abdominal wall defects. In: Callen PW (ed.). Ultrasonography in obstetrics and gynecology, 3rd ed. Philadelphia, PA: WB Saunders, 1994:370–388.

8. Nyberg DA, Mack LA. Abdominal wall defects. In: Nyberg DA, Mahony BS, Pretorius DH (eds.). Diagnostic ultrasound of fetal anomalies: Text and atlas. Chicago, IL: Year Book, 1990:395–432.

9. Emanuel PG, Garcia GI, Angtuaco TL. Prenatal detection of anterior abdominal wall defects with US. Radiographics 1995;15:517–530.

10. Filly RA. Ultrasound evaluation of the fetal neural axis. In: Callen PW (ed.). Ultrasonography in obstetrics and gynecology, 3rd ed. Philadelphia, PA: WB Saunders, 1994:189–234.

11. Nyberg DA, Mack LA. The spine and neural tube defects. In: Nyberg DA, Mahony BS, Pretorius DH (eds.). Diagnostic ultrasound of fetal anomalies: Text and atlas. Chicago, IL: Year Book, 1990:146–202.

12. Nyberg DA, Mack LA, Hirsch J, et al. Abnormalities of fetal cranial contour in sonographic detection of spina bifida: Evaluation of the "lemon" sign. Radiology 1988;167:387–392.

13. Ball RH, Filly RA, Goldstein RB, et al. The lemon sign: Not a specific indicator of meningomyelocele. J Ultrasound Med 1993;12:131–134.

14. Harmon JP, Hiett AK, Palmer CG, et al. Prenatal ultrasound detection of isolated neural tube defects: Is cytogenetic evaluation warranted? Obstet Gynecol 1995;86:595–599.

15. Czeizel AE. Prevention of congenital abnormalities by periconceptional multivitamin supplementation. BMJ 1993;306: 1645–1648.

16. Hendricks SK, Cyr DR, Nyberg DA, et al. Exencephaly: Clinical and ultrasonic correlation to anencephaly. Obstet Gynecol 1988;72:898–901.

17. Gabbe SG, Niebyl JR, Simpson JL. Obstetrics—Normal and problem pregnancies, 4th ed. New York, NY: Churchill Livingstone, 2002:516–517.

18. Callen PW. Ultrasonography in obstetrics and gynecology, 3rd ed. Philadelphia, PA: WB Saunders, 1994:445–448.

19. Hall DA, Yoder IC. Ultrasound evaluation of the uterus. In: Callen PW (ed.). Ultrasonography in obstetrics and gynecology, 3rd ed. Philadelphia, PA: WB Saunders, 1994:586–614.

20. Hertzberg BS, Kliewer MA, Farrell TA, et al. Spontaneously changing gravid cervix: Clinical implications and prognostic features. Radiology 1995;196:721–724.

21. Glazer GM, Callen PW, Filly RA. Medullary nephrocalcinosis: Sonographic evaluation. AJR Am J Roentgenol 1982;138:55–57.

22. Amis ES Jr, Newhouse JH. Essentials of uroradiology. Boston, MA: Little, Brown, 1991:216.

23. Kurtz AB, Middleton WD. Ultrasound: The requisites. St Louis, MO: Mosby, 1995:19–20.

24. Juhl JH, Crummy AB, Kuhlman JE. Paul and Juhl's essentials of radiologic imaging, 7th ed. Philadelphia, PA: Lippincott Williams & Wilkins, 1998:513.

25. Valla D, Bennamou JP. Obstruction of the hepatic veins or suprahepatic inferior vena cava. Dig Dis 1996;14:99–118.

26. Amis ES Jr, Newhouse JH. Essentials of uroradiology. Boston, MA: Little, Brown, 1991:124.

27. Bourneville DM. Sclerose tubereuse des circonvolutions cerebrales: Idiotie et epilepsie hemiplegique. Arch Int Neurol 1880;1:81–91.

28. Oesterling JE, Fishman EE, Goldman SE, et al. The management of renal angiomyolipoma. J Urol 1986;135:1121–1124.

29. Berk RN, Armbuster TG, Saltzstein SL. Carcinoma in the porcelain gallbladder. Radiology 1973;106:29–31.

30. Yoshida K, Arakawa M, Ishida S, et al. A case of hemolytic uremic syndrome associated with emphysematous cholecystitis and a liver abscess. Tohoku J Exp Med 1998;185:147–155.

31. Dodd GD III, Budzik RF Jr. Lipomatous tumors of the pelvis in women: Spectrum of imaging findings. AJR Am J Roentgenol 1990;155:317–322.

32. Backus ML, Mack LA, Middleton WD, et al. Testicular microlithiasis: Imaging appearances and pathologic correlation. Radiology 1994;192:781–785.

33. Patel MD, Olcott EW, Kerschmann RL, et al. Sonographically detected testicular microlithiasis and testicular carcinoma. J Clin Ultrasound 1993;21:447–452.

34. Weingarten BJ, Kellman GM, Middleton WD, et al. Tubular ectasia within the mediastinum testis. J Ultrasound Med 1992;11:349–353.

35. Hamm B, Fobbe F, Loy V. Testicular cysts: Differentiation with US and clinical findings. Radiology 1988;168:19–23.

36. Halpert R, Feczo P. Gastrointestinal radiology: The requisites, 2nd ed. St Louis, MO: Mosby, 1999:209–214.

37. Polak JF. The peripheral vessels. In: Rumack CM, Wilson SR, Charboneau JW (eds.). Diagnostic ultrasound. St Louis, MO: Mosby–Year Book, 1991;1:678–681.

38. Ahuja A. Parathyroid adenoma, visceral space. In: Ahuja A, Griffith J, Wong K, et al. (eds.). Diagnostic imaging: Ultrasound. Salt Lake City, UT: Amirsys, 2007:11.36–11.37.

39. Kennedy A. Polycystic ovarian syndrome. In: Ahuja A, Griffith J, Wong K, et al. (eds.). Diagnostic imaging: Ultrasound. Salt Lake City, UT: Amirsys, 2007:9.94–9.95.

40. Khalili K, Wilson SR. The biliary tree and gallbladder. In: Rumak CM, Wilson SR, Charboneau JW, et al. (eds.). Diagnostic ultrasound, 4th ed. Philadelphia, PA: Elsevier, 2011:209–213.

41. Chong WK, Shah MS. Sonography of right upper quadrant pain. Ultrasound Clin 2008;3:121–138.

42. Stavros AT. Sonographic evaluation of breast cysts. In: Breast ultrasound. Philadelphia, PA: Lippincott Williams & Wilkins, 2004:325–331.

43. Kim HS, Cha ES, Kim HH, et al. Spectrum of sonographic findings in superficial breast masses. J Ultrasound Med 2005;24:663–680.

44. Della-Giustina D, Denny M. Ectopic pregnancy. Emerg Med Clin North Am 2003;21:565–584.

45. Tay JI, Moore J, Walker JJ. Clinical review: Ectopic pregnancy. BMJ 2000;320:916–919.

46. Levine D. Ectopic pregnancy. Radiology 2007;245:385–397.

47. Venkatanarasimha N, Hilmy S, Freeman S. Testicular lipomatosis in Cowden disease. Radiology 2011;261:654–658.

48. Woodhouse JB, Ferguson MM. Multiple hyperechoic testicular lesions are a common finding on ultrasound in Cowden disease and represent lipomatosis of the testis. Br J Radiol 2006;79(946):801–803.

49. Bhatt S, Dogra VS. Role of ultrasound in testicular and scrotal trauma. Radiographics 2008;28(6):1617–1629.

50. Middleton WD, Kurtz AB, Hertzberg BS. Ultrasound: The requisites. St Louis, MO: Mosby, 2004:167–171.

51. Sebastia C, Quiroga S, Espin E, et al. Portomesenteric vein gas: Pathologic mechanisms, CT findings, and prognosis. Radiographics 2000;20:1213–1224.

52. Franken JM, Veen EJ. Hepatic portal venous gas. J Gastrointestin Liver Dis 2010;19(4):360.

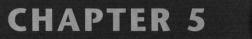

# CHAPTER 5

# NUCLEAR MEDICINE

**Marques Bradshaw / Blaine Mischen**

*The authors and editors acknowledge the contribution of the Chapter 5 authors from the second edition: Mark A. Auler, MD, and Kenneth Spicer, MD, and the Chapter 5 authors from the third edition: Beata Panzegrau, Phillip S. Davis, Leonie Gordon.*

**HISTORY:** A 68-year-old man with dementia, ataxia, and incontinence

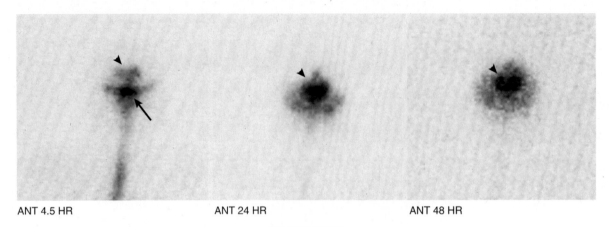

ANT 4.5 HR          ANT 24 HR          ANT 48 HR

FIGURE 5.1.1

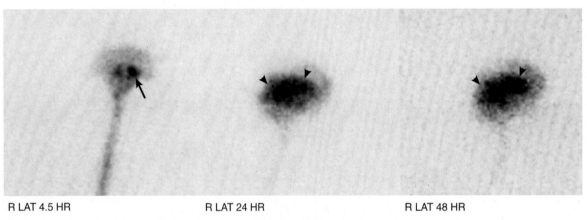

R LAT 4.5 HR          R LAT 24 HR          R LAT 48 HR

FIGURE 5.1.2

**FINDINGS:** Multiple frontal (Fig. 5.1.1) and lateral (Fig. 5.1.2) images from an indium-111 ($^{111}$In) diethylenetriamine-penta-acetic acid (DTPA) cisternography study are presented. Activity is present in the basal cisterns at 4.5 hours (*arrows*). Mild lateral ventricular activity is also seen at this time and is more prominent at 24 and 48 hours (*arrowheads*). Flow over the convexities is delayed.

**DIAGNOSIS:** Normal-pressure hydrocephalus

**DISCUSSION:** Clinically, normal-pressure hydrocephalus is characterized by the triad of ataxia, dementia, and incontinence. Cerebrospinal fluid flow reversal is useful in distinguishing this entity from other causes of dementia associated with ventriculomegaly (i.e., hydrocephalus *ex vacuo*). Surgical shunting can alleviate a patient's symptoms; however, not all patients respond to this treatment (1). The amount of response depends on the amount of activity in the ventricles compared with that over the convexities and on the duration of neurologic symptoms and signs (2).

Normally, the radiotracer reaches the basal cisterns within 1 hour after administration through lumbar puncture. Between 2 and 6 hours, the activity ascends into the interhemispheric and sylvian fissures. Radiotracer flows over the cerebral convexities by 24 hours. No lateral ventricular activity is seen under normal conditions. In classic normal-pressure hydrocephalus, radiotracer reflux into the lateral ventricles occurs and persists for 24, 48, or even 72 hours after injection.

## Aunt Minnie's Pearls

In normal-pressure hydrocephalus, radiotracer refluxes into the lateral ventricles and persists for 24, 48, or even 72 hours.

The clinical triad of dementia, ataxia, and incontinence is seen in normal-pressure hydrocephalus.

**HISTORY:** A 62-year-old man who suffered a major cerebrovascular accident

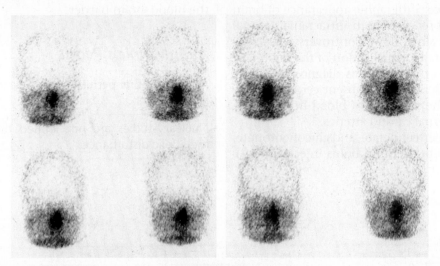

FIGURE 5.2.1

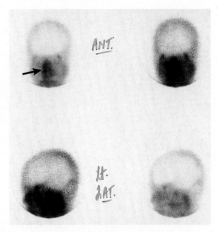

FIGURE 5.2.2

**FINDINGS:** The initial flow images from this technetium-99m ($^{99m}$Tc)–hexamethylpropylene amine oxime (HMPAO) cerebral perfusion study (Fig. 5.2.1) show that no arterial flow is present in either cerebral hemisphere. The delayed static images (Fig. 5.2.2) confirm that no cerebral activity is seen. Prominent activity is identified in the patient's face and scalp (*arrow*).

**DIAGNOSIS:** Absent cerebral perfusion

**DISCUSSION:** Although the diagnosis of brain death is made on clinical criteria, the radionuclide cerebral perfusion study is often used for confirmation. Unlike electroencephalography, radionuclide evaluation does not produce false-positive studies in patients with hypothermia or a metabolic disturbance (i.e., anoxia, uremia, hepatic encephalopathy, severe sepsis, or high doses of fentanyl, diazepam, or barbiturates) (3). The scintigraphic appearance of brain death involves absence of both intracranial arterial and major dural sinus flow. Controversy exists regarding whether faint visualization of the sagittal or transverse sinuses precludes this diagnosis (3). The hot-nose sign described with absent cerebral perfusion represents the shunting of blood from the internal to the external carotid arteries.

Unlike DTPA, pertechnetate, and glucoheptonate, HMPAO is less dependent on bolus injection (3,4).

Cerebral perfusion can be evaluated on static and on flow images because HMPAO normally crosses the blood–brain barrier.

## Aunt Minnie's Pearls

Absent cerebral perfusion can be accompanied by the hot-nose sign.

Nuclear studies are not limited by hypothermia or metabolic disturbance.

**HISTORY:** A 69-year-old woman with a history of lung cancer and increased alkaline phosphatase

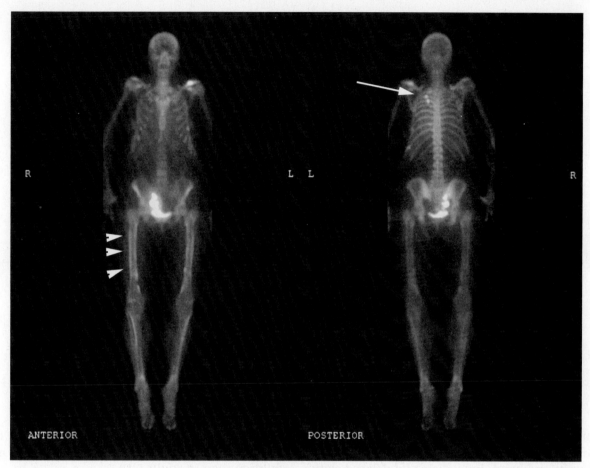

FIGURE 5.3.1

**FINDINGS:** Anterior and posterior whole-body images were obtained 3 hours after the administration of 25 mCi of $^{99m}$Tc methylene diphosphonate (MDP; Fig. 5.3.1). The bone scan demonstrates multiple rib lesions consistent with a history of previous rib fractures; the string-of-pearls sign suggests traumatic injury to the ribs (*arrow*). Increased radiotracer uptake is identified along the cortices of both femurs and tibias bilaterally (*arrowheads*). Notice the uptake within the pelvis by a renal transplant.

**DIAGNOSIS:** Hypertrophic osteoarthropathy (HOA)

**DISCUSSION:** HOA is a syndrome characterized by scintigraphic and radiographic evidence of periosteal new bone formation. Clinically, the patient presents with digital clubbing, long-bone tenderness and pain, increased soft-tissue thickness, or asymmetric, arthritis-like changes within the limb joints (5). Secondary HOA is most commonly associated with an intrathoracic neoplasm (usually a bronchogenic carcinoma) or its metastases (6). The diaphyseal and metaphyseal regions of long bones are normally involved. Characteristically, a periosteal reaction (i.e., periostosis) occurs along the shafts of the femurs, tibias, ulnas, or radii. Skeletal scintigraphy demonstrates a characteristic pattern of uptake referred to as the double-stripe or parallel-track sign (7). This refers to the symmetric, diffuse uptake of radiotracer along the medial and lateral cortices of the long bones. Less commonly involved bones are the patella, scapula, clavicle, and skull.

## Aunt Minnie's Pearls

The double-stripe or parallel-track sign is characteristic of HOA.

HOA is typically seen in lung cancer.

**HISTORY:** A 27-year-old woman with pain in the right hand who recently underwent open reduction and internal fixation of a distal right radial fracture

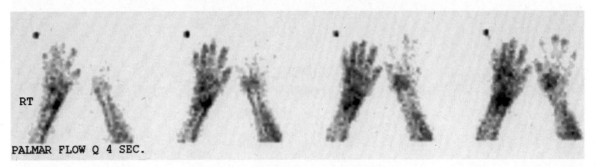

FIGURE 5.4.1

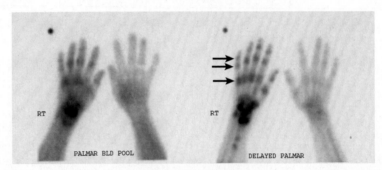

FIGURE 5.4.2

**FINDINGS:** Images from a three-phase bone scan demonstrate increased blood flow (Fig. 5.4.1) to the right wrist and hand. Immediate and delayed static images (Fig. 5.4.2) show diffuse increased bony uptake in a periarticular distribution (*arrows*). The two focal areas of abnormal increased activity in the distal right radius represent the region of fracture and operative fixation.

**DIAGNOSIS:** Reflex sympathetic dystrophy (RSD)

**DISCUSSION:** Patients with RSD (also called *complex regional pain syndrome* or *Sudeck's atrophy*) present clinically with local pain, soft-tissue swelling, and vasomotor instability of the involved extremity. The most common causes of RSD include trauma (often minor), immobilization, infection, myocardial infarction, and neurologic disease (8). Symptoms are thought to occur because of an abnormal sympathetic nervous system response to the traumatic insult (9). The disorder is less common in children than in adults (10).

Radiographically, there is periarticular soft-tissue swelling and regional osteoporosis. Classically, bone scintigraphy demonstrates increased flow and periarticular uptake in the involved extremity, with delayed images being the most sensitive for the diagnosis of reflex sympathetic dystrophy. Radionuclide imaging is not as sensitive in diagnosing this entity if symptoms have been present for >1 year because delayed images may have normal or reduced activity (11).

### Aunt Minnie's Pearl

Increased flow + periarticular uptake + patient with history of trauma and vasomotor instability = RSD.

**HISTORY:** A 69-year-old woman with an increased alkaline phosphatase level

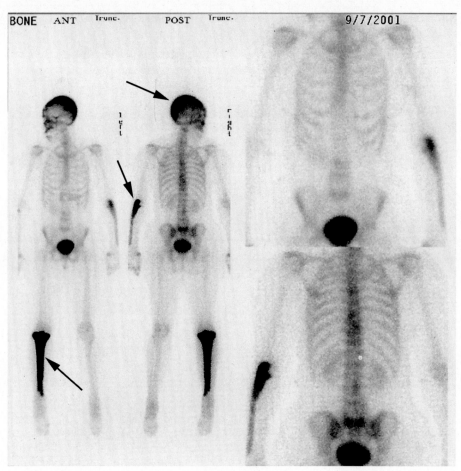

FIGURE 5.5.1

**FINDINGS:** Anterior and posterior whole-body images were obtained 3 hours after the administration of 25 mCi of $^{99m}$Tc-MDP (Fig. 5.5.1). The bone scan demonstrates intensely increased radiotracer uptake within the right tibia, left ulna, and calvarium (*arrows*).

**DIAGNOSIS:** Paget's disease

**DISCUSSION:** Paget's disease is a metabolic disorder of bone that is caused initially by excessive resorption of bone followed by irregular deposition of "new" bone. Its incidence increases with age, and 3% of individuals older than 40 years of age are believed to have the disease (12). It is twice as common in the male population, and many patients are evaluated after an increase in serum alkaline phosphatase is incidentally discovered (13).

Paget's disease can be monostotic or polyostotic and demonstrates intense radiotracer uptake within the bones involved. The characteristic uptake conforms to the shape of the bone that usually appears distorted or enlarged. The intense activity creates the appearance of an expanded cortex. Few other pathologic processes can create as intense a radiotracer uptake as Paget's disease. The pelvis (hemipelvis) is the most commonly involved bone, followed by the spine, femur, skull, tibia, clavicle, and humerus (13).

## Aunt Minnie's Pearls

Extremely intense radiotracer activity that conforms to a distorted bone in a patient that is asymptomatic with increased alkaline phosphatase = Paget's disease.

The most commonly involved bones are the pelvis, spine, skull, femur, scapula, tibia, and humerus.

**HISTORY:** An 8-year-old girl with increased serum calcium and normal parathormone level

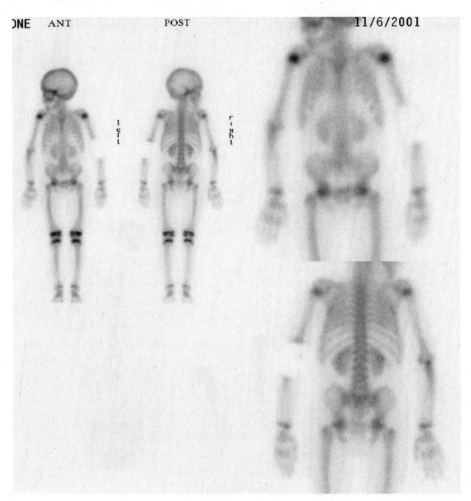

ONE ANT    POST    11/6/2001

left    right

FIGURE 5.6.1

**FINDINGS:** Anterior and posterior whole-body images were obtained 3 hours after the administration of 12.5 mCi of $^{99m}$Tc-MDP (Fig. 5.6.1). The bone scan demonstrates diffuse activity identified within both lungs.

**DIAGNOSIS:** Hypercalcemia

**DISCUSSION:** Diphosphonates are the primary ligands in skeletal scintigraphy. Extraosseous uptake of the bone-scanning agent is not unusual. The literature reports more than 20 causes of extraskeletal uptake (e.g., synovitis, bursitis, hematoma, fat necrosis, myositis ossificans, myocardial infarction, cerebral infarction, splenic infarction, effusion, ascites, edema) (14). When determining the significance of extraosseous uptake, it is important to identify the pattern of the uptake (i.e., focal or diffuse) and the structures involved.

Hypercalcemia causes a characteristic pattern of uptake within the soft tissues. Ordinarily, hypercalcemia produces diffusely increased radiotracer uptake within the lungs or stomach. Although this pattern is typical for hypercalcemia, the underlying cause can sometimes be elusive. Hypercalcemia is most commonly seen in hyperparathyroidism and neoplasms. Two other findings associated with hypercalcemia can be bilateral patellar uptake or diffuse calvarial and spinal uptake, sometimes referred to as the lollypop sign.

## Aunt Minnie's Pearls

Diffuse uptake in the lungs or stomach is typical of hypercalcemia.

Hypercalcemia is most commonly seen in hyperparathyroidism and neoplasms.

**HISTORY:** A 10-week-old infant with cholestatic jaundice

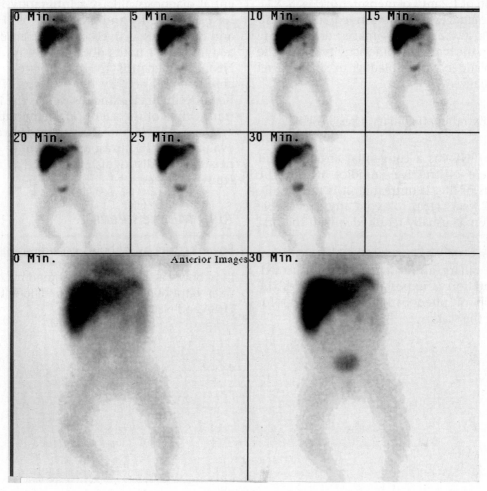

FIGURE 5.7.1

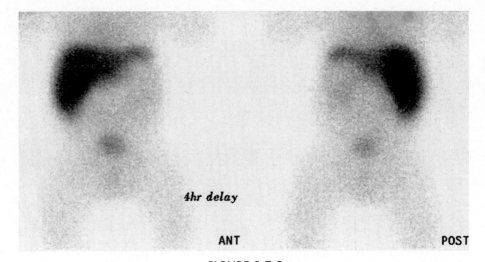

FIGURE 5.7.2

**FINDINGS:** Dynamic images of the upper abdomen were obtained at 5-minute intervals after the administration of 1.2 mCi of mebrofenin (Fig. 5.7.1). Delayed static images were performed at 2, 4, and 24 hours (Fig. 5.7.2). These images demonstrate activity within the liver and some activity within the kidney and bladder. No gallbladder or small-bowel activity is visualized.

**DIAGNOSIS:** Extrahepatic biliary atresia (EHBA)

**DISCUSSION:** EHBA is a congenital anomaly that leads to severe obstructive jaundice within the first 2 months of life. If untreated, it is universally fatal within 2 years (15). To avoid any irreversible damage, surgery is usually required within the first 60 days of life.

Biliary scans are an important diagnostic tool in excluding biliary atresia when it is suspected. Patient preparation is important and involves the administration of phenobarbital (2.5 mg/kg) for 5 days before the scan.

The demonstration of bowel activity by 24 hours effectively excludes biliary atresia from the differential diagnosis. Biliary scintigraphy is reported to have a sensitivity and specificity for EHBA of 88.2% and 88.9%, respectively (16). The absence of bowel activity by 24 hours does not always imply EHBA. Neonatal hepatitis (NH) can rarely demonstrate absent bowel activity by 24 hours. The degree of hepatocellular clearance as well as the hepatobiliary transit time of the agent can help in differentiating between EHBA and NH (16). However, further evaluation with ultrasound or biopsy is sometimes necessary to distinguish between NH and EHBA in equivocal cases.

## Aunt Minnie's Pearls

Bowel activity by 24 hours excludes biliary atresia.

If no bowel activity is demonstrated by 24 hours, consider ultrasound or biopsy to differentiate between EHBA and NH.

**HISTORY:** A 30-year-old black man with cough and hilar adenopathy

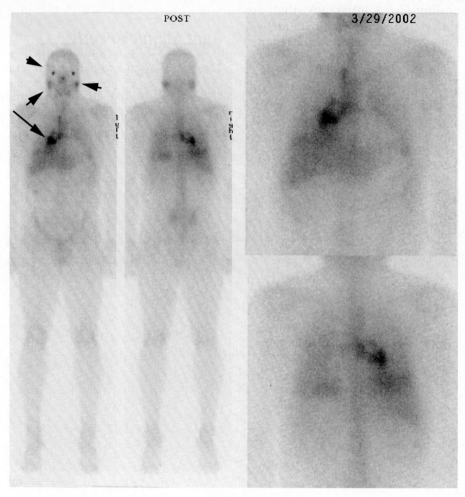

POST                          3/29/2002

left                          right

FIGURE 5.8.1

**FINDINGS:** Anterior and posterior whole-body images were obtained 48 hours after the administration of 8 mCi of gallium citrate (Fig. 5.8.1). These images demonstrate abnormal accumulation of radiotracer within the right paratracheal region and right hilum (*arrow*). Increased activity is visualized within the nasopharyngeal region and in the lacrimal and parotid glands (*arrowheads*). Some mild activity is visualized within the submandibular glands.

**DIAGNOSIS:** Sarcoidosis

**DISCUSSION:** Sarcoidosis is a chronic inflammatory disease that can involve any organ of the body.

Gallium-67 has found favor in the imaging of sarcoidosis because of its avid accumulation at the sites of active disease. To diagnose sarcoidosis, one must combine radiographic and histologic information with the clinical findings. Although a diagnosis of sarcoidosis cannot be made by gallium scan alone, it provides important information to the clinician. It can serve as a guide to appropriate biopsies in patients clinically suspected of having active disease. Gallium scintigraphy is also helpful in distinguishing between active and inactive disease based on the degree of gallium-67 uptake. Gallium-67 is taken up only by active disease and not by fibrosis. It has proved beneficial in following the progression of the disease and assessing its response to therapy.

Findings on gallium-67 scintigraphy that are characteristic for active sarcoidosis are paratracheal uptake with bilateral hilar uptake that is in the shape of the Greek letter lambda. This is known as the "lambda" sign. Prominent gallium-67 uptake in the parotid, lacrimal, and salivary glands bilaterally is referred to as the "panda" sign. This is also commonly seen in patients with active disease.

These two findings, when seen together, are highly specific for sarcoidosis (17).

## Aunt Minnie's Pearls

The lambda sign and panda sign = sarcoidosis.

Gallium-67 is the agent of choice for imaging sarcoidosis.

**HISTORY:** A 41-year-old woman with hypercalcemia and increased parathormone

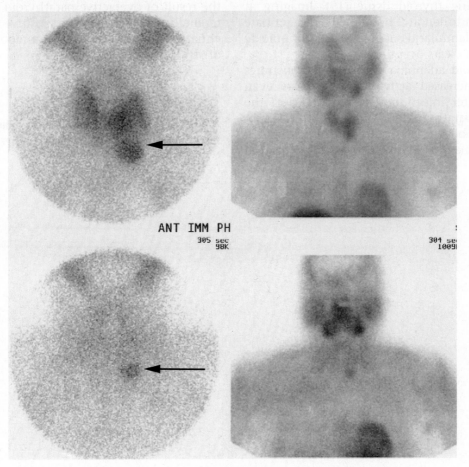

ANT IMM PH
305 sec
98K

304 sec
1009

FIGURE 5.9.1

**FINDINGS:** Anterior and anterior oblique images of the thyroid were obtained at 20 minutes after the administration of 20 mCi of $^{99m}$Tc-sestamibi (Fig. 5.9.1, *upper images*). These images demonstrate a focal area of increased radiotracer accumulation in the region of the left inferior pole of the thyroid gland (*arrow*). Anterior and anterior oblique images of the neck were obtained 2 hours after injection (Fig. 5.9.1, *lower images*) and demonstrate persistence of activity at the inferior pole of the left lobe of the thyroid while the remainder of the gland washes out (*arrow*).

**DIAGNOSIS:** Left inferior pole parathyroid adenoma

**DISCUSSION:** Parathyroid adenomas are responsible for primary hyperparathyroidism approximately 85% of the time (18). As many as 10% of these adenomas are ectopic (18). Surgery is the optimal treatment, for which accurate localization is essential. $^{99m}$Tc-sestamibi is commonly used in the evaluation of parathyroid adenomas. Sestamibi localizes to mitochondria, which is found in greater concentrations in overactive parathyroid tissue than in the normal thyroid. There is consequently slower washout of sestamibi from adenomas and hyperplastic parathyroid glands as compared with the surrounding thyroid tissue (19). Imaging at 20 minutes and then at 2 hours helps differentiate between the glandular tissues based on how quickly the radiotracer clears over time.

A parathyroid adenoma typically demonstrates a focus of increased activity that persists even at 2 hours after injection. The remainder of the thyroid and parathyroid should wash out. A subtraction method is also commonly employed in parathyroid imaging. With this method, a thyroid agent (e.g., pertechnetate) is subtracted from a sestamibi or thallium scan. Persistent activity is likely the result of overactive parathyroid tissue. The latter method is slightly more sensitive than the differential washout method, with a reported sensitivity of 90% (20).

## Aunt Minnie's Pearl

A focal hot spot that persists with delayed washout of sestamibi is characteristic of a parathyroid adenoma.

# Case 5.10

HISTORY: An infant with hypothyroidism

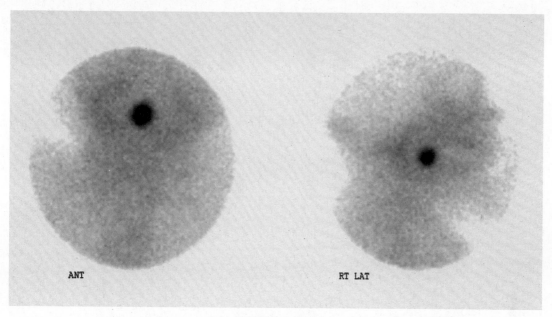

FIGURE 5.10.1

FINDINGS: A focal area of increased activity is present in the midline in the region of the tongue base on anteroposterior (*ANT*) and right lateral (*RT LAT*) views from a $^{99m}$Tc-pertechnetate thyroid scan (Fig. 5.10.1). No activity is seen in the thyroid bed.

DIAGNOSIS: Lingual thyroid

DISCUSSION: Lingual thyroid results from failure of the thyroid gland to descend during embryogenesis. The ectopic gland is typically hypofunctional. Hypothyroidism associated with ectopic thyroid tissue occurs sporadically, whereas hypothyroidism from biosynthetic defects is inherited (21).

In addition to hypothyroidism, the lingual thyroid may present as a mass in the tongue or upper neck. This abnormality must be diagnosed shortly after birth because failure to promptly begin replacement therapy adversely affects intellectual development.

## Aunt Minnie's Pearls

An ectopic or lingual thyroid is typically hypofunctional.

Screening for hypothyroidism is routine in newborns because failure to diagnose hypothyroidism may result in severe intellectual impairment.

HISTORY: A 40-year-old woman with hypertension refractory to medical therapy

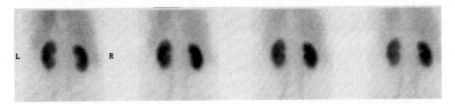

FIGURE 5.11.1

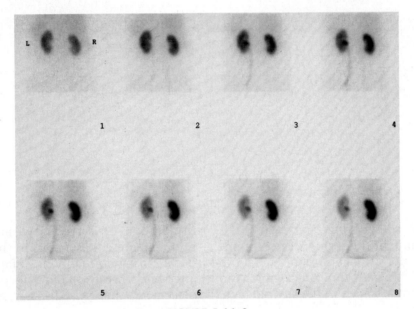

FIGURE 5.11.2

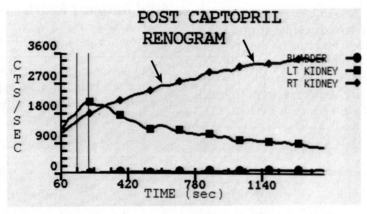

FIGURE 5.11.3

**FINDINGS:** Images acquired during a precaptopril $^{99m}$Tc-MAG3 renogram (Fig. 5.11.1) demonstrate slightly increased cortical activity retention in the right kidney. After captopril administration (Fig. 5.11.2), this asymmetry becomes pronounced. Right renal cortical activity retention is significant, and excretion of radiopharmaceutical into the collecting system is minimal. The abnormal response of the right kidney to captopril administration is also demonstrated on a time-activity curve of the renogram (Fig. 5.11.3, *arrows*).

**DIAGNOSIS:** Right renovascular hypertension

**DISCUSSION:** Renovascular hypertension is caused by hypoperfusion-induced stimulation of the renin–angiotensin system. It accounts for approximately 1% to 2% of all hypertensive patients (22). The most common causes of renal hypoperfusion are atherosclerosis and fibromuscular dysplasia. The involved kidney maintains glomerular filtration rate by compensatory vasoconstriction of the efferent arteriole by angiotensin II, the end product of the renin–angiotensin system. Captopril, an inhibitor of angiotensin-converting enzyme, prevents efferent arteriole constriction. If a hemodynamically significant lesion of the renal artery is present, the glomerular filtration rate will drop on administration of captopril compared with the precaptopril examination. Scintigraphically, this difference is seen as delayed radiotracer uptake and cortical retention (23).

### Aunt Minnie's Pearls

Renovascular hypertension is mediated by the renin–angiotensin system.

After captopril administration, delayed radiotracer uptake and cortical retention are seen in the affected kidney.

HISTORY: A decreased urine output after renal transplantation

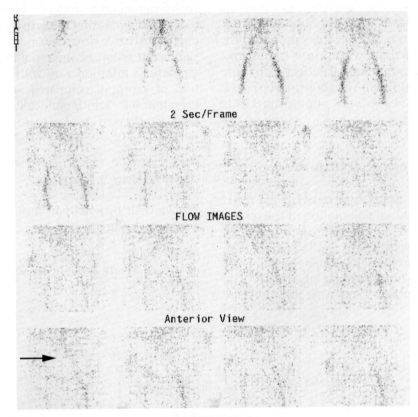

FIGURE 5.12.1

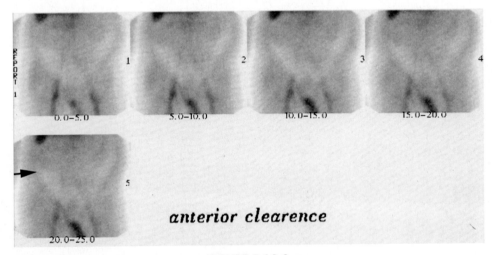

FIGURE 5.12.2

**FINDINGS:** Dynamic flow images of the lower abdomen and pelvis were obtained at 2-second-per-frame intervals after the intravenous administration of 8 mCi of $^{99m}$Tc-mertiatide (Fig. 5.12.1). These images demonstrate no flow of radiotracer to the renal transplant (*arrow*).

Dynamic clearance images reveal no uptake or excretion of the radiotracer (Fig. 5.12.2). Rather, a photopenic region (*arrow*) is visualized within the right anterior iliac fossa where the renal transplant is presumably located.

**DIAGNOSIS:** Vascular obstruction (i.e., renal artery obstruction)

**DISCUSSION:** Renal scintigraphy is valuable in the evaluation of complications associated with renal transplantation. In the immediate postoperative period (<1 week), a number of problems can occur, including hyperacute rejection, accelerated rejection, renal vein thrombosis (RVT), renal artery thrombosis (RAT), urinary leak, edema, and a hematoma. RAT and RVT are likely the result of surgical complications. The renal allograft contains no venous collaterals. A thrombus in the renal vein can result in an outflow obstruction that leads to increased impedance and ultimately to arterial compromise. RVT and RAT have the same clinical significance and can appear similar with scintigraphic examination (24).

In vascular obstruction, there is no flow, uptake, or excretion of the radiotracer, causing a photopenic defect within the expected location of the renal transplant. The defect is enhanced by normal background activity.

Hyperacute rejection would look similar, although this diagnosis is usually made in the operating room. In hyperacute rejection, preformed antibodies attack the transplanted kidney, causing vascular compromise and inhibiting flow to the kidney. The kidney turns blue immediately in the operating room.

## Aunt Minnie's Pearls

No flow, no uptake, and no excretion in the immediate postoperative period = vascular occlusion.

RAT and RVT look similar scintigraphically.

HISTORY: A 39-year-old man with an acute onset of chest pain and dyspnea

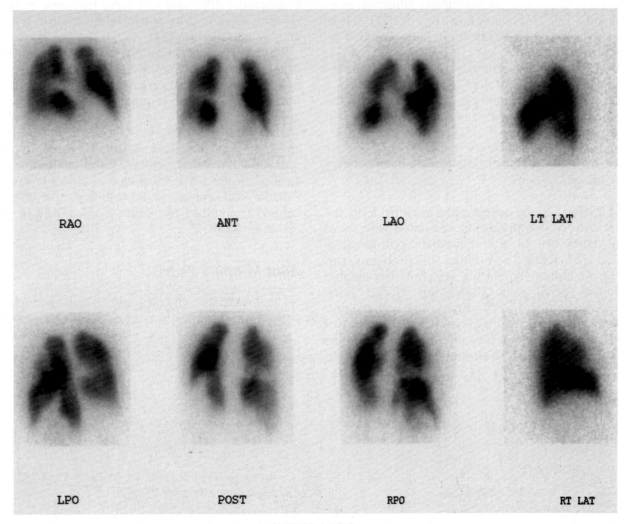

RAO     ANT     LAO     LT LAT

LPO     POST     RPO     RT LAT

FIGURE 5.13.1

FINDINGS: Pulmonary perfusion images obtained after injection of $^{99m}$Tc-MAA (Fig. 5.13.1) reveal multiple, segmental perfusion defects. Posterior ventilation images using xenon-133 ($^{133}$Xe; Fig. 5.13.2) demonstrate normal ventilation during first breath, equilibrium, and washout images.

DIAGNOSIS: Multiple pulmonary emboli

DISCUSSION: Pulmonary embolic disease is typically a sequela of deep venous thrombosis. Patients can present with a multitude of nonspecific findings, including pleuritic chest pain, hemoptysis, dyspnea, hypoxia, and tachypnea. Radiographic analysis is often nonspecific, with findings including a normal chest, atelectasis, and small pleural effusion. Less commonly, focal oligemia (i.e., Westermark sign), pulmonary artery enlargement, or a pleural-based, wedge-shaped density indicative of pulmonary infarction (i.e., Hampton's hump) can be seen.

If multiple (2) segmental ventilation–perfusion mismatches are identified in areas where there is no corresponding chest radiographic abnormality, pulmonary embolism is diagnosed with high probability

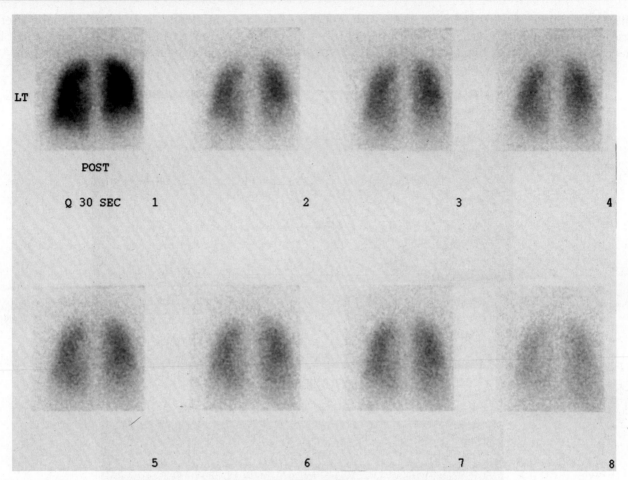

LT

POST

Q 30 SEC   1          2          3          4

5          6          7          8

FIGURE 5.13.2

in all classification schemes. In rare cases, vasculitides can produce a similar pattern with segmental mismatches in several lobes of the lung, but the patient's clinical presentation and medical history should allow accurate diagnosis of these patients. Prospective investigation of pulmonary embolism diagnosis (PIOPED) investigators have updated diagnostic criteria for probability of pulmonary embolus (25), and this source offers further discussion.

## Aunt Minnie's Pearl

If multiple (2) segmental ventilation–perfusion mismatches are identified in areas where there is no corresponding chest radiographic abnormality, pulmonary embolism is diagnosed with high probability in all classification schemes.

HISTORY: Patient A: A 62-year-old male with hypertension, hyperlipidemia, and mild coronary artery disease presenting with exertional chest pain, mild shortness of breath, and occasional palpitations. Patient B: A 49-year-old male with hypertension, diabetes, hyperlipidemia, and obesity presenting with chest pain

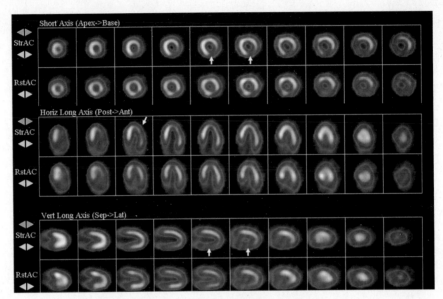

FIGURE 5.14.1

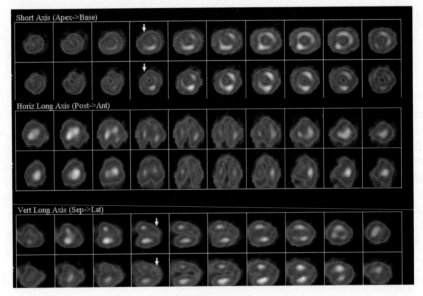

FIGURE 5.14.2

**FINDINGS:** Both patients underwent $^{99m}$Tc-sestamibi myocardial perfusion imaging with single-photon emission computed tomography (SPECT). In patient A (Fig. 5.14.1), a reversible perfusion defect involves the mid inferolateral wall (*arrows*). In patient B (Fig. 5.14.2), images reveal a fixed perfusion defect involving the apical anteroseptal region (*arrows*).

**DIAGNOSIS:** Myocardial ischemia (patient A) and infarct (patient B)

**DISCUSSION:** The three most commonly used radiopharmaceuticals for myocardial perfusion imaging are $^{99m}$Tc-sestamibi, $^{99m}$Tc-tetrofosmin, and $^{201}$Tl-chloride. $^{99m}$Tc-sestamibi is a lipophilic cation that localizes passively within the mitochondria because of a large negative transmembrane potential. Its extraction fraction is lower than that of the other agents; however, myocardial uptake is similar. Compared with $^{201}$Tl-chloride, no significant redistribution occurs. $^{99m}$Tc-tetrofosmin is similar to $^{99m}$Tc-sestamibi and has prompt myocardial uptake and rapid clearance, from the liver in particular, thus reducing artifacts from the surrounding organs. Furthermore, no significant redistribution occurs (26). $^{99m}$Tc-sestamibi and $^{99m}$Tc-tetrofosmin are newer agents and now used more frequently than $^{201}$Tl-chloride secondary to higher count rates and superior images. There is also less total radiation dose to the patient with these agents compared with $^{201}$Tl-chloride.

Radioisotope $^{201}$Tl-chloride is a potassium analog that localizes by active transport across the cell membrane. Its distribution results from initial myocardial uptake and subsequent equilibration with the blood pool. Approximately 5% of the administered dose localizes within the myocardium, with approximately 88% of the agent being extracted on the first pass (27). Myocardial perfusion imaging assesses the blood flow to the myocardial tissue. Studies are performed under resting and stress conditions. Stress may be produced mechanically, such as through exercise or by pharmacologic means (e.g., dipyridamole or adenosine, both potent vasodilators, as well as dobutamine). Areas of ischemia demonstrate a region of relatively decreased activity on poststress images, which improves on rest and redistribution images. Nonreversible abnormalities represent areas of acute or remote myocardial infarction. A third pattern of abnormal activity, known as reverse redistribution (more common with thallium), appears as relatively diminished activity on rest or redistribution images and normal on stress images. The cause of reverse redistribution is unknown, but this finding may correlate with myocardial ischemia in some patients.

Some cardiac lesions can produce positive stress tests in the absence of coronary artery disease. These lesions include mitral valve prolapse, valvular aortic stenosis, aortic regurgitation, left bundle branch block, idiopathic hypertrophic subaortic stenosis, cardiomyopathy, and hypertensive myocardial hypertrophy. Specific areas of artifact include the apex with aortic regurgitation and the septum with left bundle branch block. In idiopathic hypertrophic subaortic stenosis and hypertensive myocardial hypertrophy, increased count density in the region of the septum produces a relative decrease in the lateral wall, which can be mistaken for infarction (28).

## Aunt Minnie's Pearls

Ischemia = reversible perfusion defect.

Infarct = fixed perfusion defect.

**HISTORY:** Patient A: A 58-year-old white male with diabetes, hypertension, hyperlipidemia, and known coronary artery disease with past anterior wall myocardial infarction. Patient underwent follow-up myocardial perfusion imaging showing anteroapical scar with mild improvement of perfusion on resting images, suggesting peri-infarct ischemia. Patient denied repeat left heart catheterization and opted for nuclear viability study to assess potential benefit of revascularization. Patient B: A 66-year-old black male with hypertension, diabetes, hyperlipidemia, and multiple prior myocardial infarctions with recent chest pain and myocardial perfusion test showing inferior scar with possible peri-infarct ischemia

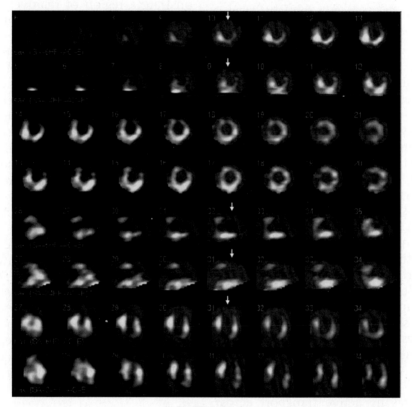

FIGURE 5.15.1

**FINDINGS:** Both patients underwent thallium ($^{201}$Tl-chloride) viability scanning with SPECT. In patient A (Fig. 5.15.1), there is viability present in the inferior, lateral, and septal walls, with extensive scar involving the anterior wall and apex (*arrows*). No improvement of the anteroapical region is seen on the 24-hour delay images, which indicates no peri-infarct ischemia—only scar tissue. In patient B (Fig. 5.15.2), viability is present throughout the myocardium with hibernating myocardium seen in the inferior wall (*arrows*) indicated by improvement of inferior wall images on 24-hour delay scan.

**DIAGNOSIS:** Anterior wall scar (Patient A) and hibernating inferior wall myocardium (Patient B)

**DISCUSSION:** Viability scanning can distinguish fixed perfusion defects seen on myocardial perfusion imaging caused by scar tissue from fixed perfusion defects caused by viable but nonfunctional myocardium such as that seen in hibernating myocardium. Hibernating myocardium is a chronic process where prolonged hypoperfusion of the myocardium secondary to significant coronary artery stenosis results in reduced cellular metabolism that does not allow normal contractility but is enough to sustain viability of the involved tissue. It is important to distinguish viable from nonviable myocardium when revascularization is being considered to restore perfusion to the affected myocardium. Revascularization of viable, hibernating myocardium can restore left ventricular function to the affected area of myocardium. However, in cases of nonviable myocardium, revascularization will not improve function of the affected myocardium. Viability scanning with $^{201}$Tl-chloride or FDG-18 PET can reveal a significant

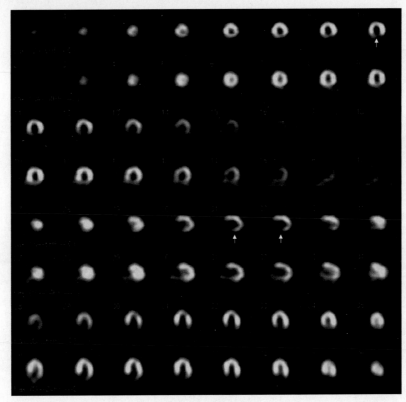

FIGURE 5.15.2

number of fixed defects to contain viable myocardium that can benefit from revascularization. Thallium viability protocols involve intravenous injection of approximately 3 mCi of $^{201}$Tl-chloride and performance of SPECT imaging approximately 15 minutes later, which provides images reflecting regional blood flow to the myocardium. Redistribution images are then obtained approximately 24 hours later (8–28 hours later) that depict viability of the myocardium. Redistribution of thallium usually begins within 4 hours but may take longer in cases of severe ischemia. Improvement of images on redistribution scan has a good positive predictive value for identifying areas of myocardium that will benefit from revascularization. The negative predictive value is not as high secondary to poor count rates. However, after the redistribution scan, a smaller dose of thallium can be reinjected, and repeat images can be obtained. Improved uptake on these repeat images also predicts improvement of function following revascularization. Persistence of a defect on these reinjection repeat images signifies a low likelihood for revascularization benefit.

FDG-18 PET scanning combined with perfusion imaging can also differentiate fixed defects owing to scar versus fixed defects resulting from viable, hibernating myocardium. Under normal conditions, fatty acids are the preferred energy substrate of the myocardium. During ischemia or high serum glucose levels, glucose becomes the predominant energy substrate. To promote glucose uptake into the heart, glucose loading is performed prior to FDG-18 infusion for viability imaging. Once euglycemia is obtained, FDG-18 is injected and scanning is performed approximately 45 minutes later. Normal subjects will have matched perfusion and FDG-18 uptake. A perfusion defect matched with decreased FDG-18 uptake indicates scar tissue. The combination of decreased perfusion with increased FDG-18 uptake indicates hibernating or severely ischemic myocardium.

## Aunt Minnie's Pearls

Viable myocardium = *Thallium*: Normal 6- and 24-hour rest images, or improvement of images on 24-hour scan (hibernating, viable myocardium). *PET FDG-18*: Perfusion defect with increased PET FDG-18 uptake (perfusion/FDG mismatch).

Nonviable myocardium = *Thallium*: Abnormal 6-hour thallium rest images with no improvement on 24-hour rest thallium scan. *PET FDG-18*: Matched perfusion and FDG-18 defects.

HISTORY: A 78-year-old man with bright red blood per rectum

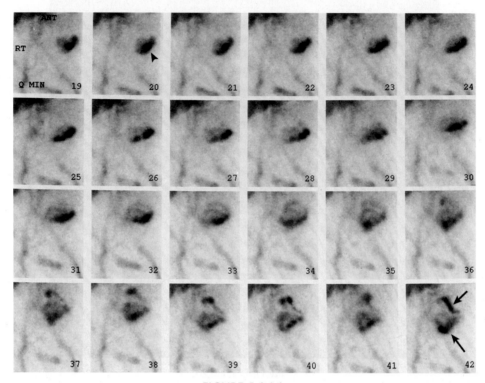

FIGURE 5.16.1

FINDINGS: Dynamic images obtained during a $^{99m}$Tc-labeled red blood cell scan (Fig. 5.16.1) reveal an abnormal focus of activity in the left lower quadrant (*arrowhead*). Activity migrated through small bowel loops during the examination (*arrows*).

DIAGNOSIS: Gastrointestinal bleeding

DISCUSSION: The principal use of the $^{99m}$Tc-labeled red blood cell scan has been in the evaluation of patients with active but not life-threatening lower gastrointestinal bleeding. This study is helpful in the detection and localization of the bleeding site. The use of this test is limited in the evaluation of upper gastrointestinal bleeding, for which fiberoptic endoscopy is more appropriate. Bleeding rates as low as 0.1 to 0.2 mL/min can be detected with $^{99m}$Tc-labeled red blood cell scintigraphy compared with 0.5 to 1.0 mL/min with angiography (29). An additional benefit is its ability to detect intermittent bleeding for up to 24 hours.

Gastrointestinal bleeding is seen as a focal area of progressively increasing activity that migrates with time as a result of bowel peristalsis. Vascular lesions that are not actively bleeding can also be detected on the flow phase. The most common causes of lower gastrointestinal bleeding include diverticulosis, neoplasia, angiodysplasia, and enterocolitis. Many diagnostic pitfalls have been identified. The more common causes are gastrointestinal activity attributable to free pertechnetate or genitourinary activity, including ectopic kidney, activity in the renal pelvis, ureter, or bladder, and genital blush (30). None of these possibilities will produce migration of activity in the bowel as seen in the index case.

## Aunt Minnie's Pearl

Focal $^{99m}$Tc-labeled red blood cell activity that migrates along the expected course of the bowel represents active gastrointestinal bleeding.

HISTORY: A 14-year-old Hispanic male with a 3-day history of crampy abdominal pain and hematochezia

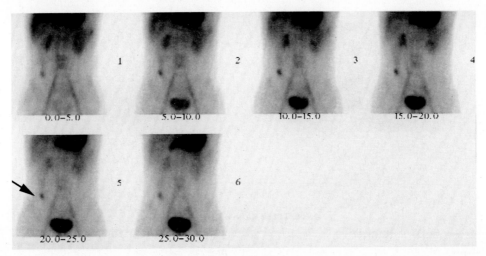

FIGURE 5.17.1

FINDINGS: Dynamic images of the abdomen were obtained at 5-minutes-per-frame intervals after the intravenous administration of 10 mCi of $^{99m}$Tc-labeled sodium pertechnetate (Fig. 5.17.1). These images reveal a focal hot spot within the right lower quadrant and normal physiologic excretion from the gastric mucosa (*arrow*).

DIAGNOSIS: Meckel's diverticulum

DISCUSSION: A Meckel's diverticulum is the vestigial remnant of the omphalomesenteric duct that is typically found within the terminal ileum. It is the most common gastrointestinal malformation, occurring in approximately 2% of the population (31). This anomaly is twice as common in the male population and generally occurs within the first 2 years of life.

The ability of $^{99m}$Tc-pertechnetate to identify this abnormality is based on the presence of ectopic gastric mucosa within the diverticulum.

The mucus-secreting cells trap pertechnetate in the same manner as normal gastric mucosa. Ulceration caused by the secretion of hydrochloric acid and pepsin from the mucosal cells ultimately results in a gastrointestinal bleed. This explains why 95% to 98% of patients with rectal bleeding are found to have ectopic gastric mucosa (32). Causes of false-positive examinations include arteriovenous malformation (AVM), intussusception, appendicitis, neoplasms, and inflammatory bowel disease (33,34).

## Aunt Minnie's Pearls

Pertechnetate scans are very sensitive for Meckel's diverticulum. Given the right clinical symptoms, they can be fairly specific as well.

Watch out for the false positives of AVM, intussusception, appendicitis, neoplasms, and inflammatory bowel disease.

HISTORY: A 13-year-old boy with a thyroid nodule discovered by physical examination

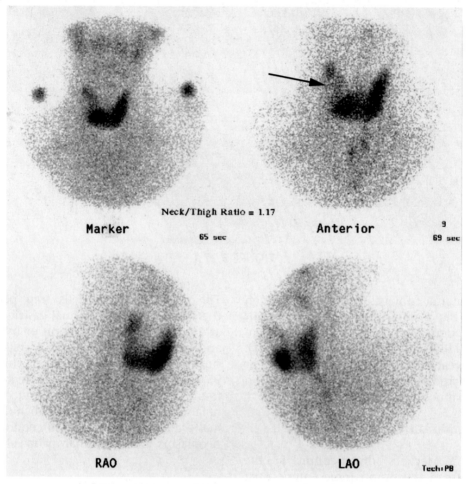

FIGURE 5.18.1

FINDINGS: Anterior and oblique pinhole images of the neck were obtained approximately 20 minutes after the administration of 15 mCi of $^{99m}$Tc-labeled sodium pertechnetate (Fig. 5.18.1). A dominant photopenic defect (*arrow*) is visualized within the superior pole of the right lobe of the thyroid gland.

DIAGNOSIS: Thyroid cancer

DISCUSSION: Although thyroid cancer typically presents as a photopenic defect or "cold nodule," most cold nodules are benign. However, as many as 25% of these cold nodules contain cancer, and further evaluation with fine-needle aspiration should be performed (35). Factors that increase the likelihood of cancer are young patients, male sex, and patients with a history of irradiation to the neck. Typically, thyroid cancers are hard to palpation and do not respond to suppression therapy.

Pertechnetate or radioiodine can be used initially to evaluate for cancer. The difference between the agents is that pertechnetate is concentrated by the thyroid and then washes out (i.e., trapped), whereas iodine-123 ($^{123}$I) is organified and remains within the thyroid. A photopenic defect is caused from a relative decrease in functioning tissue within the lesion. However, a nonfunctioning nodule can demonstrate increased uptake on pertechnetate scans in a small percentage of cancers. This leads to what is known as a discordant nodule, one that is "hot" with pertechnetate but is cold with [123]I. Hyperfunctioning nodules that demonstrate concordant findings with pertechnetate and [123]I imaging show focally increased activity and have less than 1% chance of harboring cancer (35).

### Aunt Minnie's Pearl

Cold nodules, especially in patients who are male, young, or have a history of irradiation to the neck, require further evaluation.

**HISTORY:** Two different patients treated for papillary thyroid cancer

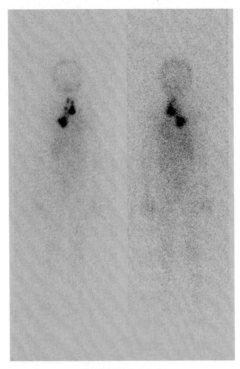

FIGURE 5.19.1

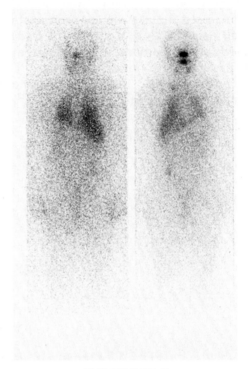

FIGURE 5.19.2

**FINDINGS:** Anterior and posterior whole-body views (Fig. 5.19.1) obtained 12 days after treatment demonstrate focal abnormal radioactivity in the neck and right upper lung.

Anterior and posterior whole-body views (Fig. 5.19.2) obtained 10 days after treatment demonstrate increased radiotracer uptake in the lungs. Physiologic radioactivity is present in the salivary glands and nasopharynx.

**DIAGNOSIS:** Thyroid carcinoma with neck lymph nodes and pulmonary metastases

**DISCUSSION:** Thyroid cancer is categorized into four major histologic types: papillary, follicular, medullary, and anaplastic. After a total thyroidectomy, radioiodine concentrates in follicular carcinoma and, to a variable degree, in papillary carcinoma. Medullary and anaplastic carcinomas do not concentrate radioiodine. Papillary carcinoma is the most common type; 30% to 55% of patients with

papillary carcinoma have local nodal metastases at the time of initial surgery. Follicular carcinoma constitutes 20% to 25% of thyroid cancers and spreads hematogenously.

Medullary carcinoma, which causes elevated serum calcitonin levels, may be found in the setting of multiple endocrine neoplasia syndromes types 2A and 2B. Approximately 50% of patients with medullary carcinoma have metastatic disease at the time of diagnosis. Anaplastic carcinomas constitute approximately 10% of thyroid cancers, and prognosis with this type of tumor is dismal (36,37). Recurrent disease is detected by monitoring thyroglobulin levels, $^{131}$I imaging, supplemented with anatomic imaging. A PET scan is also utilized, especially in evaluation of patients with non-iodine avid tumors (38).

Preparation for whole-body imaging requires withdrawal of thyroid hormone therapy for 2 to 4 weeks to allow maximal stimulation by endogenous thyroid-stimulating hormone (TSH). Use of recombinant TSH is more comfortable for patient hypothyroid preparation. Placing the patient on a low-iodide diet for the final 2 weeks is helpful in decreasing the body's iodide pool and thereby enhancing uptake of radioactive iodide. Recent TSH and thyroglobulin levels should be reviewed immediately before the patient is dosed for the total-body $^{131}$I study. Post-radioiodine treatment scan is always obtained to visualize additional foci of cancer that were not seen on 4 mCi scans.

## Aunt Minnie's Pearls

Radioiodine concentration occurs in follicular and variably in papillary carcinoma; medullary and anaplastic carcinomas do not take up radioiodine.

Inadequate endogenous TSH stimulation may result in poor tracer uptake and false-negative studies.

**HISTORY:** A 27-year-old woman with acute shortness of breath and chest pain

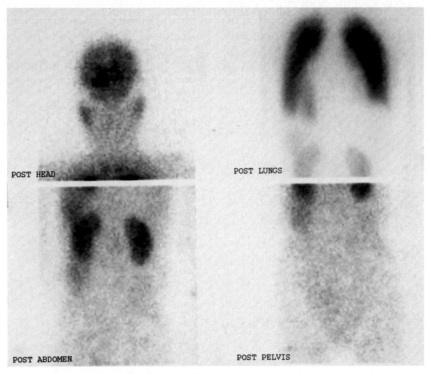

FIGURE 5.20.1

**FINDINGS:** After administration of $^{99m}$Tc-MAA to the patient, abnormal uptake is identified within the brain and kidneys (Fig. 5.20.1). Normal uptake is seen in the lungs, and the heart is markedly enlarged.

**DIAGNOSIS:** Right-to-left shunt

**DISCUSSION:** Right-to-left shunting is demonstrated by systemic embolization of $^{99m}$Tc-MAA particles as part of a pulmonary perfusion study or shunt evaluation. Normally, first-pass pulmonary uptake of $^{99m}$Tc-MAA is nearly complete because only 4% of the administered dose undergoes physiologic shunting. This small amount of physiologic shunting usually is not visually detectable (39).

Particle embolization secondary to cardiac or pulmonary shunts is most often seen in the kidneys, brain, extremities, and thyroid. Brain and extremity uptake is definitive evidence of right-to-left shunting. Care must be taken in attributing thyroid and renal uptake to a shunt because thyroid and kidney activity may be seen if free pertechnetate is present. Normal renal excretion of the radiotracer occurs as $^{99m}$Tc-MAA is metabolized (39).

## Aunt Minnie's Pearl

Brain and extremity uptake is definitive evidence of a right-to-left shunt.

**HISTORY:** A young black woman with a history of a hemolytic anemia

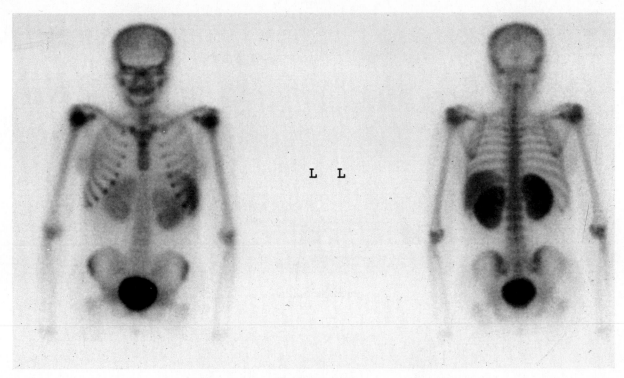

L L

FIGURE 5.21.1

**FINDINGS:** Anterior and posterior images from a whole-body bone scan (Fig. 5.21.1) reveal marked radionuclide uptake in the spleen and kidneys. The spleen appears small, whereas the kidneys are enlarged. Increased activity in the humeral heads is also identified.

**DIAGNOSIS:** Sickle cell disease

**DISCUSSION:** Sickle cell disease is a homozygous hereditary anemia that occurs because of chromosomal defect in the beta-hemoglobin chain. Red blood cells form into an abnormal sickle shape in response to low oxygen tension. Because of their abnormal shape, the sickled cells cause small-vessel occlusions that result in tissue infarction and pain crises. The spleen is usually severely affected in older patients with sickle cell disease, and the repeated infarcts lead to dystrophic calcium deposition in the organ. A characteristic appearance of a small,

densely calcified spleen can be discovered on bone scans and on radiographs or CT. Other findings on bone scan include increased or decreased activity in areas of bony infarction and increased activity in the diaphyses of the long bones caused by bone marrow expansion. The kidneys may be slightly enlarged and demonstrate increased activity, as in the index case. The cause for the abnormality in the kidneys is not completely understood, but it does not appear to correlate with altered clinical renal function (40).

## Aunt Minnie's Pearls

Markedly increased activity in a small spleen on bone scintigraphy = sickle cell disease.

Look for bone infarcts or for increased activity in the long bone diaphyses from bone marrow expansion.

HISTORY: Noncontributory

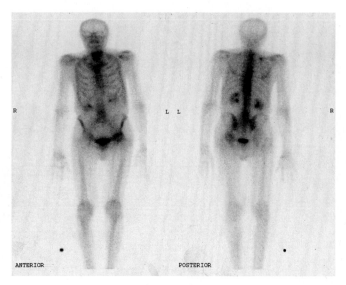

FIGURE 5.22.1

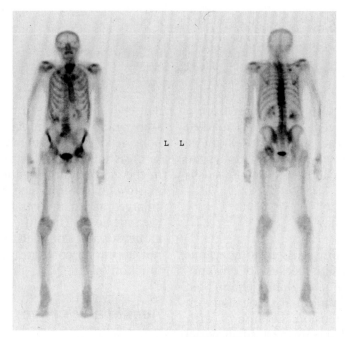

FIGURE 5.22.2

FINDINGS: The initial whole-body bone scan image (Fig. 5.22.1) demonstrates poor detail and contrast; notice the sharpness of the cobalt side marker. After technical adjustments, the repeat whole-body bone scan image (Fig. 5.22.2) shows improved detail and contrast and less soft-tissue activity.

DIAGNOSIS: Off-peak imaging with window set at the energy of the cobalt-57 (122 keV) side marker

DISCUSSION: Peaking the gamma camera is a process that involves appropriately centering the camera's single-channel analyzer windows to the radionuclide in use. Although the camera may have an automatic peaking feature, the technologist should always view the spectral display of the radionuclide being imaged to ensure that the correct energy window is selected and that it is centered on the radionuclide of interest. Off-peak imaging results from incorrect energy window selection. If the window is centered too high, available photons are excluded. If centered too low, the images contain increased amounts of scatter, which may be evident in increased visualization of soft-tissue activity. Nonuniformity also affects the response of the photomultiplier tubes, which may result in geometric hot and cold regions in the image, which correspond to the location of photomultiplier tubes (41). The camera should be peaked daily and should be on any switch to a different radionuclide (42). In the index case, the radiologist correctly identified the problem by noticing the poor resolution of the image, increased soft-tissue activity, and unusually sharp image of the cobalt marker.

## Aunt Minnie's Pearls

Off-peak imaging = incorrect energy window selection.

Peak the gamma camera daily and whenever a different radionuclide is used.

HISTORY: Quality control

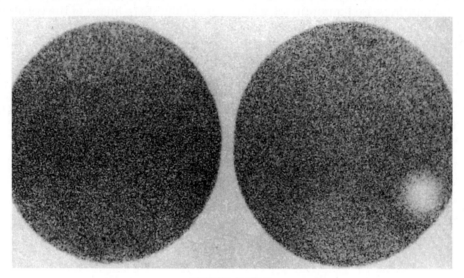

FIGURE 5.23.1

FINDINGS: Two ⁹⁹ᵐTc-pertechnetate flood-field images are submitted (Fig. 5.23.1). Image on the left demonstrates normal uniformity. The image on the right is from the same camera with a nonfunctioning photomultiplier tube.

DIAGNOSIS: Nonfunctioning photomultiplier tube

DISCUSSION: Field uniformity represents the ability of an imaging system to provide a uniform image across the entire crystal face. A properly functioning camera produces a homogeneous flood-field image or, at most, mild heterogeneity with areas of slightly increased activity corresponding to photomultiplier tubes. Drift or nonfunction of a photomultiplier tube shows as an area of decreased activity on clinical or flood-field images (43). Field uniformity is assessed daily by utilizing test images obtained with a point source or flood-field source of radioactivity; technetium or cobalt sources are commonly used. Intrinsic flood tests are performed without the collimator in place, and extrinsic flood images are obtained with the collimator attached. When the collimator is in place, only sheet sources can be used. It is important to have a general idea of how many counts are necessary to achieve a good flood image with the camera. The values needed range from a few million counts for standard cameras to >100 million counts for SPECT cameras.

## Aunt Minnie's Pearl

Field uniformity must be assessed daily.

**HISTORY:** A 56-year-old woman with dyspnea

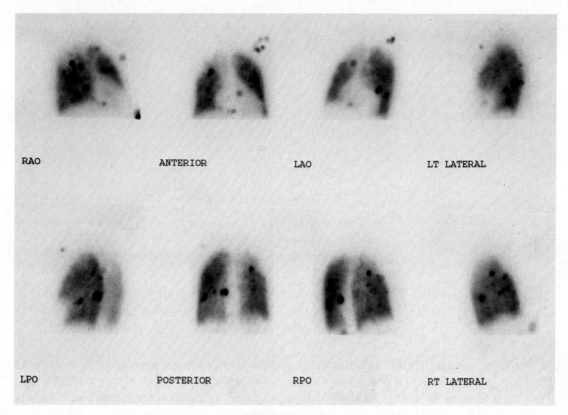

FIGURE 5.24.1

**FINDINGS:** A $^{99m}$Tc pulmonary perfusion study (Fig. 5.24.1) shows multiple abnormal foci of increased activity in both lungs.

**DIAGNOSIS:** Aggregated $^{99m}$Tc-MAA

**DISCUSSION:** Pulmonary perfusion imaging depends on capillary blockade. If blood is withdrawn into the syringe containing $^{99m}$Tc-MAA and is allowed to coagulate, the radiolabeled compound will aggregate within blood clots. Aggregation can also occur if the syringe is not agitated before injection.

The injected radiolabeled clots obstruct vessels corresponding to the size of the clot and appear as hot spots on images. The large concentrations of activity incorporated into the clots may result in a statistically significant reduction in counts to the other areas of the lung, possibly resulting in missed abnormalities (44).

## Aunt Minnie's Pearl

Aggregated $^{99m}$Tc-MAA shows up as hot spots on pulmonary perfusion imaging.

HISTORY: Noncontributory

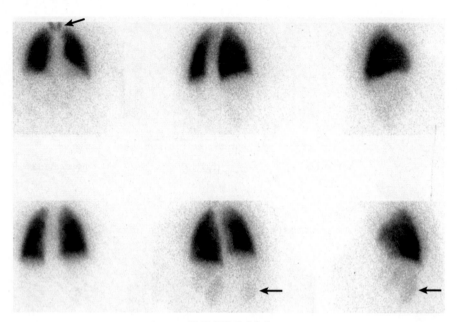

FIGURE 5.25.1

FINDINGS: Multiple images from a pulmonary perfusion study (Fig. 5.25.1) reveal normal pulmonary perfusion. However, unexpected activity is seen in the thyroid gland and faintly in the kidneys (*arrows*). A lateral static view of the head shows scalp and facial soft-tissue activity but no brain activity. This differentiates this diagnosis from the one shown in Case 5.20.

DIAGNOSIS: Radiochemical impurity; image reveals the presence of free pertechnetate

DISCUSSION: Radiochemical impurity exists when a portion of the radionuclide being imaged is in an undesired chemical form. The most common radiochemical impurity encountered in clinical practice is free pertechnetate. This impurity forms when oxygen or water is inadvertently allowed to mix with the contents of the radiopharmaceutical kit. Stannous chloride ions, needed to reduce technetium to its reactive state (from +7 to +4 valence), become oxidized by the contaminant. Oxidized technetium ions do not combine with the desired carrier molecules of macroaggregated albumin (MA), DTPA, diphosphonate, or glucoheptonate (45).

Free pertechnetate can be confirmed by thin-layer chromatography. When an organic solvent is placed on a chromatography strip with a small amount of the radiopharmaceutical, the free $^{99m}$Tc migrates with the solvent. The amount of activity that migrates divided by the total amount of activity placed on the test strip represents the fraction of free pertechnetate. The acceptable amount of radiochemical impurity is usually <5%. Another radiochemical impurity not discussed here is hydrolyzed technetium or technetium dioxide. This impurity can be discovered by performing thin-layer chromatography with a saline solvent.

## Aunt Minnie's Pearls

Suspect free pertechnetate when gastric mucosa, renal, and thyroid activity is unexpectedly seen on the nuclear medicine study.

The presence of free pertechnetate can be confirmed with thin-layer chromatography.

**HISTORY:** A patient undergoing a whole-body $^{131}$I scan

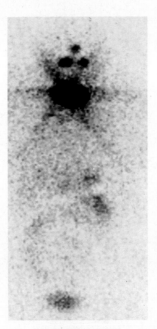

FIGURE 5.26.1

**FINDINGS:** A frontal view from the whole-body $^{131}$I scan (Fig. 5.26.1) shows a radiating star pattern of activity over the expected region of the thyroid gland.

**DIAGNOSIS:** Septal penetration

**DISCUSSION:** Just as in conventional radiography, collimators are used in nuclear medicine to absorb unwanted scattered photons before they reach the image. Scattered photons affect the scintillation camera in an area that does not correspond to their anatomic point of origin on the patient, resulting in images that are poor in resolution and contrast (46). Most modern nuclear collimators use a system of hexagonal holes bordered by septa. Normally, the photons penetrate the holes if their incident angle on the collimator is appropriate. Scattered photons encounter the collimator from an angle of incidence that makes them hit and absorb into the septa. When the scattered photons have high energy or occur in very large numbers (i.e., high photon flux), they may penetrate the thinnest portions of the septa. The characteristic six-point star pattern results because septal penetration occurs most easily through the six walls that directly face the opening of the hexagonal holes in the collimator.

Positron-emission tomography (PET) and high-dose $^{131}$I are common sources of septal penetration in clinical imaging because of the high energy and photon flux associated with them. If a low dose of $^{131}$I is used and this artifact is observed, the physician should suspect that an inappropriate collimator (low or medium energy) has been mistakenly used.

## Aunt Minnie's Pearls

Six-point star = septal penetration.

This artifact is seen with inappropriate collimator selection or whenever very high photon flux occurs.

HISTORY: A 78-year-old woman with a solitary pulmonary nodule discovered on CT

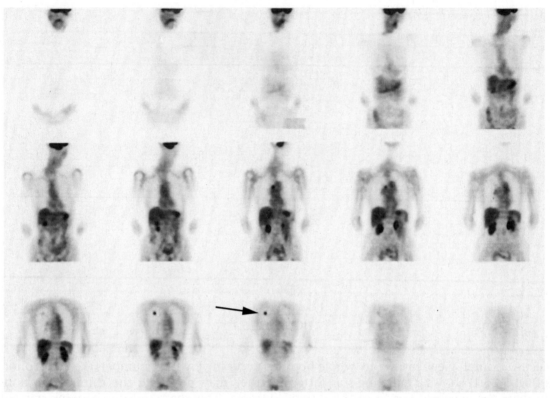

FIGURE 5.27.1

FINDINGS: Whole-body PET images were obtained approximately 45 minutes after the administration of 10 mCi of 18F-fluorodeoxyglucose (FDG; Fig. 5.27.1). This image demonstrates a focal area of increased metabolic activity within the right upper lung that corresponds to the solitary pulmonary nodule identified on prior CT. This hypermetabolic activity has a standard uptake valve (SUV) of 15.

DIAGNOSIS: Lung malignancy

DISCUSSION: A solitary pulmonary nodule (SPN) can cause quite a bit of consternation with diagnosticians and clinicians alike.

FDG–PET facilitates the evaluation of SPNs by assessing the metabolic behavior of the lesion and, from that information, determining whether the focal abnormality is benign or malignant. This examination hopes to prevent the extensive workup associated with the evaluation of an indeterminate nodule.

FDG is a glucose analog that is taken up in a similar fashion to glucose. It differs in that, once it enters the cell, it is phosphorylated, which prevents it from further metabolism. Inside the cell, FDG accumulates in proportion to glycolytic rate of the cell. Cells with high metabolic activity are more apt to be malignant. A method to quantify the degree of metabolism is the SUV. There is still debate as to the cutoff value, as the SUV is dependent on many factors such as body habitus, length of uptake period, glucose levels, and partial volumes effects (47). Also different cancers demonstrate differences in glucose metabolism. Typically, SUVs >2.5 are thought to be more suspicious of malignancy (48). FDG–PET has a reported sensitivity and specificity of 95% and 85%, respectively. It has been proved to be more accurate than conventional imaging in the detection of metastatic disease (49).

## Aunt Minnie's Pearl

Lesions with markedly abnormal metabolic activity likely represent malignancy.

HISTORY: A 52-year-old male with metastatic prostate cancer *and* new onset of back pain

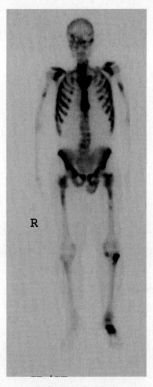

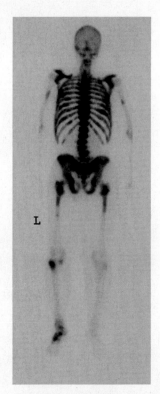

FIGURE 5.28.1

FIGURE 5.28.2

FINDINGS: Anterior and posterior whole body planar views (Figs. 5.28.1 and 5.28.2) obtained 4 hours after intravenous administration of $^{99m}$Tc-MDP demonstrate diffuse increased radiotracer uptake within the skeleton with axial predominance. No renal activity is visible.

DIAGNOSIS: Diffuse osseous prostate metastases "superscan"

DISCUSSION: The term *superscan* is applied to a bone scan with diffusely increased osseous radiotracer uptake with minimal or no urinary activity. The radiotracer uptake within skeleton is so intense that renal activity is below the windowing threshold, causing "absent kidneys sign."

Differential diagnosis of superscan includes widespread metastasis, renal osteodystrophy, severe hyperparathyroidism, osteomalacia, and Paget's disease, with the first two more common than the remaining ones. When diffuse metastatic disease is the cause, prostate and breast cancer are the most common primary malignancies.

Increased radiotracer uptake within axial and appendicular skeleton is more suggestive of hyperparathyroidism, renal osteodystrophy, or osteomalacia, whereas more intense radiotracer uptake in the axial than appendicular skeleton suggests diffuse osseous metastases.

## Aunt Minnie's Pearl

Diffusely increased radiotracer uptake predominantly in the axial skeleton, without visualization of renal activity, is suggestive of superscan owing to widespread metastases.

HISTORY: A 22-year-old runner with left leg pain for 2 weeks

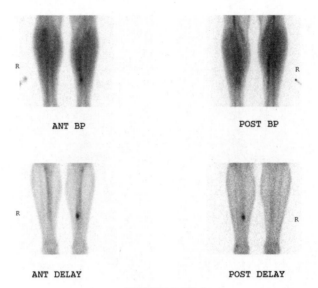

ANT BP          POST BP

ANT DELAY       POST DELAY

FIGURE 5.29.1

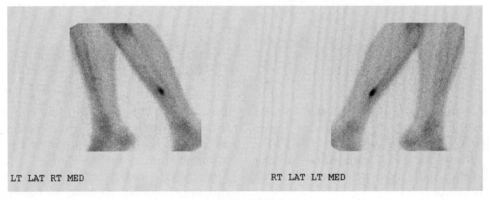

LT LAT RT MED          RT LAT LT MED

FIGURE 5.29.2

FINDINGS: Blood pool and delayed images were obtained immediately after intravenous administration of 25 mCi $^{99m}$ Tc-MDP as part of a three-phase bone scan. There is focally increased blood pool in the left distal third of the calf (Fig. 5.29.1). Delayed images demonstrate a fusiform focus of increased radiotracer uptake in the distal third of the tibia (Fig. 5.29.2).

DIAGNOSIS: Stress fracture

DISCUSSION: Stress fracture has a typical appearance on bone scan. The intense radiotracer uptake has oval or fusiform shape that parallels the long axis of the bone. It is accompanied by increased flow. Stress fracture can be visible on bone scan 1 to 2 weeks before radiographs. The stress fracture results from imbalance between reparative remodeling and repetitive injury to the bone. Healing of stress fracture takes approximately several weeks, but if not recognized early and progresses to true fracture, healing may take months. Most common sites for stress fractures are tibia (in runners), fibula, metatarsals (in recruits), and pelvis.

Differential diagnosis includes infection, metastases, or primary bone tumor, although the configuration of the radiotracer uptake and clinical scenario should point to the correct diagnosis.

## Aunt Minnie's Pearl

Intense fusiform or oval radiotracer uptake parallel to the long axis of the bone is typical of stress fracture.

## Case 5.30

**HISTORY:** A 56-year-old female with history of multiple endocrine neoplasia (MEN), status after parathyroid-ectomy, with new symptoms suggestive of gastrinoma

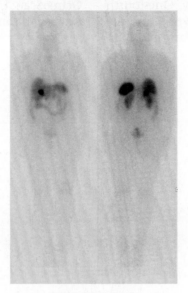

FIGURE 5.30.1

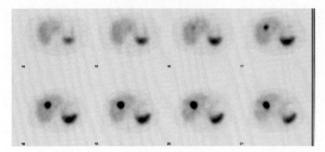

FIGURE 5.30.2

**FINDINGS:** Anterior and posterior whole-body planar views along with SPECT images of the abdomen were obtained 24 hours after administration of 5 mCi Indium Pentreotide ($^{111}$In OctreoScan). There is an intense focus of increased radiotracer uptake in the right upper quadrant, which on SPECT images is localized in the liver. Normal radiotracer uptake is present in the liver, spleen, bowel (Figs. 5.30.1 and 5.30.2).

**DIAGNOSIS:** Gastrinoma metastases

**DISCUSSION:** Somatostatin receptor imaging with $^{111}$In OctreoScan has high sensitivity for detection of most neuroendocrine tumors. The accuracy for gastrinoma approaches 95%, carcinoid 80%, pheochromocytoma and neuroblastoma >85%, and glucagonoma >70%. The exceptions are insulinoma and medullary thyroid carcinoma, with accuracy of approximately 31% and 54%, respectively. Other somatostatin receptor–positive tumors are pituitary adenoma, breast cancer, lymphoma and small-cell lung cancers. Normal $^{111}$In OcteroScan activity is identified in the blood pool, kidneys, bladder, liver, gallbladder, and spleen, with kidneys and spleen having the most intense uptake.

Primary neoplasm or metastases present as intense foci of radiotracer uptake. False-positive results can be seen in some chronic inflammatory changes such as sarcoidosis, tuberculosis, inflammatory bowel disease, and rheumatoid arthritis; however, the uptake is less intense.

Gastrinomas most commonly occur in duodenum or pancreas. In rare cases, primary tumors can be seen in the body of stomach, splenic hilum, liver, peripancreatic lymph nodes, or ovary. One-fourth of gastrinomas are related to MEN type I and are associated with hyperparathyroidism and pituitary adenomas.

## Aunt Minnie's Pearl

Intense focus of increased radiotracer uptake on [111]In OctreoScan is suggestive of neuroendocrine tumor expressing somatostatin receptors.

HISTORY: A 68-year-old with lung cancer for restaging

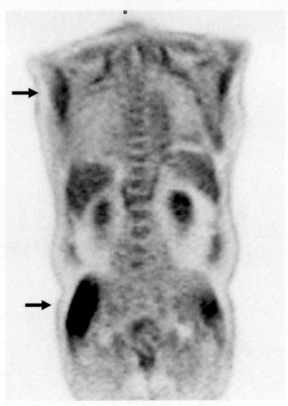

FIGURE 5.31.1

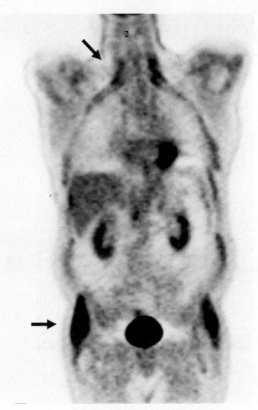

FIGURE 5.31.2

FINDINGS: Diffuse metabolic activity throughout muscles with the most intense uptake in gluteus muscles bilaterally (Figs. 5.31.1 and 5.31.2).

DIAGNOSIS: Muscular uptake on PET scan

DISCUSSION: Resting muscles use mainly free fatty acids as energy substrate. After exercise, glucose becomes the main substrate. Therefore, any physical activity, not just exercise, can cause increased metabolic uptake in the muscles. In anxious patients, tense muscles demonstrate increased FDG uptake, in the neck in particular. Speaking causes increased metabolic activity in phonation muscles, chewing in mastication muscles (50). As insulin increases the FDG uptake, diffuse muscle uptake is seen in hyperinsulinemic states, such as short fasting period or insulin administration prior to FDG injection. Several interventions are used to avoid undesirable muscle uptake: the appropriate long (approximately 8 hours) fasting time prior to administration of FDG, blood glucose level <200, muscle relaxants, warming blankets, and avoiding strenuous exercise before scan. Asymmetric, focal, and intense muscle uptake should be carefully reviewed and correlated clinically to exclude pathology.

## Aunt Minnie's Pearl

It is important to recognize physiologic muscle FDG uptake to avoid false-positive results.

HISTORY: Quality control

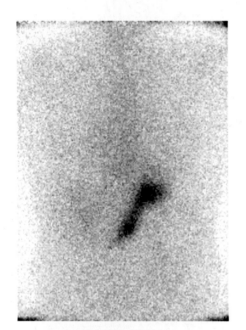

FIGURE 5.32.1

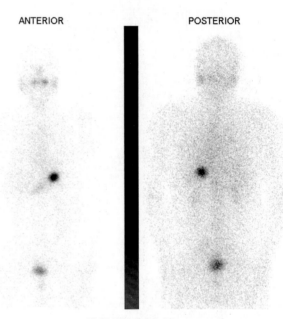

FIGURE 5.32.2

FINDINGS: Two images obtained on the same clinical visit with a follow-up whole body iodine scan for a patient who was previously treated with iodine-131 for thyroid carcinoma. The static image (Fig. 5.32.1) of the abdomen shows increased along the superior and inferior edges of the image. The whole body image (Fig. 5.32.2) demonstrates no corresponding abnormalities.

DIAGNOSIS: Edge Packing

DISCUSSION: Edge packing refers to higher sensitivity of the gamma camera near the edge of the detector resulting in increased activity along the edges or margins of the image. This results in nonuniformity of the image. If this artifact is not appropriately recognized misinterpretation of the image can occur. In this case, the whole body images do not demonstrate the same area of increased activity and should have been a clue to the presence of the artifact. State of the art gamma cameras use electronic masking to prevent the visualization of this phenomenon (51).

## Aunt Minnie's Pearls

In nuclear medicine ALWAYS consider the presence of an artifact, especially if the imaging finding does not make sense anatomically.

**HISTORY:** A 26-year-old female presents with history of thyroid cancer

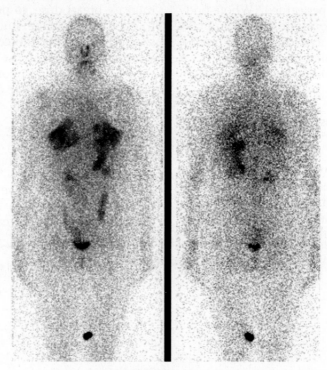

FIGURE 5.33.1

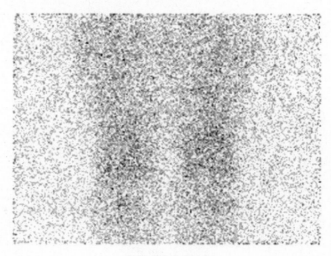

FIGURE 5.33.2

**FINDINGS:** Following the oral administration of 1 mCi of iodine-123, 24-hour whole-body and static images of the legs were performed. Whole-body images (Fig. 5.33.1) demonstrate intense uptake within both breasts as well as a focal area of intense uptake along the left leg that clears on the repeat static image (Fig. 5.33.2) (obtained after the patient cleaned her leg).

**DIAGNOSIS:** Lactating breast and contamination on the left leg

**DISCUSSION:** Iodine accumulates within the breast and will be excreted in breast milk. It is important to know whether the woman is breast feeding or plans to breastfeed. Because iodine is excreted in breast milk, administration of iodine to a patient who plans to breastfeed is prohibited. In addition, the increased engorgement of lactating breast can increase breast dose; to prevent this increased dose to the breast, iodine studies should be performed several weeks after the cessation of breast feeding. The focal area of intense uptake along the left leg was contamination as confirmed by reimaging the patient after appropriate cleansing.

## Aunt Minnie's Pearls

Breastfeeding is a contraindication to iodine therapy.

Before doing an expensive SPECT/CT to confirm a lesion consider reimaging after the patient removes clothing and cleans the area to rule out contamination.

# Case 5.34

**HISTORY:** A 48-year-old male with decreased urinary output after renal transplant

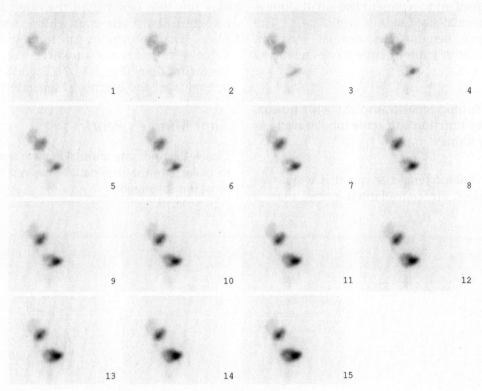

FIGURE 5.34.1

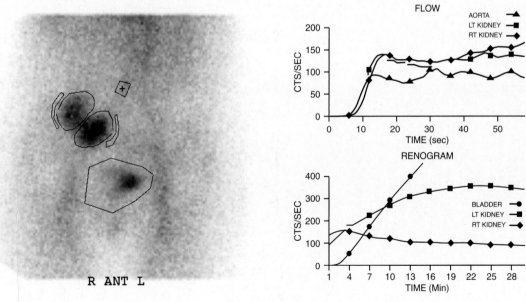

R ANT L

FIGURE 5.34.2

**FINDINGS:** The right lower quadrant transplant has an abnormal configuration. Close examination shows this transplant to represent two small kidneys rather than normal-sized kidney (Fig. 5.34.1). The superior kidney demonstrates normal washout, whereas the inferior kidney demonstrates retention of the radiotracer.

**DIAGNOSIS:** Enbloc renal transplant with normal superior kidney function and acute tubular necrosis of the inferior kidney

**DISCUSSION:** Enbloc renal transplant is when two pediatric kidneys are transplanted rather than a solitary kidney. It is important to recognize this because as this case demonstrates, one kidney may function better than the other kidney. If you recognize that there is an enbloc renal transplant place separate regions of interest around both kidneys so that renogram curves can be generated for each kidney (Fig. 5.34.2). Each kidney needs to be evaluated and diagnosed separately.

### Aunt Minnie's Pearl

Closely examine any unusual looking transplant kidney to make sure that the patient has not had an enbloc renal transplantation.

**HISTORY:** A 1-year-old with history of recurrent urinary tract infections

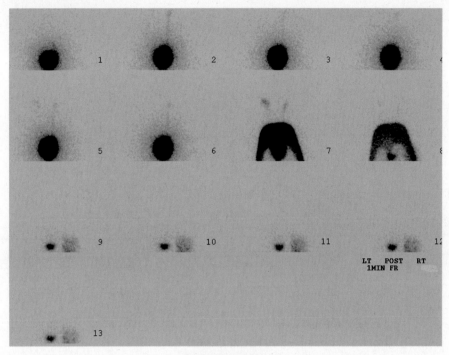

FIGURE 5.35.1

**FINDINGS:** Multiple posterior images from a radionuclide cystogram (Fig. 5.35.1) demonstrate reflux of activity bilaterally from the bladder into both renal pelvises.

**DIAGNOSIS:** Moderate bilateral vesicoureteral reflux

**DISCUSSION:** The first test that should be performed after the diagnosis of multiple urinary tract infections is a VCUG to evaluate for structural abnormalities. Subsequent follow-up exams to evaluate for degree and persistence/resolution of reflux can be performed via a radionuclide cystogram that reduces radiation dose to the patient's gonads. Radionuclide cystograms are graded as mild (reflux into the ureter), moderate (reflux into the renal pelvis), and severe (dilatation of the collecting system and dilated tortuous ureter) (52).

## Aunt Minnie's Pearl

Bladder volume can be approximated in milliliters according to the formula (age in years + 2) × 30 cm³ = bladder volume

HISTORY: A 16-year-old female with history of thyroid carcinoma

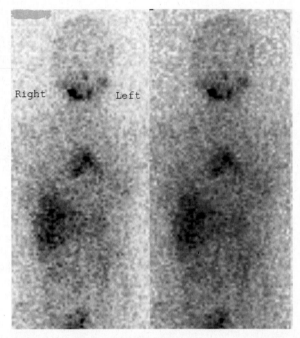

FIGURE 5.36.1

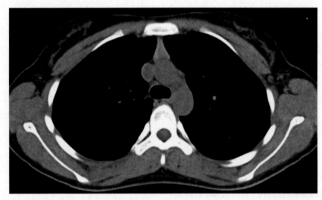

FIGURE 5.36.2

FINDINGS: Anterior and posterior whole body images demonstrate intense radioiodine uptake in an inverted V pattern within the mediastinum (Fig. 5.36.1). CT images from SPECT/CT demonstrate soft tissue density within the anterior mediastinum (Fig. 5.36.2).

DIAGNOSIS: Normal thymus

DISCUSSION: Although thyroid cancer can metastasize to the mediastinum, it is important to know what normal anatomical structures look like. Thymus uptake has been reported several times in the literature in children and young adults with

FDG. In a similar manner, radioiodine can be seen within the mediastinum secondary to normal sodium–iodine symporter within the thymus (53). In this case the normal inverted V appearance should clue you in to the diagnosis. To ease this patient's concerns SPECT/CT was performed. The CT demonstrates normal thymus within the anterior mediastinum.

## Aunt Minnie's Pearl

Normal thymic uptake can be a cause of a "false-positive" interpretation on whole body iodine scans.

**HISTORY:** A 55-year-old gentleman with decreased urinary output one week status post transplanted–kidney biopsy

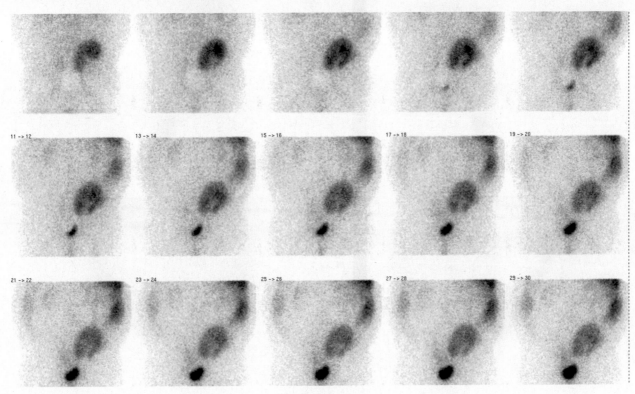

FIGURE 5.37.1

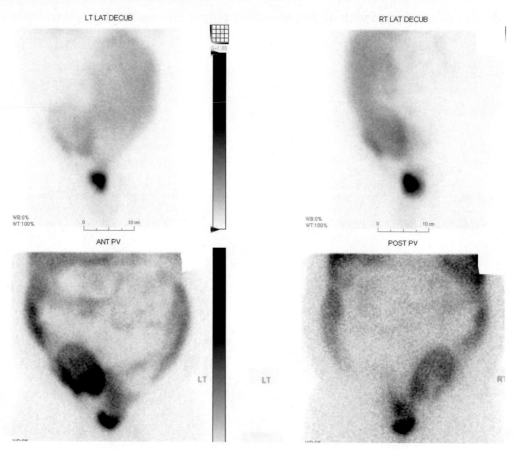

FIGURE 5.37.2

**FINDINGS:** 30-minute renogram images summed every 2 minutes demonstrate normal uptake by the renal transplant with some excretion into the urinary bladder (Fig. 5.37.1). In addition, there is extra renal activity that progressively accumulates superior and lateral to the transplanted kidney. Decubitus and postvoid images (Fig. 5.37.2) demonstrate this activity to extend into the peritoneal cavity and shift positions with change in patient positioning (right versus left decubitus).

**DIAGNOSIS:** Large urinary leak secondary to renal transplant biopsy

**DISCUSSION:** Urinary leak is typically seen within days to weeks posttransplant. In this case the urinary leak was several weeks later (past the normal time frame) and the result of biopsy of the transplanted kidney. On the initial images the accumulation superior and lateral to the transplanted kidney may be misinterpreted as bowel; however, the progressive accumulation and shifting appearance on decubitus images seals the diagnosis. Decubitus images should always be obtained when evaluating renal transplants.

## Aunt Minnie's Pearl

Decubitus images are helpful to differentiate a urinary leak from physiological bowel activity.

**HISTORY:** A 10-year-old who was incidentally found to have hypertension. Primary care physician (PCP) performed a renal ultrasound that found an adrenal mass

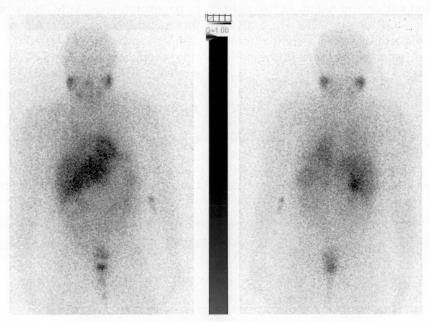

FIGURE 5.38.1

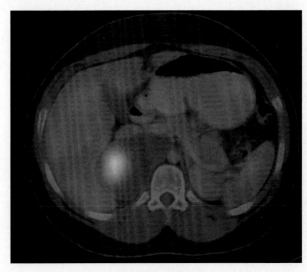

FIGURE 5.38.2

**FINDINGS:** Anterior and posterior whole body static images from an MIBG scan (Fig. 5.38.1) demonstrates a focal area of increased radiotracer accumulation within the region of the right adrenal gland. SPECT/CT fused images (Fig. 5.38.2) demonstrate a large partially necrotic right adrenal mass with intense focal uptake within the solid portion of the mass.

**DIAGNOSIS:** Ganglioneuroblastoma

**DISCUSSION:** Many residents confuse Octreotide with MIBG. MIBG can be differentiated from Octreotide by the lack of intense renal activity. Findings on planar images can be followed up with SPECT/CT for further characterization and anatomical localization. In general when evaluating for the presence of neuroblastomas, pheochromocytoma, or paragangliomas, MIBG is the study of choice as it provides full body survey. Although neuroendocrine tumors can be demonstrated on Octreotide studies, this is typically reserved for cases with high clinical suspicion with a negative MIBG scan.

## Aunt Minnie's Pearls

MIBG does not have intense renal activity.

MIBG can have heterogeneous liver activity so use caution when evaluating for liver metastasis

# REFERENCES

1. Larsson A, Moonen M, Bergh AC, et al. Predictive value of quantitative cisternography in normal pressure hydrocephalus. Acta Neurol Scand 1990;81:327–332.

2. Palmer EL, Scott JA, Strauss HW. Practical nuclear medicine. Philadelphia, PA: WB Saunders, 1992:382.

3. Laurin NR, Driedger AA, Hurwitz GA, et al. Cerebral perfusion imaging with technetium-99m HM-PAO in brain death and severe central nervous system injury. J Nucl Med 1989;30:1627–1635.

4. Wilson K, Gordon L, Selby JB Sr. The diagnosis of brain death with Tc-99m HMPAO. Clin Nucl Med 1993;18:428–434.

5. Carcassi U. History of hypertrophic osteoarthropathy (HOA). Clin Exp Rheumatol 1992;10(suppl 7):3–7.

6. Davies RA, Darby M, Richards MA. Hypertrophic pulmonary osteoarthropathy in pulmonary metastatic disease. A case report and review of the literature. Clin Radiol 1991;43:268–271.

7. Thrall JH, Ziessman HA. Nuclear medicine: The requisites, 2nd ed. St Louis, MO: Mosby, 2001:123.

8. Resnick D. Bone and joint imaging. Philadelphia, PA: WB Saunders, 1989:575–577.

9. Palmer EL, Scott JA, Strauss HW. Practical nuclear medicine. Philadelphia, PA: WB Saunders, 1992:164.

10. Goldsmith DP, Vivino FB, Eichenfield AH, et al. Nuclear imaging and clinical features of childhood reflex neurovascular dystrophy: Comparison with adults. Arthritis Rheum 1989;32:480–485.

11. O'Mara RE. Benign bone disease. In: Sandler MP, Coleman RE, Whackers FJT, et al. (eds.). Diagnostic nuclear medicine, 3rd ed. Baltimore, MD: Williams & Wilkins, 1996:693.

12. Krane SM. Paget's disease of bone. In: Braunwald E, Fauci AS, Isselbacher KJ, et al. (eds.). Harrison's principles of internal medicine, 14th ed. New York, NY: McGraw-Hill, 1998:2266–2269.

13. Roger LF. Miscellaneous conditions. In: Juhl JH, Crummy AB, Kuhlman JE (eds.). Paul and Juhl's essentials of radiologic imaging, 7th ed. Philadelphia, PA: Lippincott-Raven, 1998:237.

14. Heck LL. Extraosseous localization of phosphate bone agents. Semin Nucl Med 1980;10:311–313.

15. Bates MD, Bucuvalas JC, Alonso MH, et al. Biliary atresia: Pathogenesis and treatment. Semin Liver Dis 1998;18:281–293.

16. Verreault J, Danais S, Blanchard H, et al. Hepatobiliary scintigraphy using 99m Tc-DISIDA and obstructive cholangiopathy in children. Chir Pediatr 1987;28:1–7.

17. Sulavik SB, Spencer RP, Weed DA, et al. Recognition of distinctive patterns of gallium-67 distribution in sarcoidosis. J Nucl Med 1990;31:1909–1914.

18. Kaplan EL, Salti GI, Hara H, et al. Results and complications of the surgical treatment of primary hyperparathyroidism. Ann Ital Chir 1993;64:365–370.

19. Thrall JH, Ziessman HA. Nuclear medicine: The requisites, 2nd ed. St Louis, MO: Mosby, 2001:384–387.

20. Mettler FA, Guiberteau MT. Essentials of nuclear medicine imaging, 4th ed. Philadelphia, PA: WB Saunders, 1998:125–127.

21. Datz FL, Patch GG, Arias JM, et al. Nuclear medicine: A teaching file. St Louis, MO: Mosby, 1992:3.

22. Barron BJ, Lamk ML, Kim EE. Genitourinary nuclear medicine: II. In: Sandler MP, Coleman RE, Whackers FJT, et al. (eds.). Diagnostic nuclear medicine, 3rd ed. Baltimore, MD: Williams & Wilkins, 1996:1212.

23. Sfakinakis GN, Bourgoignie JJ. Renal scintigraphy following angiotensin-converting enzyme inhibition in the diagnosis of renovascular hypertension (captopril scintigraphy). In: Nuclear medicine annual. New York, NY: Raven, 1988:125–170.

24. Thrall JH, Ziessman HA. Nuclear medicine: The requisites, 2nd ed. St Louis, MO: Mosby, 2001:349–351.

25. Gerson MC (ed.). Cardiac nuclear medicine. New York, NY: McGraw-Hill, 1987:2–4.

26. Gottschalk A, Sostman HD, Coleman RE, et al. Ventilation–perfusion scintigraphy in the PIOPED study: part II, evaluation of the scintigraphic criteria and interpretations. J Nucl Med 1993;34:1119–1126.

27. Beller GA, Watson DD. Physiological basis of myocardial perfusion imaging with the technetium-99m agents. Semin Nucl Med 1991;21:173–181.

28. Mettler FA Jr, Guiberteau MJ. Essentials of nuclear medicine imaging, 3rd ed. Philadelphia, PA: WB Saunders, 1991:116–117.

29. Baum S. Angiography and the gastrointestinal bleeder. Radiology 1982;143:569–572.

30. Thrall JH, Ziessman HA. Nuclear medicine: The requisites. St Louis, MO: Mosby, 1995:246.

31. Isselbacher KJ, Epstein A. Diverticular, vascular, and other disorders of the intestine and peritoneum. In: Fauci AS, Braunwald E, Isselbacher KJ, et al. (eds.). Harrison's principles of internal medicine, 14th ed. New York, NY: McGraw-Hill, 1998:1648.

32. Thrall JH, Ziessman HA. Nuclear medicine: The requisites, 2nd ed. St Louis, MO: Mosby, 2001.

33. Hertzos MS, Chacko AK, Pitts CM. Leiomyoma of terminal ileum. J Nucl Med 1985;26:1278–1282.

34. Conway JJ. Radionuclide diagnosis of Meckel's diverticulum. Gastrointest Radiol 1980;5:209–213.

35. Mettler FA Jr, Guiberteau MT. Essentials of nuclear medicine imaging, 4th ed. Philadelphia, PA: WB Saunders, 1998:113–116.

36. DeLellis RA. The endocrine system. In: Cotran RS, Kumar V, Robbins SL (eds.). Robbins pathologic basis of disease, 4th ed. Philadelphia, PA: WB Saunders, 1989:1233.

37. Freitas JE, Gross MD, Ripley S, et al. Radionuclide diagnosis and therapy of thyroid cancer: Current status report. Semin Nucl Med 1985;15:106–131.

38. Shammas A, Degirmenci B, Mountz JM, et al. 18F-FDG PET/CT in patients with suspected recurrent or metastatic well-differentiated thyroid cancer. J Nucl Med 2007;48:221–226.

39. Palmer EL, Scott JA, Strauss HW. Practical nuclear medicine. Philadelphia, PA: WB Saunders, 1992:238–239.

40. Sty JR, Babbitt DP, Sheth K. Abnormal Tc-99m-methylene diphosphonate accumulation in the kidneys of children with sickle cell disease. Clin Nucl Med 1992;17:236.

41. Palmer EL, Scott JA, Strauss HW. Practical nuclear medicine. Philadelphia, PA: WB Saunders, 1992:51–52.

42. Patton JA. Quality assurance. In: Sandler MP, Coleman RE, Whackers FJT, et al. (eds.). Diagnostic nuclear medicine, 3rd ed. Baltimore, MD: Williams & Wilkins, 1996:164.

43. Thrall JH, Ziessman HA. Nuclear medicine: The requisites. St Louis, MO: Mosby, 1995:26.

44. Mettler FA Jr, Guiberteau MT. Essentials of nuclear medicine imaging, 3rd ed. Philadelphia, PA: WB Saunders, 1991:146–147.

45. Mettler FA Jr, Guiberteau MJ. Essentials of nuclear medicine imaging, 3rd ed. Philadelphia, PA: WB Saunders, 1991:34–35.

46. Sorenson JA, Phelps ME. Physics in nuclear medicine, 2nd ed. Orlando, FL: Grune & Stratton, 1987:372–374.

47. Keyes J Jr. SUV: Standard uptake or silly useless value? J Nucl Med 1995;36:1836–1839.

48. Hellwig D, Graeter TP, Ukena D, et al. 18F-FDG PET for mediastinal staging of lung cancer: Which SUV threshold makes sense? J Nucl Med 2007;48:1761–1766.

49. Coleman RE. PET in lung cancer. J Nucl Med 2001;40:814–820.

50. Jadvar H, Parker JA. Clinical PET and PET/CT. London, England: Springer, 2005:54–55.

51. Saha GB. Physics and radiobiology of nuclear medicine, 4th ed. New York, NY: Springer, 2012:140–141.

52. Mandell GA, Eggli DF, Gilday DL, et al. Society of Nuclear Medicine Procedure Guideline for radionuclide cystography in children. Version 3.0. On line society of nuclear medicine guideline. http://interactive.snm.org/docs/pg_ch32_0703.pdf.

53. Meller J, Becker W. The human sodium-iodine symporter (NIS) as a key for specific thymic iodine-131 uptake. Eur J Nucl Med 2000;27(5):473–474.

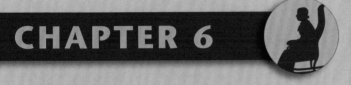

# CHAPTER 6

# NEURORADIOLOGY: BRAIN

**Timothy J. Amrhein / Usman Manzoor / Zoran Rumboldt**

*The authors and editors acknowledge the contribution of the Chapter 6A author from the third edition: Christopher K. Moses, MD.*

HISTORY: A 3-year-old boy with seizures

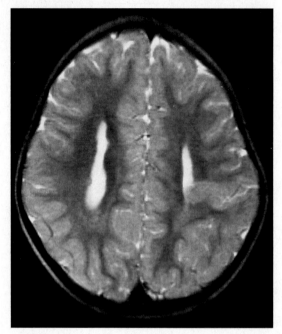

FIGURE 6.1.1

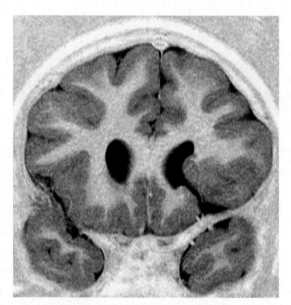

FIGURE 6.1.2

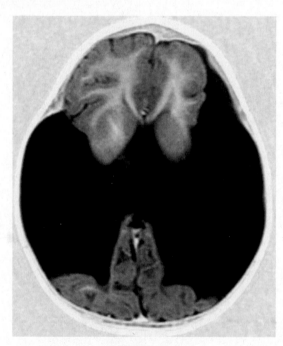

FIGURE 6.1.3

**FINDINGS:** Axial T2-weighted (Fig. 6.1.1) MR image demonstrates gray matter extending from the surface of the brain to the ependymal lining of the left lateral ventricle. Coronal T1-weighted inversion recovery image from a different patient (Fig. 6.1.2) demonstrates a gray matter–lined cleft extending from the brain surface to the left lateral ventricle. Axial T1 inversion recovery MR image in another patient (Fig. 6.1.3) demonstrates wide bilateral cerebrospinal fluid (CSF) clefts indicative of open-lip schizencephaly.

**DIAGNOSIS:** Schizencephaly (closed-lip type)

**DISCUSSION:** Schizencephaly may be close-lipped or open-lipped, unilateral or bilateral, and typically manifests with seizures and mental retardation. It is a disorder of neuronal migration caused by second-trimester insult or genetics resulting in a full-thickness communication between the brain surface (pia) and ventricular system ependyma. The cleft is lined by abnormal gray matter, which may act as a seizure focus. If the abnormal gray matter is closely apposed, the disorder is close-lipped; if unopposed, it is open-lipped.

The diagnosis is obvious in open-lipped schizencephaly—a wide CSF communication exists between the lateral ventricle and the subarachnoid space. Close-lipped schizencephaly is more subtle, and the key imaging feature is ectopic gray matter extending from the ventricular wall to the brain surface and outlining a thin, sometimes imperceptible cleft. Other clues to the diagnosis include gyri radiating into the cleft, associated subependymal heterotopias, and a dimple in the wall of the lateral ventricle. Multiplanar imaging is required, because isolated imaging in just one plane may miss the defect. Associated anomalies include absence of the septum pellucidum (90%) and septo-optic dysplasia (1,2).

## Aunt Minnie's Pearls

Close-lipped schizencephaly can be subtle—the key diagnostic feature is ectopic gray matter extending from the lateral ventricle to the brain surface outlining a thin cleft.

Multiplanar imaging is required in any child presenting with seizures to avoid the pitfall of missed schizencephaly.

HISTORY: A 15-month-old girl with seizures

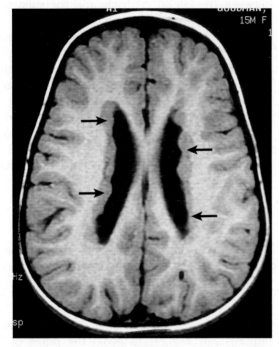

FIGURE 6.2.1

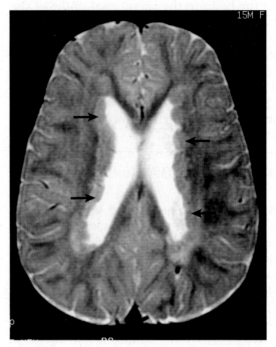

FIGURE 6.2.2

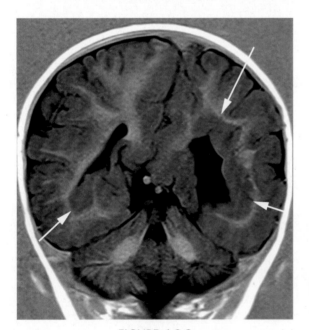

FIGURE 6.2.3

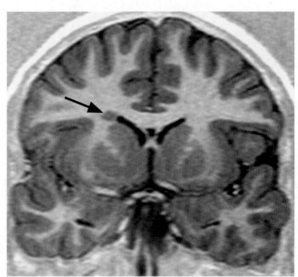

FIGURE 6.2.4

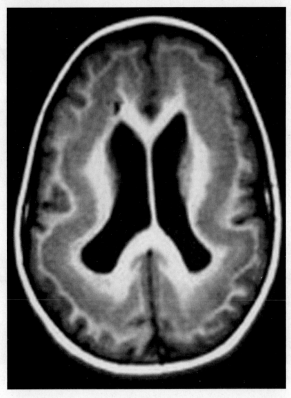

FIGURE 6.2.5

**FINDINGS:** Axial T1-weighted (Fig. 6.2.1) and T2-weighted (Fig. 6.2.2) MR images show diffuse subependymal nodules (*arrows*) lining both lateral ventricles. The nodules maintain isointensity with cortical gray matter on both pulse sequences. Coronal T1-weighted inversion recovery MR image in a different patient (Fig. 6.2.3) demonstrates large areas of gray-matter signal adjacent to the bilateral lateral ventricles (*white arrows*), consistent with multiple foci of gray-matter heterotopia. A coronal T1-weighted inversion recovery MR image from a third patient (Fig. 6.2.4) demonstrates a more subtle small focus of gray-matter heterotopia adjacent to the right lateral ventricle (*arrow*). Axial T1 inversion recovery MR image in a different patient (Fig. 6.2.5) demonstrates a band of tissue with signal characteristics of gray matter within the white matter between the cortex and the lateral ventricles, compatible with band heterotopia.

**DIAGNOSIS:** Gray-matter heterotopia

**DISCUSSION:** Gray-matter heterotopia is a relatively common congenital abnormality that results from an in utero arrest of neuronal migration. The abnormally located gray matter is usually found in the subependymal region of the lateral ventricles, around the trigones in particular. Occasionally, the heterotopias are more peripherally located near the cerebral cortex. Patients come to clinical attention because of seizures and developmental delay.

Heterotopias may be classified into three groups: subependymal heterotopia, focal subcortical heterotopia, and diffuse (band) heterotopia. The imaging hallmark is the isointensity with cortical gray matter on all imaging sequences and the lack of contrast enhancement. These characteristics allow the radiologist to distinguish this abnormality from the subependymal nodules that occur in tuberous sclerosis (1,3,4).

## Aunt Minnie's Pearl

To diagnose gray-matter heterotopia, the abnormalities must follow the signal intensity of gray matter on all pulse sequences and show no post-contrast enhancement.

**HISTORY:** Fetal MR performed for prenatal ultrasound abnormality

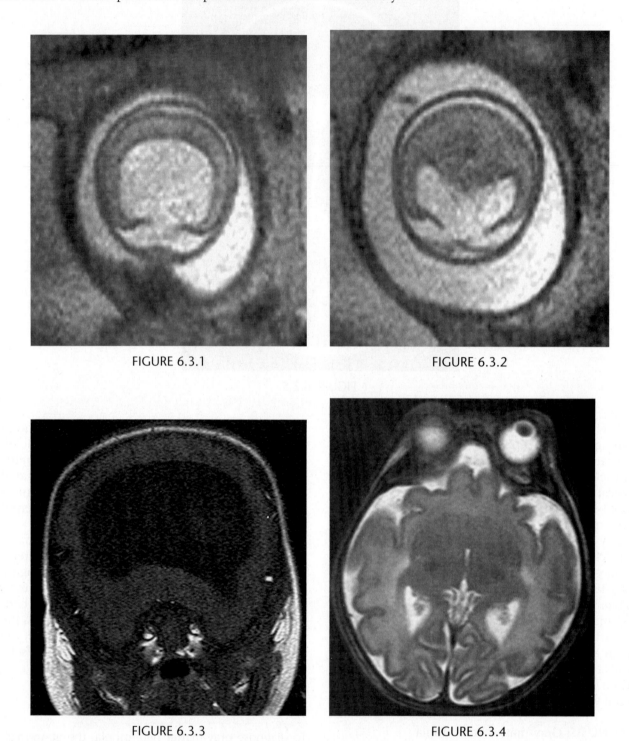

FIGURE 6.3.1

FIGURE 6.3.2

FIGURE 6.3.3

FIGURE 6.3.4

**FINDINGS:** Axial single-shot T2-weighted fetal MR images (Figs. 6.3.1 and 6.3.2) demonstrate a large monoventricle and fused cerebral hemispheres. Similar findings are identified on a coronal T1-weighted MR image in a neonate (Fig. 6.3.3). Axial T2-weighted MR image in a different patient (Fig. 6.3.4) demonstrates fused thalami and basal frontal lobes but separate occipital horns of the ventricular system and more posterior portions of cerebral hemispheres indicating lobar holoprosencephaly.

**DIAGNOSIS:** Alobar holoprosencephaly

**DISCUSSION:** Holoprosencephaly refers to a continuum of congenital malformations occurring from failure of induction of the prosencephalon and absent or incomplete cleavage of the brain into distinct cerebral hemispheres. Three subtypes have been proposed according to the severity of cerebral and facial anomalies. These include alobar, semilobar, and lobar holoprosencephaly. A rare middle interhemispheric variant has also been described, wherein the cerebral hemispheres fail to divide in the posterior frontal and parietal regions. In the most severe subtype, alobar holoprosencephaly, there is complete or near complete lack of hemispheric cleavage. A primitive midline monoventricle, fused thalami, absence of the falx cerebri, and interhemispheric fissure are the typical imaging features. Midline facial anomalies ranging from single maxillary central incisor to hypotelorism to cyclopia are usually present. A multitude of extracranial and chromosomal abnormalities may occur in association with alobar holoprosencephaly, frequently resulting in a stillborn infant or death in the neonatal period (1,5,6).

## Aunt Minnie's Pearl

Midline monoventricle with fused frontal lobes and thalami = alobar holoprosencephaly.

HISTORY: Fetal MR performed for prenatal ultrasound abnormality

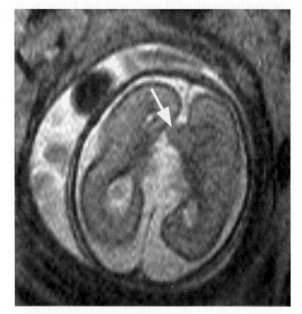

FIGURE 6.4.1

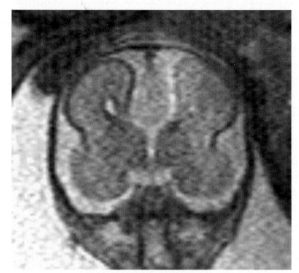

FIGURE 6.4.2

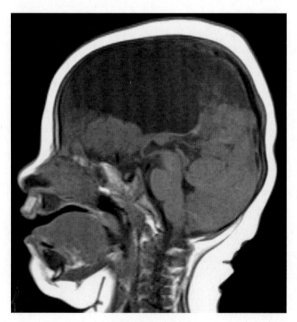

FIGURE 6.4.3

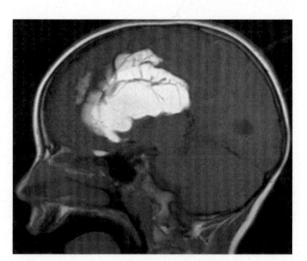

FIGURE 6.4.4

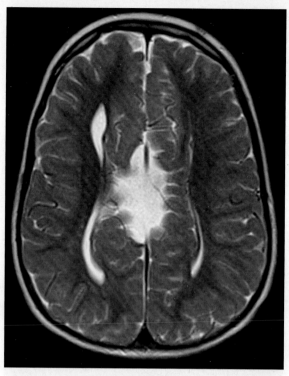

FIGURE 6.4.5

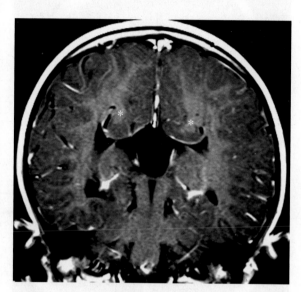

FIGURE 6.4.6

**FINDINGS:** Axial and coronal T2-weighted fetal MR image (Figs. 6.4.1 and 6.4.2) demonstrate absence of the corpus callosum and an associated interhemispheric cyst. There is also a focus of gray-matter heterotopia (*arrow*). Sagittal T1-weighted MR image in a different patient (Fig. 6.4.3) demonstrates a large interhemispheric cyst and absence of the corpus callosum. A sagittal T1-weighted image in yet another patient (Fig. 6.4.4) demonstrates a large high-signal-intensity mass representing a lipoma and absence of the corpus callosum. Finally, an axial T2-weighted image (Fig. 6.4.5) in a fourth patient demonstrates characteristic parallel configuration of the bilateral lateral ventricles. Coronal post-contrast T1-weighted image (Fig. 6.4.6) in the same patient reveals impression on the medial aspects of the bilateral lateral ventricles by abnormally configured white-matter tracts called Probst bundles (*asterisks*).

**DIAGNOSIS:** Dysgenesis of the corpus callosum with associated interhemispheric cyst

**DISCUSSION:** This case demonstrates dysgenesis of the corpus callosum with an associated interhemispheric cyst. The corpus callosum develops in an anterior-to-posterior fashion, with the posterior genu and anterior body forming first, followed by the posterior body, splenium, and rostrum. Abnormalities of the corpus callosum are often associated with other midline abnormalities such as cysts, lipomas, or abnormal anterior or hippocampal commissures. In approximately 75% of cases, callosal abnormalities are also associated with other malformations of cortical development such as heterotopia or abnormalities of sulcation; therefore it is important to carefully evaluate the brain when an abnormality of the corpus callosum is detected. The majority of patients with corpus callosum dysgenesis have decreased volume of white matter (7,8). Complete agenesis of the corpus callosum results in the development of abnormal parallel white-matter tracts called Probst bundles that run anteroposteriorly along the medial aspect of the bilateral lateral ventricles. Further, the lateral ventricles are often widely spaced and parallel in configuration.

## Aunt Minnie's Pearl

Dysgenesis of the corpus callosum is often associated with other midline abnormalities, such as cysts and lipomas, as well as other cortical abnormalities.

# Case 6.5

**HISTORY:** A 17-year-old female with headache and vomiting

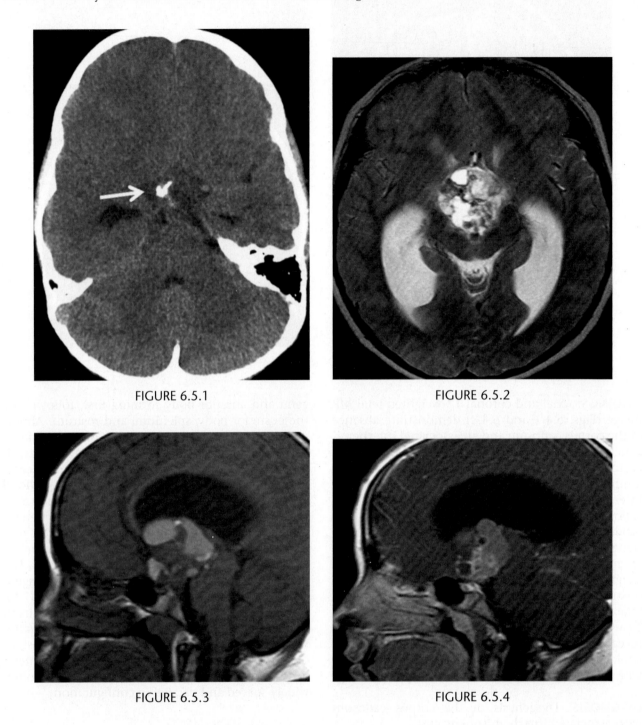

FIGURE 6.5.1

FIGURE 6.5.2

FIGURE 6.5.3

FIGURE 6.5.4

**FINDINGS:** Non-contrast axial CT image reveals a heterogeneous calcified suprasellar mass (white arrow) with solid and cystic components as well as associated hydrocephalus (Fig. 6.5.1). Axial T2-weighted image demonstrates the multilobulated nature of this mass, which contains areas of T2 hypointensity that correspond to regions of calcification identified on CT (Fig. 6.5.2). On a non-contrast sagittal T1-weighted image, the mass contains varying signal intensities ranging from isointense to adjacent gray matter to hyperintense (Fig. 6.5.3). Post-contrast T1-weighted sagittal image demonstrates a predominantly peripheral enhancement (Fig. 6.5.4).

**DIAGNOSIS:** Craniopharyngioma

**DISCUSSION:** Craniopharyngiomas are benign tumors that arise from epithelial remnants and ectopic embryonic cell rests of the Rathke's pouch. They are the most common type of non-glial–based intracranial neoplasm in the pediatric population and exhibit a bimodal age distribution with most cases occurring either between 5 and 15 years or after 50 years of age. Clinical symptoms are usually insidious owing to the relatively slow rate of tumor growth. The most common presenting symptoms are early morning headache, vomiting, visual field defects, and endocrine abnormalities.

Craniopharyngiomas are most commonly located within the suprasellar cistern with inferior extension into the sella. However, they can be located within the suprasellar space alone, the sella in isolation, or even infrasellar.

There are two distinct histopathologic subtypes of craniopharyngiomas: adamantinomatous and squamous-papillary. Adamantinomatous craniopharyngiomas occur in children (and occasionally adults) and demonstrate the following characteristic imaging features: cyst formation, calcification, and enhancement. On MRI, cystic components are usually multiple, clustered, and exhibit varied signal characteristics dependent on their relative protein content—with greater concentrations of protein resulting in increased T1 signal and concomitant T2 hypointensity. Typically, the cysts are hyperintense to CSF on fluid-attenuated inversion recovery (FLAIR) sequences. Solid components of the mass are usually isointense to brain parenchyma on T1-weighted images, iso- to hyperintense on T2-weighted images, and demonstrate heterogeneous enhancement. One may identify peripheral enhancement of the cystic components as well. On CT, the cystic components exhibit hypoattenuation. CT is very sensitive for the detection of areas of calcification (present in about 80% of cases).

The squamous-papillary subtype occurs in adults and is primarily solid with occasional mixed solid and cystic components. The cysts in this subtype are predominantly T1 hypointense and calcifications are much less common (9,10).

## Aunt Minnie's Pearls

Suprasellar cystic and solid mass with calcifications on CT.

Characteristic variations in signal intensity of multiple cysts.

**HISTORY:** A 5-year-old girl with short stature, delayed dentition, delayed skeletal maturation, and endocrine abnormalities

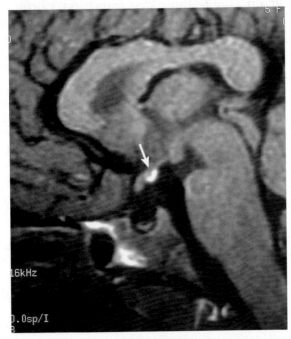

FIGURE 6.6.1

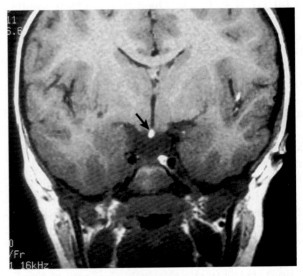

FIGURE 6.6.2

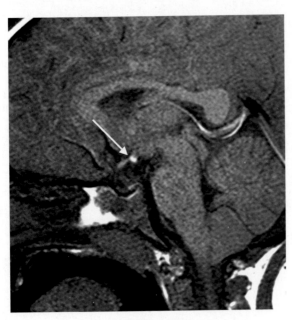

FIGURE 6.6.3

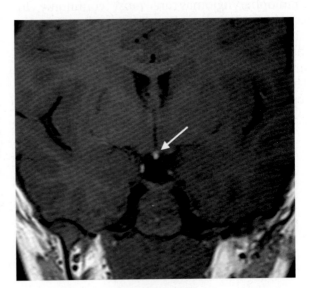

FIGURE 6.6.4

**FINDINGS:** Midline bright signal (*arrow*) is present in the region of the tuber cinereum on midline sagittal (Fig. 6.6.1) and coronal (Fig. 6.6.2) T1-weighted MR images. A small sella turcica, diminutive pituitary gland, and atretic pituitary stalk also are demonstrated. A second case from a different patient reinforces the same findings (Figs 6.6.3 and 6.6.4).

**DIAGNOSIS:** Primary panhypopituitarism with translocation of the pituitary bright spot (i.e., ectopic posterior pituitary lobe)

**DISCUSSION:** The posterior pituitary bright spot is thought to result from the inherent signal intensity of neurosecretory granules in the neurohypophysis; therefore, an ectopic bright spot may be found in any process that disrupts the transport of antidiuretic hormone from the hypothalamus to the posterior pituitary lobe. Primary panhypopituitarism occurs when the pituitary is congenitally hypoplastic or absent. In the clinical setting of panhypopituitarism, a high correlation exists between the hormonal disorder and ectopia of the neurohypophysis. Growth disturbances may dominate the clinical picture, as in the index case. Many patients have a history of traumatic or breech delivery, with the presumed association being perinatal rupture of the pituitary infundibulum. Characteristic MR findings of primary panhypopituitarism include a small sella turcica, diminutive pituitary gland, atretic pituitary stalk, and ectopic posterior pituitary bright spot (11,12).

## Aunt Minnie's Pearls

An ectopic posterior pituitary lobe arises from disruption of the normal transport of neurosecretory granules from the hypothalamus to the posterior pituitary.

Characteristic MR findings of primary panhypopituitarism include a small sella turcica, diminutive pituitary gland, atretic pituitary stalk, and ectopic posterior pituitary bright spot.

# Case 6.7

**HISTORY:** A 14-month-old male with macrocephaly, developmental delay, and seizures

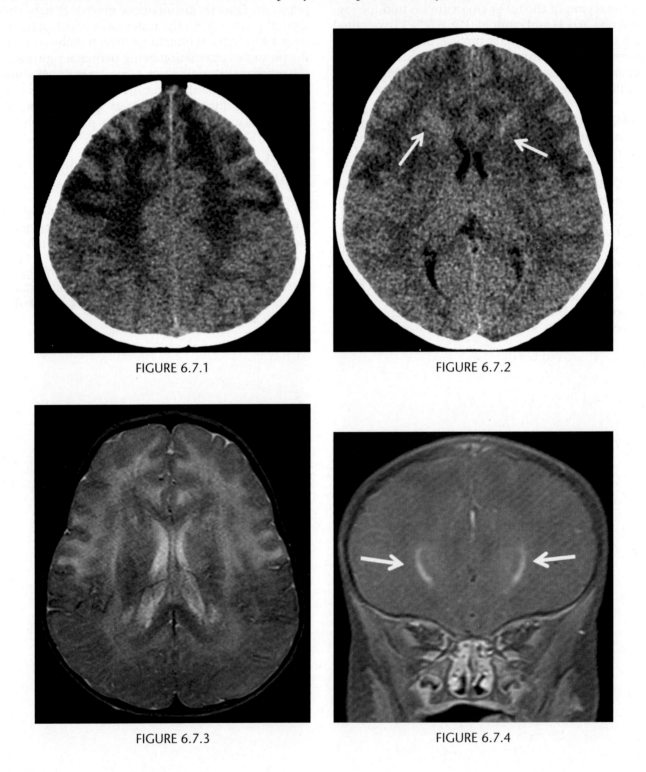

FIGURE 6.7.1

FIGURE 6.7.2

FIGURE 6.7.3

FIGURE 6.7.4

**FINDINGS:** Non-contrast CT of the brain demonstrates symmetric diffuse hypoattenuation of the bilateral frontal lobe white matter and bilateral caudate heads (Fig. 6.7.1) along with hyperdense "caps" along the bilateral frontal horns (Fig. 6.7.2, white arrows). MRI reveals symmetric T1 hypointensity and T2 hyperintensity within the bilateral frontal lobe white matter (in the regions of hypoattenuation on CT) with characteristic involvement of the subcortical U fibers as well as of the deep white-matter tracts (Fig. 6.7.3). There is mild T2 hypointensity and T1 hyperintensity of the periventricular white-matter rim anterior to the bilateral frontal horns. Postcontrast images demonstrate intense enhancement along the tips of bilateral frontal horns (Fig. 6.7.4, white arrows).

**DIAGNOSIS:** Alexander's disease (infantile form)

**DISCUSSION:** Alexander's disease (or fibrinoid leukodystrophy) is a rare disorder characterized by a mutation to the gene for glial fibrillary acidic protein (GFAP) that leads to massive deposition of Rosenthal fibers within astrocytes resulting in demyelination and rarefaction of the subependymal, subpial, and perivascular white matter with a frontal predominance. There are three distinct clinical subgroups: infantile, juvenile, and adult. The infantile form is most common and is characterized by early onset of macrocephaly, developmental delay, and seizures. Rapid progression of the disease typically leads to death within the first 2 to 3 years of life. Macrocephaly and early onset of the clinical prodrome in combination with specific imaging findings can be diagnostic in most cases. However, establishing a definite diagnosis typically requires brain biopsy or autopsy.

Characteristic imaging findings in the infantile form of Alexander disease include a predilection for the bilateral frontal lobe white matter, which manifests as hypoattenuation on CT and corresponding T2 hyperintensity on MRI. Involvement progresses posteriorly to involve the parietal white matter as well as the internal and external capsules. Not uncommonly, similar signal abnormalities can be identified within the bilateral caudate heads. The characteristic finding is T1 hyperintensity and T2 hypointensity of the periventricular frontal rim, which is hyperdense on CT and shows avid enhancement. Further distinguishing features include involvement of the subcortical U fibers early in the disease process. Alexander disease is one of the few metabolic disorders that exhibits abnormal enhancement. Involvement of brainstem and cervical cord is uncommon. Cysts may develop in affected regions of the brain in later stages of the disease (13,14).

## Aunt Minnie's Pearls

Frontal predominant white matter involvement without sparing of the subcortical U fibers.

Involvement of the caudate heads.

T1 hyperintensity, T2 hypointensity, CT hyperdensity, and enhancement within the periventricular white-matter rim anterior to the bilateral frontal horns.

HISTORY: A 16-year-old male with long-standing history of partial complex seizures

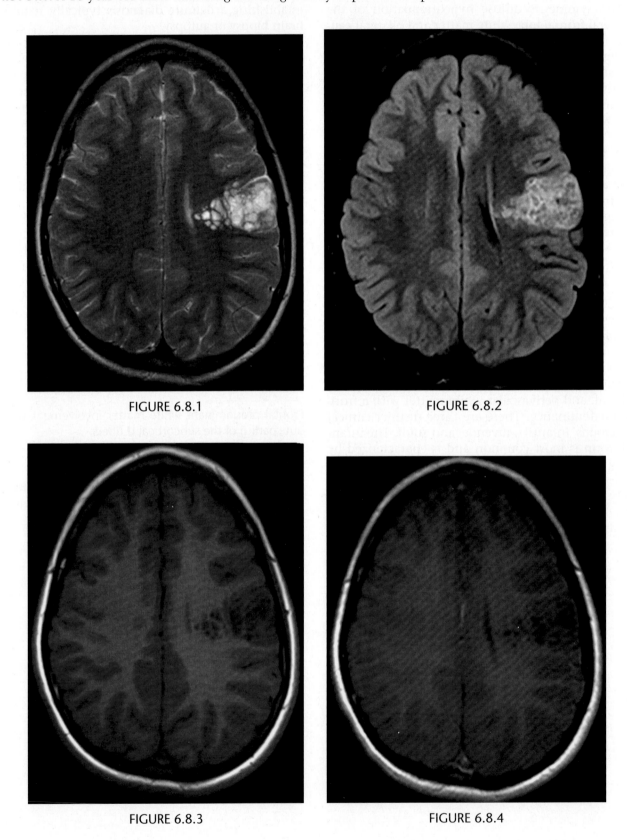

FIGURE 6.8.1

FIGURE 6.8.2

FIGURE 6.8.3

FIGURE 6.8.4

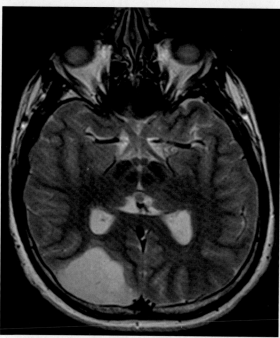

*FIGURE 6.8.5*

**FINDINGS:** Axial T2-weighted and FLAIR images reveal a well-demarcated, multilobulated, and markedly hyperintense lesion in the posterior left frontal lobe with multiple internal cystic appearing areas, giving it a "bubbly" appearance (Figs. 6.8.1 and 6.8.2). The mass is hypointense on the T1-weighted sequence and does not enhance after the administration of contrast (Figs. 6.8.3 and 6.8.4). The mass is wedge or triangular in shape with the majority centered in the cortex and the apex extending into the adjacent subcortical white matter pointing toward the ventricle. There is no associated mass effect or surrounding vasogenic edema. An axial T2-weighted image in a second patient demonstrates a mass with similar characteristics in the right occipital lobe (Fig. 6.8.5).

**DIAGNOSIS:** Dysembryoplastic neuroepithelial tumor

**DISCUSSION:** Dysembryoplastic neuroepithelial tumor (DNET, DNT) is a benign (WHO grade I), mixed glial neuronal tumor arising from the supratentorial cortex. The most common clinical presentation is that of long-standing, drug-resistant partial complex seizures in a child or a young adult. Although DNETs can occur in any part of the supratentorial cortex, they are most commonly found in the temporal lobe. Treatment requires surgical resection, which can be curative, even if incomplete.

Imaging findings are characteristic and can be diagnostic in many cases. DNETs are classically well-demarcated, multilobulated, multicystic appearing T2 hyperintense masses that arise from the cortex. Uniquely characteristic properties of DNETs are their wedge or triangular shape with the apex pointing toward the ventricles and internal "bubbly" appearance. In general, there is minimal to no associated mass effect or surrounding vasogenic edema. DNETs typically do not enhance after contrast administration; however, in around a third of cases there may be focal punctuate or peripheral enhancement. They also show high apparent diffusion coefficient (ADC) values and low relative cerebral blood volume (rCBV) on perfusion imaging. As the tumor is slow growing, it can cause remodeling or scalloping of the inner table of the adjacent calvarium in approximately 40% to 60% cases, which is best depicted on CT. The DNETs have a strong association with focal cortical dysplasia (15,16).

### Aunt Minnie's Pearl

Cortically based, wedge shaped, multilobulated, "bubbly" lesion without mass effect in a young patient with long-standing history of seizures.

HISTORY: A 14-year-old boy with seizure disorder

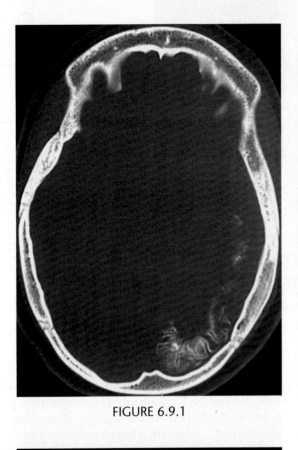

FIGURE 6.9.1

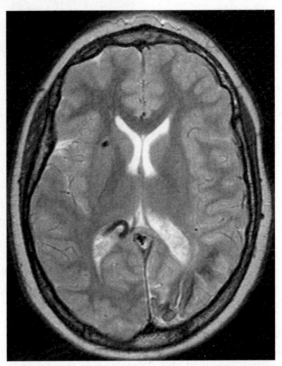

FIGURE 6.9.2

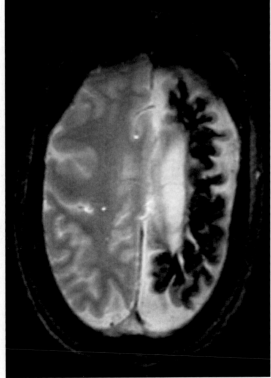

FIGURE 6.9.3

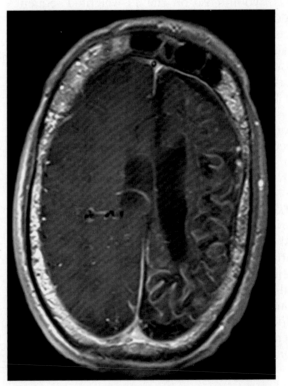

FIGURE 6.9.4

**FINDINGS:** Axial unenhanced CT scan (Fig. 6.9.1) demonstrates gyriform cortical calcifications in the temporal and occipital lobes. Axial T2-weighted MR image (Fig. 6.9.2) demonstrates gyriform low signal corresponding to the calcifications seen on the CT and volume loss of the left hemisphere, mostly within the occipital lobe. Incidentally seen are two right-sided developmental venous anomalies. Axial T2*-weighted gradient echo image in a different patient demonstrates severe atrophy of the left hemisphere with diffuse hypointensity and magnetic susceptibility artifact throughout the cortex (Fig 6.9.3). Corresponding post-contrast T1-weighted image demonstrates extensive leptomeningeal enhancement throughout the left hemisphere (Fig 6.9.4). Note the compensatory enlargement of the left frontal sinuses.

**DIAGNOSIS:** Sturge–Weber syndrome (i.e., encephalotrigeminal angiomatosis)

**DISCUSSION:** Sturge–Weber syndrome is a sporadically occurring, neurocutaneous syndrome. The hallmark of this disease is the vascular angiomatous lesion (i.e., port-wine stain or nevus flammeus) involving the face in the distribution of the trigeminal nerve and ipsilateral brain and meninges. Imaging findings include cortical calcifications, lobar atrophy with secondary calvarial changes (i.e., Dyke–Davidoff–Masson syndrome), leptomeningeal enhancement, choroid plexus angiomas, and venous abnormalities. Evaluation of patients with suspected Sturge–Weber syndrome should include contrast-enhanced MRI because the full extent of the cortical vascular lesions may not be apparent on unenhanced imaging (1,17,18).

## Aunt Minnie's Pearls

Unilateral cortical atrophy and calcifications associated with enhancing leptomeningeal and choroid plexus angiomas = Sturge–Weber syndrome.

MRI with contrast is necessary to evaluate the full extent of the disease.

HISTORY: A 21-year-old man with deafness and a recent history of double vision

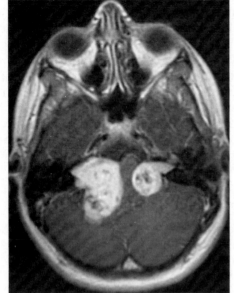

FIGURE 6.10.1

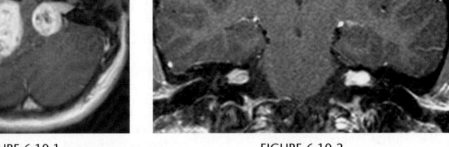

FIGURE 6.10.2

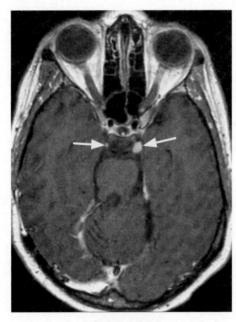

FIGURE 6.10.3

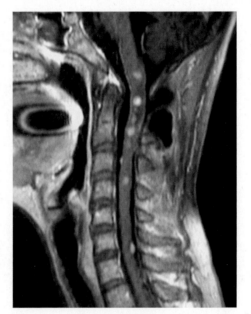

FIGURE 6.10.4

FINDINGS: Axial, T1-weighted post-contrast MR image (Fig. 6.10.1) demonstrates large bilateral avidly enhancing cerebellopontine angle masses with extension into the internal auditory canals. Coronal, T1-weighted post-contrast image in a different patient (Fig. 6.10.2) demonstrates bilateral enhancing internal auditory canal masses, compatible with vestibular schwannomas. Axial, T1-weighted post-contrast MR image in the same patient (Fig. 6.10.3) demonstrates bilateral enhancing masses (arrows) of the oculomotor nerves, left greater than right, compatible with schwannomas. Sagittal post-contrast T1-weighted image in the same patient (Fig. 6.10.4) demonstrates multiple central intramedullary nodules with avid enhancement, compatible with ependymomas. Additional enhancing extramedullary nodules are also seen representing meningiomas and schwannomas.

DIAGNOSIS: Neurofibromatosis type 2

DISCUSSION: Neurofibromatosis type 2 (NF 2) is an autosomal dominant disorder that is recognized as a distinct form of disease separated genetically, clinically, and radiographically from neurofibromatosis type 1 (NF 1). The incidence of NF 2 is approximately 1 case in 50,000 live births, compared with 1 case per 2,000 to 3,000 live births for NF 1. Bilateral vestibular schwannomas (also known as acoustic neuromas) are the hallmark of this disease, commonly manifesting during or soon after puberty. Schwannomas of other cranial and spinal nerves, intracranial and spinal meningiomas, and spinal ependymomas may also be found in these patients (1,19,20).

## Aunt Minnie's Pearls

Bilateral vestibular schwannomas = neurofibromatosis type 2.

NF 2 comprises multiple inherited schwannomas, meningiomas, and ependymomas (MISME).

HISTORY: A 17-year-old girl with mental retardation and seizures

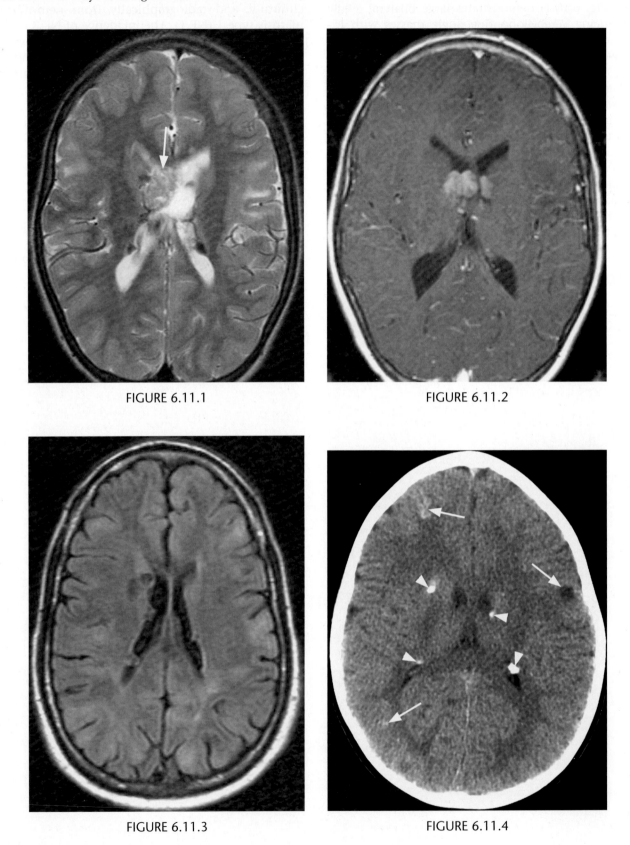

FIGURE 6.11.1

FIGURE 6.11.2

FIGURE 6.11.3

FIGURE 6.11.4

**FINDINGS:** Axial T2-weighted MR image (Fig. 6.11.1) demonstrates a large, heterogeneous mass (*arrow*) in the region of the foramen of Monro. Multiple low-signal-intensity foci are present along the subependymal surface of the lateral ventricles, and multiple foci of increased signal are seen in the subcortical white matter of the frontal lobes bilaterally. Axial post-contrast T1-weighted MR image (Fig. 6.11.2) demonstrates heterogeneous enhancement of the mass in the region of the foramen of Monro. Axial FLAIR image (Fig. 6.11.3) in a different patient demonstrates multiple foci of increased signal in the cortex and subcortical white matter consistent with tubers. Multiple low-signal subependymal nodules are also present. Axial unenhanced CT (Fig. 6.11.4) in another patient shows subependymal calcifications (*arrowheads*) and multiple high- and low-attenuating cortical and subcortical tubers (*arrows*).

**DIAGNOSIS:** Tuberous sclerosis with subependymal giant cell astrocytoma

**DISCUSSION:** Tuberous sclerosis complex (TSC) is the second most common of the neurocutaneous syndromes and is characterized by the formation of hamartomatous lesions in multiple organs. The genes responsible for TSC are tumor suppressor genes TSC1 (9q34) that encodes the protein *hamartin* and TSC2 (16p13) that encodes the protein *tuberin*. Most cases (66%) of TSC result from a spontaneous mutation, and the remainder are inherited in an autosomal dominant fashion. Although there is complete penetrance, TSC exhibits a high degree of phenotypic variability. Many patients have obvious signs at birth, whereas others remain undiagnosed for many years. In addition, approximately 20% of TSC patients do not have either of the TSC1 or TSC2 mutations. The classic clinical triad of adenoma sebaceum, seizures, and mental retardation is present only in a minority of patients with TSC.

The CNS lesions include astrocytic hamartomas of the retina, cortical tubers, and subependymal nodular hamartomas. A single cortical/subcortical lesion as seen in focal cortical dysplasia of Taylor (balloon type) is histologically the same as TSC. Approximately 15% of patients develop subependymal giant-cell astrocytomas (GCA), which are characterized as grade 1 neoplasms by the WHO. The GCAs virtually always arise near the foramen of Monro and can cause obstructive hydrocephalus. GCAs may also undergo malignant degeneration. By CT, GCA appears as an enhancing soft-tissue mass with variable calcification. MR imaging shows hypointensity to isointensity on T1-weighted images, hyperintensity on T2-weighted images, and uniform gadolinium enhancement. Even subependymal hamartomas frequently enhance on MRI, and interval increase in size is considered the only reliable sign of GCA development (18,21,22).

Lesions associated with TSC outside of the CNS include renal angiomyolipomas (AML), lymphangiomyomatosis (LAM) of the lung, and cardiac rhabdomyomas.

## Aunt Minnie's Pearls

The CNS lesions of TSC include cortical tubers, subependymal and retinal hamartomas, and GCAs. Interval increase in size of subependymal hamartomas near the foramen of Monro on MRI indicates development of GCAs.

Renal AMLs, pulmonary LAM, and cardiac rhabdomyomas are associated with TSC.

HISTORY: A 32-year-old man with ataxia, nausea, and vomiting

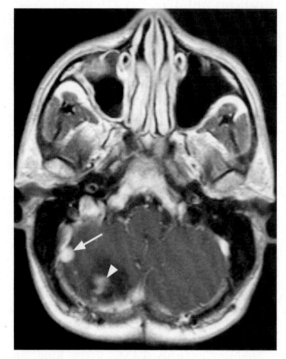

FIGURE 6.12.1

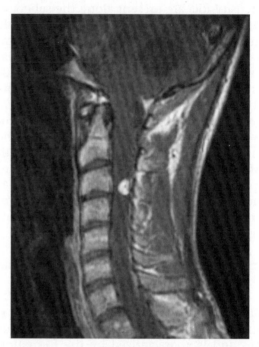

FIGURE 6.12.2

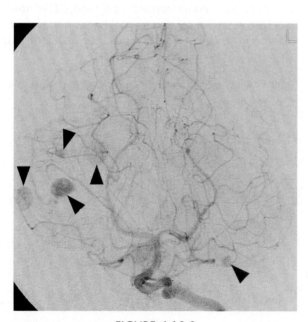

FIGURE 6.12.3

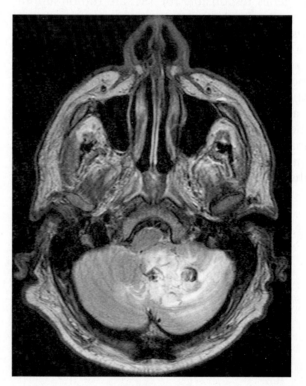

FIGURE 6.12.4

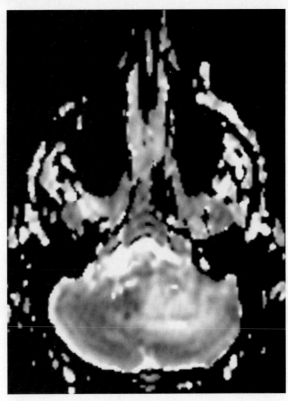

FIGURE 6.12.5

**FINDINGS:** Axial, T1-weighted post-contrast MR image (Fig. 6.12.1) demonstrates two enhancing masses in the right cerebellar hemisphere, the larger one with a cystic appearance containing a mural nodule (*arrowhead*). The other lesion is more laterally and anteriorly located (*arrow*). Sagittal post-contrast T1-weighted image through the cervical spine (Fig. 6.12.2) shows an additional enhancing lesion along the dorsal spinal cord surface. AP digital subtraction angiogram from a left vertebral injection in the same patient (Fig. 6.12.3) demonstrates multiple cerebellar hypervascular masses (*arrowheads*). Axial T2-weighted MR image in a different patient (Fig. 6.12.4) demonstrates a large mass within the left cerebellum with increased T2 signal and multiple internal flow voids. Axial ADC image through the lesion (Fig. 6.12.5) demonstrates the increased diffusion within the mass relative to the adjacent brain parenchyma.

**DIAGNOSIS:** Cerebellar hemangioblastomas in a patient with von Hippel–Lindau syndrome

**DISCUSSION:** Hemangioblastomas are rare tumors, accounting for less than 3% of all intracranial neoplasms, and typically occur in patients 20 to 50 years old. Hemangioblastomas occur sporadically or as a manifestation of von Hippel–Lindau (VHL) syndrome. VHL syndrome is inherited as an autosomal dominant disorder linked to a defect on chromosome 3. In addition to hemangioblastomas of the cerebellum, brainstem, spinal cord and other intracranial structures, lymphatic duct adenocarcinomas and non-CNS manifestations, including cysts of the kidneys, pancreas, and liver, as well as renal cell carcinoma, microcystic adenoma of the pancreas, and pheochromocytomas may be seen in patients with VHL syndrome. Hemangioblastomas in VHL syndrome are multiples in up to 40% of cases and typically present at least 10 years earlier than those occurring in patients without the syndrome. The diagnosis of VHL syndrome requires multiple hemangioblastomas or one hemangioblastoma with other visceral manifestations of the disease. More than 50% of hemangioblastomas are cystic, with a mural nodule that demonstrates intense enhancement. Owing to hypervascularity, flow voids are commonly seen either within the mass or at its periphery. In addition, on perfusion imaging, hemangioblastomas typically demonstrate increased CBV. They are one of the few benign tumors to exhibit an elevated CBV. Hemangioblastomas also show increased diffusion compared to the normal-appearing brain parenchyma. If the cyst wall is thick or enhancing, other neoplasms should be considered. A majority (around 70%) of patients with isolated cerebellar hemangioblastomas do not have VHL (18,23,24).

## Aunt Minnie's Pearls

Multiple cystic masses with an enhancing mural nodule, flow voids, or one mass with specific visceral manifestations = VHL syndrome.

Visceral manifestations of VHL syndrome = renal, pancreatic, and liver cysts, renal cell carcinoma, pheochromocytoma, and retinal hemangioblastomas.

# Case 6.13

HISTORY: A 29-month-old boy born at 36 weeks' gestation with history of neonatal intraventricular hemorrhage, seizures, and hydrocephalus, now with cerebral palsy and spastic quadriplegia

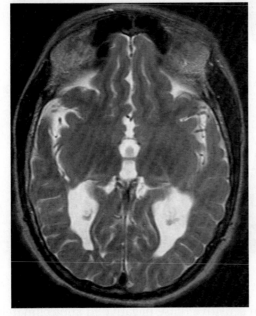

FIGURE 6.13.1

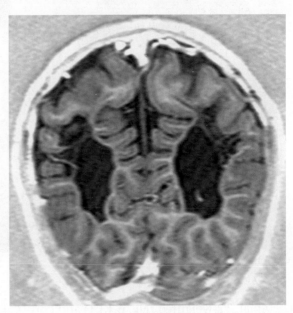

FIGURE 6.13.2

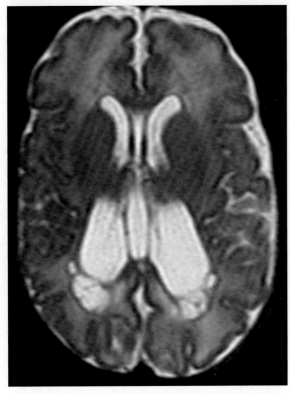

FIGURE 6.13.3

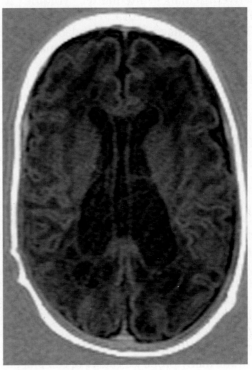

FIGURE 6.13.4

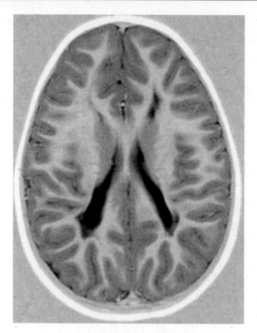

FIGURE 6.13.5

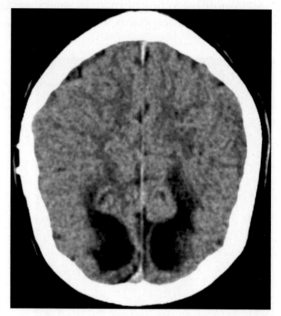

FIGURE 6.13.6

**FINDINGS:** Axial, T2-weighted (Fig. 6.13.1) and coronal T1-weighted inversion recovery (Fig. 6.13.2) MR images demonstrate irregular, "wavy" contour to the surface of dilated lateral ventricles and severe periventricular white-matter volume loss. Axial T2-weighted (Fig. 6.13.3) and T1-weighted (Fig. 6.13.4) MR images in a second patient demonstrate large cysts within the white matter posterior to enlarged bilateral lateral ventricles. Axial T1-inversion recovery MR image in a third patient (Fig. 6.13.5) demonstrates more subtle irregularity of the surface of the lateral ventricles and mild periventricular white-matter volume loss. An axial CT image from yet another patient (Fig. 6.13.6) demonstrates severe posterior white-matter volume loss.

**DIAGNOSIS:** Periventricular leukomalacia

**DISCUSSION:** Periventricular leukomalacia (PVL) is the term used to describe brain injury in premature neonates related to the susceptibility of the periventricular white matter to ischemic or infectious-inflammatory processes. Deep periventricular white matter is particularly susceptible to injury because glial cells in this area are differentiating into astrocytes and oligodendrocytes, with some in the process of myelination. The resulting dysgenetic white-matter tracts are one of the many proposed causes of cerebral palsy.

Ultrasound evaluation can show echogenic foci in the "watershed" areas of the periventricular trigones and frontal horns. Although convenient in the neonatal intensive care unit, ultrasound is not sensitive (false negative in approximately 55%) and has a high false-positive rate and low positive predictive value, with only approximately 26% of infants who have prolonged periventricular echogenicity showing significant changes on MR. This may be in part because PVL is difficult to distinguish from the normal "halo" of anisotropic myelin and vasculature in the trigonal region.

As PVL evolves and the water content of the infant brain decreases, CT and MRI can be very useful. The examiner may see hemorrhage, small cyst formation (2–3 weeks), large cyst formation (i.e., "Swiss cheese appearance"), coalescence (1–3 months), and deep white-matter hypoplasia. Although MRI can demonstrate all of these findings, CT may miss small cysts. The imaging hallmark of late PVL (synonymous with white-matter hypoplasia) is deep cortical sulci extending inward to enlarged lateral ventricles with decreased volume of white matter. Head size is normal (1,25).

## Aunt Minnie's Pearls

The CT or MRI hallmark of late PVL is deep cortical gray matter extending inward toward enlarged, usually scalloped, lateral ventricles with markedly decreased intervening white matter.

Pitfall: PVL is difficult to distinguish from the normal echogenic halo of the periventricular trigonal region on ultrasound.

**HISTORY:** An 8-year-old boy with history of head trauma

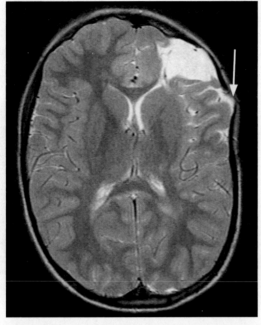

FIGURE 6.14.1

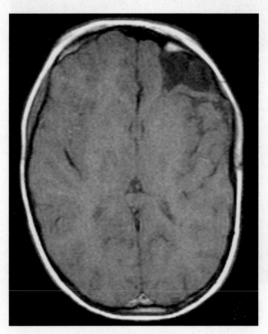

FIGURE 6.14.2

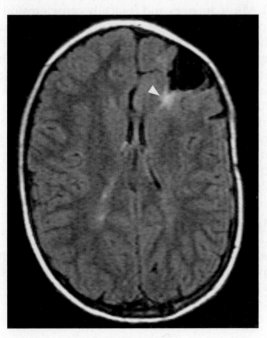

FIGURE 6.14.3

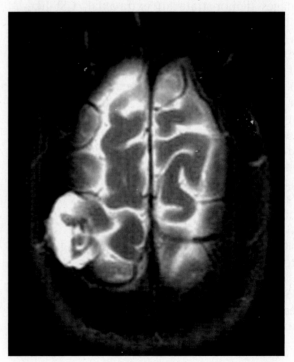

FIGURE 6.14.4

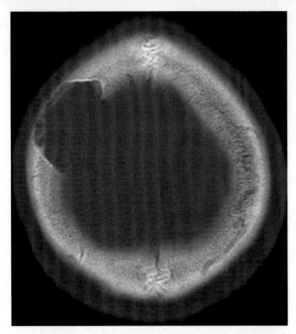

FIGURE 6.14.5

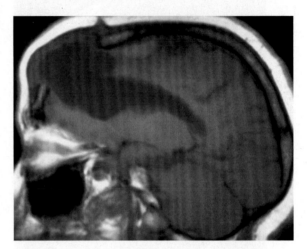

FIGURE 6.14.6

**FINDINGS:** Axial T2-weighted (Fig. 6.14.1), T1-weighted (Fig. 6.14.2) and FLAIR (Fig. 6.14.3) MR images demonstrate an extra-axial, CSF-like-intensity left frontal mass with a small area of gliosis in the adjacent brain parenchyma, best seen on the FLAIR image (*arrowhead*). There is herniation of the cystic structure through the calvarium (*arrow*). Axial T2-weighted MR image (Fig. 6.14.4) from a second patient reveals a more conspicuous CSF intensity structure herniating into the adjacent right frontal calvarium. Axial CT image (Fig. 6.14.5) from the same patient shows the effects upon the adjacent calvarium to better advantage. A sagittal T1-weighted MR image (Fig. 6.14.6) through the center of this cystic lesion demonstrates its herniation through the overlying calvarium.

**DIAGNOSIS:** Leptomeningeal cyst, growing skull fracture

**DISCUSSION:** Leptomeningeal cysts (LMCs) are rare lesions that are typically a consequence of childhood cranial fractures and may become symptomatic years later, even in adulthood. They occur in only 0.05% to 0.6% of all cranial fractures, and seizures are the most frequent symptom. LMCs are extra-axial masses that follow CSF intensity on all MR sequences and typically cause erosion of the adjacent inner table of the skull and herniate into the bone. The proposed pathogenesis includes dural tear beneath an acute fracture, followed by herniation of the arachnoid tissue through the defect. The subarachnoid adhesions then isolate the arachnoid fluid and form an encapsulated cyst, which keeps enlarging owing to CSF pulsations toward both the overlying fracture and the underlying brain. Gliosis in the adjacent brain parenchyma is also frequently found, best seen as hyperintensity on FLAIR images (26–28).

## Aunt Minnie's Pearl

Extra-axial mass that follows CSF on all pulse sequences and herniates into the adjacent skull in a patient with a history of head trauma = LMC.

**HISTORY:** A 34-year-old woman with headaches.

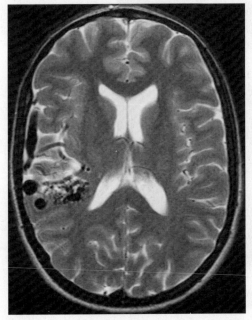

FIGURE 6.15.1

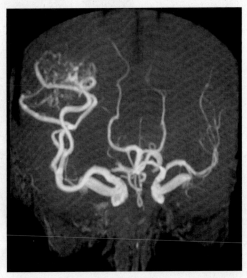

FIGURE 6.15.2

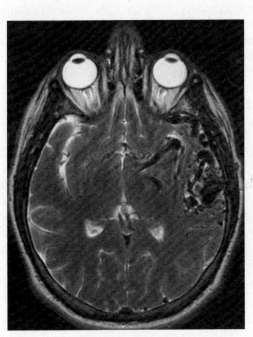

FIGURE 6.15.3

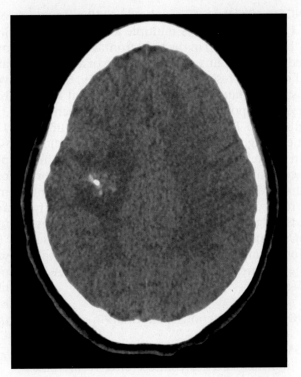

FIGURE 6.15.4

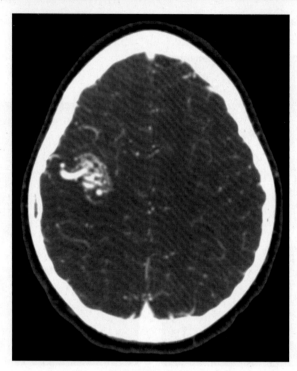

FIGURE 6.15.5

**FINDINGS:** Axial, T2-weighted MR image (Fig. 6.15.1) demonstrates multiple abnormal flow voids ("bag of worms") in the right frontal lobe, with enlarged draining veins. A 3D rendering of an unenhanced magnetic resonance angiogram (Fig. 6.15.2) demonstrates a tangle of vessels in the distal MCA territory, corresponding to the flow voids seen on the MRI. Axial, T2-weighted MR image in a different patient (Fig. 6.15.3) demonstrates multiple flow voids in the left temporal lobe with large draining veins, compatible with an arteriovenous malformation (AVM). Noncontrast CT in a third patient (Fig. 6.15.4) demonstrates an area of hyperdensity within the right centrum semiovale. Note the presence of several small foci of calcification. A corresponding CT angiogram in the same patient reveals multiple enhancing vessels consistent with an AVM (Fig. 6.15.5).

**DIAGNOSIS:** Arteriovenous malformation

**DISCUSSION:** AVMs are a tangle of abnormal blood vessels in which arteries connect directly to veins without an intervening capillary network. It is estimated that the prevalence of AVMs is 0.04% to 0.5% approximately. AVMs typically present with headache and hemorrhage (50%), seizure (25%), and focal neurologic deficit (20%–25%). The peak age of presentation is between 20 and 40 years of age. Most (85% to 90%) are located supratentorally and approximately 10% to 15% infratentorially. AVMs are classified by the Spetzler–Martin grading scale, which ranges from 1 to 5 points. Points are assigned based on size (1 for size <3 cm, 2 for sizes 3–6 cm, and 3 for size >6 cm), location (0 for noneloquent area, 1 for eloquent area of brain), and venous drainage (0 for superficial drainage, 1 for deep drainage). The points are combined to give the final grade. The goal of the grading system is to predict the risk of surgical morbidity and mortality. AVMs have a characteristic appearance on T2-weighted MR images, with a nidus of abnormal flow voids that has been described as a "bag of worms" appearance, and enlarged draining veins. Post-contrast images reveal strong enhancement of the AVM. AVMs may be seen on MR angiography, but the gold standard for characterizing AVMs is DSA to dynamically evaluate the feeding arteries, the nidus, and the draining veins (29–31).

## Aunt Minnie's Pearl

T2-weighted MRI images are virtually diagnostic of AVMs, demonstrating the nidus of the malformation with bag of worms appearance and dilated draining veins.

# Case 6.16

**HISTORY:** A 51-year-old patient with history of pontine hemorrhage 10 months ago

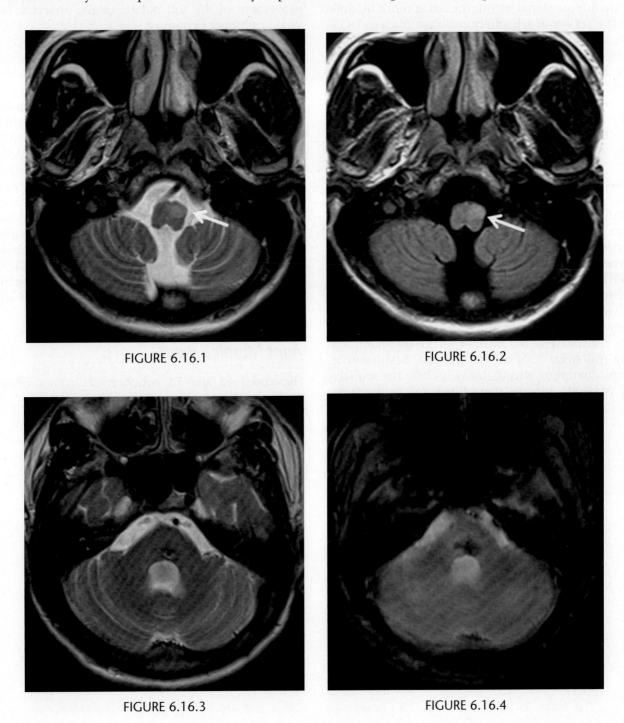

FIGURE 6.16.1

FIGURE 6.16.2

FIGURE 6.16.3

FIGURE 6.16.4

**FINDINGS:** Axial T2 and FLAIR images demonstrate hyperintense signal within the left anterior medulla in the region of left inferior olivary nucleus (ION) (Figs. 6.16.1 and 6.16.2, white arrows). In addition, the left ION is enlarged in comparison with the normal contralateral side. There was no contrast enhancement in this region (not shown). Axial T2-weighted and T2*-weighted images at the level of pons demonstrate susceptibility artifact secondary to hemosiderin deposition status post remote pontine hemorrhage (Figs. 6.16.3 and 6.16.4).

**DIAGNOSIS:** Hypertrophic olivary degeneration

**DISCUSSION:** Hypertrophic olivary degeneration (HOD) is a unique neurodegenerative process characterized by the somewhat counterintuitive hypertrophy of the affected structure, the ION. HOD occurs secondary to damage to the dentato-rubro-olivary pathway (or Guillain–Mollaret triangle) comprising white-matter tracts extending between the dentate nucleus of the cerebellum, the contralateral red nucleus of the midbrain, and the ipsilateral ION of the medulla. Brainstem lesions disrupting this pathway include the sequelae of ischemic infarct, demyelination, hemorrhage, and surgery. The most common clinical symptoms associated with HOD are rhythmic involuntary movement of the soft palate, uvula, pharynx, larynx, and upper extremity.

Characteristic imaging findings in conjunction with a suggestive clinical presentation can establish the diagnosis of HOD. CT is relatively insensitive for the detection of the subtle brainstem findings in HOD; therefore, MRI is the imaging test of choice. MR findings are dependent on the time elapsed since the causative insult. During the first 6 months, HOD manifests as T2 hyperintensity within the affected ION without definitive enlargement. Beginning at about 6 months after the insult, the ION hypertrophies and retains its T2 hyperintensity. This characteristic appearance typically persists for up to 4 years after which there is resolution of the hypertrophy with retention of the T2 hyperintensity. The above findings are present in conjunction with a causative lesion along the triangle, usually in the brainstem. There is no associated abnormal enhancement and lesions may also be bilateral (32,33).

## Aunt Minnie's Pearl

Hypertrophied and T2 hyperintense inferior olivary nucleus with a causative lesion in the brainstem.

**HISTORY:** A 16-year-old girl with seizures

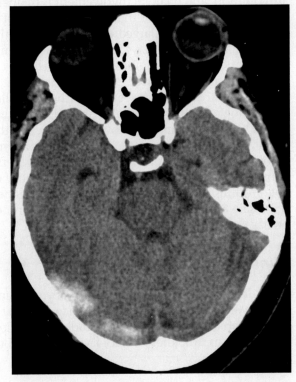

FIGURE 6.17.1

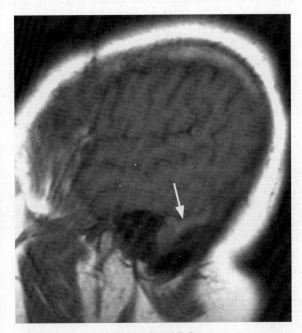

FIGURE 6.17.2

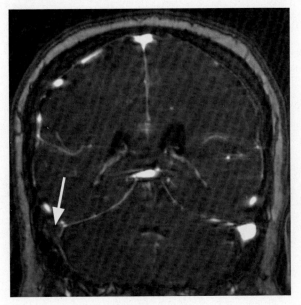

FIGURE 6.17.3

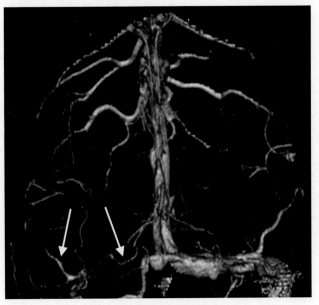

FIGURE 6.17.4

FINDINGS: Axial, noncontrast CT (Fig. 6.17.1) shows high density in the right transverse sinus. Sagittal T1-weighted MR image (Fig. 6.17.2) demonstrates high-signal intensity in the right transverse and sigmoid sinus (*arrow*). A coronal source image from post-contrast MR venogram (Fig. 6.17.3) demonstrates a filling defect (*arrow*) with absence of contrast within the right transverse sinus. A 3D rendering of CT venogram in the same patient confirms the absence of contrast opacification within the right transverse sinus (arrows) (Fig. 6.17.4).

DIAGNOSIS: Cerebral venous thrombosis

DISCUSSION: Cerebral venous thrombosis is an uncommon disorder in which the diagnosis and appropriate management are often delayed because of the nonspecific clinical manifestations. This condition is most common in infants with dehydration or septicemia. Oral contraceptives, pregnancy, diabetes, malignant neoplasms, and hematologic disorders are etiologic factors associated with venous thrombosis in adults. CT findings include hyperdense thrombus within the deep and/or cortical intracranial venous structures on noncontrast studies, which is not always present. Hypodensity representing edema or infarction may also be seen. Hemorrhagic infarcts are common, and bilateral involvement is frequently seen, particularly of the thalami. Nonfilling of the cerebral veins with enlarged collaterals is identified by angiography. MRI may be used as the definitive investigation. The thrombosed vessel becomes hyperintense on T1-weighted and T2-weighted images as the thrombus becomes replete with extracellular methemoglobin. Clot may also show loss of signal on T2*-weighted images; however, none of these signs is completely accurate for diagnosis of venous thrombosis. Absence of contrast filling, best seen on contrast-enhanced MR venogram, is the most reliable finding. Antithrombotic therapy is considered to be safe and effective treatment, even when hemorrhage is present (34,35).

## Aunt Minnie's Pearl

Hyperdensity on noncontrast CT, hyperintensity on T1-weighted images, and absence of flow on angiographic/contrast enhanced studies in the intracranial venous structures = cerebral venous thrombosis.

**HISTORY:** A 60-year-old man presenting with confusion 2 weeks after heart transplant

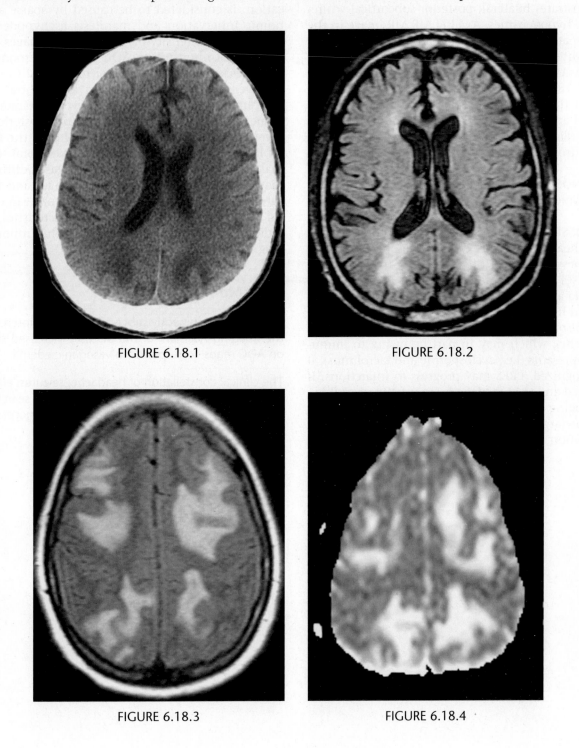

FIGURE 6.18.1

FIGURE 6.18.2

FIGURE 6.18.3

FIGURE 6.18.4

**FINDINGS:** Axial unenhanced CT (Fig. 6.18.1) demonstrates bilateral, posterior subcortical white-matter hypodensities. Axial FLAIR MR image in the same patient (Fig. 6.18.2) demonstrates bilateral hyperintense subcortical white-matter signal abnormality. Axial FLAIR MR image in a different patient (Fig. 6.18.3) demonstrates increased signal bilaterally in the cortical and subcortical regions of the frontal and parietal lobes. Corresponding ADC MR image (Fig. 6.18.4) demonstrates increased diffusion in the frontal and parietal lobes.

**DIAGNOSIS:** Posterior reversible encephalopathy syndrome (PRES)

**DISCUSSION:** PRES presents with symptoms that include headache, seizures, altered mental status, and blindness. It is most often associated with sudden increases in blood pressure as seen in cases of eclampsia and pre-eclampsia, acute glomerulonephritis, and hypertensive crisis. Various other situations may also cause PRES, most notably in transplant recipients, which may in part be owing to immunosuppresants (i.e., cyclosporine and tacrolimus). If unrecognized, PRES may progress to infarctions. If detected and treated, deficits are usually reversible.

Imaging plays an important role in early diagnosis. The target area for PRES is the posterior cerebral circulation. The resulting bilateral occipitoparietal vasogenic edema, predominantly subcortical in location, is considered to be caused by sparse autonomic innervation and manifests as hypodensity on CT, hyperintensity on T2-weighted images, and high-signal intensity on ADC maps corresponding to increased diffusion of water molecules. Cortical involvement is not uncommon and contrast enhancement is occasionally observed. Despite the name, the lesions are not necessarily posterior or reversible. They are frequently located in the frontal lobes and may be found in deep cerebral white matter and even the brainstem. Decreased diffusion may be present even in the early stages and indicates possible infarcts. Because of the protean clinical picture and subtle imaging characteristics, the radiologist may be the first to suggest this important diagnosis (36–38).

## Aunt Minnie's Pearls

Bilateral predominantly subcortical T2 hyperintensity is the imaging hallmark of the disease. Increased signal on ADC maps corresponds to vasogenic edema.

The clinical constellation of headache, seizures, altered mental status, and blindness may trigger a search for PRES. Despite the name, the lesions are not necessarily posterior or reversible.

**HISTORY:** A 58-year-old man with deafness and ataxia

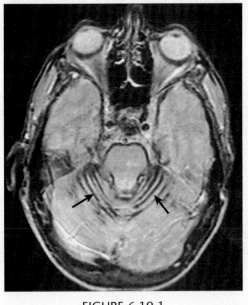

FIGURE 6.19.1

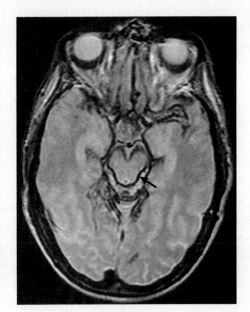

FIGURE 6.19.2

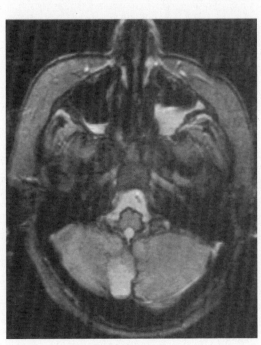

FIGURE 6.19.3

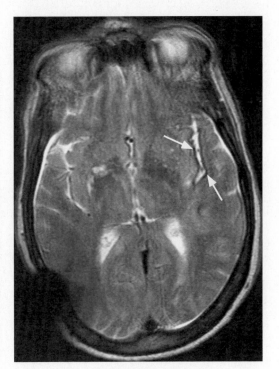

FIGURE 6.19.4

FINDINGS: Axial, T2*-weighted MR images at the level of the brainstem (Figs. 6.19.1 and 6.19.2) demonstrate low signal coating the surface of the brainstem and cerebellum (*arrows*). Axial T2*-weighted gradient echo MR image in a different patient (Fig. 6.19.3) also demonstrates low signal coating the surface of the brainstem and cerebellum. Axial T2-weighted MR image in yet another patient (Fig. 6.19.4) reveals more subtle low signal along the brain surface best seen in the left Sylvian fissure (*arrows*).

DIAGNOSIS: Superficial siderosis

DISCUSSION: Superficial siderosis is a rare disorder characterized by the deposition of hemosiderin in the leptomeninges covering the cerebrum, cerebellum, brainstem, cranial nerves, and spinal cord. Chronic subarachnoid hemorrhage is the cause of superficial siderosis, and the source of bleeding is found in less than 50% of patients. The clinical triad of sensorineural hearing loss, cerebellar ataxia, and pyramidal signs along with hemorrhagic or xanthochromic CSF permits a clinical diagnosis. MRI readily confirms the hemosiderin deposition and provides a diagnosis at an earlier stage of the disease. T2-weighted images demonstrate a rim of marked hypointensity along the surface of affected structures, which is much better demonstrated on T2*-weighted images. CT occasionally suggests the diagnosis by showing a rim of mild hyperdensity around the brainstem; however, MRI demonstrates this abnormality to a much better advantage. (39,40).

## Aunt Minnie's Pearls

A marked hypointense rim on T2-weighted, and especially T2*, MR images coating the brain and spinal cord = superficial siderosis.

The cause of this disorder is chronic subarachnoid hemorrhage.

# Case 6.20

HISTORY: A 58-year-old man with severe headaches

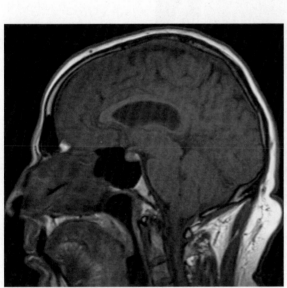

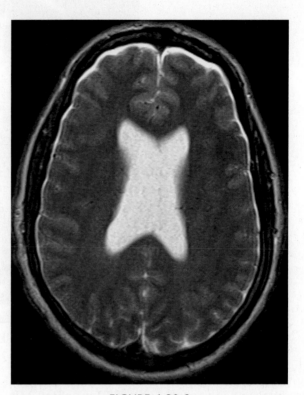

FIGURE 6.20.1

FIGURE 6.20.2

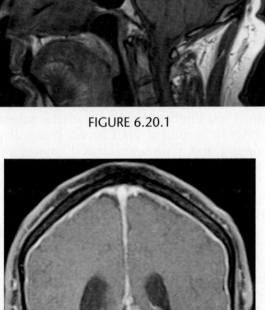

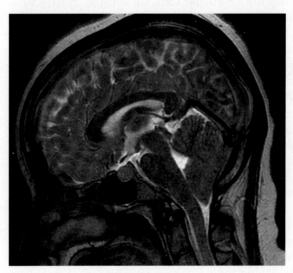

FIGURE 6.20.3

FIGURE 6.20.4

FINDINGS: Sagittal, T1-weighted (Fig. 6.20.1) MR image demonstrates narrowed distance between the mamillary bodies and superior aspect of the pons with cerebellar tonsils projecting into the foramen magnum. Axial, T2-weighted (Fig. 6.20.2) MR image demonstrates dural thickening and prominence of the extra-axial space bilaterally in both frontal regions. Coronal post-contrast T1-weighted

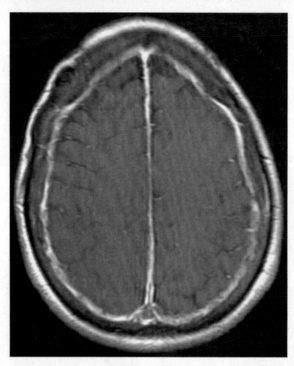

FIGURE 6.20.5

(Fig. 6.20.3) MR image demonstrates smooth, diffuse dural enhancement. Sagittal T2-weighted MR image (Fig. 6.20.4) in a different patient again demonstrates decreased distance between the mammillary bodies and the superior aspect of the pons as well as inferior cerebellar tonsillar ectopia. Note also the enlarged pituitary gland and significant narrowing of the prepontine cistern. Axial post-contrast T1-weighted MR image (Fig. 6.20.5) again demonstrates smooth diffuse pachymeningeal enhancement.

**DIAGNOSIS:** Intracranial hypotension

**DISCUSSION:** Intracranial hypotension (IH) is a clinical and pathologic entity in which imaging plays a crucial role. The common clinical presentation is positional, or orthostatic, headaches; patients develop excruciating cephalgia on standing, which is relieved only by recumbency. There are myriad other clinical findings, all of which demonstrate significant overlap with various other causes of meningeal irritation, hence the importance of radiologic evaluation.

There are several varieties of IH. The most common is spontaneous intracranial hypotension (SIH), which typically results from exertional rupture of a congenital cervicothoracic dural diverticulum, with persistent spillage of CSF into the paraspinal soft tissues. Fluid often tracks cephalad and collects in the deep nuchal region, providing a hint to the diagnosis. Post-lumbar puncture headache represents an iatrogenic version of SIH. Chronic ventricular overshunting and post-neurosurgical or posttraumatic CSF loss are other known causes of the syndrome.

CSF volume depletion invokes the Monroe–Kellie rule and produces the typical imaging features of IH: expansion of the epidural venous plexus, diffuse dural enhancement, sinking of the brain (i.e., effacement of suprasellar cisterns and inferior tonsillar migration), subdural fluid collections, and distention of the dural venous sinuses. These are best demonstrated with gadolinium-enhanced T1-weighted images, although in the acute setting, In-111 cisternography may demonstrate early systemic clearance of radiotracer in the kidneys and bladder, and the classic Christmas tree sign at the sight of rupture (41–43).

## Aunt Minnie's Pearls

Imaging findings include diffuse meningeal enhancement and "sagging brain" with effacement of suprasellar cisterns and tonsillar herniation. Subdural fluid collections may also be present.

Postural headaches in the postexertional setting suggest spontaneous intracranial hypotension.

**HISTORY:** A 36-year-old woman with headache, vertigo, nausea, and vomiting

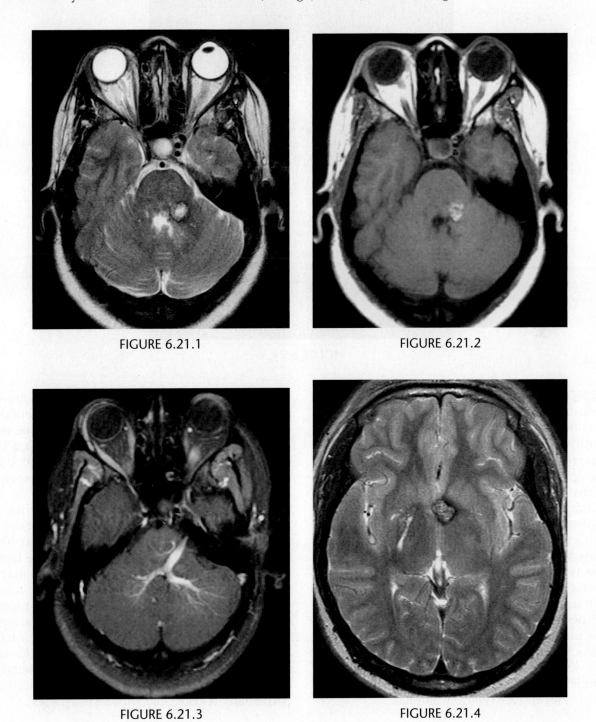

FIGURE 6.21.1                    FIGURE 6.21.2

FIGURE 6.21.3                    FIGURE 6.21.4

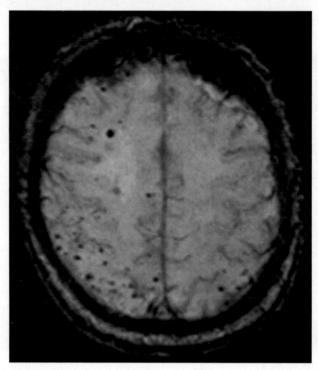

FIGURE 6.21.5

**FINDINGS:** Axial T2-weighted MR image (Fig. 6.21.1) demonstrates a heterogeneous mass within the left middle cerebellar peduncle with low-signal-intensity rim. Corresponding axial T1-weighted MR image (Fig. 6.21.2) demonstrates "popcorn-like" high-signal intensity within the mass. Axial post-contrast T1-weighted images through the same region (Fig. 6.21.3) reveal linear enhancement with a "caput medusa" appearance. Axial T2-weighted image in a different patient (Fig. 6.21.4) demonstrates a mass in the left basal ganglia with low-signal-intensity rim, consistent with a cavernoma. Axial T2*-weighted gradient echo MR image (Fig. 6.21.5) in the same patient at the level of the centrum semiovale demonstrates multiple small foci of magnetic susceptibility artifact bilaterally. Although this finding is nonspecific and could represent an alternative diagnosis (such as cerebral amyloid angiopathy), multiple cavernomas can be seen in about 10% to 20% of cases and are typically familial.

**DIAGNOSIS:** Cavernous angioma (cavernoma, cavernous malformation, cavernous hemangioma) with associated developmental venous anomaly

**DISCUSSION:** Cavernous angiomas are vascular malformations that are considered benign hamartomatous lesions with thin-walled sinusoidal vessels. Many are associated with developmental venous anomalies (DVAs), and a few cases of de novo cavernoma development next to an existing DVA have been reported. They tend to be asymptomatic but may bleed and cause headaches and seizures. These lesions are frequently sporadic but may also occur in familial forms, and in those cases tend to be multiple. Several genetic markers have been associated with familial cavernomas. Noncontrast CT may show a high-density lesion. These lesions are classically angiographically occult but may be seen if associated with a DVA. MRI is the modality of choice for diagnosis, with prominent loss of signal on T2* sequences. The lesions characteristically show both T1 and T2 heterogeneous internal "popcorn" signal intensities with a complete dark rim on T2-weighted images representing hemosiderin. Some lesions may show subtle enhancement, particularly if associated with a DVA (44,45).

### Aunt Minnie's Pearl

Nonenhancing mass with heterogeneous internal structure and complete hemosiderin ring on T2-weighted images = cavernous angioma.

**HISTORY:** A 39-year-old woman with postural headache

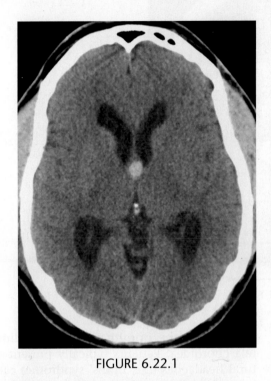

FIGURE 6.22.1

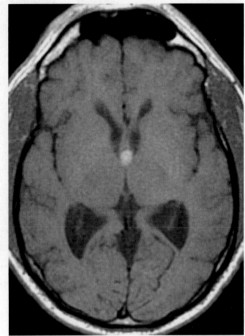

FIGURE 6.22.2

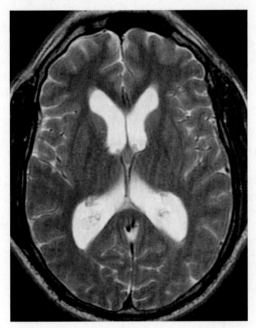

FIGURE 6.22.3

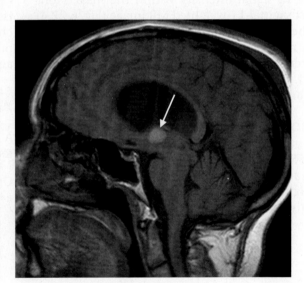

FIGURE 6.22.4

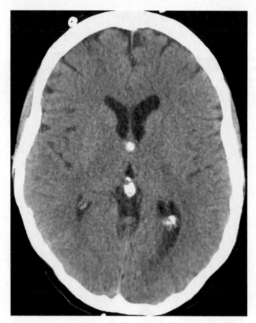

FIGURE 6.22.5

**FINDINGS:** Axial unenhanced CT image (Fig. 6.22.1) demonstrates a well-defined hyperdense midline mass in the region of the foramen of Monro, with mild prominence of the lateral ventricles. Axial T1- and T2-weighted images through the same region (Figs. 6.22.2 and 6.22.3) demonstrates increased T1 and iso T2 signal intensity within the mass. Noncontrast sagittal T1-weighted MR image (Fig. 6.22.4) from the same patient redemonstrates the T1 hyperintense mass (*arrow*). Axial unenhanced CT image in a different patient (Fig. 6.22.5) demonstrates a well-defined, hyperdense midline mass in the region of the foramen of Monro.

**DIAGNOSIS:** Colloid cyst

**DISCUSSION:** Third ventricular colloid cysts are rare masses accounting for <1% of all intracranial tumors. The origin of this benign lesion remains controversial, although a widely accepted theory suggests an origin from the primitive neuroepithelium of the tela choroidea. Patients typically present with postural headaches (i.e., Bruns' syndrome) caused by a ball-valve effect at the foramen of Monro, with associated obstructive hydrocephalus. Acute ventricular obstruction resulting in death has been reported. Colloid cysts usually do not enhance and are either isodense or hyperdense to brain on CT. The signal characteristics on MR vary, but the most common appearance is a hyperintense mass on T1-weighted images caused by the high cholesterol content (46,47).

## Aunt Minnie's Pearls

A hyperdense midline mass on noncontrast CT in the region of the foramen of Monro = colloid cyst.

On T1-weighted MRI, a colloid cyst usually presents as a high-signal-intensity mass.

**HISTORY:** A 9-year-old boy with precocious puberty

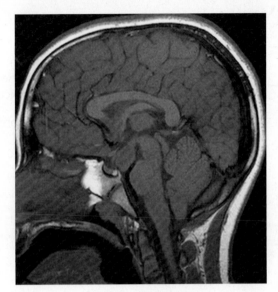

FIGURE 6.23.1

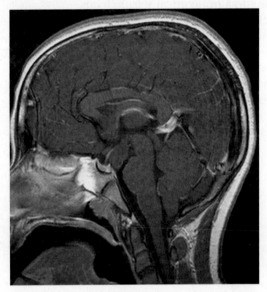

FIGURE 6.23.2

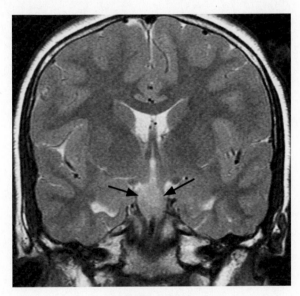

FIGURE 6.23.3

**FINDINGS:** Sagittal, T1-weighted MR images before and after contrast (Figs. 6.23.1 and 6.23.2) demonstrate nonenhancing mass between the pituitary stalk and mamillary bodies in the region of the tuber cinereum. Coronal T2-weighted image in the same patient (Fig. 6.23.3) demonstrates a high-signal-intensity mass (*arrows*) in the region of the tuber cinereum and along the walls of the third ventricle in the hypothalamus.

**DIAGNOSIS:** Hypothalamic hamartoma (HH), or hamartoma of tuber cinereum

**DISCUSSION:** Hypothalamic hamartomas (HHs) are congenital, nonneoplastic lesions classically associated with "gelastic" or laughing seizures. Patients may also display central precocious puberty (CPP) or be entirely asymptomatic. The clinical presentation is often dependent on lesion anatomy, with small, pedunculated

HHs producing CPP and large, sessile HHs producing gelastic seizures. HH produces a specific type of epilepsy owing to a noncortical seizure focus.

Magnetic resonance imaging shows a mass, sometimes reaching 4 cm in diameter, which projects from the tuber cinereum or mamillary bodies into the suprasellar or interpeduncular cisterns. HH follows signal intensity of gray matter on T1-weighted sequences, is of iso-to-hyperintense T2 signal, and does not enhance. Hypothalamic astrocytoma may have a similar imaging appearance. Because of its often pedunculated and noncortical location,

transcallosal neurosurgical resection can produce cure with minimal morbidity (48,49).

### Aunt Minnie's Pearls

A nonenhancing mass iso-to-hyperintense on T2-weighted images that is located between the mamillary bodies and pituitary infundibulum is typical.

HH is associated with gelastic seizures and precocious puberty.

HISTORY: A 36-year-old woman with intermittent headaches

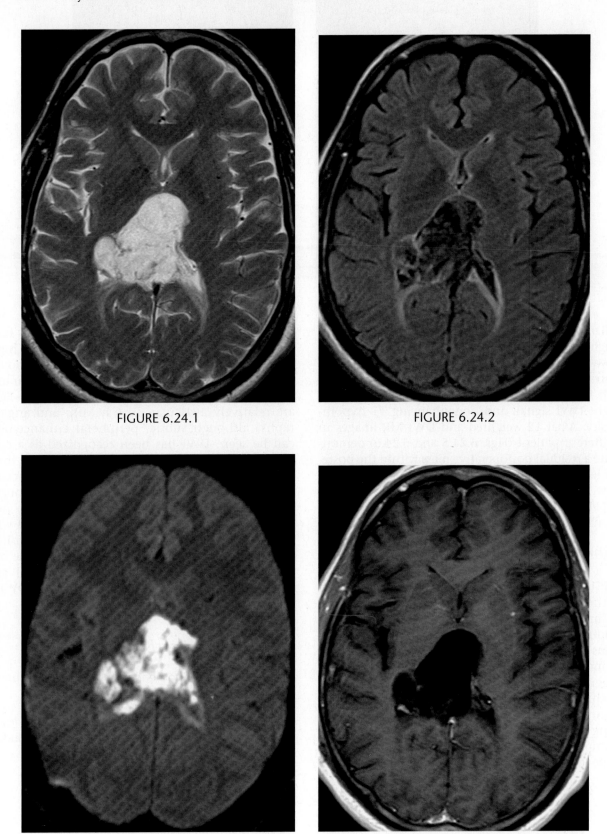

FIGURE 6.24.1

FIGURE 6.24.2

FIGURE 6.24.3

FIGURE 6.24.4

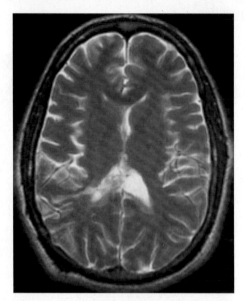

FIGURE 6.24.5

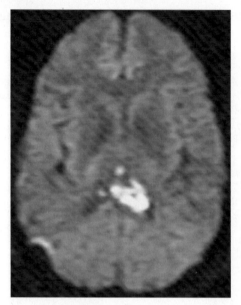

FIGURE 6.24.6

**FINDINGS:** Axial T2-weighted, FLAIR, diffusion-weighted imaging (DWI), and post-contrast T1-weighted MR images (Figs. 6.24.1 to 6.24.4) demonstrate an extra-axial mass in the suprapineal recess with T2 hyperintensity, heterogeneous FLAIR signal, bright DWI signal, and nonenhancing T1 hypointensity. Axial T2-weighted and DWI MR images in a different patient (Figs. 6.24.5 and 6.24.6) demonstrate a residual postoperative mass within the posterior left lateral ventricle that is not visualized on the T2-weighted image (nor was it seen on T1-weighted and FLAIR images) but is very conspicuous as hyperintensity on DWI consistent with epidermoid.

**DIAGNOSIS:** Epidermoid cyst (primary cholesteatoma)

**DISCUSSION:** Epidermoid cysts arise from normal epithelial cells that are present during neural tube closure. Growth results from the accumulation of products owing to the desquamation of the squamous epithelium lining the mass, and thus epidermoids are slowly growing lesions. A frequent imaging conundrum is the differentiation between arachnoid cysts and epidermoid tumors, which share common anatomic distributions and imaging features by CT and conventional MRI. For example, both can occur in the cerebellopontine angle or suprasellar or parasellar region and in the perimesencephalic cisterns. Both entities have low-signal intensity on T1-weighted and high-signal intensity on T2-weighted images, although epidermoids often have a "dirty" CSF appearance with internal heterogeneity on FLAIR images. Both are relatively avascular on CT, MRI, and angiography, although subtle, peripheral enhancement can be seen. DWI has been recognized as a convenient and reliable discriminator between these two lesions. Epidermoids are bright on DWI resulting from a combination of "T2 shine-through" and diffusion of water molecules similar to normal brain parenchyma, as can be confirmed with the ADC map. Arachnoid cysts predictably follow CSF, becoming dark on DWI. The appearance of a smooth round lesion mimicking CSF on CT and "conventional" MR images but bright on DWI is diagnostic of epidermoid (50–52).

## Aunt Minnie's Pearls

CSF-like extra-axial non-enhancing mass that is bright on DWI = epidermoid.

Non-contrast–enhancing unilocular extra-axial lesion that follows CSF on all imaging modalities, including DWI, is diagnostic of an arachnoid cyst.

HISTORY: A 16-year-old boy with recent history of headaches, nausea, vomiting, and ataxia

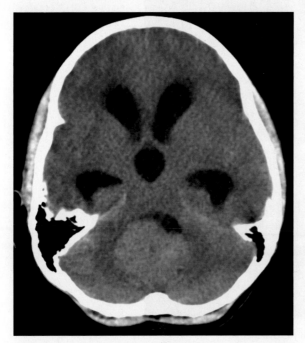

FIGURE 6.25.1

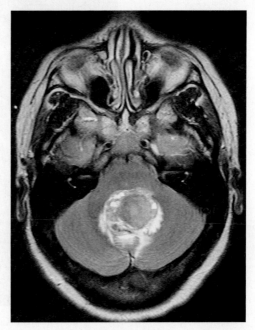

FIGURE 6.25.2

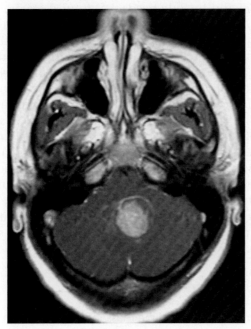

FIGURE 6.25.3

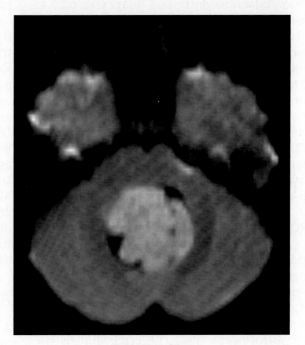

FIGURE 6.25.4

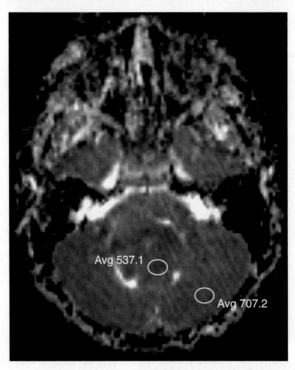

FIGURE 6.25.5

**FINDINGS:** Axial noncontrast CT image (Fig. 6.25.1) demonstrates a hyperdense mass arising from the cerebellar vermis that expands the fourth ventricle and causes hydrocephalus. Axial T2-weighted and post-contrast T1-weighted images (Figs. 6.25.2 and 6.25.3) reveal a low-signal-intensity mass with dense post-contrast enhancement. Axial DWI (Fig. 6.25.4) in the same patient demonstrates hyperintensity with corresponding low signal on the ADC map (Fig. 6.25.5), consistent with relatively low diffusion of water molecules. Note that the mass contains lower values on the ADC map than the adjacent normal-appearing brain parenchyma.

**DIAGNOSIS:** Medulloblastoma

**DISCUSSION:** Medulloblastoma is a highly malignant neuroepithelial tumor found predominantly in the posterior fossa. It is the most common malignant CNS tumor and one of the most common tumors seen in the posterior fossa in children, after pilocytic astrocytoma (PA). The cerebellum is the most common location, and most (>75%) are located in the vermis. Lateral locations are more common in older children and adults. Symptoms are usually brief and include headache, truncal ataxia, spasticity, and sixth nerve palsy. These masses are usually hyperdense on noncontrast CT. On MRI, these tumors show relatively lower-signal intensity than the adjacent normal brain parenchyma on ADC maps, indicating decreased diffusion of water molecules, at least in part caused by densely packed small blue cells. This is in contrast with PAs, which are very bright on ADC maps. On T1- and T2-weighted images, both tumors may show variable signal intensities and amounts of post-contrast enhancement. Medulloblastomas may be indistinguishable from atypical teratoid rhabdoid tumors (ATRTs), usually diagnosed in infants. A diagnosis of medulloblastoma necessitates MR imaging of the entire spine to exclude drop metastases (53,54).

### Aunt Minnie's Pearl

A hyperdense, midline mass in the cerebellum in a pediatric patient on noncontrast CT and with low diffusion on MRI = medulloblastoma (or ATRT).

**HISTORY:** A 10-year-old girl with fever and headache

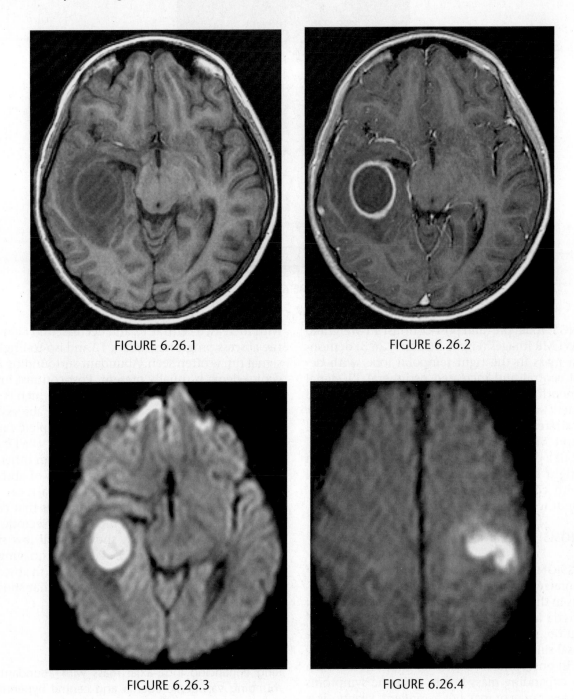

FIGURE 6.26.1

FIGURE 6.26.2

FIGURE 6.26.3

FIGURE 6.26.4

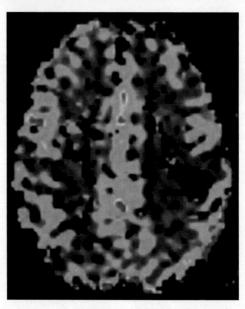

FIGURE 6.26.5

**FINDINGS:** Axial pre- and post-contrast T1-weighted and DWI MR images (Figs. 6.26.1 to 6.26.3) demonstrate a mass in the right temporal lobe, with decreased central and increased peripheral T1 signal and smooth, dense, peripheral enhancement and prominent surrounding vasogenic edema. The mass demonstrates very bright central DWI signal. Axial DWI and MR perfusion images (Figs. 6.26.4 and 6.26.5) in a different patient demonstrate an area of very bright DWI signal in the posterior left frontal lobe with correspondingly decreased relative CBV consistent with an abscess.

**DIAGNOSIS:** Brain abscess

**DISCUSSION:** Brain abscesses account for up to 5% of all cerebral masses and are the most common focal infections in the CNS. They are most commonly caused by bacteria and may arise from hematogenous dissemination, meningitis, or direct extension from the paranasal sinuses or mastoids. Symptoms are usually abrupt in onset and are related to mass effect from a rapidly expanding mass lesion. Systemic symptoms such as fever may or may not be present. Diagnosis is predominantly with MRI, which demonstrates a mass with increased central T2 and decreased T1 signal. As the abscess progresses, a dark T2 and iso-to-bright T1 signal rim is often seen. Abundant surrounding vasogenic edema is usually present. Post-contrast images show ring enhancement of the lesion, which is nonspecific. Some features such as thinner abscess wall closest to the ventricle and smooth complete capsule suggest abscess but are not always seen. DWI can be used to reliably differentiate abscess from other ring enhancing lesion. The central portions of abscesses are very hyperintense on DWI and dark on ADC maps, owing to thick, proteinacious pus that causes restricted diffusion of water molecules. Necrotic metastatic tumors, conversely, show central low signal on DWI, comparable to CSF. Perfusion imaging can also be utilized and show decreased CBV in abscesses, as opposed to peripherally neoplasms that show increased CBV (55–57).

### Aunt Minnie's Pearl

Ring enhancing intra-axial mass with abundant surrounding vasogenic edema and central hyperintense signal on DWI = cerebral abscess.

**HISTORY:** A 69-year-old man with progressive generalized weakness, aphasia, and dementia

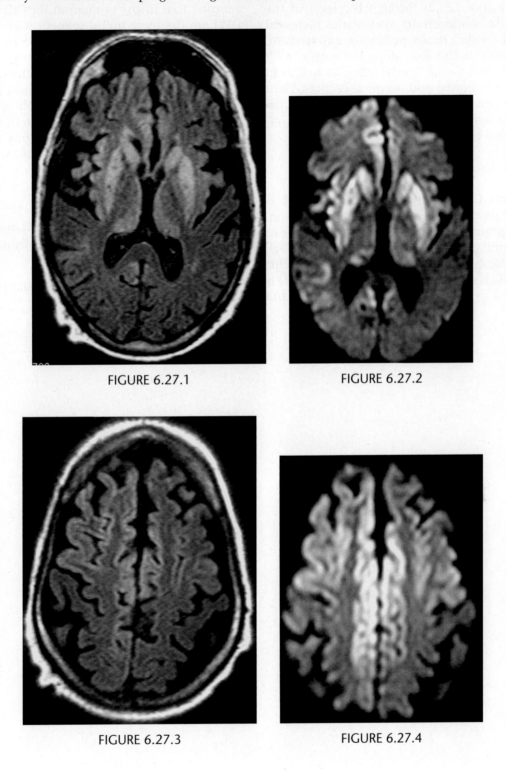

FIGURE 6.27.1

FIGURE 6.27.2

FIGURE 6.27.3

FIGURE 6.27.4

**FINDINGS:** Axial FLAIR and DWI MR images (Figs. 6.27.1 and 6.27.2) through the level of the basal ganglia demonstrate symmetric increased signal in the caudate heads, putamina, and thalami. Increased signal is also seen along the cortex of bilateral insula and mesial frontal lobes, as well as in the posterior temporal and occipital cortices, right greater than left. Axial FLAIR and DWI more superiorly in the same patient (Figs. 6.27.3 and 6.27.4) reveal bilateral cortical hyperintensity.

**DIAGNOSIS:** Creutzfeldt–Jakob disease

**DISCUSSION:** Creutzfeldt–Jakob disease (CJD) is a rare, fatal disease categorized generally as a subacute spongiform encephalopathy and occurring in sporadic, familial, and variant forms. The etiology of the disease is thought to be abnormal proteins (prions), which are transmissible. Clinically, CJD is characterized by rapidly progressive dementia and generalized myoclonus. MRI is the single best diagnostic tool in the evaluation for CJD. FLAIR and DWI are the most useful sequences and have a reported accuracy of approximately 95 percent. Imaging in the acute phase demonstrates hyperintense signal on both FLAIR and DWI in the cortex, striatum, and thalamus. Extensive cortical hyperintensity involving both cerebral hemispheres on DWI is essentially pathognomonic for CJD. In later phases of the disease, there is cortical atrophy and the hyperintense signal on DWI disappears (57–59).

## Aunt Minnie's Pearls

Hyperintense signal on FLAIR and DWI in the striatum, thalami, and cortex bilaterally in a patient with rapidly progressive dementia = CJD.

MRI is the single best diagnostic modality for diagnosis.

**HISTORY:** A 49-year-old man with refractory complex partial seizures

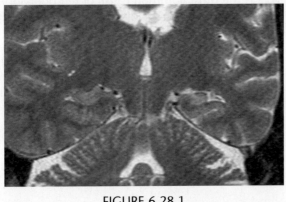

FIGURE 6.28.1

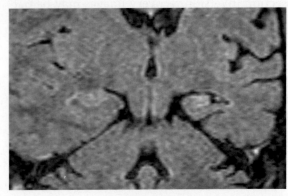

FIGURE 6.28.2

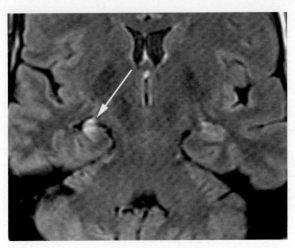

FIGURE 6.28.3

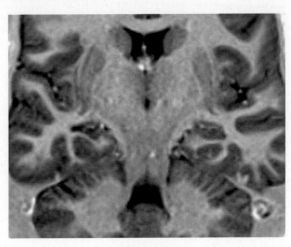

FIGURE 6.28.4

**FINDINGS:** Coronal FLAIR and T2-weighted MR images (Figs. 6.28.1 and 6.28.2) demonstrate increased signal, atrophy, and loss of the normal internal architecture within the left hippocampus. Coronal FLAIR and T1-weighted inversion recovery MR images (Fig. 6.28.3 and 6.28.4) in another patient demonstrate T2 hyperintensity (Fig. 6.28.3, *arrow*) and atrophy within the right hippocampus compatible with mesial temporal sclerosis.

**DIAGNOSIS:** Mesial temporal sclerosis or hippocampal sclerosis

**DISCUSSION:** Mesial temporal sclerosis (MTS) is the most common cause of temporal lobe epilepsy, which is frequently refractory to antiepileptic medication and therefore treated surgically. Presurgical evaluation is multispecialty and multimodality, incorporating clinical findings, neuropsychologic testing, structural imaging (high-resolution coronal MRI), functional neuroimaging (fMRI, SPECT, PET), MR spectroscopy (MRS), electroencephalography (ictal and interictal), and intracarotid amobarbital (Wada) testing. The goal of these techniques is to noninvasively detect unilateral MTS, identify nearby eloquent brain tissue, and plan the surgery accordingly. If bitemporal MTS is found, depth electrodes or other invasive monitoring must be placed to further map the cortex.

The condition MTS affects the hippocampus, the medial temporal lobe terminus of the limbic system. Specifically, subfields CA1, CA3, and CA4 show cell loss histologically, with relative sparing of subfield CA2. MRI can demonstrate volume loss (visual or volumetric) with hyperintensity of the hippocampus on T2-weighted or FLAIR sequences. Coronal, thin-section inversion recovery images may be particularly useful. Functional MRI is useful for mapping eloquent cortex, whereas SPECT and PET show ictal hyperperfusion and interictal hypoperfusion. MRS demonstrates a decrease in the NAA/Cho+Cr ratio. Wada testing selectively anesthetizes each hemisphere and evaluates language and memory function before temporal lobe resection (60–62).

## Aunt Minnie's Pearls

MTS is the most common cause of temporal lobe epilepsy, and the workup is directed at noninvasively detecting unilateral disease.

The primary radiologic contribution to the diagnosis of MTS is coronal, thin-section, high-resolution T2-weighted (including FLAIR images) MRI, which shows volume loss and high signal in the hippocampus.

**HISTORY:** A 45-year-old male alcoholic with ataxia and ophthalmoplegia

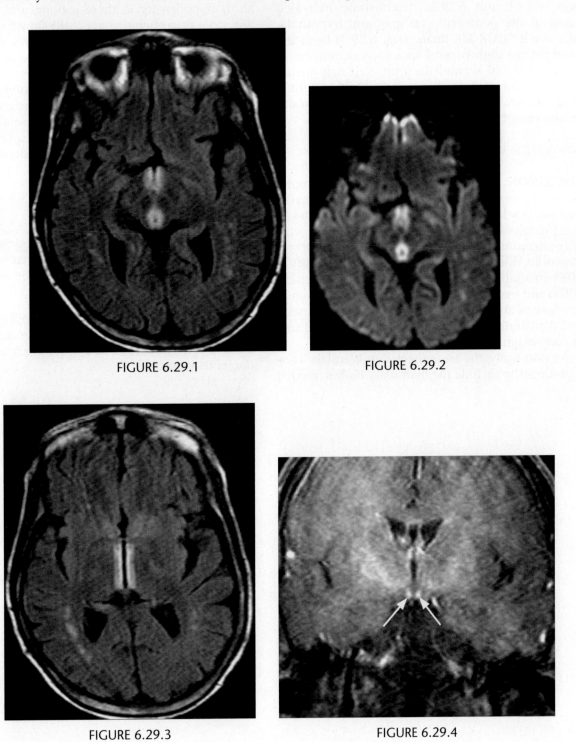

FIGURE 6.29.1

FIGURE 6.29.2

FIGURE 6.29.3

FIGURE 6.29.4

**FINDINGS:** Axial FLAIR and DWI MR images (Figs. 6.29.1 and 6.29.2) demonstrate increased signal in the periaquaductal gray and hypothalamus. Axial FLAIR MR image (Fig. 6.29.3) from the same patient slightly more superiorly demonstrates increased signal around the third ventricle in the hypothalamus. Coronal post-contrast T1-weighted image with fat saturation (Fig. 6.29.4) demonstrates enhancement of the mamillary bodies (*arrows*).

**DIAGNOSIS:** Wernicke's encephalopathy

**DISCUSSION:** The classic triad of ophthalmoplegia (with nystagmus), ataxia, and mental status changes is seldom seen in patients with Wernicke's encephalopathy, who most commonly present with only altered mental status. Early treatment with intravenous thiamine is essential because mortality is >10% in adults. Owing to the vague clinical presentation and frequency of confounding factors such as alcoholism and Korsakoff's psychosis (i.e., amnesia and confabulation), imaging can play a crucial role in early diagnosis.

Anatomically, the areas affected in Wernicke's encephalopathy include the mamillary bodies, medial thalami, and periaquaductal gray matter. CT may show hypodensity in these regions, and occasionally (5%) microhemorrhage. MRI shows symmetric increase in signal on T2-weighted, DWI, and FLAIR images. Contrast has a limited role because lesions fail to enhance in 50% of acute cases. A late finding on imaging studies is mamillary body atrophy. Wernicke's encephalopathy is underdiagnosed in the pediatric age group, where the mortality rate is 42 percent. Children usually do not display the classic triad, often have an underlying malignancy, and are almost always female (63,64).

## Aunt Minnie's Pearls

Symmetric lesions of the mamillary bodies, medial thalami, and periaquaductal gray matter suggest Wernicke's encephalopathy and may be a lifesaving finding.

Absence of the classic triad of ophthalmoplegia, ataxia, and altered mental status should not preclude the diagnosis of Wernicke's or the intravenous administration of thiamine.

**HISTORY:** A 28-year-old white woman with history of numbness and weakness

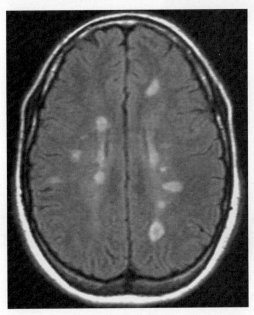

FIGURE 6.30.1

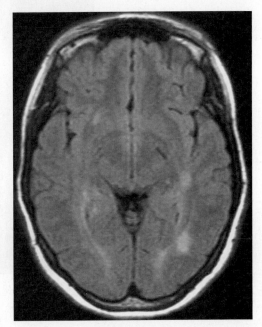

FIGURE 6.30.2

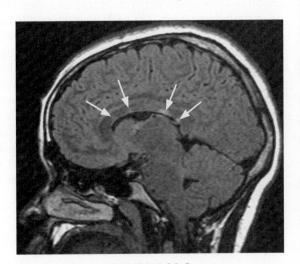

FIGURE 6.30.3

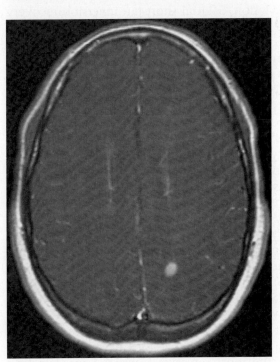

FIGURE 6.30.4

**FINDINGS:** Axial FLAIR MR images (Figs. 6.30.1 and 6.30.2) demonstrate multiple foci of hyperintensity in the periventricular regions bilaterally, several of which are oriented perpendicular to the axis of the ventricles. Lesions are also seen along the optic radiations. Sagittal FLAIR MR image (Fig. 6.30.3) demonstrates multiple foci of hyperintense signal (*arrows*) within the corpus callosum. Axial

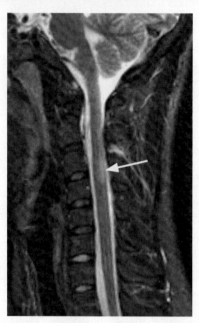

FIGURE 6.30.5

post-contrast T1-weighted MR image (Fig. 6.30.4) demonstrates enhancement of a left parietal white-matter lesion. Sagittal short-tau inversion recovery (STIR) T2-weighted MR image of the cervical spine (Fig. 6.30.5) demonstrates a focus of hyperintense intramedullary signal (*arrow*) posteriorly at the C3–C4 level, without cord expansion.

DIAGNOSIS: Multiple sclerosis

DISCUSSION: Multiple sclerosis (MS) is an inflammatory, autoimmune disease characterized by demyelination and axonal injury with multiple CNS lesions separated in both space and time. MS may present with any neurologic deficit, but most commonly weakness, parasthesias, vertigo, and visual or urinary disturbances. The natural history typically manifests as unpredictable relapsing and remitting symptoms. There is no single test that is diagnostic of MS, including MRI. The sensitivity of diagnosing MS within the first year after a single attack is 94%, with a specificity of 83 percent. The principles of MS diagnosis are based on showing dissemination of white-matter lesions in space and time. MR is the most sensitive technique for detecting MS lesions. MR typically demonstrates low T1 and high T2 signal abnormalities in the periventricular white matter, which are characteristically oriented perpendicular to the ventricles (Dawson's fingers), ovoid lesions, corpus callosum lesions, and spinal cord involvement. Active lesions enhance with gadolinium contrast agents and may be bright on DWI. When evaluating patients for MS, it is helpful to perform dedicated coronal sequences for evaluation of the optic nerves, as optic neuritis may be the first presentation of MS. McDonald's criteria should be used when evaluating patients for MS. Any three of the four following criteria constitute MR findings compatible with MS: (1) one gadolinium-enhancing lesion or nine T2-hyperintense lesions when there is no enhancing lesion, (2) with at least one infratentorial lesion, (3) at least one juxtacortical lesion, and (4) at least three periventricular lesions. A spinal cord lesion may be substituted for a brain lesion. According to the revised criteria dissemination in space requires at least one T2 lesion in at least two of four locations (juxtacortical, periventricular, infratentorial, and spinal cord) and dissemination in time requires a new T2 lesion on a follow-up scan. The sensitivity of diagnosing MS in patients with isolated clinical syndromes was found to be 72% with an 87% specificity (65,66).

### Aunt Minnie's Pearls

Multiple periventricular white-matter lesions oriented perpendicular to the ventricles (Dawson's fingers) and involving corpus callosum = MS.

Enhancing lesions suggest active demyelinating plaques.

**HISTORY:** Elderly diabetic patient with sudden development of involuntary, abnormal movement of the left arm and leg

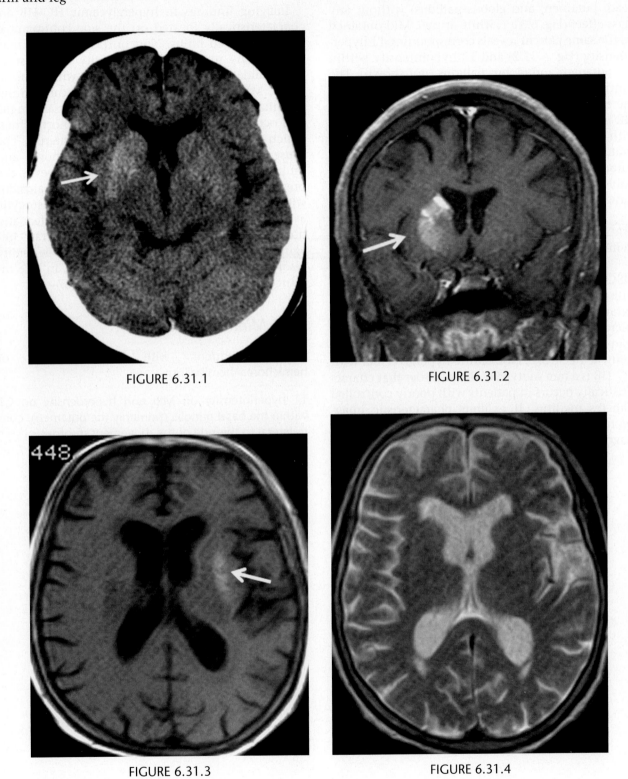

FIGURE 6.31.1

FIGURE 6.31.2

FIGURE 6.31.3

FIGURE 6.31.4

**FINDINGS:** Non-enhanced CT demonstrates right basal ganglia hyperdensity (involving the caudate head, putamen, and globus pallidus) without any mass effect (Fig. 6.31.1, white arrow). MRI obtained on the same patient reveals corresponding T1 hyperintensity (Fig. 6.31.2) and T2 hypointensity within the putamen and globus pallidus (not shown). The contralateral basal ganglia and the remainder of the brain parenchyma are normal in appearance. MR images from a different patient, who presented with right-sided involuntary movements, demonstrate unilateral T1 hyperintensity within the left putamen (Fig. 6.31.3, white arrow) without appreciable associated abnormal signal on the FLAIR (not shown) and T2-weighted (Fig. 6.31.4.) sequences.

**DIAGNOSIS:** Nonketotic hyperglycemia with Hemichorea–Hemiballismus

**DISCUSSION:** Hemichorea–hemiballism (HC–HB) is a disorder characterized by sudden onset of involuntary movements involving one half of the body. There are numerous reported causes of HC–HB, many of which are irreversible, the most common being acute stroke. Nonketotic hyperglycemia with HC–HB is a rare subtype of this disorder that characteristically occurs in patients with poorly controlled diabetes mellitus. It exhibits characteristic imaging findings that can greatly aid in establishing the diagnosis. Early recognition of this condition is of paramount importance as appropriate serum glucose control can reverse the patient's symptoms.

Imaging findings in hyperglycemic HC–HB are characteristically located on the side contralateral to the involved limbs. Noncontrast brain CT may demonstrate unilateral hyperdensity in the striatum (caudate nucleus and putamen), without mass effect. MRI is more sensitive with typical findings of unilateral T1 hyperintensity in the basal ganglia and occasional associated T2 signal abnormalities, which may be either hypo- or hyperintense. The cause of the MR signal changes is unknown and multiple theories have been proposed; however, the prevailing theory is one of metabolic impairment within the basal ganglia that leads to gemistocytic astrocyte accumulation. There is no mass effect and no abnormal enhancement on post-contrast imaging. The basal ganglia hyperintensity generally resolves within a few months; however, in rare instances it may persist for several years (67–69).

## Aunt Minnie's Pearls

Diabetic patient with acute onset of hemichorea–hemiballism.

T1 hyperintensity on MRI and hyperdensity on CT within the basal ganglia (primarily the putamen), contralateral to the side of the movement disorder.

# REFERENCES

1. Osborn AG, Blaser SI, Castillo M, et al. Congenital malformations. In: Osborn AG, Blaser SI, Castillo M, et al. (eds.). Diagnostic imaging: Brain. Salt Lake City: Amyrsis, 2004:I-1-4–I-1-119.
2. Oh KY, Kennedy AM, Frias AE, et al. Fetal schizencephaly: Pre- and postnatal imaging with a review of the clinical manifestations. Radiographics 2005;25:647–657.
3. Barkovich JA. Morphologic characteristics of subcortical heterotopia: MR imaging study. AJNR Am J Neuroradiol 2000; 21:290–295.
4. Mitchell LA, Simon EM, Filly RA, et al. Antenatal diagnosis of subependymal heterotopia. AJNR Am J Neuroradiol 2000; 21:296–300.
5. Simon EM, Barkovich AJ. Holoprosencephaly: New concepts. Magn Reson Imaging Clin N Am 2001;9:149–164, viii–ix.
6. Simon EM, Hevner R, Pinter JD, et al. The middle interhemispheric variant of holoprosencephaly. AJNR Am J Neuroradiol 2002;23:151–155.
7. Barkovich AJ, Simon EM, Walsh CA. Callosal agenesis with cyst. A better understanding and new classification. Neurology 2001;56:220–227.
8. Hetts SW, Sherr EH, Chao S, et al. Anomalies of the corpus callosum: An MR analysis of the phenotypic spectrum of associated malformations. AJR Am J Roentgenol 2006;187: 1343–1348.
9. Curran JG, O'Connor E. Imaging of craniopharyngioma. Childs Nerv Syst 2005;21:635–639.
10. Sartoretti-Schefer S, Wichmann W, Aguzzi A, et al. MR differentiation of adamantinous and squamous-papillary craniopharyngiomas. AJNR Am J Neuroradiol 1997;18:77–87.
11. Elster AD. Modern imaging of the pituitary. Radiology 1993; 187:1–14.
12. Argyropoulou MI, Kiortsis DN. MRI of the hypothalamic–pituitary axis in children. Pediatr Radiol 2005;35:1045–1055.
13. Trommer BL, Naidich TP, Dal Canto MC, et al. Noninvasive CT diagnosis of infantile Alexander's disease: Pathologic correlation. J Comput Assist Tomogr 1983;7:509–516.
14. Van der Knaap MS, Naidu S, Breiter SN, et al. Alexander disease: Diagnosis with MR imaging. AJNR Am J Neuroradiol 2001;22:541–552.
15. Ostertun B, Wolf HK, Campos MG, et al. Dysembryoplastic neuroepithelial tumors: MR and CT evaluation. AJNR Am J Neuroradiol 1996;17:419–430.
16. Fernandez C, Girard N, Paz Paredes A, et al. The usefulness of MR imaging in the diagnosis of dysembryoplastic neuroepithelial tumor in children: A study of 14 cases. AJNR Am J Neuroradiol 2003;24:829–834.
17. Juhász C, Haacke EM, Hu J, et al. Multimodality imaging of cortical and white matter abnormalities in Sturge–Weber syndrome. AJNR Am J Neuroradiol 2007;28:900–906.
18. Smirniotopoulos JG. Neuroimaging of the phakomatoses: Sturge–Weber syndrome, tuberous sclerosis, von Hippel–Lindau syndrome. Neuroimaging Clin N Am 2004;14: 171–183.
19. Rodriguez D, Poussaint TY. Neuroimaging findings in neurofibromatosis type 1 and 2. Neuroimaging Clin N Am 2004; 14:149–170.
20. Ruggieri M, Iannetti P, Polizzi A, et al. Earliest clinical manifestations and natural history of neurofibromatosis type 2 (NF2) in childhood: A study of 24 patients. Neuropediatrics 2005;36:21–34.
21. Baskin HJ. The pathogenesis and imaging of tuberous sclerosis complex. Pediatr Radiol 2008;38:936–952.
22. Hirfanoglu T, Gupta A. Tuberous sclerosis complex with a single brain lesion on MRI mimicking focal cortical dysplasia. Pediatr Neurol 2010;42:343–347.
23. Slater A, Moore NR, Huson SM. The natural history of cerebellar hemangioblastomas in von Hippel–Lindau disease. AJNR Am J Neuroradiol 2003;24:1570–1574.
24. Quadery FA, Okamoto K. Diffusion-weighted MRI of haemangioblastomas and other cerebellar tumours. Neuroradiology 2003;45:212–219.
25. Nagae LM, Hoon AH Jr, Stashinko E, et al. Diffusion tensor imaging in children with periventricular leukomalacia: Variability of injuries to white matter tracts. AJNR Am J Neuroradiol 2007;28:1213–1222.
26. Gean AD. Leptomeningeal cyst. In: Gead AD (ed.). Imaging of head trauma. New York, NY: Raven Press, 1994:381–385.
27. Ersahin Y, Gülmen V, Palali I, et al. Growing skull fractures (craniocerebral erosion). Neurosurg Rev 2000;23:139–144.
28. Houra K, Beros V, Sajko T, et al. Traumatic leptomeningeal cyst in a 24-year-old man: Case report. Neurosurgery 2006; 58:E201.
29. Castillo M. Cerebral vascular malformations. In: Castillo M (ed.). Neuroradiology (Third Series) test and syllabus. Reston, VA: American College of Radiology, 2006:25–35.
30. Hadizadeh DR, Falkenhausen M, Gieseke J, et al. Cerebral arteriovenous malformations: Spetzler–Martin classification at subsecond-temporal-resolution four-dimensional MR angiography compared with that at DSA. Radiology 2007;246: 205–213.
31. Söderman M, Andersson T, Karlsson B, et al. Management of patients with brain arteriovenous malformations. Eur J Radiol 2003;46:195–205.
32. Kitajima M, Korogi Y, Shimomura O, et al. Hypertrophic olivary degeneration: MR imaging and pathologic findings. Radiology 1994;192:539–543.
33. Goyal M, Versnick E, Tuite P, et al. Hypertrophic olivary degeneration: Metaanalysis of the temporal evolution of MR findings. AJNR Am J Neuroradiol 2000;21:1073–1077.
34. Leach JL, Fortuna RB, Jones BV, et al. Imaging of cerebral venous thrombosis: Current techniques, spectrum of findings, and diagnostic pitfalls. Radiographics 2006;26:S19–S43.
35. Poon CS, Chang JK, Swarnkar A, et al. Radiologic diagnosis of cerebral venous thrombosis: Pictorial review. AJR Am J Roentgenol 2007;189(suppl 6):S64–S75.
36. McKinney AM, Short J, Truwit CL, et al. Posterior reversible encephalopathy syndrome: Incidence of atypical regions of involvement and imaging findings. AJR Am J Roentgenol 2007;189:904–912.
37. Bartynski WS, Boardman JF, Zeigler ZR, et al. Posterior reversible encephalopathy syndrome in infection, sepsis, and shock. AJNR Am J Neuroradiol 2006;27:2179–2190.
38. Bartynski WS, Boardman JF. Distinct imaging patterns and lesion distribution in posterior reversible encephalopathy syndrome. AJNR Am J Neuroradiol 2007;28:1320–1327.
39. Kumar N. Superficial siderosis. Arch Neurol 2007;64:491–496.
40. Pyhtinen J, Pääkkö E, Ilkko E. Superficial siderosis in the central nervous system. Neuroradiology 1995;37:127–128.
41. Farb RI, Forghani R, Lee SK, et al. The venous distension sign: A diagnostic sign of intracranial hypotension at MR imaging of the brain. AJNR Am J Neuroradiol 2007;28:1489–1493.
42. Smirniotopoulos JG, Murphy FM, Rushing EJ, et al. Patterns of contrast enhancement in the brain and meninges. Radiographics 2007;27:525–551.
43. Yousry I, Förderreuther S, Moriggl B, et al. Cervical MR imaging in postural headache: MR signs and pathophysiological implications. AJNR Am J Neuroradiol 2001;22:1239–1250.
44. Bertalanffy H, Benes L, Miyazawa T, et al. Cerebral cavernomas in the adult. Review of the literature and analysis of 72 surgically treated patients. Neurosurg Rev 2002;25:1–53.
45. Vilanova JC, Barceló J, Smirniotopoulos JG, et al. Hemangioma from head to toe: MR imaging with pathologic correlation. Radiographics 2004;24:367–385.

46. Armao D, Castillo M, Chen H, et al. Colloid cyst of the third ventricle: Imaging–pathologic correlation. AJNR Am J Neuroradiol 2000;21:1470–1477.

47. Sener RN. Colloid cyst: Diffusion MR imaging findings. J Neuroimaging 2007;17:181–183.

48. Freeman JL, Coleman TC, Wellard RM, et al. MR imaging and spectroscopic study of epileptogenic hypothalamic hamartomas: Analysis of 72 cases. AJNR Am J Neuroradiol 2004;25:450–462.

49. Lefton DR, Pinto RS, Silvera VM, et al. Radiologic features of pediatric thalamic and hypothalamic tumors. Crit Rev Diagn Imaging 2000;41:237–278.

50. Hakyemez B, Aksoy U, Yildiz H, et al. Intracranial epidermoid cysts: Diffusion-weighted, FLAIR and conventional MR findings. Eur J Radiol 2005;54:214–220.

51. Forghani R, Fard R, Kiehl TR, et al. Fourth ventricle epidermoid tumor: Radiologic, intraoperative, and pathologic findings. Radiographics 2007;27:1489–1494.

52. Tsuruda JS, Chew WM, Moseley ME, et al. Diffusion-weighted MR imaging of the brain: Value of differentiating between extraaxial cysts and epidermoid tumors. AJNR Am J Neuroradiol 1990;11:925–931.

53. Koeller KK, Rushing EJ. Medulloblastoma: A comprehensive review with radiologic–pathologic correlation. Radiographics 2003;23:1613–1637.

54. Rumboldt Z, Camacho DLA, Lake D, et al. Apparent diffusion coefficients for differentiation of cerebellar tumors in children. AJNR Am J Neuroradiol 2006;27:1362–1369.

55. Reddy JS, Mishra AM, Behari S, et al. The role of diffusion-weighted imaging in the differential diagnosis of intracranial cystic mass lesions: A report of 147 lesions. Surg Neurol 2006;66:246–250.

56. Bükte Y, Paksoy Y, Genç E, et al. Role of diffusion-weighted MR in differential diagnosis of intracranial cystic lesions. Clin Radiol 2005;60:375–383.

57. Rumboldt Z, Thurnher MM, Gupta RK. Central nervous system infections. Semin Roentgenol 2007;42:62–91.

58. Kallenberg K, Schulz-Schaeffer WJ, Jastrow U, et al. Creutzfeldt–Jakob disease: Comparative analysis of MR imaging sequences. AJNR Am J Neuroradiol 2006;27:1459–1462.

59. Young GS, Geschwind MD, Fischbein NJ, et al. Diffusion-weighted and fluid-attenuated inversion recovery imaging in Creutzfeldt–Jakob disease: High sensitivity and specificity for diagnosis. AJNR Am J Neuroradiol 2005;26:1551–1562.

60. Bronen RA, Fulbright RK, Kim JH, et al. A systematic approach for interpreting MR imaged of the seizure patient. AJR Am J Radiol 1997;169:241–247.

61. Hayman LA, Fuller GN, Cavazos JE, et al. The hippocampus: Normal anatomy and pathology. AJR Am J Radiol 1998; 171:1139–1146.

62. Urbach H. Imaging of the epilepsies. Eur Radiol 2005;15: 494–500.

63. Sechi G, Serra A. Wernicke's encephalopathy: New clinical settings and recent advances in diagnosis and management. Lancet Neurol 2007;6:442–455.

64. Zuccoli G, Gallucci M, Capellades J, et al. Wernicke encephalopathy: MR findings at clinical presentation in twenty-six alcoholic and nonalcoholic patients. AJNR Am J Neuroradiol 2007;28:1328–1331.

65. Ge Y. Multiple sclerosis: The role of MR imaging. AJNR Am J Neuroradiol 2006;27:1165–1176.

66. Swanton JK, Rovira A, Tintore M, et al. MRI criteria for multiple sclerosis in patients presenting with clinically isolated syndromes: A multicentre retrospective study. Lancet Neurol 2007;6:677–686.

67. Lee EJ, Choi JY, Lee SH, et al. Hemichorea–hemiballism in primary diabetic patients: MR correlation. J Comput Assist Tomogr 2002;6:905–911.

68. Oh SH, Lee KY, Im JH, et al. Chorea associated with nonketotic hyperglycemia and hyperintensity basal ganglia lesion on T1-weighted brain MRI study: A meta-analysis of 53 cases including four present cases. J Neurol Sci 2002;200: 57–62.

69. Cherian A, Thomas B, Baheti NN, et al. Concepts and controversies in nonketotic hyperglycemia-induced hemichorea: Further evidence from susceptibility-weighted MR imaging. J Magn Reson Imaging 2009;29:699–703.

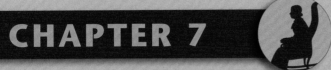

# CHAPTER 7

# NEURORADIOLOGY: HEAD AND NECK

Lubdha M. Shah / Richard H. Wiggins, III

**HISTORY:** A 40-year-old man with neck swelling.

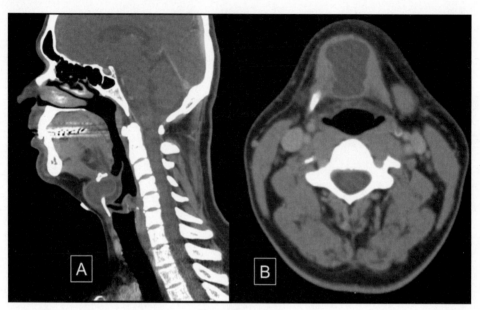

FIGURE 7.1.1

**FINDINGS:** Sagittal reconstruction post-contrasted CT of the cervical soft tissues demonstrates a well-circumscribed homogeneous midline cystic lesion, between the hyoid bone and the thyroid cartilage without surrounding aggressive features (Fig. 7.1.1A). Axial standard algorithm CECT image at a level between the hyoid and thyroid cartilage shows the midline well-circumscribed mass embedded within the anterior strap musculature (Fig. 7.1.1B).

**DIAGNOSIS:** Thyroglossal duct cyst.

**DISCUSSION:** In the third week of fetal life, the thyroid primordium originating at the level of the foramen cecum descends in the neck. It penetrates through the underlying mesoderm of the tongue and floor of mouth musculature, passes anterior to the hyoid bone and laryngeal cartilages, and reaches its final position anterior to the thyrohyoid membrane and strap muscles by the seventh week of gestation (1). This thyroid anlage is connected to the tongue by the thyroglossal duct (TGD), which normally involutes by eighth to tenth week of gestation. Portions of the thyroglossal duct may persist and secretions from the epithelial lining may give rise to a cystic lesion, known as a thyroglossal duct cyst (TGDC) (2). The thyroglossal duct is closely associated with the hyoid bone, which explains why most TGD cysts are located at the level of the hyoid bone (15%) or in the strap muscles immediately inferior to it (65%) (3,4).

This cystic lesion is located either midline at the level of the hyoid bone or slightly off midline within the strap muscles. It has well-circumscribed smooth margins with homogeneous low fluid-like attenuation on CT. Internal areas of high attenuation may be due to increased protein content, possibly due to prior infection. There may be peripheral rim enhancement (5). Similarly, on MRI the signal intensity is fluid-like: T1 hypointense and T2 hyperintense. A thick enhancing rim may be due to infection/inflammation.

## Aunt Minnie's Pearls

The thyroglossal duct cyst is one of the most common incidental lesions found on cervical soft tissue CT studies.

If you look closely, you will frequently see small cystic lesions near the hyoid bone, often with a small osseous defect in the midline of the bone.

If there is irregular nodularity or weird chunky calcifications associated with the cyst, be sure to consider a thyroid carcinoma.

**HISTORY:** 37-year-old man with right jaw mass.

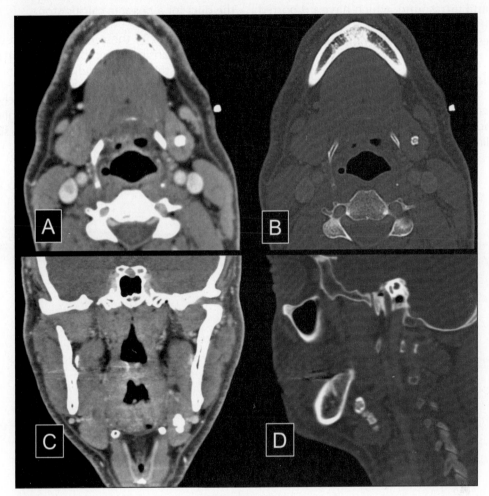

FIGURE 7.2.1

**FINDINGS:** Axial standard (A) and bone (B) algorithm images obtained at a level immediately below the mandible demonstrates a focal high density lesion within the left submandibular gland (SMG) (Fig. 7.2.1). The gland itself shows no inflammatory changes. A small radiodense marker on the skin surface overlying the mass demarcates the location of the patient's pain. The coronal (C) standard algorithm image and the oblique sagittal (D) bone algorithm images show that there are several lesions extending along the expected course of the left SMG duct.

**DIAGNOSIS:** Submandibular gland lithiasis.

**DISCUSSION:** Sialolithiasis occurs in the submandibular gland 80% of the time (6) in part due to its anatomy. The submandibular gland has a wider lumen but tighter orifice. It also lies in a dependent position with uphill course of the submandibular duct (Wharton's duct) (7). Wharton's duct extends from the submandibular gland to the posterior edge of the mylohyoid muscle. It then curves around the muscle and enters the sublingual space on the surface of the mylohyoid muscle and drains into the sublingual papilla (8). The viscous secretions are also contributory to the formation of sialoliths. Obstruction of a duct by a calculus can result in painful swelling of the submandibular gland due to secretion and stasis of saliva. Different imaging modalities can be used to evaluate the large salivary glands including conventional sialography, ultrasonography, computed tomography (CT), digital sialography, and digital subtraction sialography. However, approximately 10% to 20% of sialoliths in the submandibular gland or duct are not radiopaque and, therefore, are not visible on radiographs (8). In addition, phlebolithiasis and hemangiomas with calcifications or calcified lymph nodes may mimic sialoliths on radiographs. Calculi are readily detected by CT and ultrasound, which have a reported high sensitivity and specificity (9,10). Newer imaging techniques include MR sialography (8).

## Aunt Minnie's Pearls

Calcifications can be found anywhere along the course of the submandibular gland duct, extending along the ipsilateral sublingual space.

If there are inflammatory changes seen to the SMG itself, you should look along the expected course of the duct for a possible calcific stone.

It is important in these cases to try to differentiate a mass lesion arising within the gland from inflammatory changes of the entire gland.

An obstructed SMG duct can lead acutely to abnormal enhancement and enlargement of the gland early, and fatty replacement and decrease gland size in chronic cases.

**HISTORY:** 55-year-old man with persistent hoarseness.

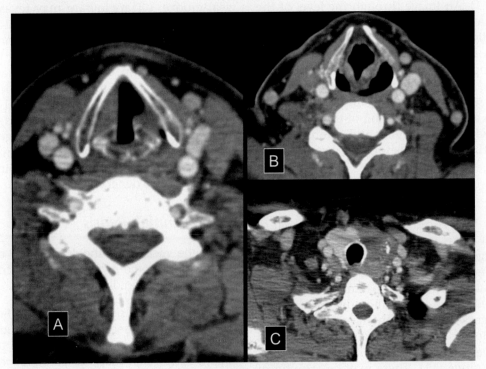

FIGURE 7.3.1

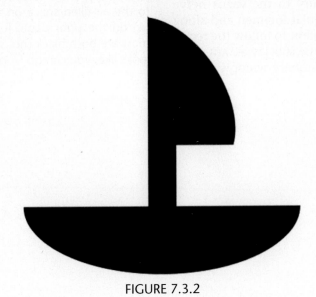

FIGURE 7.3.2

**FINDINGS:** Multiple axial post-contrasted standard algorithm CT images through the cervical soft tissues (Fig. 7.3.1). An image through the level of the vocal cords demonstrates asymmetry of the vocal cords with slight widening of the thyroarytenoid groove (A). A slightly higher axial image (B) shows thickening and anteromedialization of the left aryepiglottic fold and enlargement of the pyriform sinus. A lower section through the thyroid gland (C) demonstrates an aggressive lesion of the left lobe of the thyroid with heterogeneity and extension posteriorly into the left tracheoesophageal groove.

**DIAGNOSIS:** Vocal cord paralysis (VCP).

**DISCUSSION:** VCP is caused by the dysfunction of the ipsilateral vagus nerve (cranial nerve 10) or recurrent laryngeal nerve. On CT and magnetic resonance imaging (MRI) of the neck, one should look for a constellation of findings: paramedian position of the affected vocal cord, ballooning of the ipsilateral laryngeal ventricle, anteromedial rotation of the arytenoid cartilage, medially displaced and thickened aryepiglottic fold and an enlarged ipsilateral pyriform sinus (11). There may be atrophy of the cricoarytenoid cartilage (12).

Look for a lesion or injury to the vagus nerve from the medulla to the jugular foramen and along the carotid space. It is important to follow the recurrent laryngeal nerves from the subclavian artery on the right and the aortopulmonary window on the left. Also, remember that the recurrent laryngeal nerves ascend to the larynx in the tracheoesophageal groove. CT angiogram may reveal an internal carotid artery dissection. Additional cranial neuropathies may be present depending on the location of the injury/lesion. If there is loss of the ipsilateral pharynx sensation, cranial nerve 9 may be affected. Denervation of the ipsilateral sternocleidomastoid and trapezius is suggestive of cranial nerve 11 injury. The lesion/injury in these cases may be anywhere from the brainstem to the jugular foramen. If a lesion affects cranial nerve 12 in the superior carotid space to the level of the hyoid bone, there may be tongue denervation.

## Aunt Minnie's Pearls

While the vocal cords should normally be symmetric, there can be some asymmetry of the cords with motion or vocalization during the CT scan.

The spinnaker sail sign is the primary finding of cord paralysis, and the secondary signs include those listed above. I often have to draw a picture to explain the spinnaker sail sign shape to our land-locked residents and fellows. So here is a picture of a black spinnaker sail just for you (Fig. 7.3.2) (I made it myself) to compare to the air-filled space on axial section in Figure 7.3.1 (A) on the prior page. Just imagine the sail and the mast are both black (no, seriously, that's really what it looks like; you can go Google it for yourself).

**HISTORY:** A 63 year-old man with left cheek nontender mass.

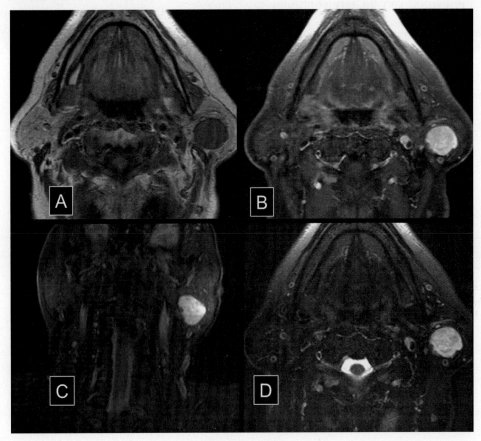

FIGURE 7.4.1

**FINDINGS:** Multiple MRI images through the face show a well-circumscribed lesion within the left parotid gland. This lesion has low T1 signal intensity before contrast (A) and avidly enhances following contrast administration (B) (Fig. 7.4.1). The coronal T2 FSE with FS (C) and the axial STIR (D) both show very bright T2 signal intensity of this lesion, even brighter than that of the cerebrospinal fluid (CSF) on the T2 FSE FS image. There are no surrounding inflammatory or aggressive changes, and no other lesions are seen.

**DIAGNOSIS:** Benign mixed tumor

**DISCUSSION:** Benign Mixed Tumor (aka BMT, pleomorphic adenoma) is the most common epithelial tumor of the parotid gland, comprising 60% to 70% of all salivary gland tumors (13). They can arise from the superficial or deep lobe of the parotid gland in middle-aged patients (slight female preponderance) and tend to be asymptomatic. These lesions are typically solitary, well-circumscribed and slow-growing. Larger masses may have a lobulated contour. The tumor matrix may show calcification or ossification (14), and rarely, these tumors can contain fat (15). On MRI, these lesions have a characteristic T2 hyperintense signal due to the myxoid material; it tends to be as bright as the CSF but may sometimes be heterogeneous due to small areas of fibrosis or calcification. With contrast administration, these lesions show patchy enhancement. These lesions displace adjacent structures, such as compressing muscles toward the mandibular ramus rather than invading them (16).

## Aunt Minnie's Pearls

Lesions within the parotid can be very confusing to evaluate.

The most common mass within the parotid is simply a lymph node, while the most common pathologic lesion is a BMT. These can become large as they slowly grow with benign surrounding changes.

A large benign appearing mass in the deep spaces of the cervical soft tissues that crosses the stylomandibular tunnel (the space between the mandible and the styloid process) is usually a BMT, especially if it is very bright on the T2 imaging— as bright as CSF.

HISTORY: A 55-year-old woman with pancreatic cancer on chemotherapy through a right chest Chemo-Port complains of right neck edema and pain.

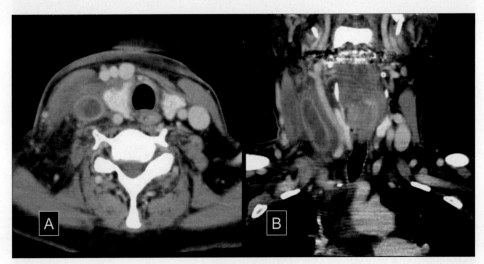

FIGURE 7.5.1

FINDINGS: Post-contrasted axial (A) and coronal (B) CT images through the cervical soft tissues show inflammatory changes within the right neck (Fig. 7.5.1). There are several round structures anterior to the right thyroid lobe with density similar to the main cervical vessels. There appears to be a fluid collection with surrounding enhancement lateral to the right lobe of the thyroid gland and the right common carotid artery. The coronal (B) image shows this tubular lesion to extend superiorly and inferiorly within the right neck.

DIAGNOSIS: Internal jugular vein septic thrombophlebitis.

DISCUSSION: Septic thrombophlebitis refers to venous thrombosis associated with inflammation in the setting of bacteremia (17). It may be associated with use of central venous devices and intravenous therapy. Neoplastic disease often creates a thrombogenic state, through inflammation mediators, tumor necrosis factor, platelet activation, as well as a procoagulant substances released by tumor cells. Furthermore, long indwelling lines increase risk for thrombosis, reported in 0.06% to 32% of patients, although the risk changes with type of catheter, neoplasm, chemotherapy regimes and radiation (18). The thrombus can become infected with persistent bacteremia and septic embolization may occur. Septic thrombophlebitis should be suspected in patients with persistent bacteremia after 72 hours of appropriate antimicrobial therapy, particularly in the setting of an intravascular catheter. Histologic findings consist of inflammation and suppuration within the vein wall. Thrombus with or without pus may be seen within the vein lumen, with evidence of perivascular inflammation. The diagnosis may be made based on culture data together with radiographic evidence of thrombosis. On contrast-enhanced CT, one may detect an intraluminal filling defect in venous structure with a catheter. The proximal or distal segment of vein may opacify with contrast. There is perivascular fat stranding and hazy enhancement of the surrounding tissues. Treatment with only antimicrobials is rarely effective for controlling infection. It is important to remove the focus of infection (e.g., intravenous catheter). Anticoagulation and in some cases a more aggressive approach such as resection of the affected vein (19) or thrombectomy (20) may be needed.

## Aunt Minnie's Pearls

The clinical history here gives the case away, but also reminds of us the importance of clinical information when reading head and neck studies.

Head and neck cases should never be read without clinical history, and that clinical information may completely change the way studies are interpreted.

The anterior collateral venous vasculature in this case also helps to make the diagnosis of jugular vein thrombosis, and the surrounding inflammatory changes tell you that it is thrombophlebitis.

**HISTORY:** A 23-year-old woman with right facial swelling and pain.

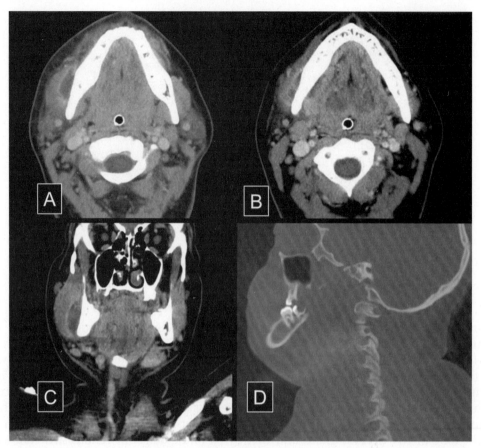

FIGURE 7.6.1

**FINDINGS:** Axial post-contrasted CT images through the mandible (A) and at a level through the bottom of the mandible (B) show a fluid collection within the right masticator space, within the right masseter muscle, and wrapping around the bottom of the mandible (Fig. 7.6.1). The coronal (C) reconstruction image shows how the fluid collection wraps around the mandible inferiorly. The sagittal reconstruction (D) with bone window to the right of midline shows the right-sided teeth.

**DIAGNOSIS:** Odontogenic abscess.

**DISCUSSION:** An odontogenic abscess most often involves the masticator space but can extend into the adjacent submandibular space. Bone algorithm on CT may show the dental caries and/or the periodontal disease as indicated by periapical lucency with osseous erosion. There may also be periosteal elevation if there is associated osteomyelitis. Contrast-enhanced CT is helpful to delineate the peripherally enhancing abscess and associated phlegmon in the masticator space. The muscles of mastication may be edematous and swollen. Be sure to evaluate the suprazygomatic masticator space as well as the infrazygomatic masticator space for the full extent of the infection.

The acute dental abscess is usually polymicrobial comprising facultative anaerobes, such as viridans group streptococci and the *Streptococcus anginosus* group, with predominantly strict anaerobes, such as anaerobic cocci, *Prevotella* and *Fusobacterium* species (21). Patients often present with trismus. Despite some reports of increasing antimicrobial resistance in isolates from acute dental infection, the vast majority of localized dental abscesses respond to surgical treatment, with antimicrobials limited to spreading and severe infections.

Odontogenic source of infection may spread to maxillary sinus or cervical soft tissues by direct extension. Hematogenous spread to distant sites such as the brain is also possible (22).

# Case 7.6 (Continued)

## Aunt Minnie's Pearls

The masticator space is one of the more confusing spaces of the suprahyoid neck, as it includes the muscles of mastication as well as a portion of the posterior mandible, which can have its own differentials, as well as being included in facial bone differentials.

The most common pathology of the masticator space is the odontogenic abscess.

A fluid collection adjacent to the mandible should always prompt a thorough evaluation of the adjacent teeth, which are often ignored on imaging studies.

The teeth are also important with sinus disease, as the odontogenic origin of maxillary sinus disease is commonly missed, so be sure to also look for lucencies around the tooth roots.

HISTORY: A 71-year-old man with tenderness and swelling over the right angle of the mandible.

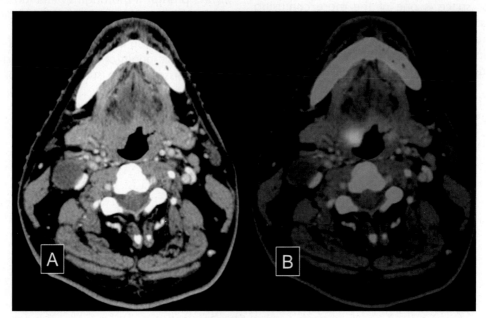

FIGURE 7.7.1

FINDINGS: Axial post-contrasted CT image immediately below the mandible (A) and fused PET/CT image at the same level (B) show a simple appearing cystic mass at the right angle of the mandible (Fig. 7.7.1). The fused PET/CT image shows increased uptake within the right lateral and inferior base of the tongue, but no increased uptake within the cystic lesion.

DIAGNOSIS: Squamous cell carcinoma necrotic lymph node.

DISCUSSION: A cystic rounded lesion along the anterior margin of the sternocleidomastoid muscle may represent a congenital lesion such as a second branchial cleft cyst in a **young** patient. However, in an **older** patient, it may represent a necrotic lymph node (LN) with the primary lesion located at the base of the tongue or in the palatine tonsils.

Although there are various reports of different size criteria for diagnosing metastatic lymphadenopathy, the literature trend indicates that smaller criteria have been suggested because of the substantial false negatives for the diagnosis of nodal metastasis. Other morphologic imaging features should be evaluated. For instance, a metastatic LN has a more rounded morphology rather than the kidney bean shape of a normal LN (23). Metastatic LN, particularly from squamous cell carcinoma (SCC), may show heterogeneous enhancement due to medullary necrosis (24). In fact, any node with central necrosis is considered metastatic from SCC, regardless of its size. Other imaging features of metastatic lymphadenopathy include extracapsular spread and carotid artery invasion. A patient's prognosis is reduced by 50% when there is extracapsular spread (24). On CT, extracapsular spread is suspected when the border of the LN is irregular and hazy with infiltration into the adjacent structures. Loss of the fatty plane between a suspicious LN and the carotid artery and the degree of tumor surrounding the arterial circumference are indicative of carotid artery invasion (25).

### Aunt Minnie's Pearls

This case highlights an important discussion on clinical information when reading studies. When you see a well-circumscribed cystic lesion at the angle of the mandible, the age of the patient determines the leading differential consideration.

In a child, you should be thinking about the branchial cleft cyst, **but** in a patient over 60, you should be thinking about a SCC node, and the primary is almost always at either the ipsilateral palatine tonsil or the base of the tongue.

You should be suspicious even if it looks like a very simple cyst and there are no surrounding aggressive features to suggest extracapsular spread and no nodularity. It doesn't matter how benign it looks, if the patient is over 60, it is a SCC node, **NOT** a congenital cyst. This is a very important discussion because those diagnoses are treated so differently. Importantly, there are increasing numbers of HPV positive SCC cases in younger patients, sometimes in their 40s.

**HISTORY:** A 58-year-old man with nontender left neck mass.

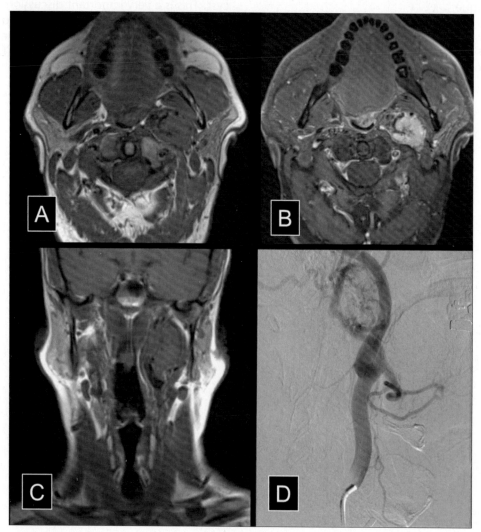

FIGURE 7.8.1

**FINDINGS:** Axial T1 precontrast (A) and correlating post contrast (B) image through the same level show an avidly enhancing lesion within the left cervical soft tissues (Fig. 7.8.1). The coronal T1 precontrasted image (C) shows multiple flow voids within the lesion. The catheter angiography image (D) from a left common carotid injection shows a vascular blush and splaying of the ICA and the ECA.

**DIAGNOSIS:** Carotid body tumor

**DISCUSSION:** Carotid body (CB) paragangliomas (aka carotid body tumor, glomus caroticum) are vascular masses arising from the carotid body paraganglia. These highly vascular masses splay the external and internal carotid arteries and demonstrate intense rapid enhancement on CT and MRI. Although typically unilateral, they can be bilateral in 5% to 10% of cases (26). Lesions larger than 2 cm may exhibit a "salt and pepper" appearance on T1-weighted MRI. The "salt" is T1 hyperintensity due to subacute hemorrhage. The "pepper" is T1/T2 hypointense serpentine vascular flow voids. CB paragangliomas are slightly hyperintense to muscle on T2-weighted images. Catheter angiography will reveal a lesion splaying the ECA and ICA with a prolonged tumor blush and early draining veins. The lesion is most often supplied by the ascending pharyngeal artery or ascending cervical artery. As the lesion enlarges, it will encase, but not narrow the ICA and ECA. CB paragangliomas have somatostatin surface receptors to which indium-111 octreotide, a nuclear medicine somatostatin analog, will attach and show focal radiotracer uptake.

Paragangliomas may be hereditary and may be part of genetic syndromes such as Von Hippel–Lindau syndrome, neurofibromatosis type I (von Recklinghausen disease), MEN 2A and MEN 2B. Look for multiple lesions as 2% to 10% of sporadic paragangliomas are multicentric, while 25% to 75% are multiple in familial cases (26). These can occur at the contralateral carotid bifurcation, in the high carotid space approximately 2 cm below the jugular foramen (glomus vagale), at the jugular foramen (glomus jugulare), and at the cochlear promontory (glomus tympanicum).

The typical patient is middle-aged and presents with a painless slow-growing, pulsatile mass. Clinical manifestations include hoarseness of voice, lower cranial nerve palsies, pulsatile tinnitus, and other neuro-otologic symptoms (27).

## Aunt Minnie's Pearls

Paragangliomas are usually found in the abdomen, with less than 5% within the head and neck, but these are the most clinically symptomatic. Paragangliomas can occur at several locations within the cervical soft tissues. When they occur at the carotid bifurcation, they are called carotid body tumors.

Again, to emphasize, paragangliomas within the carotid sheath or space that are centered 2 cm below the skull base are called glomus vagale tumors. If the paraganglioma is centered at the jugular foramen, they are called jugular paragangliomas. Smaller paragangliomas found on the cochlear promontory are called glomus tympanicum tumors. These are all the same pathology, but are given different names based on their location.

**HISTORY:** A 63-year-old woman with neck pain.

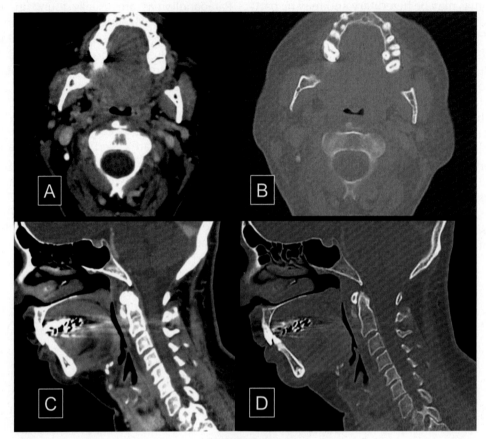

FIGURE 7.9.1

**FINDINGS:** Axial post-contrasted standard (A) and correlating bone algorithm (B) CT images demonstrate a calcific density anterior to the C2 vertebral body (Fig. 7.9.1). The sagittal standard (C) and bone algorithm (D) reconstructed CT images show the density anterior to C2 as well as prevertebral fluid tracking inferiorly, posterior to the airway. The fluid causes prominence of the prevertebral soft tissues.

**DIAGNOSIS:** Longus colli tendinitis

**DISCUSSION:** Acute longus colli tendinitis (aka acute retropharyngeal tendonitis, calcific tendonitis of the longus coli) is an inflammatory process related to calcium hydroxyapatite deposition in the superior oblique fibers of the longus colli muscles (28). The longus colli muscle extends from the anterior arch C1 to the T3 vertebrae. The clinical picture can be confusing as patients present with acute neck pain, stiffness, odynophagia, low-grade fever and mild leukocytosis (29). Imaging, particularly CT, can help make the diagnosis by identifying characteristic, amorphous calcification in the proximal fibers of the longus colli, which lie inferior to the anterior arch of the atlas. These calcifications coupled with a nonenhancing smooth, lenticular prevertebral fluid collection/effusion is considered nearly pathognomonic of this entity (28).

## Aunt Minnie's Pearls

When fluid is seen within the cervical soft tissues, it is important to differentiate an abscess from other pathologies.

For cervical soft tissue CT studies, it is always important to set the window and level settings so that air is a different density from fat, as where there is air and where there is fat is critical for several cervical pathologies.

The presence of fluid within the prevertebral soft tissues is an example of the importance of this differentiation, as benign fluid and a retropharyngeal abscess are very different clinical entities.

Benign fluid at this location can be seen with longus colli tendonitis as well as jugular vein thrombosis and thrombophlebitis.

An abscess at this location can be dangerous as the prevertebral space lies immediately anterior to the danger space (even sounds bad), which is a potential space and a potential route of spread of pathology inferiorly into the mediastinum.

HISTORY: A 57-year-old woman with dizziness.

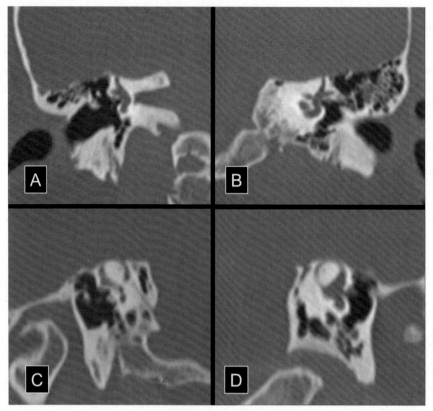

FIGURE 7.10.1

FINDINGS: A CT of the temporal bones with bilateral coronal (A and B) and the bilateral short axis (C and D) bone algorithm non contrasted images demonstrate absence of bone over the bilateral superior semicircular canals (Fig. 7.10.1). The short axis reconstructions are generated simply by going superiorly on the axial sections to the top of the temporal bone, and then connecting the dots of the fluid filled semicircular canals. These are helpful to show the semicircular canals in profile.

DIAGNOSIS: Superior semicircular canal dehiscence

DISCUSSION: Semicircular canal dehiscence is the extreme thinning or absence of the bony roof over the semicircular canal. This is best seen as ≥ 2 mm dehiscence of the roof on high resolution CT of the temporal bones in the coronal and Poschl or short axis views (perpendicular to the long axis of the petrous bone). There may be associated thinning of the tegmen tympani. Semicircular canal dehiscence causes vestibular and auditory symptoms and signs as a consequence of the third mobile window in the inner ear created by the dehiscence (30). Common symptoms include sound and pressure induced vestibular symptoms and eye movements (31). Tullio phenomenon of vertigo and nystagmus due to loud noises can be seen. Of note, there can be asymptomatic thinning of the bone over the semicircular canal or posterior semicircular canal. A defect in the osseous semicircular canal can also cause apparent conductive hearing loss (32).

## Aunt Minnie's Pearls

If you look closely, you can find semicircular canal dehiscence more frequently than you would guess. Similar to spinal degenerative changes, the imaging finding does not always match the clinical presentation. These patients will not always have Tullio phenomenon clinically.

If you do a study for possible semicircular canal dehiscence, remember to also look at the posterior semicircular canal for possible thinning near the inferior petrosal vein or other anomalous draining veins.

HISTORY: A 52-year-old woman with right papilledema.

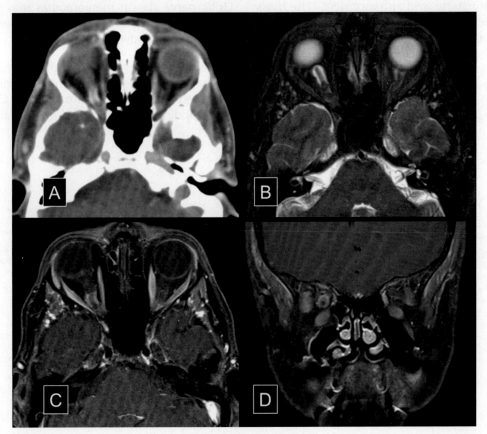

FIGURE 7.11.1

FINDINGS: Axial post-contrasted standard algorithm CT (A) image through the orbits shows linear high density medial and lateral to the right optic nerve (Fig. 7.11.1). Correlating axial T2 FSE fat saturated image (B) shows very prominent CSF anterior to the high density seen on CT along the optic nerve and low signal intensity where the high density was seen on the CT. Axial post-contrasted fat saturated T1 image (C) and coronal post-contrasted fat saturated T1 image (D) show enhancement surrounding the right optic nerve correlating to the high density on CT.

DIAGNOSIS: Optic nerve sheath meningioma

DISCUSSION: These benign tumors arise in middle-aged patients (slight female predominance) from the dural sheath around the optic nerve. There is an association with neurofibromatosis type 2 (33). Patients present with proptosis, progressive visual loss, color vision defects and afferent papillary defects. On CT, optic nerve meningiomas may show "tram-track" calcification. Calcification may be demonstrated in optic nerve sheath meningiomas in 20% to 50% of cases (34). Similarly, this sign can be seen with enhanced T1-weighted MRI with fat-saturation. This MRI tram-track sign is composed of two enhanced areas of tumor separated from each other by the negative defect of the optic nerve (34). The lesions are isointense to brain on T1- and T2-weighted MRI and demonstrate avid enhancement. The mass effect from the meningioma may result in the dilatation of the optic nerve sheath posterior to the globe resulting in the appearance of a peri-optic cyst. Meningiomas have been described as involving the orbit in 1% of cases (35). Optic nerve sheath meningiomas arise from meningothelial cells of the arachnoid situated along the optic nerve sheath.

## Aunt Minnie's Pearls

Optic nerve sheath meningiomas may be seen with NF-2, so look for other MISME lesions such as schwannomas and ependymomas.

MRI is better for evaluation of these lesions, but if you are having trouble determining a meningioma from optic nerve glioma or other pathology, CT can be useful for findings the "tram-track" calcifications.

HISTORY: A 50-year-old woman with weakness.

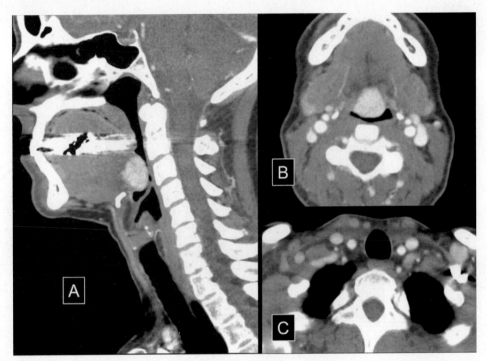

FIGURE 7.12.1

FINDINGS: Sagittal reconstructed image (A) from a post-contrasted CT with standard algorithm shows a high density mass within the base of the tongue at the midline. Axial post-contrasted image at the level of the mandible (B) shows the lesion to be well-circumscribed and without surrounding aggressive features. An image from a lower level through the neck at the level of the clavicles (C) shows that something is missing (Fig. 7.12.1).

DIAGNOSIS: Lingual thyroid

DISCUSSION: Ectopic lingual thyroid is rare embryological anomaly, which originates from failure of the thyroid gland to descend from the foramen caecum to its normal eutopic pre-laryngeal site. The tongue is the most frequent ectopic location of the thyroid gland (90% of cases); the clinical incidence of lingual thyroid varies between 1:3,000 and 1:10,000 (36). It occurs more frequently in females, with a female to male ratio 4:1 (37). Most ectopic thyroids are asymptomatic, and no therapy is necessary. Symptoms are related to the growth of the thyroid tissue, causing dysphagia, dysphonia with stomatolalia, bleeding or dyspnea (38). In about 70% to 75% of the patients with lingual thyroid, there is an absence of normal thyroid gland (39).

Lingual thyroid appears as a well-circumscribed rounded midline lesion at the base of the tongue, usually at the site of the foramen cecum. Its imaging features are similar to that of normal thyroid gland with high density on noncontrasted CT. It shows avid enhancement and uptake on Tc-99m pertechnetate scans.

## Aunt Minnie's Pearls

The base of the tongue is the most common location of an ectopic thyroid, and in those cases, it is usually the only functioning thyroid. Therefore, in these cases when you see a high density lesion within the midline base of the tongue, it is important to look and see if there is any normal thyroid gland in the expected thyroid bed.

These lesions have a very benign appearance, not an aggressive invasive appearance like a SCC of the base of the tongue. Additionally, there will be no lymphadenopathy seen. These rare lesions can increase in size during puberty, and a thyroid carcinoma arising from a lingual thyroid is extremely rare.

**HISTORY:** Sensorineural hearing loss in a child.

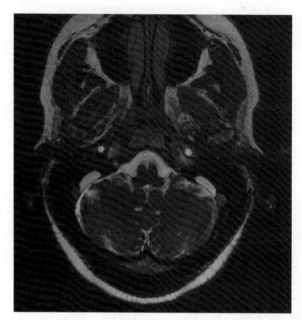

FIGURE 7.13.1

**FINDINGS:** Axial thin section T2 weighted image through the skull base shows bilateral cystic structures along the posterior temporal bones with signal intensity similar to CSF (Fig. 7.13.1). These are immediately medial to the sigmoid sinuses and have a benign homogeneous appearance. There is a septation (black line) between these cystic structures and the posterior fossa CSF.

**DIAGNOSIS:** Large endolymphatic sac anomaly (LESA)

**DISCUSSION:** LESA is a congenital enlargement of the inner ear endolymphatic system. On MRI, this is identified as an enlarged endolymphatic sac(s), and on CT, there is corresponding enlargement of the vestibular aqueduct(s). The endolymphatic duct and sac are readily visible on T2-weighted MRI (40). Look for enlargement of the bony vestibular aqueduct diameter greater than 1.5 mm on CT halfway between the crus communis and the intracranial aperture of the aqueduct (41). In general, the vestibular aqueduct should not be greater in size than the adjacent SCC. LESA is the most common cause of congenital sensorineural hearing loss (SNHL) (42), and it is the most commonly identified radiographic abnormality of the inner ear (43). The classic scenario is progressive SNHL in a child or young adult, which is exacerbated by minor trauma.

## Aunt Minnie's Pearls

LESA is the most common congenital anomaly found on temporal bone imaging.

These cases are thought to present with SNHL after relatively minor trauma because of a fragile cochlea. You should look for the endolymphatic duct and sac (the duct is actually only a few mm, the rest is actually the sac) in the axial series of both CT and MRI near the level of the vestibule.

Some people like to use different words for things so that others can't figure out what they are talking about in medicine, so if you happen to hear someone say large vestibular aqueduct syndrome (LVAS) that is the same thing as LESA. Some people will use LVAS for the findings on CT and LESA for the same findings on MRI.

If you are interested in the seventh week gestation arrested development leading to this abnormality, go find an embryology book.

**HISTORY:** A 22-year-old woman with balance problems.

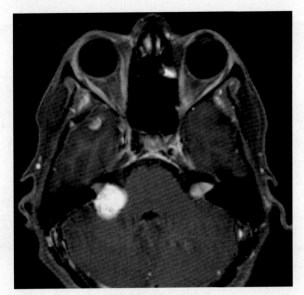

FIGURE 7.14.1

**FINDINGS:** Axial post-contrasted T1 image with fat saturation through the level of the orbits demonstrates enhancing lesions in both internal auditory canals (Fig. 7.14.1). The lesion on the right is larger and has more extension into the cerebellopontine angle (CPA), with mass effect on the adjacent brain.

**DIAGNOSIS:** Bilateral vestibular schwannomas in neurofibromatosis type 2

**DISCUSSION:** Vestibular schwannoma is the most common CPA mass. These lesions commonly arise from the inferior vestibular division of the eighth cranial nerve, accounting for 80% to 90% of all CPA tumors (44). Sensorineural hearing loss is the most common result, though rarely, they can cause facial nerve palsy. The presence of bilateral vestibular schwannomas in a child or young adult is highly suggestive of neurofibromatosis type 2.

Vestibular schwannomas are well-demarcated from the adjacent brain parenchyma and CSF. They appear isointense to brain on T1-weighted MRI and hyperintense on T2-weighted MRI. They typically enhance intensely though larger lesions may show intramural cyst and internal T2/ GRE hypointensity related to hemosiderin. Most vestibular schwannomas often arise near the Obersteiner-Redlich zone, which marks the transition from glial cells to Schwann cells and from the central to the peripheral nervous system (45). When small, they conform to the tubular shape of the internal auditory canal. The mass takes on the classic "ice cream cone"

appearance as it enlarges and bulges into the CPA. Thin-section T2 images and heavily weighted T2 sequences, such as construction interference steady state (CISS), are helpful in identifying a fundal cap of CSF between the lateral portion of the lesion and the cochlear canal. This is important as a 2 mm or greater fundal cap will enable a hearing preservation surgical approach.

## Aunt Minnie's Pearls

It is thought that bilateral vestibular schwannomas = NF2, but it is important to remember possible facial nerve involvement in these cases. Sometimes the enhancing lesion within the IAC is actually a facial nerve schwannoma rather than a vestibular schwannoma. That is why evaluation of the labyrinthine segment of the facial nerve is important in these cases to differentiate between the two pathologies.

Since the vestibulocochlear nerve fibers are more sensitive than the facial nerve fibers, a facial nerve schwannoma within the IAC may compress the cochlear nerve, causing the patient to present with hearing loss, instead of facial nerve symptoms. In such cases, the clinical findings are misleading.

Remember that NF2 is the MISME disease so look around for other lesions. If you remembered that, you might have gotten extra Aunt Minnie points for noticing the small meningioma in the anterior right middle cranial fossa on this case!

**HISTORY:** A 85-year-old man with slowly progressive conductive hearing loss.

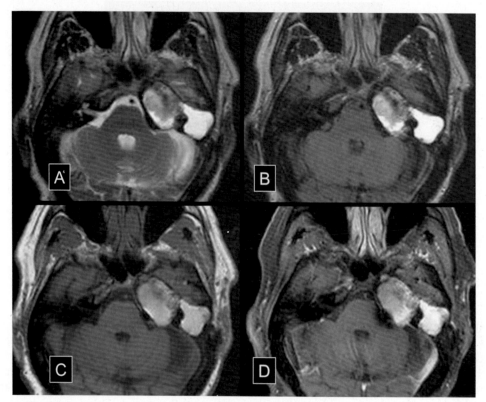

FIGURE 7.15.1

**FINDINGS:** Multiple axial MRI sections through the temporal bones at the same level show an expansile lesion on the left involving the left mastoid, middle ear cavity, and petrous apex. The axial T2 (A) and FLAIR (B) images show bright signal intensity within the lesion predominantly laterally. There are surrounding benign changes without brain vasogenic edema. The axial T1 precontrast (C) and correlating axial T1 post-contrasted fat saturation (D) images show that there is similar bright T1 signal intensity with no enhancement of the lesion (Fig. 7.15.1).

**DIAGNOSIS:** Cholesterol granuloma

**DISCUSSION:** A cholesterol granuloma (CG) (aka chocolate cyst or blue-dome cyst) is a complicated inflammatory process of the otomastoid space due to chronic inflammation. This specialized granulation tissue is prone to hemorrhage with resultant chronic blood products and cholesterol crystals, which further aggravate the inflammatory process. CGs most often occur in the middle ear cavity but may occur anywhere along the tympanic cleft (42). Lesions of the petrous apex may present with sensorineural hearing loss, tinnitus, and/or multiple cranial nerve palsies depending on the size and location of the lesion. A CG appears as a smooth expansile mass of the petrous apex or otomastoid space on CT. There may be focal areas of bony wall dehiscence. On MRI, the lesion displays T1 and T2 hyperintense signal due to the presence of chronic blood products and fluid debris (46). There may be a peripheral T2 hypointense rim due to hemosiderin. CGs may show peripheral enhancement due to granulation tissue but do not demonstrate central enhancement (42).

## Aunt Minnie's Pearls

These lesions may be found incidentally when small. When they are centered within the petrous apex, it is important to look for expansile changes and loss of the osseous trabecula to try to differentiate these lesions from benign fluid or a congenital cholesteatoma.

In those cases, the MRI is important for differentiation with benign bright T2 and dark T1 signal intensity (SI) indicating fluid, while restricted diffusion suggests cholesteatoma, and bright T1 and T2 SI points to CG. This case also highlights the importance of the pre-contrasted T1 images, which show that the lesion is not actually enhancing.

Caution to those of you that like to first jump to the post-contrasted images. For head and neck cases, the pre-contrasted T1 is often more important than the post-contrasted images, especially within the cervical soft tissues, where the normal extracranial fat helps define pathologies.

HISTORY: A 53-year-old man with bilateral hearing loss.

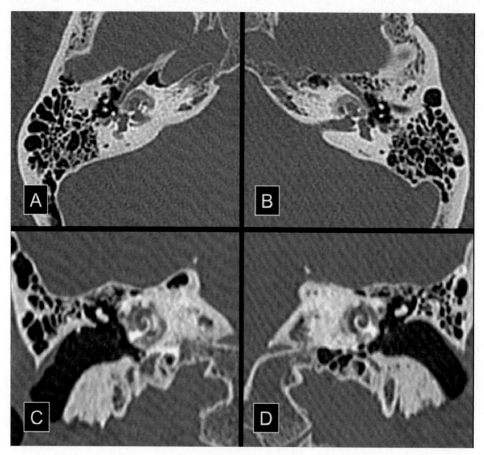

FIGURE 7.16.1

FINDINGS: Temporal bone CT case with bilateral axial (A and B) and coronal (C and D) images show patchy lucencies surrounding the cochleas bilaterally (Fig. 7.16.1).

DIAGNOSIS: Otosclerosis

DISCUSSION: In otosclerosis (aka otospongiosis), normal dense endochondral bone of the otic capsule is replaced with vascular spongy bone. There is a continuum from the more localized fenestral otospongiosis (FO) involving the oval window at the medial wall of the tympanic cavity and the round window to a lesser extent and the more extensive cochlear form. Cochlear otospongiosis (CO) (or retrofenestral otosclerosis) involves the bones surrounding the cochlea and is almost always accompanied by FO. Submillimter CT of the temporal bones with multiplanar reconstruction is best for delineating these osseous changes. The hypodense plaque lateral to the oval window (fissula ante fenestram) is a pathognomic finding of FO. There is resultant narrowing of the oval window. With CO, there are multiple foci of demineralization surrounding the cochlea. FO presents with progressive conductive hearing loss while CO present with mixed conductive and sensorineural hearing loss. It is bilateral 80% of the time and presents in the second and third decades (42).

## *Aunt Minnie's Pearls*

What is usually seen on imaging is the otospongiotic phase of otosclerosis, unfortunately another poorly named medical pathology. So may be more accurate to call it otospongiosis instead.

Symmetric and midline things are often the hardest to identify in the neuro world, but the bone surrounding the otic capsule (cochlea and vestibule) is the highest density bone in the body, so we should always see bright white bone surrounding those structures.

MRI may actually show enhancement surrounding the otic capsule, so this can be confusing if you only have an MRI and no CT studies to compare.

If that enhancement is actually within the otic capsule instead of surrounding it, think about labyrinthitis instead of otospongiosis.

# REFERENCES

1. Moore KL. The developing human, 3rd ed. Philadelphia, PA: Saunders, 1988.
2. Allard RH. The thyroglossal cyst. Head Neck Surg 1982; 5(2):134–146.
3. Filston HC. Common lumps and bumps of the head and neck in infants and children. Pediatr Ann 1989;18(3):180–182, 184, 186.
4. Koeller KK, Alamo L, Adair CF, et al. Congenital cystic masses of the neck: radiologic-pathologic correlation. Radiographics 1999;19(1):121–146; quiz 152–153.
5. Reede DL, Bergeron RT, Som PM. CT of thyroglossal duct cysts. Radiology 1985;157(1):121–125.
6. Gritzmann N. Sonography of the salivary glands. AJR Am J Roentgenol 1989;153(1):161–166.
7. Yousem DM, Kraut MA, Chalian AA. Major salivary gland imaging. Radiology 2000;216(1):19–29.
8. Jager L, Menauer F, Holzknecht N, et al. Sialolithiasis: MR sialography of the submandibular duct—an alternative to conventional sialography and US? Radiology 2000;216(3): 665–671.
9. Avrahami E, Englender M, Chen E, et al. CT of submandibular gland sialolithiasis. Neuroradiology 1996;38(3):287–290.
10. Yoshimura Y, Inoue Y, Odagawa T. Sonographic examination of sialolithiasis. J Oral Maxillofac Surg 1989;47(9):907–912.
11. Hutchins T. Vocal cord paralysis. In: Diagnositc imaging: head and neck, 2nd ed. Salt Lake City, UT: Amirsys, 2011.
12. Romo LV, Curtin HD. Atrophy of the posterior cricoarytenoid muscle as an indicator of recurrent laryngeal nerve palsy. AJNR Am J Neuroradiol 1999;20(3):467–471.
13. Christe A, Waldherr C, Hallett R, et al. MR imaging of parotid tumors: typical lesion characteristics in MR imaging improve discrimination between benign and malignant disease. AJNR Am J Neuroradiol 2011;32(7):1202–1207.
14. Silver AR, Som PM. Salivary glands. Radiol Clin N Am 1998; 36:941–966.
15. Shah GV. MR imaging of salivary glands. Neuroimag Clin N Am 2004;14:777–808.
16. Joe VQ, Westesson PL. Tumors of the parotid gland: MR imaging characteristics of various histologic types. AJR Am J Roentgenol 1994;163(2):433–438.
17. Mermel LA, Allon M, Bouza E, et al. Clinical practice guidelines for the diagnosis and management of intravascular catheter-related infection: 2009 Update by the Infectious Diseases Society of America. Clin Infect Dis 2009;49(1):1–45.
18. Van Rooden CJ, Tesselaar ME, Osanto S, et al. Deep vein thrombosis associated with central venous catheters—a review. J Thromb Haemost 2005;3(11):2409–2419.
19. Andes DR, Urban AW, Acher ChW, et al. Septic thrombosis of basilic, axillary, and subclavian veins caused by a peripherally inserted central venous catheter. Am J Med 1998,105:446–450.
20. Kniemeyer HW, Grabitz K, Buhl R, et al. Surgical treatment of septic deep venous thrombosis. Surgery 1995,118:49–53.
21. Robertson D, Smith AJ. The microbiology of the acute dental abscess. J Med Microbiol 2009;58(Pt 2):155–162.
22. Antunes AA, de Santana Santos T, de Carvalho RW, et al. Brain abscess of odontogenic origin. J Craniofac Surg 2011; 22(6):2363–2365.
23. Som PM, Curtin HD, Mancuso AA. An imaging-based classification for the cervical nodes designed as an adjunct to recent clinically based nodal classifications. Arch Otolaryngol Head Neck Surg 1999;125(4):388–396.
24. van den Brekel MW, Stel HV, Castelijns JA, et al. Cervical lymph node metastasis: assessment of radiologic criteria. Radiology 1990;177(2):379–384.
25. Yousem DM, Hatabu H, Hurst RW, et al. Carotid artery invasion by head and neck masses: prediction with MR imaging. Radiology 1995;195(3):715–720.
26. Davidson H. Carotid body paraganglioma. In: Diagnostic imaging: head and neck, 2nd ed. Salt Lake City, UT: Amirsys, 2011.
27. Rao AB, Koeller KK, Adair CF. From the archives of the AFIP. Paragangliomas of the head and neck: radiologic-pathologic correlation. Armed Forces Institute of Pathology. Radiographics 1999;19(6):1605–1632.
28. Eastwood JD, Hudgins PA, Malone D. Retropharyngeal effusion in acute calcific prevertebral tendinitis: diagnosis with CT and MR imaging. AJNR Am J Neuroradiol 1998;19(9): 1789–1792.
29. Ring D, Vaccaro AR, Scuderi G, et al. Acute calcific retropharyngeal tendinitis. Clinical presentation and pathological characterization. J Bone Joint Surg Am 1994;76(11):1636–1642.
30. Minor LB. Clinical manifestations of superior semicircular canal dehiscence. Laryngoscope 2005;115(10):1717–1727.
31. Mong A, Loevner LA, Solomon D, et al. Sound- and pressure-induced vertigo associated with dehiscence of the roof of the superior semicircular canal. AJNR Am J Neuroradiol 1999; 20(10):1973–1975.
32. Curtin HD. Superior semicircular canal dehiscence syndrome and multi-detector row CT. Radiology 2003;226(2):312–314.
33. Dutton JJ. Optic nerve sheath meningiomas. Surv Ophthalmol 1992;37(3):167–183.
34. Kanamalla US. The optic nerve tram-track sign. Radiology 2003;227(3):718–719.
35. Ortiz O, Schochet SS, Kotzan JM, et al. Radiologic-pathologic correlation: meningioma of the optic nerve sheath. AJNR Am J Neuroradiol 1996;17(5):901–906.
36. Benhammou A, Bencheikh R, Benbouzid MA, et al. Ectopic lingual thyroid. B-ENT. 2006;2(3):121–122.
37. Toso A, Colombani F, Averono G, et al. Lingual thyroid causing dysphagia and dyspnoea. Case reports and review of the literature. Acta Otorhinolaryngol Ital 2009;29(4):213–217.
38. Mussak EN, Kacker A. Surgical and medical management of midline ectopic thyroid. Otolaryngol Head Neck Surg 2007; 136(6):870–872.
39. Akyol MU, Ozcan M. Lingual thyroid. Otolaryngol Head Neck Surg 1996;115(5):483–484.
40. Harnsberger HR, Dahlen RT, Shelton C, et al. Advanced techniques in magnetic resonance imaging in the evaluation of the large endolymphatic duct and sac syndrome. Laryngoscope 1995;105(10):1037–1042.
41. Valvassori GE, Clemis JD. The large vestibular aqueduct syndrome. Laryngoscope 1978;88(5):723–728.
42. Davidson H. Imaging of the temporal bone. Neuroimaging Clin N Am 2004;14:721–760.
43. Mafee MF, Charletta D, Kumar A, et al. Large vestibular aqueduct and congenital sensorineural hearing loss. AJNR Am J Neuroradiol 1992;13(2):805–819.
44. Mark AS. Vestibulocochlear system. Neuroimaging Clin N Am 1993;3:153–170.
45. St Martin MB, Hirsch BE. Imaging of hearing loss. Otolaryngol Clin North Am 2008;41(1):157–178, vi–vii.
46. Chaljub G, Vrabec J, Hollingsworth C, et al. Magnetic resonance imaging of petrous tip lesions. Am J Otolaryngol 1999;20(5):304–313.

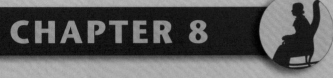

# CHAPTER 8

# NEURORADIOLOGY: SPINE IMAGING

**Daniel B. Nissman / Matthew S. Chin**

*The authors and editors acknowledge the contribution of the Chapter 11 author from the second edition: Mauricio Castillo, MD and the Chapter 6C author from the third edition: Donna R. Roberts*

**HISTORY:** A 16-year-old male presents with intermittent lower back pain. Scoliosis on physical examination

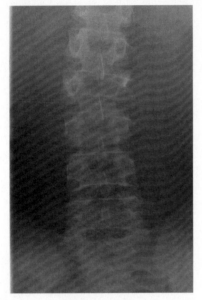

FIGURE 8.1.1

FIGURE 8.1.2

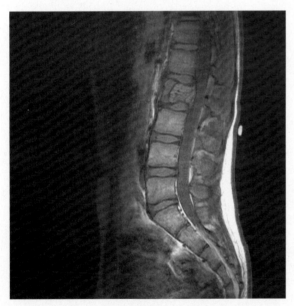

FIGURE 8.1.3

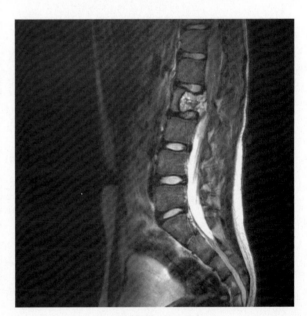

FIGURE 8.1.4

**FINDINGS:** Frontal radiograph (Fig. 8.1.1) shows an expanded left L2 transverse process with soft-tissue calcification adjacent to it. Subsequent axial CT image (Fig. 8.1.2) demonstrates a lytic lesion in the L2 vertebral body with a sclerotic rim, extending into the posterior elements. On T1-weighted, T2-weighted, and contrast-enhanced magnetic resonance imaging (MRI) sagittal images (Figs. 8.1.3 to 8.1.5), the heterogeneously enhancing, expansile,

L2 vertebral body lesion is causing partial vertebral body collapse and spinal canal stenosis.

**DIAGNOSIS:** Spinal osteoblastoma

**DISCUSSION:** Osteoblastomas are rare, benign primary neoplasms of spine and long bones, accounting for 1% of primary bone tumors (1,2). Forty percent occur in the spine, usually the posterior

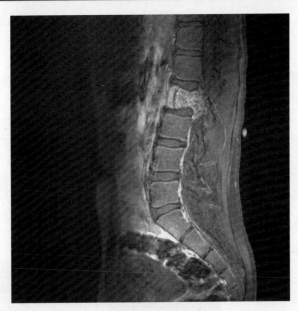

FIGURE 8.1.5

elements, with an additional 17% diagnosed in the sacrum. Secondary aneurysmal bone cysts are seen between 6% and 10% of osteoblastoma cases (1,3).

Spinal osteoblastomas are usually diagnosed in young adults (mean age: 20) and have a male predominance (2:1). Symptoms at presentation include back pain or neurological problems. Painful scoliosis may also result from these lesions.

Similar to osteoid osteomas, these lesions comprise osteoid and primitive woven bone, yet differ given their ability to grow >2 cm (average size: 3.2 cm) (1). Unlike osteoid osteomas, they may display rapid resorption of bony cortex, with extension into the surrounding soft tissues. Malignant osteoblastomas have also been reported—with characteristics similar to osteosarcomas (osteoblastoma-like osteosarcoma) (4,5). These malignant-type osteoblastomas demonstrate greater recurrence at prior excision sites as well as disease metastatic to the lungs (6).

Radiographic appearances of osteoblastomas vary (7). The most common pattern is a lytic lesion with multiple small calcifications and a thin sclerotic rim. These lesions may also appear completely lucent with minimal central calcifications. Pseudomalignant features may be present in 25% of the cases, including cortical thinning, expansion of the bone, and the presence of a soft-tissue mass (8). Given the nonspecific radiographic findings, further imaging studies are usually warranted.

CT scans allow characterization of the lesion's nidus, matrix mineralization, and extent of involvement. With MRI, osteoblastomas have hypointense T1-weighted and hypo-to-hyper-intense T2-weighted signal, relative to bone marrow, based on the amount of ossified matrix material (7). Although limited in its visualization of subtle calcifications, MR allows better visualization of any soft-tissue edema or masses. Percutaneous biopsy will often be performed prior to definitive treatment.

Surgery (curettage or wide excision) is the primary treatment modality. Wide excision is chosen for cases with biopsy or radiographic features of the more aggressive variant. High recurrence rates (up to 24%) have been reported with curettage—significantly less with en bloc resections (1,6). As a result, a wider excision than simple curettage of the lesion may be chosen even in those without more aggressive features. Radiation therapy is controversial, especially given reports of radiation-induced sarcomas, yet utilized in fast growing or recurrent disease (9,10). Few case studies proposed a potential benefit of chemotherapy in aggressive lesions (11,12). Associated aneurysmal bone cysts are usually treated with excision and/or embolization.

## Aunt Minnie's Pearls

Although rare, spine osteoblastomas should be considered when a lucent, sclerotic, or mixed lesion is seen within the spine, the posterior elements in particular.

CT and MRI play complementary roles in its characterization.

Treatment involves curettage or wide surgical excision.

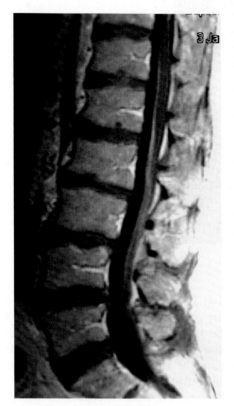

FIGURE 8.2.1

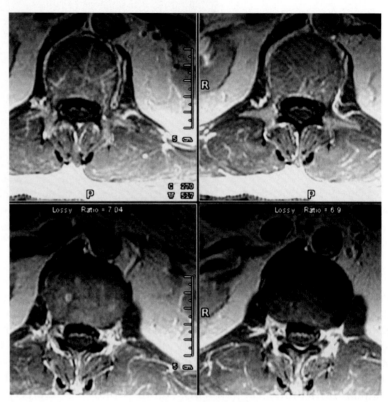

FIGURE 8.2.2

**FINDINGS:** Post-contrast, sagittal (Fig. 8.2.1), and axial (Fig. 8.2.2), T1-weighted images of the lumbar spine show contrast enhancement of the ventral roots of the cauda equina.

**DIAGNOSIS:** Guillain–Barré syndrome (GBS)

**DISCUSSION:** The diagnosis of GBS is based on clinical features, including weakness, sensory loss, pain, and hypoflexia, or areflexia in the lower extremities. Similar to poliomyelitis, the disease progresses cephalad. After days or weeks, the symptoms plateau and may regress. Some patients show brainstem involvement and may necessitate respiratory support.

Cerebrospinal fluid (CSF) analysis shows only elevated proteins. Current research shows that there are variants of GBS (13). The most common is an acute, inflammatory, demyelinating polyneuropathy (AIDP) for which pathologic examination shows lymphocyte and macrophage infiltration of peripheral nerves with segmental demyelination. Two other subtypes of GBS are acute motor and sensory axonal neuropathy (AMSAN) and acute motor axonal neuropathy (AMAN). These two are known as acute axonal forms, demonstrate marked wallerian degeneration, and have poor prognosis. AIDP is the most common form of GBS in North America and Europe (13). The incidence of AIDP is 1 to 2 cases per 100,000 persons per year, with males affected more often (14). Most cases of AIDP are sporadic, but a preceding infectious episode is common (15). AMAN and AMSAN are more common in the Far East, affect younger patients and occur more frequently during the summer months (14,16). AMAN is, in particular, associated with a recent infection with *Campylobacter jejuni* (15). The mainstay of treatment is supportive therapy, and other treatments such as plasma exchange, intravenous immunoglobulin, and corticosteroids have shown some efficacy in treating GBS (13). The prognosis is usually good, but 7% to 15% of patients have substantial neurologic deficits. The incidence of death is 5% (16). Overall, 80% of patients recover.

Unenhanced, T1-weighted images may show slightly high signal in the spinal nerve roots (17) but are nearly always normal (18–20). Nerve root enhancement is seen in patients with GBS (17, 20–23). The syndrome has a predilection for the proximal nerve roots (16). Enhancement of the anterior nerve roots without enhancement of the posterior nerve roots suggests GBS, especially in patients without sensory changes (17). Occasionally, the anterior gray-matter horns within the conus medullaris may show enhancement.

## Aunt Minnie's Pearls

Nerve root enhancement in a patient with an acute onset of rapidly progressive lower-extremity weakness along with appropriate laboratory findings suggest the diagnosis of GBS.

Enhancement of only the anterior rootlets of the proximal cauda equina is generally seen in GBS and in other polio-like variants.

HISTORY: A 47-year-old woman with midthoracic pain, a chronic cough, weight loss, and night sweats

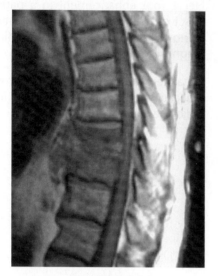

FIGURE 8.3.1

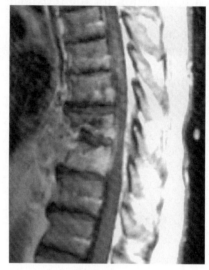

FIGURE 8.3.2

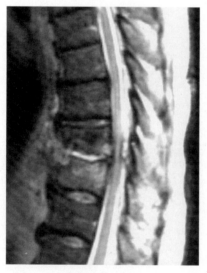

FIGURE 8.3.3

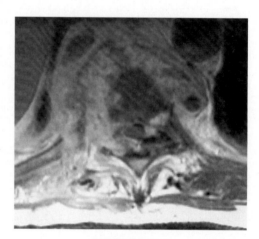

FIGURE 8.3.4

FINDINGS: A sagittal, pre-contrast, T1-weighted MR image (Fig. 8.3.1); corresponding post-contrast image (Fig. 8.3.2); sagittal, T2-weighted image (Fig. 8.3.3); and axial, post-contrast, T1-weighted image (Fig. 8.3.4) show that the disc space at the T9 to T10 level is mostly preserved. There is end-plate erosion and erosion of the anterior-inferior corner of T9 and of the anterior-superior corner of T10. An enhancing soft-tissue mass is recognized under the anterior longitudinal ligament. The axial image shows extension into the paravertebral regions and epidural space. There is cord compression.

DIAGNOSIS: Tuberculosis of the spine (i.e., Pott disease)

DISCUSSION: Approximately 3% to 5% of tuberculosis cases involve the skeleton in HIV-negative patients, and 60% of cases are skeletal in HIV-positive patients (24). In cases of skeletal tuberculosis, the spine is most commonly involved. Spinal tuberculosis occurs in 50% of patients with skeletal involvement (25). Untreated spinal tuberculosis can lead to extensive bone destruction and possible compression of the spinal cord. Compared with pyogenic spondylitis, spinal tuberculosis more commonly leads to paraplegia. The relatively common involvement of the neural arches in tuberculosis contributes to cord compression (24). Spinal tuberculosis usually results from a hematogenous spread to the spine or from direct extension from a paraspinal abscess. Spinal tuberculosis more commonly involves the thoracic and lumbar regions (26,27). Vertebral body destruction begins anteriorly at the superior and inferior end plates, and sclerosis may be seen. Infection spreads under the anterior or posterior longitudinal ligaments.

More than two vertebrae are involved in >50% of patients. Bony erosion anteriorly leads to wedging of the vertebral body, and when multiple segments are involved, kyphosis occurs. Radiographs show indistinctness of the end plates, narrowing of the disc space, and loss of vertebral body height. Erosions and sclerosis of the vertebral body may be seen. Involvement of an entire vertebral body may occur and lead to complete collapse, resulting in a vertebra plana. Large paraspinal abscesses can be seen in the psoas muscles. Occasionally, an abscess may contain a bone sequestrum. Although the focus of infection is usually the anterior portion of the vertebral bodies (27), posterior spinal tuberculosis occurs with an incidence of about 2% to 10% (28). MRI is the preferred modality for evaluating spinal tuberculosis. T1-weighted images show low signal within the vertebral body, and T2-weighted images show high signal owing to bone marrow edema. A thick rim of enhancement around paraspinal and intraosseous abscesses is typical of tuberculosis (26,29). Cold abscesses are usually disproportionately large when compared with the degree of bone involvement. Abscesses tend to be more prominent in children. When tuberculosis involves only a disc, differentiation from a pyogenic infection is not possible. Brucellosis has imaging features similar to those of tuberculosis but more often involves the lumbosacral junction.

Treatment of spinal tuberculosis is predicated on eradication of the infection and correction of any spinal deformity, particularly kyphosis. Spinal tuberculosis can be successfully treated with chemotherapy alone (30). In patients where surgery is indicated, in particular those with kyphotic deformity, anterior or posterior stabilization instrumentation can be placed. Involvement of no more than two vertebral bodies can be stabilized using anterior instrumentation, the first reported method for treating tuberculous involvement of the spine. Multisegment involvement is likely best treated with posterior instrumentation (31).

## Aunt Minnie's Pearls

Large paraspinal abscesses with a thick rim of enhancement accompanied by little bone destruction, particularly in children, suggest tuberculosis.

Isolated destruction of the posterior elements particularly in the cervical region accompanied by adenopathy or abscesses is typical of tuberculosis.

Fluid collections under the anterior or posterior (or both) longitudinal ligaments with involvement of only the anterior aspect of one or more vertebral bodies are suggestive of tuberculosis.

**HISTORY:** A 34-year-old man with AIDS and back pain (Figs. 8.4.1 to 8.4.3). Another patient is illustrated in Figures 8.4.4 and 8.4.5

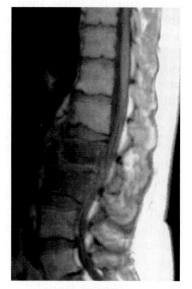

FIGURE 8.4.1

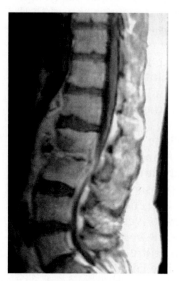

FIGURE 8.4.2

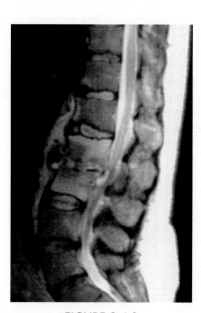

FIGURE 8.4.3

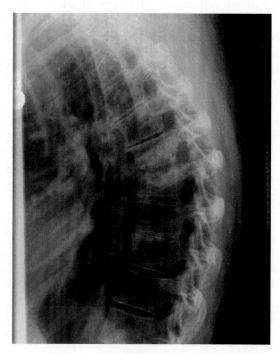

FIGURE 8.4.4

**FINDINGS:** A sagittal, T1-weighted MR image (Fig. 8.4.1); post-contrast, T1-weighted image (Fig. 8.4.2); and a T2-weighted image (Fig. 8.4.3) show a narrowed L2–L3 disc space with erosion of the end plates. The bone marrow of L2 and L3 has abnormal signal intensity. There is a small, rim-enhancing area of low-signal intensity posterior to the abnormal disc, resulting in narrowing of the spinal canal. On the T2-weighted images, the abnormal disc is bright. Lateral radiograph of the

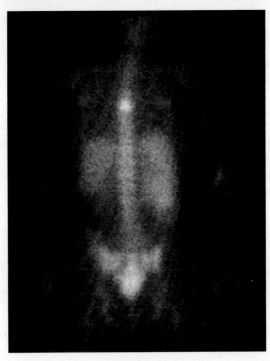

FIGURE 8.4.5

thoracic spine (Fig. 8.4.4) demonstrates marked end plate destruction centered at a midthoracic disc level. Posterior planar image from a gallium-67 scan (Fig. 8.4.5) demonstrates a corresponding focus of intense radiotracer uptake.

**DIAGNOSIS:** Discitis with epidural abscess (first patient) and discitis alone (second patient)

**DISCUSSION:** Discitis is an inflammatory process of the intervertebral disc spaces, usually of the lumbar spine. Variable symptoms include fever, abdominal pain, limp, refusal to walk or sit up, and pain in the back, hip, or knee. In adults, infection usually begins at the vertebral body end plates and spreads to the adjacent disc. The opposite occurs in children, whose intervertebral discs are vascularized, with infection spreading to vertebral bodies from an infected disc. An immunocompromised state, advanced age, diabetes mellitus, systemic infection, and genitourinary infection or surgical manipulation predispose to osteomyelitis and discitis (32). *Staphylococcus aureus* is the most common bacterial cause of spinal osteomyelitis, but other common pathogens include *Streptococcus, Enterobacter, Escherichia coli,* tuberculosis, *Klebsiella,* and *Salmonella* (32–34). Radiographs are negative early, but bone scan results are generally positive. MRI is probably the imaging method of choice and allows early identification of the infection and delineation of paraspinal or epidural abscesses in more advanced cases (35). On MRI, the affected disc is always bright on T2-weighted images; degenerated discs are dark on T2-weighted images. The adjacent end plates show low-intensity T1 signal and high-intensity T2 signal. After contrast is given, the disc and adjacent vertebrae enhance. Involvement of other vertebrae begins generally at the level of the canal for the basivertebral vein and is clearly seen on sagittal T2 images. Epidural abscesses usually are found at the level of the infected disc and are seen as masses that enhance peripherally and compress the thecal sac. Occasionally, at the level of an epidural abscess, the spinal cord shows high-intensity T2 signal, probably caused by venous congestion and edema. Diffusion-weighted imaging demonstrates restricted diffusion in pyogenic abscesses of the spine as it does in the brain.

Radionuclide imaging in spinal infections are mostly performed with technetium-99m-labeled diphosphonate bone scans or gallium-67 citrate. Both of these modalities are highly sensitive for infection in the spine but lack specificity. Gallium-67 scans are preferred over indium-111–labeled white blood cells, which have better diagnostic performance outside the spine because the white blood cells have difficulty reaching the site of infection. Improved specificity can be obtained when gallium-67 scans are interpreted with a three-phase bone scan. Infections are considered to be present when the activity on the gallium-67 scan is greater than that of the bone scan (36). Although MRI has better performance characteristics in the initial diagnostic workup, radionuclide imaging is more specific in the postsurgical and posttreatment setting (37).

Identification of the causative organism is essential to the proper treatment of discitis osteomyelitis. In the absence of positive blood cultures, percutaneous biopsy of the affected disc and end plates is needed to establish a diagnosis. Unfortunately, approximately only 50% of biopsy specimens yield a positive result. Some have advocated repeat biopsy in these situations (38). Treatment for epidural abscess is surgical evacuation.

## Aunt Minnie's Pearls

MRI allows early identification of infection and delineation of paraspinal or epidural abscesses. The affected disc always has high signal intensity on fluid-sensitive images.

In the postsurgical and posttreatment settings, radionuclide imaging is more specific for infection than MRI.

Percutaneous biopsy is essential to establish the identity of the infecting organism(s) in the absence of positive blood cultures.

In children, discitis is an inflammatory process centered on a lumbar intervertebral disc. Children between the ages of 6 months to 4 years are more frequently affected.

**HISTORY:** A 10-year-old girl after a motor vehicle crash, during which she was wearing only a lap seat belt (Figs. 8.5.1 and 8.5.2). Figures 8.5.3 to 8.5.5 are from a different patient with the same mechanism of injury

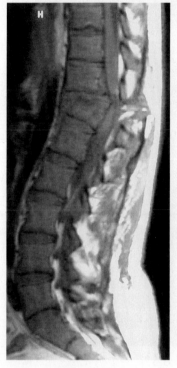

FIGURE 8.5.1

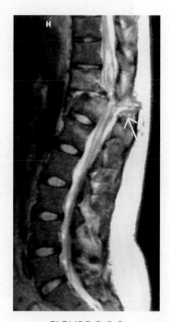

FIGURE 8.5.2

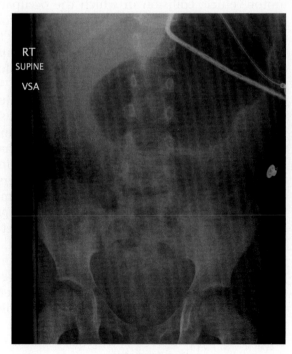

FIGURE 8.5.3

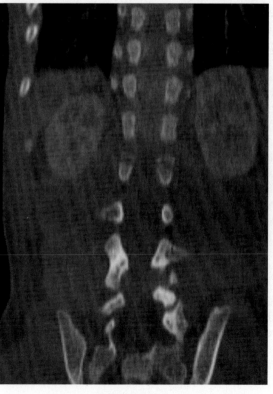

FIGURE 8.5.4

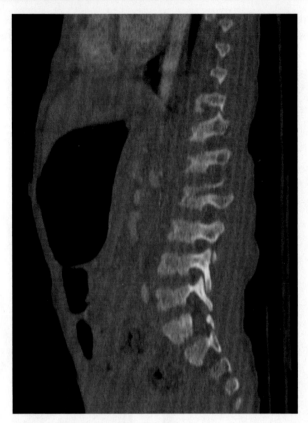

FIGURE 8.5.5

**FINDINGS:** Sagittal, T1-weighted (Fig. 8.5.1), and T2-weighted (Fig. 8.5.2) images show a fracture dislocation through the T12–L1 level. There is wedge compression deformity of L1 and displacement of bone fragments into the canal, resulting in compression of the spinal cord. The T2-weighted image shows edema of the involved vertebrae and of the cord. Notice the posterior extension (Fig. 8.5.2, *arrow*) of the fracture. A frontal radiograph of the lumbar spine (Fig. 8.5.3) in a different patient demonstrates a transverse fracture through the vertebral body and pedicles of L2. Coronal CT reformat (Fig. 8.5.4) in this patient demonstrates the same findings. The sagittal CT reformat (Fig. 8.5.5) shows the extension of the fracture line through the posterior elements, including the pedicles.

**DIAGNOSIS:** Chance-type fracture

**DISCUSSION:** The Chance fracture, or transverse spinal fracture, is created by forceful hyperflexion of the body against a rigid object some distance anterior to the spine acting as an axis of rotation. Hyperflexion creates a distraction force, resulting in a transverse fracture through the posterior elements and the vertebral body. Chance-type fractures generally occur in the setting of a head-on motor vehicle collision in which the occupant is wearing only a lap-type seat belt or as a consequence of horseback riding accidents. Chance fractures are part of the seat belt syndrome comprising spine injuries in combination with intra-abdominal injuries. In one series of Chance fractures, 44% of patients had substantial intra-abdominal injuries (39). In children presenting with the seat belt sign, 78% had intestinal injuries (40). If an abdominal wall contusion is present in the setting of a Chance fracture, one multicenter study (41) found intra-abdominal injury in 85% of patients. Conversely, they also found that the absence of an abdominal wall contusion was associated with a low chance of intra-abdominal injury (14%). Chance fractures usually involve the thoracolumbar junction, but these fractures can occur anywhere in the thoracic and lumbar spine (39,42). Chance fractures are unstable, but neurological injury occurs infrequently. In a series of 19 patients, 27.7% had neurologic findings (43).

Radiographic findings of Chance fractures can be subtle. Acutely, these fractures may be missed. Pedicles and spinous processes should be examined closely for a break in their cortex indicating fracture. In the lateral view, the fracture may be visualized. Extension of the fracture through the vertebral body may result in irregularity of the superior or inferior end plates. A widened space between the spinous processes with anterior angulation of the vertebral body is suspicious for a Chance fracture. CT findings may also be subtle. In a review of CT scans obtained during a 4-year period, it was found that lap belt–associated injuries of the lumbar spine were missed in five patients (44). Because these fractures occur along the transverse plane, they may be missed on CT scans acquired in the axial projection. Sagittal reconstructions may identify these fractures more clearly. MRI shows the fracture line to have high T2 signal, bone marrow edema, and in many cases, injury to the distal cord and the conus medullaris.

A spectrum of injuries owing to the flexion–distraction mechanism seen in the Chance fracture occurs, ranging from predominantly bony injury to only soft-tissue injury (disc and ligaments). Injuries with an injury pattern different from the classic Chance fracture are known as Chance-type or Chance equivalent fractures (45).

In children, Chance fracture equivalents involving the inferior or superior end plate also occur. The end plates act like physes and may be preferentially injured. In one series, two-thirds of cases involved the end plates, whereas only one-third demonstrated the classic fracture pattern (46).

## Aunt Minnie's Pearl

In any trauma patient with abdominal bruising from a seat belt, search carefully for lumbar spine fractures and intra-abdominal injuries.

# Case 8.6

**HISTORY:** Young patient with left upper-extremity weakness after a motorcycle accident

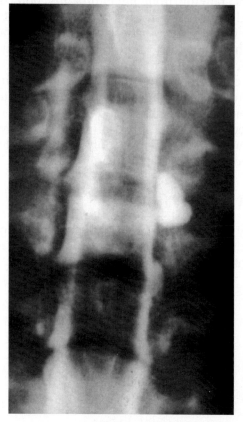

FIGURE 8.6.1

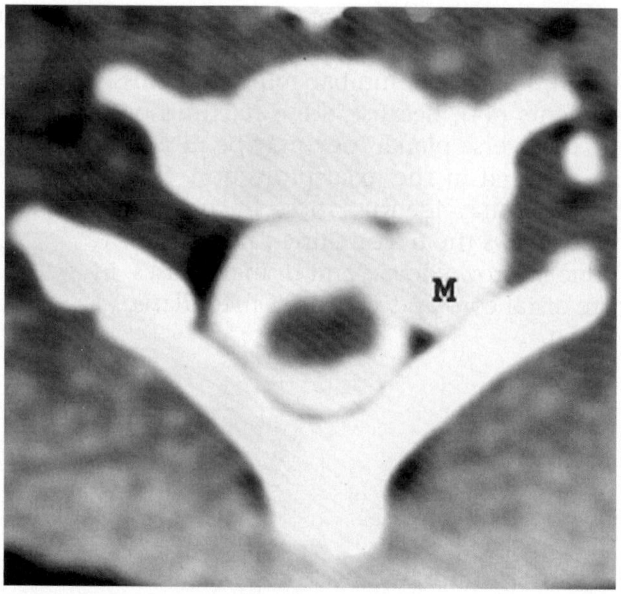

FIGURE 8.6.2

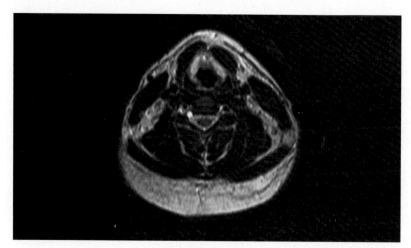

FIGURE 8.6.3

**FINDINGS:** Frontal view from a cervical myelogram (Fig. 8.6.1) shows a small, contrast-filled, abnormal structure in the lower cervical spine. The postmyelogram axial CT view (Fig. 8.6.2) confirms the presence of the lesion (*M*). In another patient with right upper-extremity weakness also after a motorcycle accident, an axial T2-weighted MR image (Fig. 8.6.3) shows absence of the right exiting nerve root with a cystic structure in its expected location.

**DIAGNOSIS:** Cervical pseudo-meningocele owing to traumatic nerve root avulsion

**DISCUSSION:** Nerve root avulsions result from severe traction on the exiting nerve roots. They are seen most commonly in the cervical spine in association with traction injuries of the arm but can occur in the lumbosacral region with lumbosacral or pelvic fractures. The typical appearance on myelography, CT myelography, or MRI is that of an absent exiting nerve root at the level of the neural foramen (47,48). The avulsed nerve root often retracts laterally, leaving a CSF-filled cavity or pseudomeningocele in the lateral aspect of the spinal canal extending into the neural foramen and occasionally extraforaminally into the surrounding paraspinous soft tissues. Although pseudo-meningoceles typically fill with contrast introduced into the subarachnoid space, they can occasionally become walled off and manifest as extradural cystic masses. The absence of pseudo-meningoceles on myelography or CT myelography therefore does not exclude an avulsed nerve root. A T2-weighted MR image can demonstrate all pseudo-meningoceles. In rare cases, pseudo-meningocele formation may be associated with spinal cord herniation (49–51). Although many nerve root avulsions occur in association with motor vehicle accidents, they also occur during birth from excessive traction on the shoulder (52). With complete nerve root avulsion, nerve regeneration is impossible. However, through recent advancements in surgical techniques, it is possible with microsurgery to reinnervate the brachial plexus by nerve transfer from other peripheral nerves (53).

## Aunt Minnie's Pearls

Severe traction injuries of the arm can lead to nerve root avulsion and pseudo-meningocele formation.

Traumatic avulsions of the cervical nerve roots are more common in newborns and in young men (who are more prone to motor vehicle accidents).

HISTORY: Two patients with cervical spine trauma after motor vehicle collision

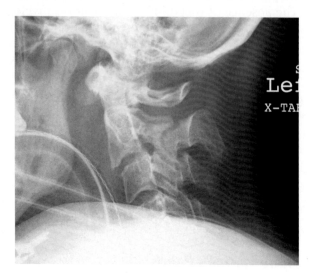

FIGURE 8.7.1

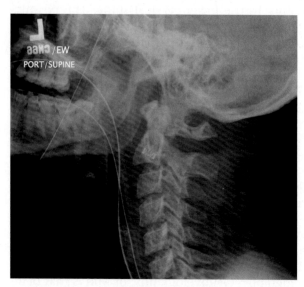

FIGURE 8.7.2

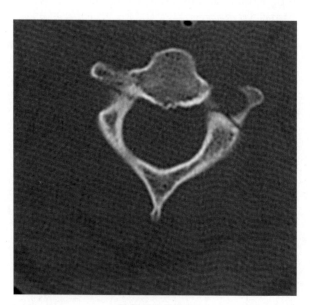

FIGURE 8.7.3

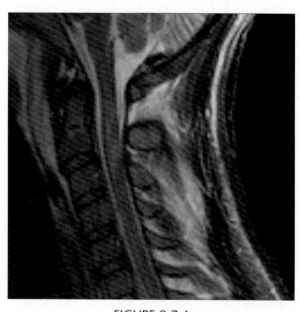

FIGURE 8.7.4

FINDINGS: A lateral radiograph of the cervical spine in one patient (Fig. 8.7.1) demonstrates a bilaminar fracture of the axis with 3-mm anterolisthesis of C2 on C3. In the other patient, lateral radiograph of the cervical spine (Fig. 8.7.2) demonstrates posterior angulation of C2 in relation to C3 with anterolisthesis of 2 mm of C2 on C3. In this same patient, an axial CT image (Fig. 8.7.3) demonstrates bilateral pedicle fractures with involvement of the left transverse foramen. A sagittal T2-weighted MR image

(Fig. 8.7.4) demonstrates edema of the spinal cord at the level of the body of C2.

DIAGNOSIS: Traumatic spondylolisthesis of the axis (hangman's fracture)

DISCUSSION: Traumatic spondylolisthesis of the axis (TSA) is a bilateral fracture of the posterior elements of the C2 vertebra that comprise the neural arch. The degree of instability of the injury is related to the degree of disruption of the anterior longitudinal ligament and the C2/C3 disc.

Termed a "hangman's fracture" by Schneider et al. (54), owing to the similarity of the fracture pattern seen in judicial hangings, the mechanism and expected injuries in TSA are quite different from that seen in judicial hangings. Today, motor vehicle accidents, falls, and diving accidents are the most common situations resulting in this type of injury. The most common mechanism is hyperextension with axial compression. Hyperflexion also plays a role, particularly in the more severe injuries. In contrast, the mechanism in judicial hangings using a submental knot is hyperextension with distraction.

A number of radiographic classification systems based on the lateral cervical spine radiograph have been developed to predict degree of instability. The presumption is that a nondisplaced fracture indicates that the anterior longitudinal ligament and disc are intact and that as displacement and angulation increase, the degree of disruption of these structures increases thereby leading to increasing instability. In the two most widely used systems, those of Effendi et al. (55) and Levine and Edwards (56), fractures are graded from 1 to 3 with grade 3 representing the most unstable injury. In both, a type 3 TSA indicates bilateral jumped facets. As positioning after trauma can artifactually reduce the grade of injury, clinical judgment should also be used to determine the degree of instability.

The role of imaging is to determine the type of injury and the presence of complications (57). The lateral cervical spine radiograph is usually sufficient to make the diagnosis of a TSA. The primary role of computed tomography is to evaluate for potential vertebral artery injury and to help identify additional fractures. MRI is used to identify or confirm injury to the spinal cord depending on the clinical situation. Occasionally, lateral flexion and extension radiographs may be of use in determining the stability of the fracture.

Treatment is based on the determination of stability as determined by the classification system in use and the clinical picture (58). Those fractures deemed stable are treated with external fixation: rigid collar or halo vest. Those fractures deemed unstable are treated with anterior cervical fusion.

### Aunt Minnie's Pearls

Traumatic spondylolisthesis of the axis is commonly the result of hyperextension injuries with axial compression. Flexion plays more of a role in severe injuries.

The mechanism in judicial hangings with a submental knot is hyperextension with distraction.

Potential complications include vertebral artery injury and spinal cord injury.

HISTORY: A 35-year-old man with a 3-month history of low back pain and saddle-like distribution anesthesia (Figs. 8.8.1 and 8.8.2). Figures 8.8.3 to 8.8.5 show an example of another subtype of this diagnosis. (Case courtesy of Dr. Aquilla Turk, III)

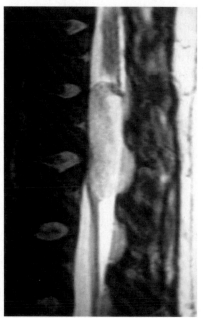

FIGURE 8.8.1

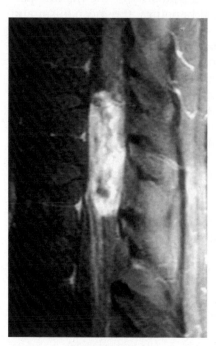

FIGURE 8.8.2

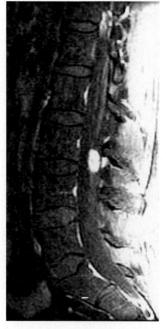

FIGURE 8.8.3

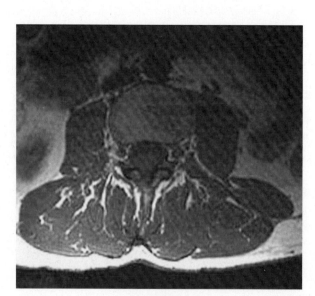

FIGURE 8.8.4

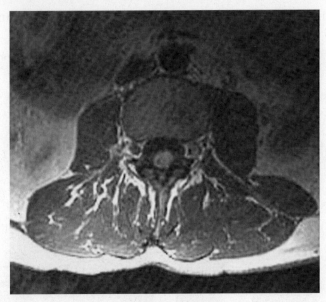

FIGURE 8.8.5

**FINDINGS:** Sagittal, T2-weighted (Fig. 8.8.1) and post-contrast, T1-weighted (Fig. 8.8.2) images show an enhancing mass in the region of the conus medullaris with some enhancement of the distal nerve roots. In a different patient, a sagittal T1-weighted post-contrast (Fig. 8.8.3) image shows an enhancing lesion within the distal cord also at the level of the conus medullaris. Axial T1-weighted pre-contrast (Fig. 8.8.4) and post-contrast (Fig. 8.8.5) images demonstrate this lesion to be intramedullary.

**DIAGNOSIS:** Spinal cord ependymoma, myxopapillary ependymoma

**DISCUSSION:** Ependymomas are the most common intramedullary tumors in adults, followed by astrocytomas and hemangioblastomas (59). In children, astrocytomas are more common than ependymomas (60). Ependymomas arise from ependymal cells lining the central spinal canal and usually cause symmetric expansion of the cord. Eighty percent of cord ependymomas have associated cysts (61). These are considered to be reactive cysts and are not lined by neoplastic cells but by gliosis. Sixty-seven percent of intramedullary ependymomas occur in the cervical region (62), with extension of the solid portion of the tumor for an average of four vertebral body segments (61,63,64). Unlike astrocytomas that demonstrate infiltrative pathology, ependymomas are generally well-circumscribed lesions, making surgical resection possible (65,66). The myxopapillary variant of ependymoma generally involves the filum terminale (65). Clinically, these patients present with nonspecific back pain or focal neurologic symptoms.

Ependymomas are isointense to hypointense on unenhanced, T1-weighted images and enhance after gadolinium administration (63,64). Sharply marginated enhancement is typical of ependymomas, and this correlates surgically with the margins of the tumor (61). Ependymomas can hemorrhage, and if bleeding occurs along the periphery of the tumor, a hypointense hemosiderin ring will be seen on T2-weighted images. Ependymomas may show blood-fluid levels in their cysts. It has been reported that cervical ependymomas are more likely to hemorrhage (63). Myxopapillary ependymomas have a typical sausage shape, are located in the proximal filum terminale, do not bleed, may extend into the nerve roots of the cauda equina or the conus medullaris, and show enhancement.

## Aunt Minnie's Pearls

A well-enhanced, sharply marginated, centrally located lesion, in the cervical spine in particular, is most likely an ependymoma.

A spinal cord tumor containing a rim of chronic blood products or intratumoral blood is most often an ependymoma.

A sausage-shaped, enhancing tumor in the filum terminale is nearly always an ependymoma. The differential diagnosis includes astrocytoma, paraganglioma, and metastasis.

**HISTORY:** A 26-year-old female presents with recurrent lower back pain, extending into bilateral thighs

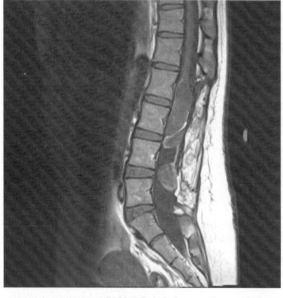

FIGURE 8.9.1

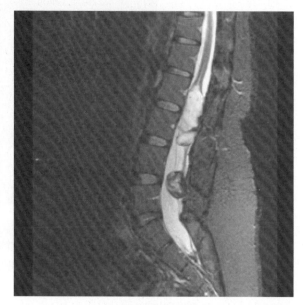

FIGURE 8.9.2

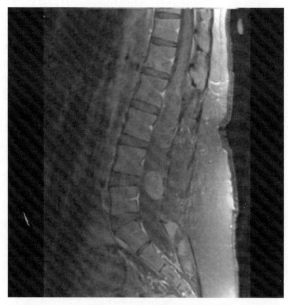

FIGURE 8.9.3

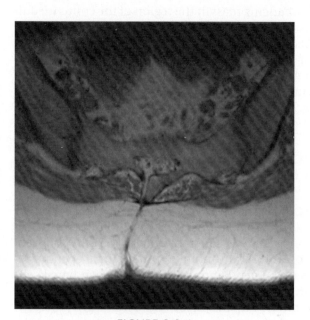

FIGURE 8.9.4

**FINDINGS:** Sagittal T1-weighted, T2-weighted, and contrast-enhanced images show two heterogeneous, low signal on T1-weighted images, predominantly high signal on T2-weighted images, enhancing intradural round lesions at the level of L4–L5 and the conus with a thin filum terminale connecting them (Figs. 8.9.1 to 8.9.3). Additional axial T2-weighted image of the sacrum (Fig. 8.9.4) demonstrates a subcutaneous dermal sinus tract.

**DIAGNOSIS:** Spinal dermoid

**DISCUSSION:** Spinal dermoids are rare, slow-growing dysontogenic tumors that arise from ectopic ectoderm and mesoderm embryonic rests inclusion within the spinal canal at the time of neural tube closure (third–fifth weeks of fetal life) (67). Accounting for approximately 1% to 2% of intraspinal tumors, they occur predominantly in the lumbosacral region (60%), followed by the thoracic region (10%)—usually residing in an intradural, extramedullary location (68,69). Approximately 20% of spinal dermoids are associated with a dermal sinus tract (67).

With a slight increased predominance in males, spinal dermoids are usually diagnosed between second and third decades (70). Symptoms result from the lesion's location, owing to its compressive effect on adjacent structures. The most common presenting symptom is lower back or sciatic pain. Spinal dermoids and tethered cord have been associated with progressive lower neurologic and bladder dysfunction—including postoperative cases of myelomeningocele repair (71). Excluding spina bifida repair, acquired dermoid cysts have also occurred with other procedures (e.g., spinal surgery or lumbar puncture)—likely a result from implantation of epidermal tissue into the subdural space. Rupture of these lesions may cause seizures, chemical (aseptic) meningitis, or arachnoiditis—owing to the spread of lipid droplets throughout the subarachnoid spaces (72).

The combination of fluid, fat, solid tissue, and calcium is diagnostic of a dermoid tumor (67,73). Based on its composition, these lesions have a heterogeneous appearance on MRI. High signal on T1-weighted images correlates with fatty secretions of sebaceous glands or cholesterol from degenerating epithelial cells. However, the intensity of the dermoid cystic components varies, usually hypointense on T1-weighted and iso- to hyperintense on T2-weighted sequences, relative to the spinal cord. Noncontrasted CT easily confirms the presence of fat and calcifications within the lesion. Fat-fluid levels are occasionally seen on CT. In addition to spina bifida, vertebral anomalies associated with spinal dermoids, radiographs may also demonstrate erosion (scalloping) of the posterior vertebral body walls and widened interpedicular widths (74).

There is presentation and imaging overlap between spinal epidermoids and dermoids. Neuroenteric or arachnoid cysts should also be considered in the differential; however, they are more easily differentiated from dermoids.

Surgery is the primary treatment modality, with good outcomes upon excision. Malignant transformation of spinal dermoids is extremely rare (75). Steroids may be beneficial for treatment of meningitis-type symptoms.

## Aunt Minnie's Pearls

Although rare, spinal dermoids should be considered in spina bifida patients or young adults with intraspinal masses.

CT and MRI imaging play complementary roles in its characterization, particularly MRI given its superior visualization of other spinal structures.

**HISTORY:** A 38-year-old man with progressive weakness of the legs

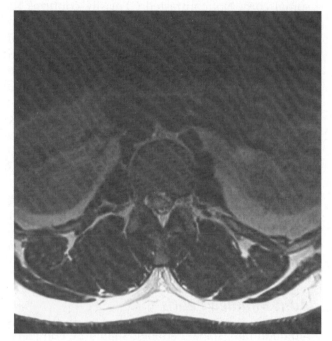

FIGURE 8.10.1

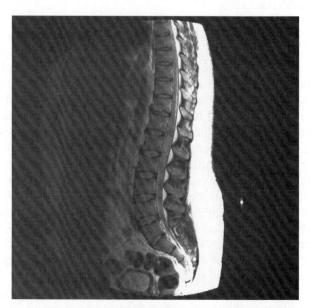

FIGURE 8.10.2

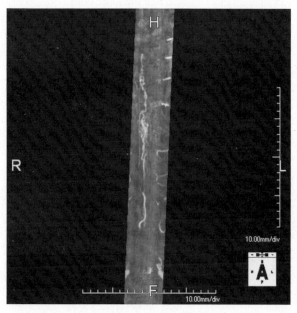

FIGURE 8.10.3

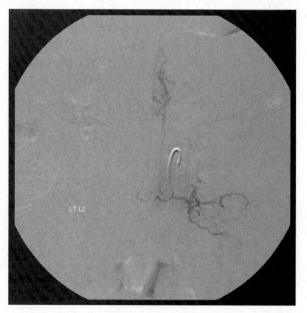

FIGURE 8.10.4

## Case 8.10 (Continued)

**FINDINGS:** Axial (Fig. 8.10.1) and sagittal T2-weighted (Fig. 8.10.2) images of the spine show abnormal increased T2-weighted signal associated with the conus medullaris consistent with venous congestion. In addition, there are multiple prominent intradural, extramedullary flow voids. A 3D reconstruction from MR angiography of the spine (Fig. 8.10.3) shows the anterior spinal artery arising at the L2 level and extends superiorly to the level of T12. The artery then feeds an arteriovenous malformation. Multiple irregular draining veins are also seen extending superiorly and inferiorly. These findings were confirmed at catheter angiography (Fig. 8.10.4) (Case courtesy of Dr. Vittoria Spampinato).

**DIAGNOSIS:** Spinal arteriovenous malformation

**DISCUSSION:** Vascular malformations of the spinal cord have been classified according to the anatomic location and characteristics of the malformation nidus (shunt). Intramedullary, pial, and mixed lesions occur. In one classification scheme, type 1 malformations are glomus-like, with a small, compact nidus and a few feeding vessels. Type II malformations are juvenile and have a larger nidus with multiple feeders from the anterior and posterior spinal arteries. Type III malformations, which can be seen in association with Cobb syndrome, are metameric, with an extensive lesion extending outside the cord and involving the meninges, epidural space, and the adjacent vertebral body. These lesions are congenital. A similar lesion is the dural arteriovenous fistula (dAVF) with a direct communication between arteries and draining veins and no intervening nidus. The dAVFs are the most common spinal vascular malformations, found in a slightly older patient population and are more likely acquired lesions (76,77).

Patients with spinal arteriovenous malformation (AVMs) present with progressive neurologic deficits. Acute deficits may occur after hemorrhage of the lesion, leading to hematomyelia or subarachnoid hemorrhage, which has a high mortality rate. Additional pathology includes venous congestion, mass effect, and "steal phenomena" (76). Spinal AVMs may also undergo spontaneous thrombosis. Myelography usually demonstrates enlarged, tortuous vessels on the surface of the spinal cord associated with these vascular malformations. On MRI, these vessels appear as serpentine flow voids (78). Abnormal cord signal occurs if there has been intramedullary hemorrhage or ischemia or infarction from chronic venous congestion resulting in edema. All symptomatic arteriovenous dural fistulas result in high-intensity T2 signal in the spinal cord. Although dynamic gadolinium-enhanced MRA has been shown to be useful in the evaluation of spinal AVMs (79–81), spinal arteriography remains the gold standard. Therapy comprises intravascular embolization and surgery (82,83).

## Aunt Minnie's Pearls

In the presence of hematomyelia, a spinal vascular malformation should be sought.

With AVFs, MRI shows high-intensity T2 signal in the cord and enlarged blood vessels (draining veins) on the surface of the cord.

With AVMs, MRI shows a nidus containing flow voids inside the cord.

HISTORY: Patient on long-term steroid therapy presenting with lower thoracic back pain

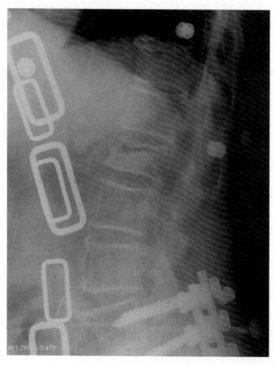

FIGURE 8.11.1

FINDINGS: The lateral radiograph (Fig. 8.11.1) shows a wedge compression fracture of L1. The vertebral body contains a gas-filled cleft.

DIAGNOSIS: Vertebral osteonecrosis (i.e., Kümmell disease)

DISCUSSION: Kümmell disease refers to osteonecrosis of a collapsed vertebral body. The most common cause of vertebral body osteonecrosis is posttraumatic, typically following an osteoporotic vertebral body compression fracture. However, other causes may lead to osteonecrosis first prior to vertebral body collapse, including neurologic, vasomotor, and nutritional deficiencies as well as administration of exogenous steroids.

Theoretically, an episode of trauma leads to ischemia and delayed vertebral body collapse. An association between vertebral body ischemia and the presence of gas (nitrogen) within the vertebral body, also known as an intravertebral vacuum cleft, is characteristic of this entity. A radiographic and histologic study of patient's undergoing kyphoplasty for vertebral compression fractures found that the intravertebral vacuum cleft has a sensitivity of 85% and a specificity of 99% for osteonecrosis (84). In an analysis of 1,272 patients, near equally divided among patients with osteoporotic vertebral fractures, spinal infections, spinal metastases, and multiple myeloma, Feng et al., demonstrated that the vacuum phenomenon was seen in 18.9% in patients with osteoporotic fractures, 6.4% in patients with multiple myeloma, and in only one patient with tuberculous spondylitis (85). With the exception of the patient with the spinal infection, the morphology of the vacuum phenomenon was that of a linear cleft. In the case of the infection, the intravertebral gas had a more bubble-like and diffused appearance. It is important to recognize the linear cleft of intravertebral gas because this finding effectively excludes metastatic disease or infectious involvement of the vertebral body (86,87). Radiographically, the cleft appears as a radiolucent transverse band in the centrum of the collapsed vertebra or adjacent to one of its end plates. The cleft may increase in size with spinal extension and be inhomogeneous on CT scans. On MRI, the intravertebral cleft appears as a linear signal void on T1-weighted and T2-weighted sequences. Prolonged positioning of the patient in a supine position during MRI may lead to displacement of the gas within the cleft by fluid, with high-intensity T2 signal appearing on delayed sequences. When seen centrally in the vertebrae, this change appears to be specific for osteonecrosis also (88).

## Aunt Minnie's Pearls

A linear cleft of gas seen in the centrum of a collapsed vertebral body is diagnostic of vertebral osteonecrosis.

The cleft of gas effectively excludes metastasis and infection, although, it is seldom seen in multiple myeloma.

HISTORY: A 71-year-old male presented with intermittent, yet worsening lower back and buttock pain. Physical examination demonstrated "fullness" in skin in the coccygeal region.

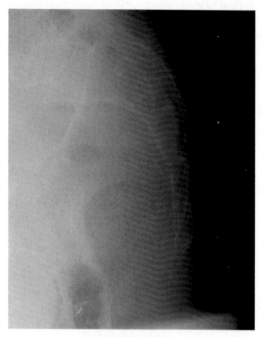

FIGURE 8.12.1

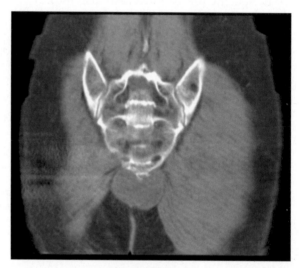

FIGURE 8.12.2

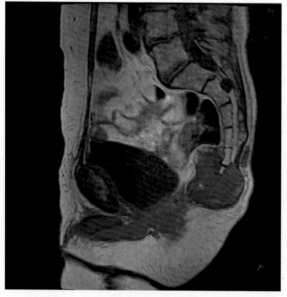

FIGURE 8.12.3

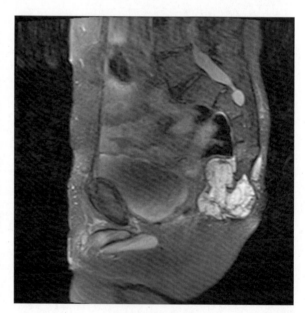

FIGURE 8.12.4

FINDINGS: Lateral lumbar radiograph (Fig. 8.12.1) shows ill-defined soft tissue opacity overlying the distal coccyx with tiny calcifications in it. A coronal CT image of the pelvis (Fig. 8.12.2) demonstrates a partially calcified soft-tissue mass slightly eroding into the adjacent coccygeal bone. Sagittal T1-weighted, T2-weighted, and contrast-enhanced images show predominantly low T1 and high T2 signal intensity heterogeneously enhancing lobulated mass encompassing the coccyx (Figs. 8.12.3 to 8.12.5).

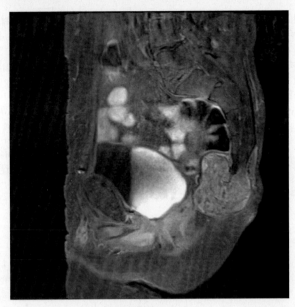

FIGURE 8.12.5

**DIAGNOSIS:** Sacrococcygeal chordoma

**DISCUSSION:** Chordomas are rare, accounting for ~2% to 4% of bone tumors and 20% of primary spine tumors (89,90). Arising from notochordal remnants, these slow-growing lesions develop along the axial skeleton—usually involving the sacrum and coccyx (50% of reported cases), skull base (35%), or mobile spine (15%, most commonly the C2 vertebral body) (2).

Rare in children, these lesions are typically diagnosed in the sacrococcygeal region between 40 and 60 years of age—presenting 10 to 20 years earlier in cases that involve the skull base. Chordomas are more common in males (2:1 ratio). Symptoms at the time of presentation greatly depend on tumor location. They usually present with back pain owing to bone destruction and compression of adjacent structures. Additional symptoms may include constipation, peri-rectal or lower extremity paresthesia, neurogenic bladder, or fecal incontinence.

Chordomas in the sacrococcygeal region classically present with lytic destruction of several sacral vertebrae, combined with a soft-tissue mass anterior to the sacrum. Surprisingly, the intervertebral discs and posterior elements are usually spared. The reported radiographic findings of bone expansion, rarefaction, calcification, and trabeculation associated with chordomas (91) are nonspecific and other entities—including chondrosarcoma, lymphoma, plasmacytoma, teratoma, and metastases—should be considered during diagnostic workup.

Radiographs consistently underestimate a tumor's soft-tissue component. Therefore, CT and MRI are recommended for better delineation of its extra-vertebral extent. On CT, chordomas appear as centrally located, well-circumscribed, expansive, enhancing soft-tissue masses with intratumoral calcifications or bone fragments (2). Up to 50% of chordoma have intratumoral calcifications (92).

Given potential extension into the epidural space or adjacent structures, MRI is frequently obtained owing to its greater soft tissue contrast properties. On MRI, sacrococcygeal chordomas are lobulated tumors, with low-to-intermediate T1-weighted and high T2-weighted signal intensity on pre-contrast sequences—exhibiting a heterogeneous honeycomb enhancement pattern on post-contrast T1-weighted images (2,92,93). Chordomas may demonstrate high T1-weighted intensity owing to high protein content. Blooming artifact on gradient echo sequences results from intralesional hemorrhage.

The primary treatment for chordoma is surgery. En-bloc surgical resection may be followed by radiation, in cases of incomplete removal. For nonsurgical candidates (with large invasive tumors), radiotherapy may suppress or slow down tumor growth. Despite slow growth, chordomas have a poor long-term prognosis, which varies depending on degree of resection (94,95). The overall median survival time is 7 to 9 years—less in patients with metastatic disease at time of diagnosis. The instances of metastatic disease range between 30% and 43% in the literature (96,97). The most common sites of metastatic disease are adjacent pelvic lymph nodes, the lungs, or bones—usually treated with either surgery or radiotherapy. Chemotherapy may have a beneficial role in these patients, based on active ongoing multicenter clinical trials (98).

## Aunt Minnie's Pearls

Consider chordomas for midline sacrococcygeal masses, particularly adults.

Although usually visualized on radiographs as a destructive lesion, CT and MRI imaging are essential for adequate evaluation of the soft tissue component.

Although slow growing, chordomas have a high recurrence rate and intermediate survival rate despite treatment.

**HISTORY:** Elderly Japanese man with progressive myelopathy (Figs. 8.13.1 and 8.13.2). Another case is illustrated in Figures 8.13.3 and 8.13.4.

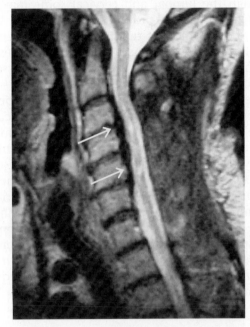

FIGURE 8.13.1

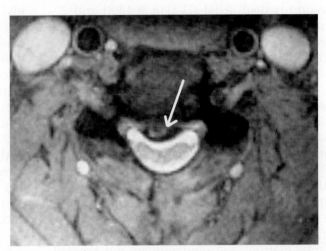

FIGURE 8.13.2

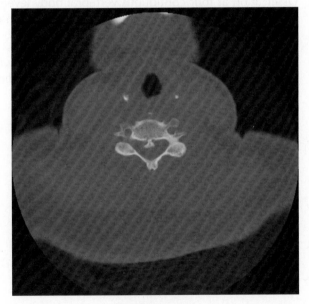

FIGURE 8.13.3

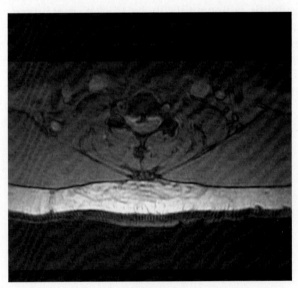

FIGURE 8.13.4

FINDINGS: A sagittal, T2-weighted (Fig. 8.13.1) image shows a thick, dark, linear structure (*arrows*) posterior to the C2–C6 vertebrae. This results in narrowing of the spinal canal and compression of the cord, which also contains abnormally high signal intensity. On an axial, T2-weighted image (Fig. 8.13.2), the thickened ligament (*arrow*) is seen narrowing the canal and compressing the cord. In the second patient, axial CT (Fig. 8.13.3) and T2-weighted (Fig. 8.13.4) images demonstrate a central ossified structure projecting posteriorly from the vertebral body resulting in effacement of the ventral thecal sac and flattening of the cord.

DIAGNOSIS: Ossification of the posterior longitudinal ligament in the setting of diffuse idiopathic skeletal hyperostosis (DISH) in the first patient and in isolation in the second patient

DISCUSSION: DISH, or Forestier disease, is a bone-forming diathesis (enthesopathy) affecting 10% to 20% of the elderly population. It is not considered an arthropathy because the articular cartilage, adjacent bone marrow, and synovium are not affected. Although DISH has been called senile ankylosing spondylitis, it has no association with HLA-B27 antigen and is easily differentiated from ankylosing spondylitis radiographically by thicker, more disorganized paravertebral excrescences; lucency between the excrescences and the vertebral bodies; and no involvement of the posterior elements (99,100).

The spine-related findings of DISH are normal mineralization, flowing ossification of the ligaments of at least four contiguous vertebral bodies, and preservation of the disc or joint space. The middle-to-lower thoracic spine is most commonly affected, although the lumbar and cervical spine may also be involved. Other prominent findings of DISH include ossification at tendinous and ligamentous insertions without intrinsic joint abnormalities and the absence of apophyseal joint ankylosis or sacro-iliac joint disease.

The posterior longitudinal ligament may be calcified or ossified. In Western countries, ossification of the posterior longitudinal ligament is commonly associated with DISH, whereas in Eastern countries, it may occur in an isolated form. The most common symptom is that of a myelopathy generally resulting from narrowing of the cervical canal to <10 mm in its anteroposterior dimension. Surgery is the mainstay of management for symptomatic disease. Disease spanning just one or two segments can be treated via an anterior approach with corpectomy, whereas longer segment disease requires decompressive laminectomy (101).

## Aunt Minnie's Pearls

Ossification at four contiguous vertebral body levels + preservation of the disc space + no ankylosis in an elderly patient = DISH.

DISH is a common disease found in patients with ossification of the cervical posterior longitudinal ligament.

## Case 8.14

**HISTORY:** A 32-year-old man with chronic low back pain and right footdrop (Figs. 8.14.1 and 8.14.2). Figure 8.14.3 is another patient with the same pathology.

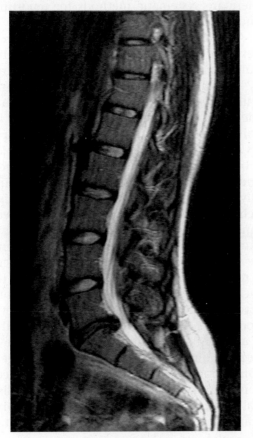

FIGURE 8.14.1

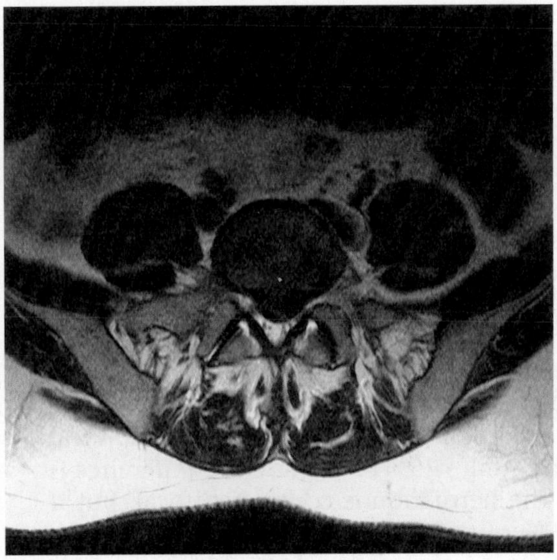

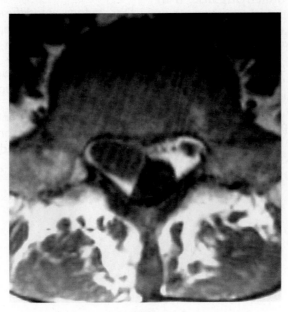

FIGURE 8.14.2

FIGURE 8.14.3

**FINDINGS:** A sagittal, T2-weighted image (Fig. 8.14.1) shows a dark epidural abnormality at the L5–S1 disc space that projects posteriorly and narrows the spinal canal. An axial, T2-weighted image (Fig. 8.14.2) of the same patient shows that the abnormality is contiguous with the disc. The degree of narrowing of the canal is better appreciated in this image. In a different patient with the same type of pathology, an axial, T1-weighted image (Fig. 8.14.3) shows a hypointense lesion in the right lateral recess of S1.

**DIAGNOSIS:** Central disc herniation (first patient) and sequestered herniated disc fragment (second patient)

**DISCUSSION:** Standard nomenclature for describing disc pathology was introduced in 2001 and should be used in imaging reports (102). Extension of disc material beyond the vertebral end plates for >50% of the disc circumference is defined as a bulge. A disc bulge is usually circumferential and symmetric but can be asymmetric as commonly seen in scoliosis. It may result from generalized relaxation of the annulus fibrosus and radial tears and is very common at the L5–S1 level. A localized extension of disc material beyond the limits of the intervertebral disc space is called disc herniation, which can be focal or broad-based. If <25% of the disc circumference is involved, the herniation is considered focal, but if 25% to 50% of the disc circumference is involved, the herniation is broad-based. A disc herniation may be considered a disc protrusion if it has a wide margin of attachment to the underlying disc. If in any plane, including the sagittal plane, the size of the disc fragment is wider than its base, then it is considered an extrusion. The location of the herniation is described as central, right or left central, foraminal, or extraforaminal. A herniation may become separated from the original disc, becoming a sequestration or free fragment. A free disc fragment extends through a tear in the posterior longitudinal ligament and may remain localized or migrate superiorly or inferiorly within the ventral epidural space. In addition to disc herniations, other degenerative changes of the spine include osteophytes, facet joint disease, and thickened ligamentum flavum. These can also result in compressive sequeale and there are systematic methods for reporting spinal and neuroforaminal stenosis (103).

An MRI study of 60 asymptomatic volunteers between the ages of 20 and 50 years found a disc bulge in 62% of subjects and a disc protrusion in 67% of subjects. Disc extrusions and free fragments with nerve root compression were found in 18% of the subjects and may be more predictive of low back pain (104). Similar findings were seen in a study of 98 asymptomic subjects: 52% of the subjects had a bulge at least one level, 27% had a protrusion, and 1% had an extrusion (105). Treatment is usually initially conservative; however, there is current debate in the literature concerning the adequacy of randomized, controlled trials in assessing the efficacy of treatment approaches (106). Failure to relieve symptoms or recurrent symptoms after surgery is referred to as failed back syndrome, and its causes include recurrent disc herniation, scar formation, arachnoiditis, and surgery at the wrong level. Postoperative MRI is usually equivocal initially, but it is useful in differentiating recurrent disc herniation from epidural scar 6 to 8 weeks after surgery. After contrast administration, peripheral enhancement is consistent with herniation because the disc material is not perfused; however, granulation tissue and scar demonstrate prominent enhancement.

## Aunt Minnie's Pearls

Disc bulges are diffuse and result in stenosis when accompanied by osteophytes, degenerative facet joint disease, and thickened ligamentum flavum.

Disc herniations are focal or broad-based, and many patients respond to conservative treatment.

Postoperative recurrent or residual disc herniations show no significant or peripheral contrast enhancement, whereas scar and granulation tissue show prominent enhancement.

## Case 8.15

**HISTORY:** A 40-year-old man with neck pain (Figs. 8.15.1 to 8.15.3). Two more patients with the same diagnosis, one with low back pain (Fig 8.15.4) and the other with cauda equina syndrome (Figs. 8.15.5 and 8.15.6).

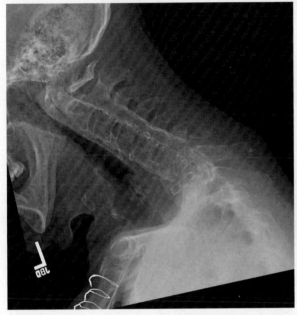

FIGURE 8.15.1

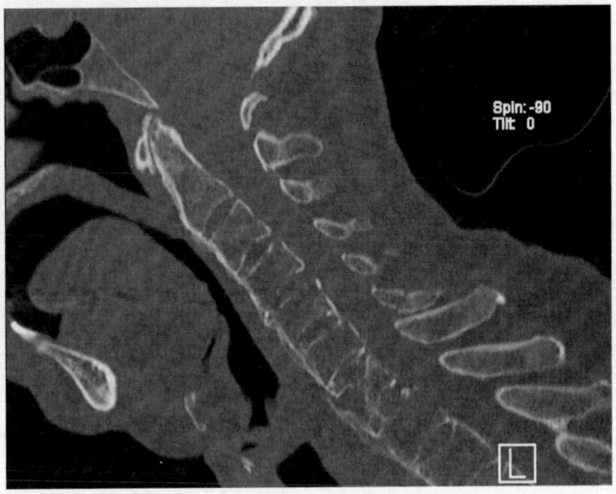

FIGURE 8.15.2

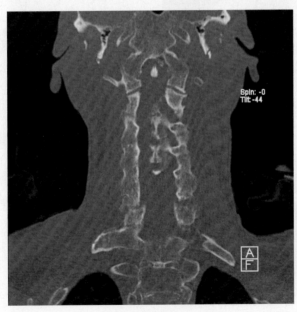

FIGURE 8.15.3

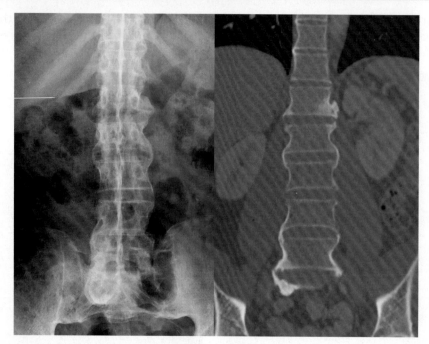

FIGURE 8.15.4

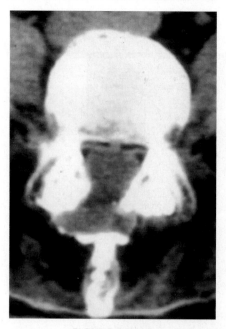

FIGURE 8.15.5

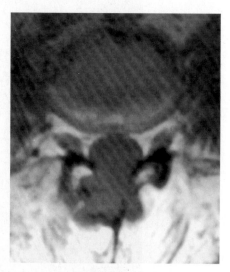

FIGURE 8.15.6

**FINDINGS:** Lateral cervical spine radiograph (Fig. 8.15.1) demonstrates delicate syndesmophytes bridging the cervical vertebral bodies and fusion of the facet joints. A fracture through the C6/C7 level is present. The sagittal CT reformat (Fig. 8.15.2) illustrates the gracile syndesmophytes anteriorly and a fracture through the C6 spinous process and the superior body of C7. The coronal CT reformat (Fig. 8.15.3) demonstrates the multilevel fusion of the facets and the fracture through the C6/C7 level. Frontal lumbar spine radiograph (Fig. 8.15.4, *left*) and select coronal reformat from an abdominal CT (Fig. 8.15.4, *right*) in the second patient demonstrate thin syndesmophytes spanning the lateral aspects of the lumbar vertebral bodies, best seen at the L2/L3 level. In the third patient, axial CT (Fig. 8.15.5) and T1-weighted MR images (Fig. 8.15.6) show CSF-filled diverticula eroding the posterior elements.

**DIAGNOSIS:** Ankylosing spondylitis

**DISCUSSION:** Ankylosing spondylitis is a seronegative spondyloarthropathy associated with HLA-B27. This entity affects men 3 to 10 times more often than women, with an age of onset between 15 and 35 years (107). Imaging findings include bilateral, symmetric sacroiliac joint erosions and sclerosis progressing to complete fusion late in the disease. Fine, marginal syndesmophytes (i.e., ossification of the outer fibers of the annulus fibrosus) ascend the spine, giving the appearance of a "bamboo" spine. Typically, spinal changes follow sacroiliac disease (107). Erosions occur at the corners of vertebral bodies, leading to "squared vertebral bodies." The presence of destructive changes at the superior and inferior portions of the vertebral bodies is known as a Romanus lesion and is an early sign of ankylosing spondylitis. The erosions later become sclerotic, giving the appearance of "shiny corners" (108).

The spine in ankylosing spondylitis patients is prone to injury. Minor stress or trauma may result in fractures through the intervertebral disc or through the vertebral bodies adjacent to the end plates and can extend through the posterior elements (109,110). Delayed identification and treatment of these fractures, with continued motion, leads to the formation of pseudoarthrosis at the fracture site. If the fracture occurs through the cervical spine, instability with cord compression may result, leading to severe neurologic complications.

A 10-year retrospective review of spinal cord injury in patient's with ankylosing spondylitis by Thumbikat et al. (111) noted that most of these patients were able to walk after the initial injury and then subsequently declined neurologically. In particular, overcorrection of the exaggerated kyphosis that develops in ankylosing spondylitis was identified as the cause of subsequent neurologic decline in 40%. In one patient, this occurred during positioning for an MR scan. Another cause for delayed neurologic decline was the presence of a spinal epidural hematoma.

In the setting of trauma, initial radiographs may be difficult to interpret or nondiagnostic owing to severe osteopenia and obscuration of the cervicothoracic junction. As a result, one can have a low threshold for performing CT (112) and possibly MRI.

Late in the disease, additional MR findings may include erosion of the posterior vertebral elements, dural diverticula, and arachnoiditis (i.e., nerve root clumping and cord tethering). A sterile discitis known as an Anderson lesion can occur. The cause of these late findings is unknown, but decreased elasticity of the meninges combined with ligamentous inflammation has been proposed as leading to chronic arachnoiditis and diverticula formation (113–115).

## Aunt Minnie's Pearls

Fine, confluent syndesmophytes are characteristic of ankylosing spondylitis.

In the setting of trauma, one can have a low threshold for CT and possible MRI of the spine.

Causes of subsequent neurological deterioration after the initial injury include iatrogenic overcorrection of the patient's normal hyperkyphosis (including positioning for imaging exams) and spinal epidural hematoma.

On MRI, chronic cases of ankylosing spondylitis can have prominent dural diverticula, clumping of nerve roots, and tethering of the spinal cord.

**HISTORY:** A 28-year-old male presented with neck pain, persisting after a recent motor vehicle collision. (This case courtesy of Dr. Mauricio Castillo)

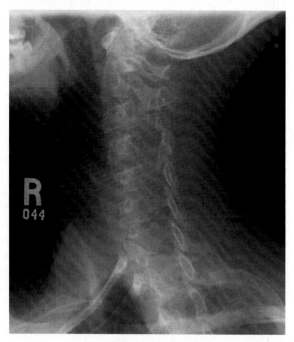

FIGURE 8.16.1

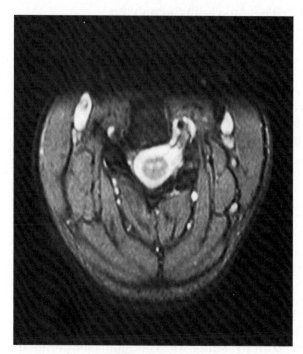

FIGURE 8.16.2

**FINDINGS:** Right posterior oblique cervical spine radiograph (Fig. 8.16.1) shows a widened left neural foramen and a nonvisualized left pedicle with well-corticated, smooth appearance of adjacent osseous structures. An axial T2-weighted image (Fig. 8.16.2) shows absence of the left pedicle, enlarged left neural foramen, and hypertrophy of the contralateral articulating facets.

**DIAGNOSIS:** Congenital absence of the pedicle (pedicle agenesis)

**DISCUSSION:** Absence of a cervical spine pedicle is a rare congenital anomaly (116,117) that results from early developmental failure in formation or subsequent ossification of a vertebral chondrification center during the fourth to eighth weeks of gestation. Recognition of this entity is important as misdiagnosis may result in unnecessary invasive interventions (116–118). In one study, 18% of patient with pedicle agenesis received inappropriate therapy (halo immobilization, surgical exploration, or radiation) owing to an initial misdiagnosis of trauma or neoplasm (117).

The most frequent region of pedicle agenesis is the cervical spine, followed by the lumbar and thoracic spine. The C6 vertebra is the most commonly reported cervical site, with L4 being the most site of occurrence in the lower spine (119). In symptomatic cases, presenting symptoms are usually neck pain radiating to the back and shoulders, or upper extremity sensory deficits.

Radiographic signs of pedicle agenesis on the AP radiograph include loss of the pedicle contour, apparent separation of the ipsilateral transverse process from the vertebral body, and deviation of the spinous process away from the affected side. On the oblique radiograph (Fig. 8.16.1), the left neuroforamen appears enlarged owing to the absent pedicle. The presence of compensatory hypertrophy and sclerosis of the contralateral pedicle supports a diagnosis of unilateral pedicle agenesis. Additional articular pillar dysplasia and spinal segmentation anomalies may also be present (117,118,120).

In cases of a radiographically nonvisualized unilateral pedicle, one should consider other benign (aneurysmal bone cyst, osteoblastoma, or osteoid osteoma) and malignant (metastases or myeloma) lesions. In cases of minimal compensatory hypertrophy in the contralateral pedicle, metastatic disease will often be the primary consideration until it is excluded with further workup. Additional considerations for an absent pedicle include erosion from a spinal canal or bone tumor, tortuous vessel, or extradural cyst (meningocele).

Despite pedicle agenesis, the spine is considered stable as the anterior column and ipsilateral posterior elements are intact. If there is uncertainty regarding the diagnosis of pedicle agenesis, computed tomography, with or without 3D reconstructions, should be performed. In cases of metastatic disease or primary neoplasm of bone, a nuclear bone scan will demonstrate intense uptake in the region of the interest (121,122). High radionuclide uptake on bone scan in the contralateral pedicle would be seen in pedicle agenesis, owing to stress hypertrophy (119).

Treatment of pedicle agenesis is conservative. Complications are rare, usually sequelae of nerve compression.

## Aunt Minnie's Pearls

Pedicle agenesis is a rare, congenital anomaly, which should be considered in the presence of contralateral compensatory pedicle hypertrophy.

Appropriate knowledge and awareness of such an anomaly can prevent inappropriate management.

**HISTORY:** A 2-month-old girl with a subcutaneous mass on her back

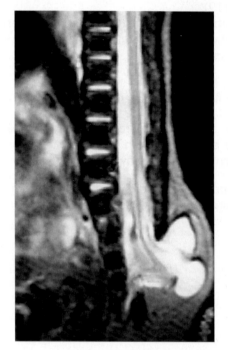

FIGURE 8.17.1

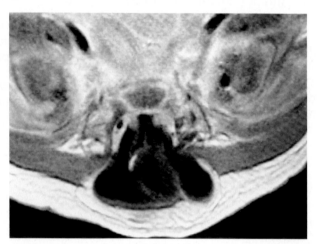

FIGURE 8.17.2

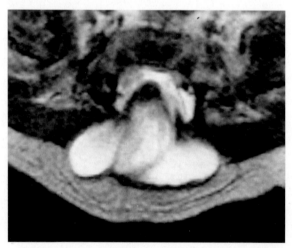

FIGURE 8.17.3

**FINDINGS:** A sagittal, T2-weighted image (Fig. 8.17.1); axial, T1-weighted image (Fig. 8.17.2); and axial, T2-weighted image (Fig. 8.17.3) show a fluid-filled meningocele at the posterior sacrum. The sac contains portions of unfolded spinal cord and nerve roots. The spinal cord is dysplastic and tethered. There is a posterior spinal bifida, and the mass is covered by subcutaneous fat.

**DIAGNOSIS:** Lipomyelomeningocele

**DISCUSSION:** Spinal dysraphisms can be divided into open and closed types, depending on whether neural tissue is exposed or covered by skin (123–125). For example, myelomeningoceles and myeloceles are open dysraphisms. Lipomyelomeningoceles and lipomyelocele are examples of closed spinal defects.

These probably arise from premature disjunction of the neuroectoderm from cutaneous ectoderm, with entrapped ectodermal elements differentiating into lipomatous tissue. Lipomyelomeningoceles account for 20% of skin-covered lumbosacral masses and up to one-half of occult spinal dysraphisms (126). The spinal cord is dorsally contiguous, with a lipomatous mass that extends to the subcutaneous tissues. Nerve roots do not course through the fatty mass, which is dorsal to the cord and extradural in location. In lipomyelomeningoceles, the dysplastic and unfolded spinal cord, called the placode, lies superficial to the level of the bony defect owing to expansion of the subarachnoid space ventrally (127). In a lipomyelocele, the placode lies inside of the spinal canal and therefore deep to the bony defect. A tethered cord is almost always present, and up to 25% of patients have associated hydrosyringomyelia (128). Skin tags or dimples, dermal sinuses, and other cutaneous defects are found in up to 50% of patients. Lipomyelomeningoceles should be differentiated from the less common intraspinal lipomas, because the clinical outcome after surgery is better for intraspinal lipomas (129,130). This disorder is not associated with the Chiari II malformation, a congenital hind brain malformation associated with open spinal defects.

## Aunt Minnie's Pearls

A lipomyelomeningocele is a closed spinal dysraphism in which the distal spinal cord is contiguous dorsally with a large fatty mass.

A tethered cord, hydrosyringomyelia, and cutaneous abnormalities are common findings associated with lipomyelomeningocele.

This lesion is not associated with the Chiari II malformation.

HISTORY: A 20-year-old woman with mild lower-extremity weakness

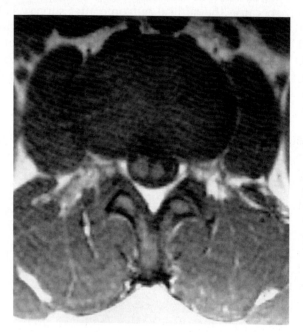

FIGURE 8.18.1

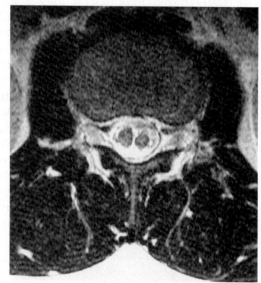

FIGURE 8.18.2

FINDINGS: Axial, T1-weighted (Fig. 8.18.1) and T2-weighted (Fig. 8.18.2) images show that the spinal cord is divided by a fluid-filled cleft. The left hemicord is smaller than the right one.

DIAGNOSIS: Diastematomyelia

DISCUSSION: Diastematomyelia is a closed dysraphism in which the spinal cord is divided into two hemicords by a sagittal cleft (131). This congenital anomaly most commonly occurs in the female population (80%–85%) and usually involves the low thoracic or upper lumbar regions (132). The term *split cord malformation* also applies to this spectrum of abnormalities, the outcome of which is determined by the fate of intervening primitive streak tissue (127). In one-half of the cases, each hemicord has its own dural sac i.e., type 1); in the other half, (i.e., type 2) the hemicords share a common dural sac (133). If the primitive streak tissue forms a bony or cartilaginous spur, the hemicords will be contained within two dural sacs. If a fibrous septum develops or the primitive streak tissue is resorbed, the hemicords will be contained within one dural sac (127). A fibrous or bony spur separating the two hemicords is present in 50% of cases and is multiple in about 6% of cases (134). Evaluation of the bony spur and associated bony abnormalities, including scoliosis and vertebral segmentation anomalies, is best accomplished with CT (135,136). MRI is useful in demonstrating associated spinal anomalies, including Chiari II malformation, tethered cord, and hydromyelia (which may be confined to one hemicord). Treatment is surgical, with removal of the bony spur, which may tether the cord.

## Aunt Minnie's Pearl

Diastematomyelia is a closed dysraphic state in which the spinal cord is divided into two hemicords by a sagittal cleft.

**HISTORY:** A 1-month-old girl with clubfeet and bladder incontinence

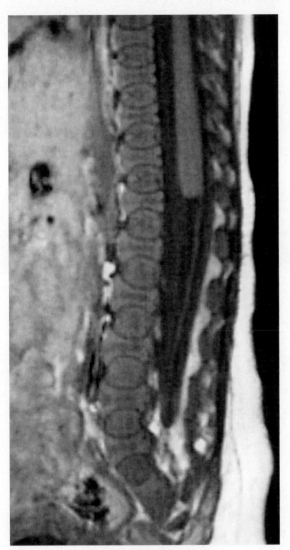

FIGURE 8.19.1

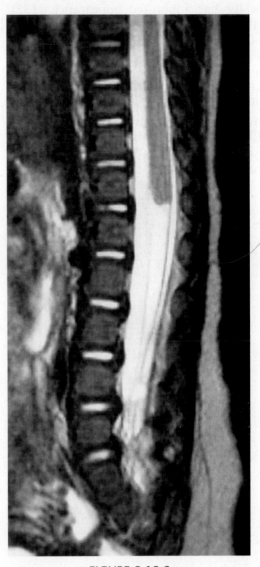

FIGURE 8.19.2

**FINDINGS:** Sagittal, T1-weighted (Fig. 8.19.1), and T2-weighted (Fig. 8.19.2) images show a conus medullaris that is truncated, a sparse cauda equina, and only one sacral vertebrum.

**DIAGNOSIS:** Caudal regression syndrome with partial sacral agenesis

**DISCUSSION:** The caudal regression syndrome is a congenital anomaly in which there is abnormal formation of the lower portion of the spine and spinal cord (60). There is a spectrum of abnormalities with various degrees of lumbosacral hypoplasia or aplasia, ranging from only partial malformation of the sacrum to fused lower extremities (i.e., sirenomelia or mermaid syndrome; 123–125). The caudal regression syndrome is frequently associated with abnormalities of the genitourinary system and with lower-extremity sensory and motor abnormalities. Caudal regression syndrome can be seen as part of other syndromic complexes such as VACTERL (vertebral abnormality, anal imperforation, cardiac malformation, tracheoesophageal fistula, renal abnormalities, limb abnormalities), OEIS association (omphalocele, exstrophy of the cloaca, imperforate anus, spinal anomalies), and the Currarino triad (partial sacral agenesis, anorectal malformation, and presacral mass) (127).

A high percentage of infants with this condition are born to diabetic mothers. The distal spinal cord typically has a blunted appearance (137). Occasionally, the cord is tethered at the level where the spine terminates, and a blunted (or truncated) conus medullaris is not seen. The cause of this condition is unknown but appears to be the result of some disturbance in the mechanism of retrogressive differentiation that is responsible for the formation of the conus medullaris and the cauda equine (138,139). Because the notochord, which is responsible for the formation of the distal spinal column, is affected, the distal spinal cord, the sacrum, and coccyx also fail to form normally. Motor impairment may occur, but sensation is usually relatively spared (140).

## Aunt Minnie's Pearls

In the presence of a truncated-appearing conus medullaris, always count the sacral segments (there should be five).

The caudal regression syndrome is rare, and many patients are the offspring of diabetic mothers.

**HISTORY:** A 59-year-old man with a known disorder and new right-sided weakness

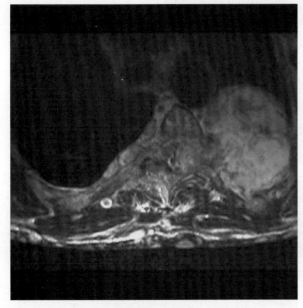

FIGURE 8.20.1

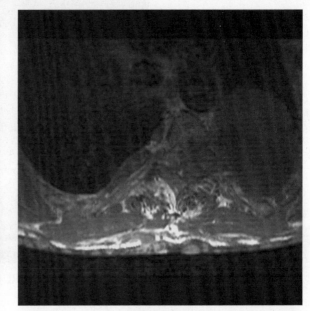

FIGURE 8.20.2

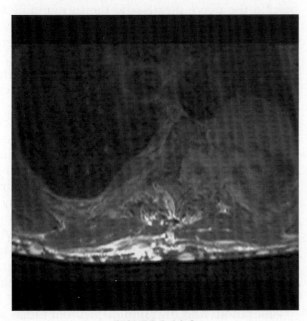

FIGURE 8.20.3

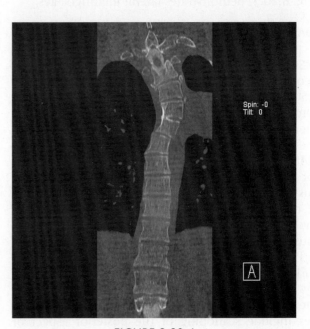

FIGURE 8.20.4

**FINDINGS:** Axial T2-weighted (Fig. 8.20.1), T1-weighted (Fig. 8.20.2), and T1-weighted post-contrast (Fig. 8.20.3) images demonstrate a large heterogeneous mass with both intraspinal and paraspinal extension widening the neural foramen and displacing the thoracic cord to the right. The mass demonstrates heterogeneous enhancement. Also noted are innumerable subcutaneous lesions. A sagittal reconstruction obtained as part of a CT myelogram (Fig. 8.20.4) demonstrates levoscoliosis of the thoracic spine as well as the mass seen on the axial MR images centered at the apex of the scoliotic

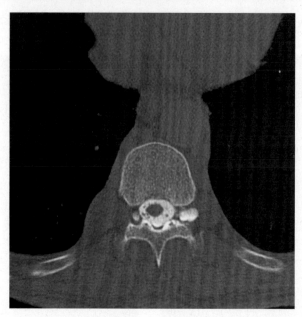

FIGURE 8.20.5

deformity. An axial image from the CT myelogram (Fig. 8.20.5) demonstrates lateral meningoceles.

**DIAGNOSIS:** Neurofibromatosis type 1 (NF1)

**DISCUSSION:** NF1 is the most common neurocutaneous syndrome, with an incidence of 1 in every 2,500 to 5,000 individuals (141–147). It is an autosomal dominant disorder caused by a mutation in the NF1 tumor suppressor gene located on chromosome 17, which codes for the protein neurofibromin (148). A list of clinical criteria has been established for the diagnosis of NF1, and including cutaneous lesions, nervous system tumors, Lisch nodules of the iris, osseous lesions, and a first-degree relative with the disorder. Two or more of these criteria must be met for the diagnosis (141).

Prominent spinal involvement can be seen in NF1 patients. The most common skeletal abnormality in NF1 is scoliosis most commonly involving the thoracic region. Other bony spinal abnormalities include scalloping of the posterior aspect of vertebral bodies, posterior element hypoplasia, and bony remodeling caused by compression from expanding soft-tissue tumors. Spinal tumors include neurofibromas (the characteristic lesion of NF1), schwannomas, and intrinsic spinal cord tumors. Neurofibromas can be localized, diffuse, or plexiform. Some consider plexiform neurofibromas pathognomonic of NF1 (143), which occur in ~50% of patients with NF1 (146). These benign tumors diffusely involve a long segment of a nerve and its branches in a tortuous manner and can extend beyond the nerve sheath into the surrounding tissues (143). The natural history of most tumors is slow growth, but degeneration into malignant nerve sheath tumors is the dreaded complication with a 7% to 13% lifetime risk in NF1 patients (146). Other spinal abnormalities seen in NF1 include dural ectasia and lateral meningoceles.

On plain-film, scoliosis, vertebral body scalloping, dysplastic posterior elements, widened interpedicular distances, and neuroforaminal enlargement can be seen (144). A "ribbon" deformity of the ribs can also be seen owing to multiple neurofibromas of intercostal nerves. CT imaging is useful in evaluating vertebral anomalies and bony changes associated with adjacent tumor growth. CT myelography may be helpful in assessing lateral meningoceles. MRI, however, is the optimal technique for evaluating the soft-tissue abnormalities of NF1.

Paraspinous and intraspinous neurofibromas are well visualized on MR. Although commonly asymptomatic in NF1, in the younger patients in particular, spinal neurofibromas can be seen at all segments of the spine at imaging (149). Spinal tumors in NF1 are primary intraforaminal extending into the canal but can also be intradural and seldom intramedullary (149). When small, tumors can be seen as nodules along the nerve roots of the cauda equina, but as they enlarge, they can widen the neural foramen and expand outside the canal in a "dumbbell" pattern (150). Tumors may also displace and compress the cord and cauda equina. On T1-weighted images, the tumors have signal intensity similar to muscle and they are hyperintense on T2-weighted images (143). Contrast enhancement is variable. Signs suggestive of malignant degeneration include new neurological symptoms associated with a lesion, increase in the size of a previously stable neurofibroma, and central necrosis with irregular peripheral enhancement (143).

## Aunt Minnie's Pearls

The majority of neurofibromas are solitary and not associated with NF1.

The majority of spinal nerve sheath tumors in NF1 are asymptomatic, particularly in children.

A previously stable lesion that becomes symptomatic or increases in size should raise suspicion for malignant degeneration.

# Case 8.21

**HISTORY:** Two young patients (Fig. 8.21.1 is one patient and Figs. 8.21.2 and 8.21.3 are another patient) with weakness in all extremities, but predominantly in the lower ones

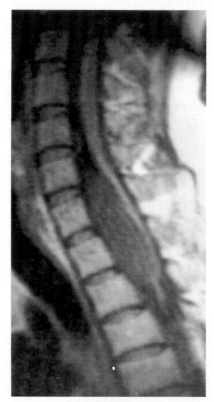

FIGURE 8.21.1

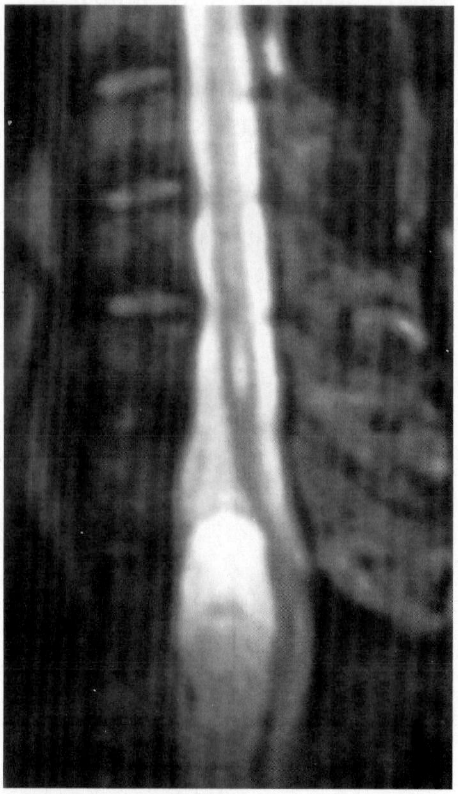

FIGURE 8.21.2

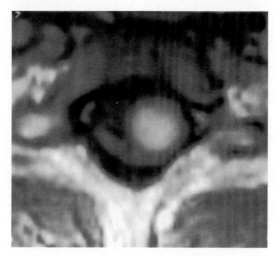

FIGURE 8.21.3

**FINDINGS:** A sagittal, T1-weighted image (Fig. 8.21.1) shows a low-intensity mass anterior to a compressed spinal cord at the C6–T2 levels. There is widening of the canal and scalloping of the posterior surface of the vertebral bodies in the region of the mass. In a different patient, a sagittal, T2-weighted image (Fig. 8.21.2) shows a hyperintense mass in the lower cervical spinal canal. The mass results in a wide canal and compression of the cord. There is fusion of the vertebral bodies anterior to the mass. An axial, T1-weighted image (Fig. 8.21.3) in the same patient shows that the mass is hyperintense.

**DIAGNOSIS:** Neurenteric cysts

**DISCUSSION:** About the third week of development, the amniotic cavity and the yolk sac are temporarily connected by the neurenteric canal that allows for transient contact of the endoderm with the neural ectoderm, which later forms the notochord. Incomplete separation of the notochord from the endoderm (precursor of the foregut) may result in formation of neurenteric cysts (151). These cysts are rare but have a fairly typical imaging appearance. Histologically, neurenteric cysts are derived from the gastrointestinal or respiratory tract. The cysts may be lined with mucus-secreting columnar epithelia resembling the lining of the gastrointestinal tract or pseudostratified ciliated epithelium resembling the respiratory tract lining (152). The cysts are usually found in the cervical or thoracic regions or in the posterior cranial fossa and are intradural, extramedullary masses. Neurenteric cysts may manifest at any time, depending on the severity of associated congenital malformations and the degree of compression of the spinal cord. In numerous cases, cyst decompression has provided dramatic resolution of symptoms such as paresthesias or paraplegia (151).

In 50% of cases, radiographs demonstrate vertebral anomalies such as fusion abnormalities or anterior or posterior spinal dysraphism (152). Other findings include widening of the spinal canal, diastematomyelia, and the Klippel–Feil anomaly. CT myelography generally demonstrates an intradural, extramedullary mass located in the ventral epidural space (153). MRI better delineates the contents of the cyst. Because of the high protein content of the cyst, T1 and T2 relaxation times are shortened. On T1-weighted sequences, neurenteric cysts demonstrate signal intensity higher than CSF. They are also bright on T2-weighted images (152,154).

## Aunt Minnie's Pearl

When vertebral body anomalies are seen along with cystic intraspinal masses, include neurenteric cysts in the differential diagnosis.

HISTORY: A 53-year-old woman on chronic steroid treatment with low back pain

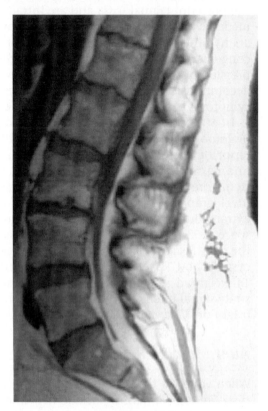

FIGURE 8.22.1

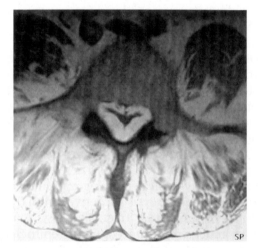

FIGURE 8.22.2

FINDINGS: Sagittal (Fig. 8.22.1) and axial (Fig. 8.22.2), T1-weighted images of the lumbar spine demonstrate circumferential, high signal–intensity tissue surrounding the distal thecal sac and compressing the nerve roots.

DIAGNOSIS: Epidural lipomatosis

DISCUSSION: Epidural lipomatosis comprises excessive accumulation of unencapsulated fatty tissue in the epidural space, generally in the thoracic or lumbar regions. Patients are usually on high-dose steroid therapy, are morbidly obese, or have endocrinopathies such as Cushing syndrome, although the disease may be idiopathic (155). The majority of patients with epidural lipomatosis are asymptomatic or have alternate explanations for their symptoms (156). For those who are symptomatic, the presenting symptom is usually chronic back pain; however, radiculopathies and myelopathy can occur (157). Treatment can be medical or surgical. Decreasing steroid dosages and instituting weight management have been effective for some patients (158). Decompressive surgery has also been

successful at alleviating symptoms (155,159–161). Epidural lipomatosis generally does not occur in the cervical region unless it were to exist elsewhere too in the spine (156,161). In the thoracic region, fat accumulates more dorsally, whereas in the lumbar region, fat accumulation is circumferential (161).

In a recent meta-analysis of all 104 cases (156), the distribution of epidural lipomatosis was dependent on the underlying etiology. In steroid-induced lipomatosis, 56% of patients demonstrated increased epidural fat only in their thoracic spine, 33% only in the lumbar spine, and 11% affecting both thoracic and lumbar spines. Lipomatosis in the setting of obesity, however, favored the lumbar spine in 70% and the thoracic spine in only 30%. In idiopathic cases, 50% of patients had their disease localized to the lumbar spine, 38% to the thoracic spine, and 12% affecting both the thoracic and lumbar spines. Furthermore, it was noted was that success of therapy was dependent on the underlying etiology. In steroid-induced lipomatosis, both decompressive surgery and medical therapy had a success rate of 77%. In obesity-related lipomatosis, treatment with weight management alone had improvement in symptoms in 82%. Decompressive surgery was successful in 67%. In the idiopathic group, decompressive surgery had a success rate of 94%. None in this group received conservative management.

On imaging, abnormal soft tissue, which follows the signal intensity characteristics of fat, is seen in the epidural space in the thoracic or lumbar regions. CT demonstrates fatty, low-density tissue filling the epidural space with impression on the thecal sac (160). This may extend for several vertebral levels. On MRI, the fat does not enhance, is homogeneous (a difference between normal fat and angiomyolipomas and angiolipomas), and decreases in signal intensity with the use of fat-suppression techniques. Furthermore, the normal width of the epidural fat is between 3 and 5 mm. More than 6 mm may be considered abnormal. However, there is only a loose link between the thickness of epidural fat and the presence of symptoms, as many asymptomatic people have an epidural fat thickness >6 mm (162). Extension of the fat into the neural foramina correlates with the presence of radiculopathy. In the distal lumbar spine, the lipomatosis surrounds the nerve roots.

## Aunt Minnie's Pearls

Epidural fat wider than 6 mm and extending for long segments is typical of epidural lipomatosis. Be sure to evaluate the spine for other causes of back pain as many individuals with an abnormal amount of epidural fat have alternate explanations for back pain.

Epidural lipomatosis is common dorsally in the thoracic region and circumferentially in the lumbar spine.

The signal intensity of epidural lipomatosis is nulled in fat-suppression sequences.

**HISTORY:** A 58-year-old female presents with lower back pain

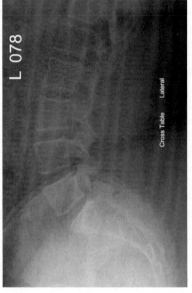

FIGURE 8.23.1

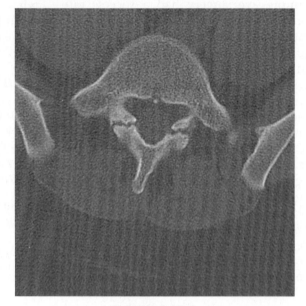

FIGURE 8.23.2

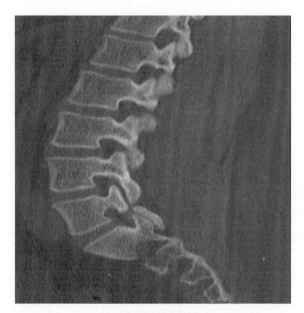

FIGURE 8.23.3

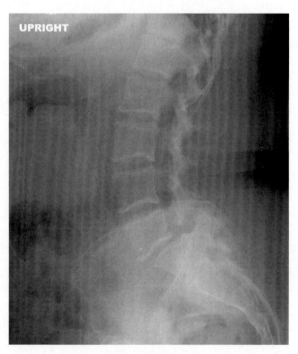

FIGURE 8.23.4

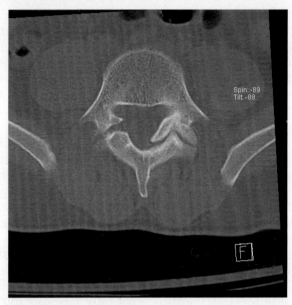

FIGURE 8.23.5

**FINDINGS:** Lateral radiograph (Fig. 8.23.1) and axial/sagittal CT images (Figs. 8.23.2 and 8.23.3) of the lumbar spine demonstrate a lucency through the L5 pars interarticularis bilaterally. In a second patient, a lateral radiograph (Fig. 8.23.4) demonstrates a grade 1 anterolisthesis of L5 on S1 owing to bilateral pars interarticularis defects. The axial CT image through the L5 pars interarticularis in a third patient (Fig. 8.23.5), demonstrates differing appearances of the two pars interarticularis defects.

**DIAGNOSIS:** Bilateral pars interarticularis defects (isthmic spondylolysis)

**DISCUSSION:** Isthmic spondylolysis is an osseous defect of the pars interarticularis, which represents the confluence of the pedicle, lamina, and articular facets. With a general population prevalence of 3% to 6%, spondylolysis is a relatively common condition (163–165). More common in males (2:1) and adolescents or young competitive athletes, it is frequently seen at the level of L5, followed by L4. Although unilateral cases have been reported, most patients have bilateral pars interarticularis defects (166).

Spondylolysis may be asymptomatic, discovered incidentally. When symptomatic, it usually presents with back pain or radiculopathy. Likely a combination of a congenitally dysplastic pars interarticularis and repetitive micro-trauma leading to a stress fracture, spondylolysis may progress to spondylolytic spondylolisthesis (167,168).

With spondylolysis, the posterior elements including the inferior articular processes separate from their anterior counterparts—the vertebra body, pedicle, transverse process, and superior articular processes. On imaging, spondylolysis may present as a hairline fracture, fibrous ankylosis, or a pseudoarthrosis.

Imaging is utilized to detect pars interarticularis defects, establish prognosis, and guide treatment. Radiographs are usually sufficient for the initial diagnosis of spondylolysis or spondylolisthesis. Easily visualized on a lateral radiograph of good quality, oblique projections demonstrate the classic linear lucency in the "neck" of the pars interarticularis—appearing like a lucent collar on the neck of the "Scottie dog."

Usually reserved for equivocal cases, surgical planning or posttreatment follow-up, CT with multiplanar reformatting is the most accurate imaging modality for pars interarticularis defect detection and healing assessment (169,170). Depending on slice thickness, the pars interarticularis defect may not be readily apparent on axial images. Therefore, the presence of other signs, specifically an enlarged vertebral canal or peri-articular process callus, can aid in diagnosis. Sagittal CT reconstructions can easily confirm pars interarticularis defects.

The appearance of pars interarticular defects may differ from side to side in people with bilateral spondylolysis. The degree of healing and stress response may differ leading to situations where one side has an overt defect and the contralateral side has a more sclerotic appearance (166).

Given suboptimal visualization of bones, MRI is reserved for patients, mainly children, with continued back pain yet no clear radiographic or CT findings of spondylolysis (165,170–172). STIR or T2-weighted fat-suppressed sequences are utilized, given their optimal visualization of bone edema. On sagittal images, wedging of the posterior vertebral body and displacement of the posterior elements is usually demonstrated, in patients with minimally subluxed spondylolysis or spondylolisthesis. Furthermore, MRI is superior in the assessment of the disc material, nerve root, and fibrous tissue in these patients. Hollenberg et al. have proposed a classification system for spondylolysis based on marrow signal and the appearance of the pars interarticularis cortical margin (173). Radionuclide bone scintigraphy has been used in the past but has lost favor owing to a relatively high degree of radiation exposure and lack of sensitivity and specificity (166).

Some clinicians would advocate the use of MRI as a secondary imaging modality (over CT), given its lack of ionizing radiation. However, the concomitant presence of degenerative changes in the adjacent facets may limit visualization of isthmic spondylolysis.

Based on work by Wiltse et al., spondylolisthesis is classified by etiology: isthmic (pars interarticularis defects), degenerative, traumatic (excludes pars interarticularis defects), pathologic, dysplastic, or iatrogenic (postsurgical) (174). Spondylolisthesis is also graded, based on the degree of the slippage of one vertebral body, relative to its caudal counterpart. Every 25% increment or fraction thereof of anterior displacement relative to the caudal vertebral body anteroposterior length represents an increase in the grade: grades 1 to 4.

Treatment depends on patient demographics and symptoms, chronicity of the findings, and degree of spondylolisthesis. With spondylolysis or mild spondylolisthesis, most cases are treated conservatively—usually a hard brace for a few months (165,175). In competitive athletes and patients with neurological symptoms or high-grade spondylolisthesis, surgical fusion may be required (176,177).

## Aunt Minnie's Pearls

Pars interarticularis osseous defects are common, present early in life, are usually bilateral, and may progress to spondylolisthesis.

Cross-sectional imaging, CT and/or MRI, may be necessary in equivocal, pediatric, or neurologically symptomatic cases.

Most cases can be treated with observation or brace immobilization, but surgical intervention may be required in severe cases or professional athletes.

# REFERENCES

1. Lucas DR, Unni KK, McLeod RA, et al. Osteoblastoma: Clinico-pathologic study of 306 cases. Hum Pathol 1994;25:117–134.
2. Llauger J, Palmer J, Amores S, et al. Primary tumors of the sacrum: Diagnostic imaging. AJR Am J Roentgenol 2000;174:417–424.
3. Martinez V, Sissons HA. Aneurysmal bone cyst. A review of 123 cases including primary lesions and those secondary to other bone pathology. Cancer 1988;61(11):2291–2304.
4. Bertoni F, Unni KK, McLeod RA, et al. Osteosarcoma resembling osteoblastoma. Cancer 1985;55:416–426.
5. Bertoni F, Bacchini P, Donati D, et al. Osteoblastoma-like osteosarcoma. The Rizzoli Institute experience. Mod Pathol 1993;6:707–716.
6. Berry M, Mankin H, Gebhardt M, et al. Osteoblastoma: A 30-year study of 99 cases. J Surg Oncol 2008;98:179–183.
7. Kroon HM, Schurmans J. Osteoblastoma: Clinical and radiologic findings in 98 new cases. Radiology 1990;175:783–790.
8. McLeod RA, Dahlin DC, Beabout JW. The spectrum of osteoblastoma. AJR Am J Roentgenol 1976;126:321–325.
9. Kan P, Schmidt MH. Osteoid osteoma and osteoblastoma of the spine. Neurosurg Clin N Am 2008;19:6570.
10. Boriani S, Amendola L, Bandiera S, et al. Staging and treatment of osteoblastoma in the mobile spine: A review of 51 cases. Eur Spine J 2012;21(10):2003–2010.
11. Camitta B, Wells R, Segura A, et al. Osteoblastoma response to chemotherapy. Cancer 1991;68:999–1003.
12. Berberoglu S, Oguz A, Aribal E, et al. Osteoblastoma response to radiotherapy and chemotherapy. Med Pediatr Oncol 1997;28:305–309.
13. Lindenbaum Y, Kissel JT, Mendell JR. Treatment approaches for Guillain–Barré syndrome and chronic inflammatory demyelinating polyradiculoneuropathy. Neurol Clin 2001;19:187–204.
14. Barohn RJ, Saperstein DS. Guillain–Barré syndrome and chronic inflammatory demyelinating polyneuropathy. Semin Neurol 1998;18:49–61.
15. Cosi V, Versino M. Guillain–Barré syndrome. Neurol Sci 2006;27:S47–S51.
16. Goetz CG, Pappert EJ. Textbook of clinical neurology, 1st ed. Philadelphia, PA: WB Saunders, 1999.
17. Byun WM, Park WK, Park BH, et al. Guillain–Barré syndrome: MRI findings of the spine in eight patients. Radiology 1998;208:137–141.
18. Crino PB, Zimmerman R, Laskowitz D, et al. Magnetic resonance imaging of the cauda equina in Guillain–Barré syndrome. Neurology 1994;44:1334–1336.
19. Iwata F, Utsumi Y. MRI in Guillain–Barré syndrome. Pediatr Radiol 1997;27:36–38.
20. Perry JR, Fung A, Poon P, et al. Magnetic resonance imaging of nerve root inflammation in the Guillain–Barré syndrome. Neuroradiology 1994;36:139–140.
21. Georgy BA, Chong B, Chamberlain M, et al. MR of the spine in Guillain–Barré syndrome. AJNR Am J Neuroradiol 1994;15:300–301.
22. Morgan GW, Barohn RJ, Bazan C III, et al. Nerve root enhancement with MRI in inflammatory demyelinating polyradiculoneuropathy. Neurology 1993;43(pt 1):618–620.
23. Patel H, Garg BP, Edwards MK. MRI of Guillain–Barré syndrome. J Comput Assist Tomogr 1993;17:651–652.
24. Moon MS. Tuberculosis of the spine. Controversies and a new challenge. Spine 1997;22:1791–1797.
25. Moore SL, Rafii M. Imaging of musculoskeletal and spinal tuberculosis. Radiol Clin North Am 2001;39:329–342.
26. Shanley DJ. Tuberculosis of the spine: Imaging features. AJR Am J Roentgenol 1995;164:659–664.
27. Weaver P, Lifeso RM. The radiological diagnosis of tuberculosis of the adult spine. Skeletal Radiol 1984;12:178–186.
28. Abdelwahab IF, Camins MB, Hermann G, et al. Vertebral arch or posterior spinal tuberculosis. Skeletal Radiol 1997;26:737–740.
29. Sharif HS. Role of MRI in the management of spinal infections. AJR Am J Roentgenol 1992;158:1333–1345.
30. Kamara E, Mehta S, Brust JCM, et al. Effect of delayed diagnosis on severity of Pott's disease. Int Orthop 2012;36:245–254.
31. Luk KDK. Commentary: Instrumentation in the treatment of spinal tuberculosis, anterior or posterior? Spine J 2011;11:726–733.
32. Friedman JA, Maher CO, Quast LM, et al. Spontaneous disc space infections in adults. Surg Neurol 2002;57:81–86.
33. Fernandez M, Carrol CL, Baker CJ. Discitis and vertebral osteomyelitis in children: An 18-year review. Pediatrics 2000;105:1299–1304.
34. Kothari NA, Pelchovitz DJ, Meyer JS. Imaging of musculoskeletal infections. Radiol Clin North Am 2001;39:653–671.
35. Afshani E, Kuhn JP. Common causes of low back pain in children. Radiographics 1991;11:269–291.
36. Ziessman HA, O'Malley JP, Thrall JH. Nuclear medicine: The requisites, 2nd ed. Philadelphia, PA: Elsevier Mosby, 2006.
37. Prandini N, Lazzeri E, Rossi B, et al. Nuclear medicine imaging of bone infections. Nucl Med Comm 2006;27:633–644.
38. Gouliouris T, Aliyu SH, Brown NM. Spondylodiscitis: Update on diagnosis and management. J Antimicrob Chemother 2010;65(suppl 3):iii11–iii24.
39. Gumley G, Taylor TK, Ryan MD. Distraction fractures of the lumbar spine. J Bone Joint Surg Br 1982;64:520–525.
40. Vandersluis R. The seatbelt syndrome. J Can Med Assoc 1987;137:1023–1024.
41. Tyroch AH, McGuire AL, McLean SF, et al. The association between Chance fractures and intra-abdominal injuries revisited: A multicenter review. Am Surg 2005;71(5):434–438.
42. Bernstein MP, Mirvis SE, Shanmuganathan K. Chance-type fractures of the thoracolumbar spine: Imaging analysis in 53 patients. AJR Am J Roentgenol 2006;187:859–868.
43. Gertzbein SD, Court-Brown CM. Flexion–distraction injuries of the lumbar spine. Mechanisms of injury and classification. Clin Orthop Relat Res 1988;227:52–60.
44. Taylor GA, Eggli KD. Lap-belt injuries of the lumbar spine in children: A pitfall in CT diagnosis. AJR Am J Roentgenol 1988;150:1355–1358.
45. Groves CJ, Cassar-Pullicino VN, Tins BJ, et al. Chance-type flexion–distraction injuries in the thoracolumbar spine: MR imaging characteristics. Radiology 2005;236:601–608.
46. De Gauzy JS, Jouve J-L, Violas P, et al. Classification of Chance fracture in children using magnetic resonance imaging. Spine 2007;32(2):E89–E92.
47. Hashimoto T, Mitomo M, Hirabuki N, et al. Nerve root avulsion of birth palsy: Comparison of myelography with CT myelography and somatosensory evoked potential. Radiology 1991;178:841–845.
48. Pétras A, Sobel DF, Mani JR, et al. CT myelography in cervical nerve root avulsion. J Comput Assist Tomogr 1985;9:275–279.
49. DaSilva VR, Al-Gahtany M, Midha R, et al. Upper thoracic spinal cord herniation after traumatic nerve root avulsion. Case report and review of the literature. J Neurosurg 2003;99(suppl 3):306–309.
50. Tanaka M, Ikuma H, Nakanishi K, et al. Spinal cord herniation into pseudomeningocele after traumatic nerve root avulsion: Case report and review of the literature. Eur Spine J 2007;17(suppl 2):263–266.
51. Yokota H, Yokoyama K, Noguchi H, et al. Spinal cord herniation into associated pseudomeningocele after brachial plexus avulsion injury: Case report. Neurosurgery 2007;60(1):E205; discussion E205.
52. Miller SF, Glasier CM, Griebel ML, et al. Brachial plexopathy in infants after traumatic delivery: Evaluation with MRI. Radiology 1993;189:481–484.

53. Walker AT, Chaloupka JC, de Lotbiniere AC, et al. Detection of nerve rootlet avulsion on CT myelography in patients with birth palsy and brachial plexus injury after trauma. AJR Am J Roentgenol 1996;167:1283–1287.

54. Schneider RC, Livingston KE, Cave AJE, et al. "Hangman's fracture" of the cervical spine. J Neurosurg 1965;22:141–154.

55. Effendi B, Roy D, Cornish B, et al. Fracture of the ring of the axis: A classification based on the analysis of 131 cases. J Bone Joint Surg 1981;63B:319–327.

56. Levine AM, Edwards CC. The management of traumatic spondylolisthesis of the axis. J Bone Joint Surg Am 1985;67A:217–226.

57. Mirvis SE, Young JWR, Lim C, et al. Hangman's fracture: Radiologic assessment in 27 cases. Radiology 1987;163:713–717.

58. Li X, Dai L, Lu H, et al. A systematic review of the management of hangman's fractures. Eur Spine J 2006;15:257–269.

59. Masaryk TJ. Neoplastic disease of the spine. Radiol Clin North Am 1991;29:829–845.

60. Barkovich AJ. Pediatric neuroimaging, 3rd ed. Philadelphia, PA: Lippincott Williams & Wilkins, 2000.

61. Patel U, Pinto RS, Miller DC, et al. MR of spinal cord ganglioglioma. AJNR Am J Neuroradiol 1998;19:879–887.

62. Koeller KK, Rosenblum RS, Morrison AL. Neoplasms of the spinal cord and filum terminale: Radiologic–pathologic correlation. Radiographics 2000;20:1721–1749.

63. Fine MJ, Kricheff II, Freed D, Epstein FJ. Spinal cord ependymomas: MRI features. Radiology 1995;197:655–658.

64. Miyazawa N, Hida K, Iwasaki Y, et al. MRI at 1.5 T of intramedullary ependymoma and classification of pattern of contrast enhancement. Neuroradiology 2000;42:828–8232.

65. Burger PC, Scheithauer BW. Tumors of the central nervous system: Atlas of tumor pathology. Washington, DC: Armed Forces Institute of Pathology, 1994.

66. McCormick PC, Torres R, Post KD, et al. Intramedullary ependymoma of the spinal cord. J Neurosurg 1990;72:523–532.

67. McAdams HP, Erasmus JJ. Mediastinum. In: Haaga JR, Lanzieri CF, and Gilkeson RC (eds.). CT and MR imaging of the whole body, vol. 1, 4th ed. Philadelphia, PA: Mosby, 2003:959–960.

68. Lunardi P, Missori P, Gagliardi FM, et al. Long-term results of the surgical treatment of spinal dermoid and epidermoid tumors. Neurosurgery 1989;25:860–864.

69. Graham DV, Tampieri D, Villemure JG. Intramedullary dermoid tumor diagnosed with the assistance of magnetic resonance imaging. Neurosurgery 1988;23:765–777.

70. Hagga JR, Lanzieri CF, Gilkeson RG, et al. Pediatric head and neck imaging. In: Egelhoff JC (ed.). CT and MR imaging of the whole body, vol 1, 4th ed. St. Louis, MO: Mosby-Elsevier Science, 2003.

71. Scott RM, Wolpert SM, Bartoshesky LE, et al. Dermoid tumors occurring at the site of previous myelomeningocele repair. J Neurosurg 1986;65:779–783.

72. Cha JG, Paik SH, Park JS, et al. Ruptured spinal dermoid cyst with disseminated intracranial fat droplets. Br J Radiol 2006;79:167–169.

73. Do-Dai DD, Brooks MK, Goldkamp A, et al. Magnetic resonance imaging of intramedullary spinal cord lesions: A pictorial review. Curr Probl Diagn Radiol 2010;39:160–185.

74. Wakely SL. The posterior vertebral scalloping sign. Radiology 2006;239:607–609.

75. Kudo N, Hasegawa K, Ogose A, et al. Malignant transformation of a lumbar intradural dermoid cyst. J Orthop Sci 2007;12:300–302.

76. Krings T, Thron AK, Geibprasert S, et al. Endovascular management of spinal vascular malformations. Neurosurg Rev 2010; 33:1–9.

77. Thron A. Spinal dural arteriovenous fistulas. Radiologe 2001; 41:955–960.

78. Osborn AG. Diagnostic neuroradiology, 1st ed. St. Louis, MO: Mosby, 1994.

79. Pui MH. Gadolinium-enhanced MR angiography of spinal arteriovenous malformation. Clin Imaging 2004;28(1):28–32.

80. Ali S, Cashen TA, Carroll TJ, et al. Time-resolved spinal MR angiography: Initial clinical experience in the evaluation of spinal arteriovenous shunts. AJNR Am J Neuroradiol 2007;28(9):806–810.

81. Mull M, Nijenhuis RJ, Backes WH, et al. Value and limitations of contrast-enhanced MR angiography in spinal arteriovenous malformations and dural arteriovenous fistulas. AJNR Am J Neuroradiol 2007;28(7):1249–1258.

82. Guimaraens L, Arbelaez A, Sola-Martinez T, et al. Image-guided interventions in the spine and spinal cord. In: Castillo M (ed.). Spinal imaging. Philadelphia, PA: Hanley & Belfus, 2001:169–185.

83. Nichols DA, Rufenacht DA, Jack DR Jr, et al. Embolization of spinal dural arteriovenous fistula with polyvinyl alcohol particles: Experience in 14 patients. AJNR Am J Neuroradiol 1992;13:933–940.

84. Libicher M, Appelt A, Berger I, et al. The intravertebral vacuum phenomenon as specific sign of osteonecrosis in vertebral compression fractures: Results from a radiological and histological study. Eur Radiol 2007;17:2248–2252.

85. Feng S-W, Chang M-C, Wu H-T, et al. Are intravertebral vacuum phenomena benign lesions? Eur Spine J 2011;20:1341–1348.

86. Bhalla S, Reinus WR. The linear intravertebral vacuum: A sign of benign vertebral collapse. AJR Am J Roentgenol 1998;170:1563–1569.

87. Brower AC, Downey EF Jr. Kümmell disease: Report of a case with serial radiographs. Radiology 1981;141:363–364.

88. Malghem J, Maldague B, Labaisse MA, et al. Intravertebral vacuum cleft: Changes in content after supine positioning. Radiology 1993;187:483–487.

89. McMaster ML, Goldstein AM, Bromley CM, et al. Chordoma: Incidence and survival patterns in the United States, 1973-1995. Cancer Causes Control 2001;12(1):1–11.

90. Kelley SP, Ashford RU, Rao AS, et al. Primary bone tumours of the spine: A 42-year survey from the Leeds Regional Bone Tumour Registry. Eur Spine J 2007;16(3):405–409.

91. Cable DC, Moir C. Pediatric sacrococcygeal chordomas: A rare tumor to be differentiated from sacrococcygeal teratoma. J Pediatr Surg 1997;32:759–761.

92. Maclean FM, Soo MY, Ng T. Chordoma: Radiological–pathological correlation. Australas Radiol 2005;49:261–268.

93. Sung MS, Lee GK, Kang HS, et al. Sacrococcygeal chordoma: MR imaging in 30 patients. Skeletal Radiol 2005;34:87–94.

94. Chugh R, Tawbi H, Lucas DR, et al. Chordoma: The nonsarcoma primary bone tumor. Oncologist 2007;12:1344–1350.

95. Park L, Delaney TF, Liebsch NJ, et al. Sacral chordomas: Impact of high-dose proton/photon-beam radiation therapy combined with or without surgery for primary versus recurrent tumor. Int J Radiat Oncol Biol Phys 2006;65:1514–1521.

96. Chambers PW, Schwinn CP. Chordoma. A clinicopathologic study of metastasis. Am J Clin Pathol 1979;72:765–776.

97. Higinbotham NL, Phillips RF, Farr HW, et al. Chordoma. Thirty-five-year study at Memorial Hospital. Cancer 1967; 20:1841–1850.

98. Casali PG, Stacchiotti S, Sangalli C, et al. Chordoma. Curr Opin Oncol 2007;19:367–370.

99. Brower AC. Arthritis in black and white, 2nd ed. Philadelphia, PA: WB Saunders, 1996.

100. Sartoris DJ. Musculoskeletal imaging: The requisites, 1st ed. St. Louis, MO: Mosby, 1996.

101. Mizuno J, Nakagawa H. Ossified posterior longitudinal ligament: Management strategies and outcomes. Spine J 2006; 6(suppl):282–288.

102. Fardon DF, Milette PC. Combined Task Forces of the North American Spine Society, American Society of Nomenclature and Classification of Lumbar Disc Pathology. Recommendations of the Combined Task Forces of the North American Spine Society, American Society of Spine Radiology, and American Society of Neuroradiology. Spine 2001;26:E93–E113.

103. Renfrew D. Atlas of spine imaging. Philadelphia, PA: WB Saunders, 2003.

104. Weishaupt D, Zanetti M, Hodler J, et al. MRI of the lumbar spine: Prevalence of intervertebral disk extrusion and sequestration, nerve root compression, end plate abnormalities, and osteoarthritis of the facet joints in asymptomatic volunteers. Radiology 1998;209:661–666.

105. Jensen MC, Brant-Zawadzki MN, Obuchowski N, et al. Magnetic resonance imaging of the lumbar spine in people without back pain. N Engl J Med 1994;331(2):69–73.

106. Katz JN, Harris MB. Clinical practice. Lumbar spinal stenosis. N Engl J Med 2008;358(8):818–825.

107. Resnick D. Inflammatory disorders of the vertebral column: Seronegative spondyloarthropathies, adult-onset rheumatoid arthritis, and juvenile chronic arthritis. Clin Imaging 1989;13:253–268.

108. Barozzi L, Olivieri I, De Matteis M, et al. Seronegative spondyloarthropathies: Imaging of spondylitis, enthesitis and dactylitis. Eur J Radiol 1998;27(suppl 1):12–17.

109. Karasick D, Schweitzer ME, Abidi NA, et al. Fractures of the vertebrae with spinal cord injuries in patients with ankylosing spondylitis: Imaging findings. AJR Am J Roentgenol 1995;165:1205–1208.

110. Shih TT, Chen PQ, Li YW, et al. Spinal fractures and pseudoarthrosis complicating ankylosing spondylitis: MRI manifestation and clinical significance. J Comput Assist Tomogr 2001;25:164–170.

111. Thumbikat P, Hariharan RP, Ravichandran G, et al. Spinal cord injury in patients with ankylosing spondylitis: A 10-year review. Spine 2007;32(26):2989–2995.

112. Gonzalez-Beicos A, Nunez DB Jr, Fung AW, et al. Trauma to the ankylotic spine: Imaging spectrum of vertebral and soft tissue injuries. Emerg Radiol 2007;14:371–378.

113. Bilgen IG, Yunten N, Ustun EE, et al. Adhesive arachnoiditis causing cauda equina syndrome in ankylosing spondylitis: CT and MRI demonstration of dural calcification and a dorsal dural diverticulum. Neuroradiology 1999;41:508–511.

114. Charlesworth CH, Savy LE, Stevens J, et al. MRI demonstration of arachnoiditis in cauda equina syndrome of ankylosing spondylitis. Neuroradiology 1996;38:462–465.

115. Ginsburg WW, Cohen MD, Miller GM, et al. Posterior vertebral body erosion by arachnoid diverticula in cauda equina syndrome: An unusual manifestation of ankylosing spondylitis. J Rheumatol 1997;24:1417–1420.

116. Hadley LA. Congenital absence of pedicle from the cervical vertebra. AJR Am J Roentgenol 1946;55:193–197.

117. Wiener MD, Martinez S, Forsberg DA. Congenital absence of a cervical spine pedicle: Clinical and radiologic findings. AJR Am J Roentgenol 1990;155:1037–1041.

118. Sheehan J, Kaptain G, Sheehan J, et al. Congenital absence of a cervical pedicle: Report of two cases and review of the literature. Neurosurgery. 2000;47:1439–1442.

119. Yochum TR, Rowe LJ (eds.). Congenital anomalies and normal skeletal variants. Essentials of skeletal radiology, 3rd ed. Baltimore, MD: Lippincott Williams & Wilkins, 2005: 290,308–309.

120. Danziger J, Jackson H, Bloch S. Congenital absence of a pedicle in a cervical vertebra. Clin Radiol 1975;26:53–56.

121. Martin NL, Preston DF, Robinson RG. Osteoblastomas of the axial skeleton shown by skeletal scanning: Case report. J Nucl Med 1976;17:187–189.

122. Hudson TM. Scintigraphy of aneurysmal bone cysts. AJR Am J Roentgenol 1984;142:761–776.

123. Tortori-Donati P, Fondelli MP, Rossi A, et al. Segmental spinal dysgenesis: Neuroradiologic findings with clinical and embryologic correlation. AJNR Am J Neuroradiol 1999;20: 445–456.

124. Tortori-Donati P, Rossi A, Cama A. Spinal dysraphism: A review of neuroradiological features with embryological correlations and proposal for a new classification. Neuroradiology 2000;42:471–491.

125. Tortori-Donati P, Rossi A, Biancheri R, et al. Magnetic resonance imaging of spinal dysraphism. Top Magn Reson Imaging 2001;12:375–409.

126. Naidich TP, McLone DG, Mutleur S. A new understanding of dorsal dysraphism with lipoma (lipomyeloschisis): Radiological evaluation and surgical correction. AJNR Am J Neuroradiol 1983;4:103–116.

127. Rossi A, Biancheri R, Cama A, et al. Imaging in spine and spinal cord malformations. Eur J Radiol 2004;50(2):177–200.

128. Brophy JD, Sutton LN, Zimmerman RA, et al. Magnetic resonance imaging of lipomyelomeningocele and tethered cord. Neurosurgery 1989;25:336–340.

129. Bulsara KR, Zomorodi AR, Villavicencio AT, et al. Clinical outcome differences for lipomyelomeningoceles, intraspinal lipomas, and lipomas of the filum terminale. Neurosurg Rev 2001;24:192–194.

130. Pierre-Kahn A, Zerah M, Renier D, et al. Congenital lumbosacral lipomas. Childs Nerv Syst 1997;13:298–334; discussion 335.

131. Hilal SK, Marton D, Pollack E. Diastematomyelia in children: Radiographic study of 34 cases. Radiology 1974;112:609–621.

132. Byrd SE, Darling CF, McLone DG. Developmental disorders of the pediatric spine. Radiol Clin North Am 1991;29: 711–752.

133. Pang D, Dias MS, Ahab-Barmada M, et al. Split cord malformation: Part I. A unified theory of embryogenesis for double spinal cord malformations. Neurosurgery 1992;31(3):451–480.

134. Ozek MM, Pamir MN, Ozer AF, et al. Correlation between computed tomography and magnetic resonance imaging in diastematomyelia. Eur J Radiol 1991;13:209–214.

135. Kurihara N, Takahashi S, Ogawa A, et al. CT and MR findings in diastematomyelia, with embryogenetic consideration. Radiat Med 1992;10:73–77.

136. Skalej M, Duffner F, Stefanou A, et al. 3D spiral CT imaging of bone anomalies in a case of diastematomyelia. Eur J Radiol 1999;29:262–265.

137. Barkovich AJ, Raghavan N, Chuang S, et al. The wedge-shaped cord terminus: A radiographic sign of caudal regression. AJNR Am J Neuroradiol 1989;10:1223–1231.

138. Pang D. Sacral agenesis and caudal spinal cord malformations. Neurosurgery 1993;32(5):755–778; discussion 778–779.

139. Nievelstein RA, Valk J, Smit LM, et al. MR of the caudal regression syndrome: Embryologic implications. AJNR Am J Neuroradiol 1994;15:1021–1029.

140. Mihmanli I, Kurugoglu S, Kantarci F, et al. Dorsolumbosacral agenesis. Pediatr Radiol 2001;31:286–288.

141. National Institutes of Health. Neurofibromatosis. Conference statement, National Institutes of Health Consensus Development Conference. Arch Neurol 1988;45(5):575–578.

142. Upadhyaya M, Osborn MJ, Maynard J, et al. Mutational and functional analysis of the neurofibromatosis type 1 (NF1) gene. Hum Genet 1997;99(1):88–92.

143. Murphey MD, Smith WS, Smith SE, et al. From the archives of the AFIP. Imaging of musculoskeletal neurogenic tumors: Radiologic–pathologic correlation. Radiographics 1999;19(5):1253–1280.

144. Restrepo CS, Riascos RF, Hatta AA, et al. Neurofibromatosis type 1: Spinal manifestations of a systemic disease. J Comput Assist Tomogr 2005;29(4):532–539.

145. Tsirikos AI, Saifuddin A, Noordeen MH. Spinal deformity in neurofibromatosis type-1: Diagnosis and treatment. Eur Spine J 2005;14(5):427–439.

146. Ferner RE. Neurofibromatosis 1 and neurofibromatosis 2: A twenty-first century perspective. Lancet Neurol 2007;6(4): 340–351.

147. Ferner RE, Huson SM, Thomas N, et al. Guidelines for the diagnosis and management of individuals with neurofibromatosis 1. J Med Genet 2007;44(2):81–88.

148. Messiaen LM, Callens T, Mortier G, et al. Exhaustive mutation analysis of the NF1 gene allows identification of 95% of mutations and reveals a high frequency of unusual splicing defects. Hum Mutat 2000;15(6):541–555.

149. Thakkar SD, Feigen U, Mautner VF, et al. Spinal tumors in neurofibromatosis type 1: An MRI study of frequency, multiplicity and variety. Neuroradiology 1999;41(9):625–629.

150. Barkovich AJ. Pediatric neuroimaging. Philadelphia, PA: Lippincott Williams & Wilkins, 2005.

151. Brooks BS, Duvall ER, el Gammal T, et al. Neuroimaging features of neurenteric cysts: Analysis of nine cases and review of the literature. AJNR Am J Neuroradiol 1993;14: 735–746.

152. Geremia GK, Russell EJ, Clasen RA. MRI characteristics of a neurenteric cyst. AJNR Am J Neuroradiol 1988;9:978–980.

153. Aoki S, Machida T, Sasaki Y, et al. Enterogenous cyst of cervical spine: Clinical and radiological aspects (including CT and MRI). Neuroradiology 1987;29:291–293.

154. Yang S, Liu HM. MRI of a multiple component craniocervical neurenteric cyst. Eur J Radiol 1996;22:138–140.

155. Hierholzer J, Benndorf G, Lehmann T, et al. Epidural lipomatosis: Case report and literature review. Neuroradiology 1996;38:343–348.

156. Fogel GR, Cunningham PY, Esses SI. Spinal epidural lipomatosis: Case reports, literature review and meta-analysis. Spine J 2005;5:202–211.

157. Lisai P, Doria C, Crissantu L, et al. Cauda equina syndrome secondary to idiopathic spinal epidural lipomatosis. Spine 2001;26:307–309.

158. Borstlap AC, van Rooij WJ, Sluzewski M, et al. Reversibility of lumbar epidural lipomatosis in obese patients after weight-reduction diet. Neuroradiology 1995;37:670–673.

159. Lee M, Lekias J, Gubbay SS, et al. Spinal cord compression by extradural fat after renal transplantation. Med J Aust 1975;1:201–203.

160. Randall BC, Muraki AS, Osborn RE, et al. Epidural lipomatosis with lumbar radiculopathy: CT appearance. J Comput Assist Tomogr 1986;10:1039–1041.

161. Zentner J, Buchbender K, Vahlensieck M. Spinal epidural lipomatosis as a complication of prolonged corticosteroid therapy. J Neurosurg Sci 1995;39:81–85.

162. Pinkhardt EH, Sperfeld A-D, Bretschneider V, et al. Is spinal epidural lipomatosis an MRI-based diagnosis with clinical implications? A retrospective analysis. Acta Neurol Scand 2008;117(6):409–414. 10.1111/j.1600-0404.2007.00964.x.

163. Roche MA, Rowe GG. The incidence of separate neural arch and coincident bone variations: A survey of 4200 skeletons. Anat Rec 1951;109:233–252.

164. Beutler WJ, Fredrickson BE, Murtland A, et al. The natural history of spondylolysis and spondylolisthesis: 45-year follow-up evaluation. Spine 2003;28:1027–1035.

165. Leone A, Cianfoni A, Cerase A, et al. Lumbar spondylolysis: A review. Skeletal Radiol 2011;40:683–700.

166. Rothman SL, Glenn WV. CT multiplanar reconstruction in 253 cases of lumbar spondylolysis. AJNR Am J Neuroradiol 1984;5:81–90.

167. Troup JD. Mechanical factors in spondylolisthesis and spondylolysis. Clin Orthop 1976;147:59–67.

168. Fredrickson BE, Baker D, McHolick WJ, et al. The natural history of spondylolysis and spondylolisthesis in children and adolescents. J Bone Joint Surg Am 1984;66:699–707.

169. Grogan JP, Hemminghytt S, Williams AL, et al. Spondylolysis studied with computed tomography. Radiology 1982;145:737–742.

170. Campbell RS, Grainger AJ, Hide IG, et al. Juvenile spondylolysis: A comparative analysis of CT, SPECT and MRI. Skeletal Radiol 2005;34:63–73.

171. Jinkins JR, Matthes JC, Sener RN, et al. Spondylolysis, spondylolisthesis, and associated nerve root entrapment in the lumbosacral spine: MR evaluation. AJR Am J Roentgenol 1992;159:799–803.

172. Ulmer JL, Mathews VP, Elster AD, et al. MR imaging of lumbar spondylolysis: The importance of ancillary observations. AJR Am J Roentgenol 1997;169:233–239.

173. Hollenberg GM, Beattie PF, Meyers SP, et al. Stress reactions of the lumbar pars interarticularis: The development of a new MRI classification system. Spine 2002;27:181–186.

174. Wiltse LL, Newman PH, Macnab I. Classification of spondylolysis and spondylolisthesis. Clin Orthop Relat Res 1976; 117:23–29.

175. Steiner ME, Micheli LJ. Treatment of symptomatic spondylolysis and spondylolisthesis with the modified Boston brace. Spine 1985;10:937–943.

176. Cheung EV, Herman MJ, Cavalier R, et al. Spondylolysis and spondylolisthesis in children and adolescents. II. Surgical management. J Am Acad Orthop Surg 2006;14:488–498.

177. Reitman CA, Esses SI. Direct repair of spondylolytic defects in young competitive athletes. Spine J 2002;2:142–144.

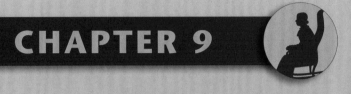

# CHAPTER 9

# THORACIC RADIOLOGY

**Lejla Aganovic / Timothy Singewald / James G. Ravenel**

*The authors and editors acknowledge the contribution of the Chapter 7 author from the second edition: Caroline Chiles, MD.*

HISTORY: A 25-year-old woman with recurrent pneumonia

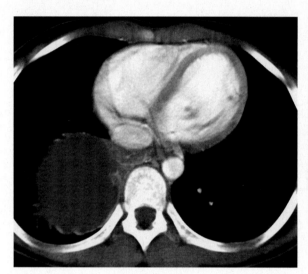

FIGURE 9.1.1

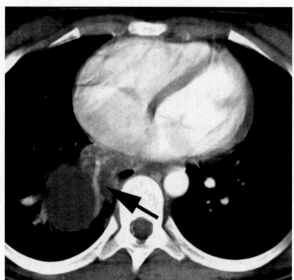

FIGURE 9.1.2

FINDINGS: A part-solid and cystic mass is visible in the posterior basal segment of the right lower lobe on contrast-enhanced CT (Figs. 9.1.1 and 9.1.2) of the chest. There is a large systemic vessel coursing through the mass (Fig. 9.1.2, *arrow*).

DIAGNOSIS: Intralobar bronchopulmonary sequestration

DISCUSSION: Bronchopulmonary sequestration is a rare pulmonary lesion in which a portion of lung is set apart from the rest of the lung and receives systemic arterial supply. There are two types of sequestration: intralobar and extralobar. Characteristics of intralobar sequestration include systemic arterial supply and pulmonary venous drainage from a portion of lung with no connection to the tracheobronchial tree, whereas an extralobar sequestration has a separate pleural covering, systemic arterial supply, and systemic venous drainage (1). Some believe that some intralobar sequestrations may be acquired rather than congenital lesions given that they are typically detected incidentally and at an older age than extralobar sequestration. Approximately 50% intralobar sequestrations are diagnosed before the age of 20 and the diagnosis is seldom reported after the age of 40 (2).

It is most common for the intralobar sequestrations to occur in the posterior basal segments of the lower lobes. Although the systemic supply is usually from the aorta, arteries to an intralobar sequestration may arise from the diaphragm, chest wall, or abdomen. Typical radiographic features include focal consolidation that may contain cystic areas or gas. In addition, there may be emphysema distal to the lesion (1). In most cases the systemic arterial supply is identifiable although CT angiography may be necessary to document the course and location of the vessel.

## Aunt Minnie's Pearls

Intralobar bronchopulmonary sequestration has systemic arterial supply and pulmonary venous drainage and may be discovered as an incidental finding.

Extralobar bronchopulmonary sequestration has a pleural covering, systemic arterial supply, and systemic venous drainage—usually in left lower lobe and generally associated with other congenital anomalies.

HISTORY: A 64-year-old farmer with shortness of breath

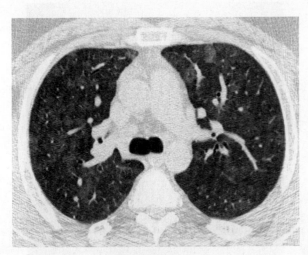

FIGURE 9.2.1

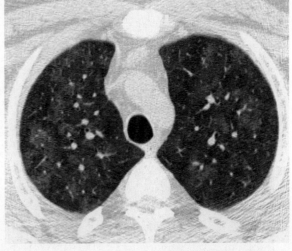

FIGURE 9.2.2

FINDINGS: Axial high resolution computed tomography (HRCT) images (Figs. 9.2.1 and 9.2.2) through chest demonstrate multiple ill-defined centrilobular nodules throughout the lungs.

DIAGNOSIS: Subacute hypersensitive pneumonitis

DISCUSSION: Hypersensitivity pneumonitis is an allergic lung disease caused by inhalation of antigens contained in a variety of organic dusts (3). Radiographic and pathologic abnormalities that are seen in patients with hypersensitive pneumonitis (HP) are quite similar, regardless of the organic antigen responsible. These abnormalities can be classified into acute, subacute, and chronic stages. In the acute phase diffuse ill-defined airspace consolidation can be seen on chest radiograph and chest CT. After resolution of acute abnormalities a fine nodular pattern is often visible on radiographs. Typical findings of subacute HP on HRCT include patchy ground-glass opacities,

small ill-defined centrilobular nodules, or both (4). The nodules are typically smaller than 4 mm and involve all lung zones to a similar extent with relative sparing of the fissures and pleural surfaces. Chronic hypersensitivity pneumonitis is characterized by the presence of fibrosis, although findings of active disease may also be present. Findings in fibrosis include intralobular interstitial thickening, irregular interfaces, irregular interlobular septal thickening, honeycombing, and traction bronchiectasis.

## Aunt Minnie's Pearls

Diffuse centrilobular nodules in a person exposed to organic dust are characteristic of subacute hypersensitive pneumonitis.

Nodules of subacute hypersensitivity pneumonitis typically spare the periphery of the lung.

HISTORY: A 23-year-old woman with chronic cough

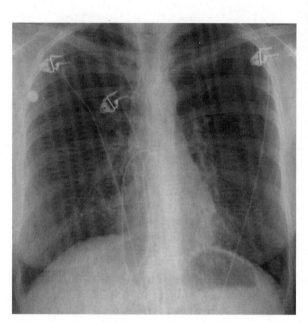

FIGURE 9.3.1

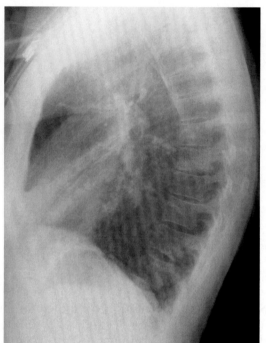

FIGURE 9.3.2

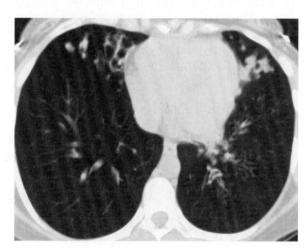

FIGURE 9.3.3

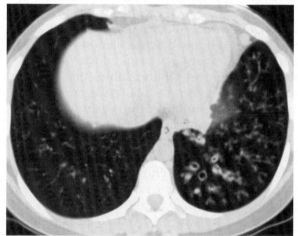

FIGURE 9.3.4

**FINDINGS:** Posteroanterior (PA; Fig. 9.3.1) and lateral (Fig. 9.3.2) views of the chest show coarse tubular opacities at both lung bases. The CT reveals varicoid and cystic bronchiectasis within the right middle lobe and lingula (Fig. 9.3.3) and left lower lobe (Fig. 9.3.4) associated with branching tubular opacities (mucoid impaction) and air trapping.

**DIAGNOSIS:** Primary ciliary dyskinesia (PCD)

**DISCUSSION:** PCD is primarily an autosomal recessive inherited disorder that includes a heterogeneous group of ultrastructural defects involving the axoneme or central functional element of the cilia. Functionally, these disturbances result in reduced or disorganized beating of the ciliated epithelial cells or, in some cases, complete immotility. The ineffectual beating or immotility of cilia results in accumulation of mucus resulting in recurrent infections of the upper and lower respiratory tracts (5). In some cases there is inversion of the normal anatomic structures of the thorax and abdomen, situs inversus universalis, or partialis; PCD with situs inversus universalis is known by the eponym, Kartagener syndrome.

Bronchiectasis is a common sequela of PCD, typically involving the dependent zones including the lower lobes, right middle lobe, and/or the lingular segments of the left upper lobe. Chest radiographs may demonstrate overinflation, bronchial wall thickening, and bronchial dilation. Bronchiectasis can be quite subtle on conventional radiographs and may appear as parallel linear CT demonstrates bronchiectasis, that is often varicoid or cystic in the lower lobes, with or without right middle lobe or lingular involvement and relative sparing of the upper lobes (6).

### Aunt Minnie's Pearl

Bronchiectasis in PCD is basal predominant, distinguishing it from the typical pattern seen in cystic fibrosis.

**HISTORY:** Mass on chest x-ray

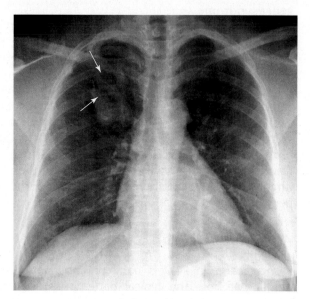

FIGURE 9.4.1

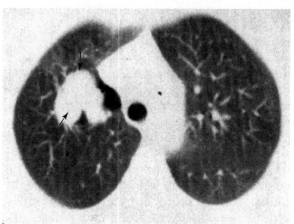

FIGURE 9.4.2

**FINDINGS:** Right upper lobe mass with finger-like projections superiorly (Fig. 9.4.1, *arrows*). CT images (Fig. 9.4.2) reveal a V-shaped tubular mass with distal air trapping (*arrows*).

**DIAGNOSIS:** Congenital bronchial atresia

**DISCUSSION:** Bronchial atresia is an uncommon congenital anomaly that is usually detected as an incidental finding in adults. The apicoposterior segment of the left upper lobe is most commonly affected followed by the right upper lobe, middle lobe, and lower lobes (7,8). The lung develops normally in a position distal to the atretic bronchus and is ventilated by collateral air drift (8,9). Airways distal to the atretic segmental bronchus continue to produce mucus, which leads to mucoid impaction or mucocele formation within the bronchus. The affected lobe appears hyperaerated and is both oligemic and hyperlucent (8,9). Bronchial atresia is generally asymptomatic and requires no further treatment although it should be distinguished from obstructing neoplasm.

## Aunt Minnie's Pearl

Findings of bronchial atresia result from mucoid impaction distal to atretic bronchus and hyperexpanded lobe; usually apicoposterior segment of left upper lobe.

# Case 9.5

Dysphagia in a 30-year-old man

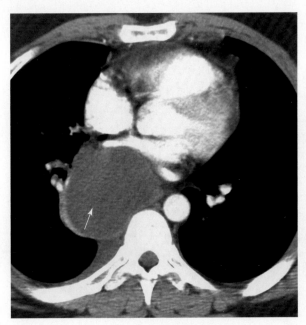

FIGURE 9.5.1

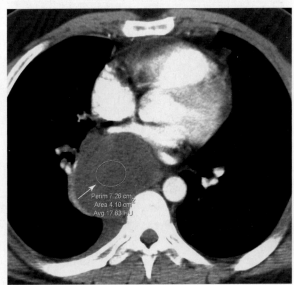

FIGURE 9.5.2

**FINDINGS:** Axial CT images (Figs. 9.5.1 and 9.5.2) show a large, sharply marginated, fluid density subcarinal mass (*arrows*).

**DIAGNOSIS:** Bronchopulmonary–foregut cyst

**DISCUSSION:** A bronchopulmonary–foregut cyst is a developmental anomaly that is lined by columnar epithelium, and is filled with either clear serous or thick mucoid material (9). The distinction between cyst of bronchial or foregut origin may not be evident until resection. Although most bronchopulmonary–foregut cysts are asymptomatic and incidentally discovered on routine chest radiographs, they may become infected, resulting in symptoms. Large bronchopulmonary–foregut cysts within the mediastinum can create symptoms related to compression of the trachea and esophagus, including dyspnea and dysphagia.

Bronchopulmonary–foregut cysts can occur anywhere in the mediastinum and are usually round or ovoid masses near the carina (9). Congenital cysts may be easier to categorize when there is only one evident site of origin, that is, bronchogenic cysts may be intrapulmonary, whereas foregut cysts may be found along the lower esophagus.

On CT images, bronchogenic cysts typically appear as homogeneous water-attenuation masses. When the fluid contains calcium oxalate, proteinacious material, or hemorrhage, the contents of the cysts may have higher attenuation and may mimic soft tissue masses (10). On T1-weighted MR images, the bronchogenic cyst may have low-signal intensity, or it may have high-signal intensity if the contents of the cysts are proteinacious. On T2-weighted images, the cyst has homogeneously high attenuation (10).

Bronchogenic cysts are often treated by surgical excision to relieve or avoid symptoms of compression or infection. An alternative to surgery is needle aspiration of the mediastinal cyst and may be done via a trans-esophageal approach (11).

## Aunt Minnie's Pearls

Bronchopulmonary–foregut cysts are typically mediastinal and may be water attenuation or higher on CT.

The tissue of origin of a mediastinal cyst may be difficult to accurately predict when in the upper mediastinum or subcarinal recess.

**HISTORY:** A 36-year-old female with recurrent pneumothoraces

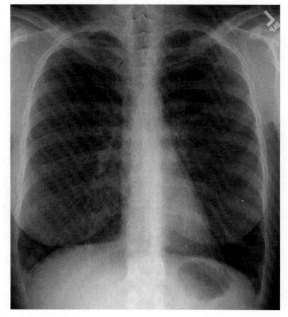

FIGURE 9.6.1

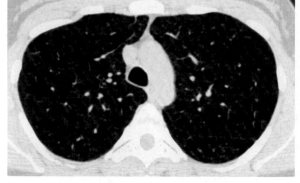

FIGURE 9.6.2

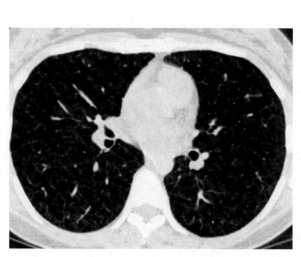

FIGURE 9.6.3

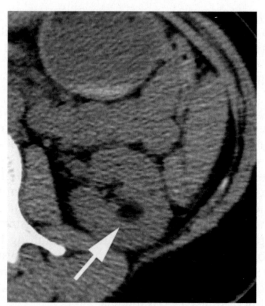

FIGURE 9.6.4

**FINDINGS:** Frontal chest radiograph (Fig. 9.6.1) reveals overinflated lungs and subtle fine reticular opacities and cystic lucencies. HRCT through upper and mid lungs demonstrates numerous discrete round cystic spaces of varying sizes that have barely perceptible walls (Figs. 9.6.2 and 9.6.3). Non contrast image through the left kidney demonstrates fat containing lesion (Fig. 9.6.4, *arrow*).

**DIAGNOSIS:** Lymphangioleiomyomatosis (LAM) with angiomyolipoma of the kidney

**DISCUSSION:** LAM is a rare, idiopathic disorder that almost exclusively affects women of childbearing age. Pathologic findings in LAM are characterized by diffuse interstitial proliferation of smooth muscle cells in the lungs. Patients typically present with dyspnea and recurrent pneumothoraces. The most commonly described radiographic manifestation of LAM is a pattern of generalized, symmetric, reticular, or reticulonodular opacities, seen in approximately 80% to 90% of affected patients (12). It is postulated that these reticular and reticulonodular opacities result from the visualization of numerous superimposed cyst walls. Lung volumes are normal to increased.

Typical CT and HRCT findings of LAM include diffuse bilateral thin-walled cysts surrounded by normal intervening lung parenchyma, affecting all zones equally. The cysts range from 2 to 5 mm in diameter but have been reported to be as large as 25 mm. Cystic changes of LAM are apparent on conventional chest CT; however, individual cysts, their extent, and distribution are better seen at HRCT (12). Other features of LAM include adenopathy, pleural effusions, and pneumothoraces.

Abdominal findings can be present in >70% of patients with LAM (13). The most common finding is renal angiomyolipoma that can occur in up to 50% of patients with LAM. Some investigators claim that isolated pulmonary LAM and LAM associated with renal angiomyolipomas are a forme fruste of tuberous sclerosis.

## Aunt Minnie's Pearls

Diffuse bilateral thin-walled cysts throughout the lungs in women of childbearing age are diagnostic of LAM.

Extrathoracic related findings are present in >70% of cases.

**HISTORY:** A 36-year-old woman with mental status changes

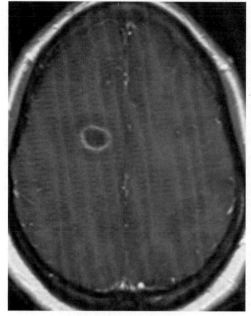

FIGURE 9.7.1

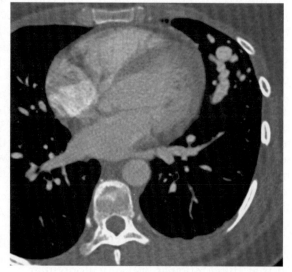

FIGURE 9.7.2

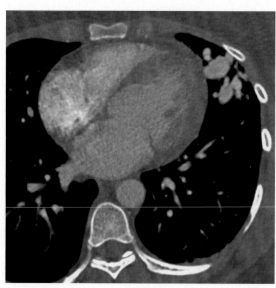

FIGURE 9.7.3

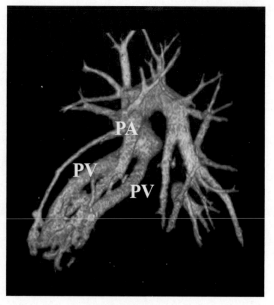

FIGURE 9.7.4

**FINDINGS:** Gadolinium-enhanced MR image reveals ring enhancing right parietal lesion (Fig. 9.7.1). Contrast-enhanced CT reveals a tangle of large enhancing vessels in the lingula (Figs. 9.7.2 and 9.7.3). Three-dimensional volume–rendered image (Fig. 9.7.4) shows the architecture to better advantage (*PA* = pulmonary artery; *PV* = draining pulmonary veins).

**DIAGNOSIS:** Pulmonary arteriovenous malformation (PAVM) with cerebral abscess

**DISCUSSION:** PAVMs are abnormal communications between pulmonary arteries and pulmonary veins. The majority of PAVM are congenital in origin. Although the exact pathogenesis is unknown, a popular hypothesis is incomplete resorption of vascular septae in the lungs (14). PAVM may also be acquired as a result of pulmonary right-to-left shunting in association with various conditions including hepatic cirrhosis, mitral stenosis, and trauma, among others. PAVMs can be divided into two types. Simple PAVM is a single large pulmonary artery to pulmonary vein communication, which is usually nonseptate. Complex PAVM has multiple feeding arteries and draining veins, usually with a septate aneurysmal communication between arteries and veins (15). Because the normal pulmonary capillary bed is bypassed, untreated arteriovenous malformations may cause dyspnea and cyanosis as a result of the pulmonary to systemic shunt and cerebrovascular ischemia and infarction, as well as brain abscess, as a result of the passing of emboli and bacteria directly into the systemic circulation (16,17). A cerebral event (stroke or abscess) as in this case may be the initial clinical manifestation of a PAVM.

Contrast-enhanced CT has been shown to be the standard in diagnosis of PAVM as well as treatment planning. The typical appearance is either blood vessels connected to a serpiginous mass or a homogenous, delimited mass of several centimeters in diameter. CT has been shown to be superior in sensitivity to pulmonary angiography, particularly with thin sections and multi-planar reformations through the absence of lesion superimposition on CT as well as detect other small PAVMs. Maximum intensity projection (MIP) images can be particularly helpful in displaying the entire AVM as well as its architecture (18). Pulmonary angiography, however, is still necessary to determine the full architecture of a PAVM, and for treatment with embolization.

Approximately 70% of cases with PAVM are associated with Osler–Weber–Rendu Syndrome, also known as Hereditary hemorrhagic telangiectasia, an autosomal dominant disorder associated with multiple organ arteriovenous malformations (14).

### Aunt Minnie's Pearl

Approximately 70% of patients with a PAVM have hereditary hemorrhagic telangiectasia.

**HISTORY:** A 61-year-old woman with cough and dyspnea

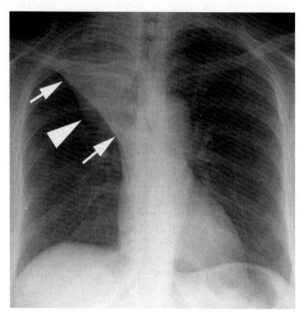

FIGURE 9.8.1

**FINDINGS:** On the frontal chest radiograph (Fig. 9.8.1), there is superior retraction of the right hilum and minor fissure (*arrows*), with mass causing a reverse-S configuration (*arrowhead*).

**DIAGNOSIS:** Right upper lobe collapse caused by primary lung neoplasm—"S sign of Golden"

**DISCUSSION:** In 1925, Golden described the orientation of the minor fissure in patients with upper lobe collapse caused by a central mass (19). The medial aspect of the minor fissure outlines the inferior margin of the mass; the lateral aspect of the minor fissure moves superiorly as the right upper lobe collapses, producing a reverse-S appearance. Additional signs of volume loss in the right upper lobe include rightward shift of the trachea and mediastinum, elevation of the right hemidiaphragm with a juxtaphrenic peak, with resulting hyperexpansion of the right middle and lower lobes, and crowding of the ribs (20,21).

Lobar collapse in an adult is often the result of an endobronchial lesion. In the outpatient setting, the primary consideration is a neoplasm until proven otherwise, whereas a mucus plug is a common cause of lobar collapse in the hospitalize patient. Collapse may also occur as a result of extrinsic compression of the bronchus or by a bronchial stricture. The appearance of the collapse can be a clue to the cause. A relatively straight margin can be seen with collapse owing to mucus plugging or other small endobronchial lesion, whereas larger lesions produce a focal convexity in the fissure as in this case.

## Aunt Minnie's Pearl

The S sign of Golden indicates right upper lobe collapse caused by central mass.

HISTORY: A 57-year-old woman with a history of breast carcinoma

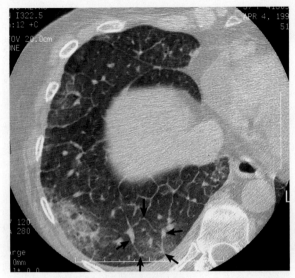

FIGURE 9.9.1

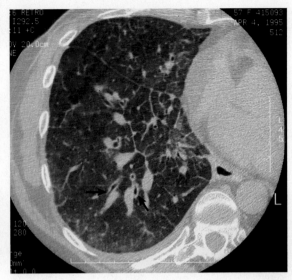

FIGURE 9.9.2

FINDINGS: Axial HRCT images of right lung (1-mm collimation, high spatial frequency algorithm, targeted image) show thickening of the interlobular septa throughout the right lung. Polygonal structures represent secondary pulmonary lobules outlined by thickened septa (Fig. 9.9.1, *arrows*). The bronchovascular bundles seen tangentially and in cross-section are thickened (Fig. 9.9.2, *arrows*).

DIAGNOSIS: Lymphangitic carcinomatosis

DISCUSSION: Lymphangitic spread of tumor in the lung is a relatively rare metastatic pattern, typically to the result of adenocarcinomas. The tumor cells are deposited in the lung periphery by hematogenous dissemination and then, rather than forming the typical nodule, infiltrate the pulmonary lymphatics and interlobular septa growing back toward the hila, producing thickening of the interlobular septa and peribronchovascular interstitium (22). Occasionally, the spread of lymphoma can also occur along pulmonary lymphatics, extending peripherally from a central lesion. Although pulmonary sarcoidosis may mimic this radiographic appearance, the patient's clinical presentation and past medical history should allow for confident distinction of the two. In particular, the presence of unilateral disease or pleural effusion strongly favors lymphangitic carcinoma (23). When in doubt the diagnosis can be confirmed by bronchoscopy with trans-bronchial biopsy. It is important to remember that lung cancer and treatment of lung cancer with radiation therapy may lead to central venous and lymphatic obstruction that may result in interstitial opacities (24). This local phenomenon should not be confused with lymphangitic carcinomatosis and the inappropriate use of this term can have grave implications with the misclassification of staging leading to inappropriate therapy.

## Aunt Minnie's Pearl

Lymphangitic carcinomatosis refers to hematogenous dissemination of tumor with growth toward the hila along the pulmonary interstitium.

**HISTORY:** A 35-year-old woman with cough

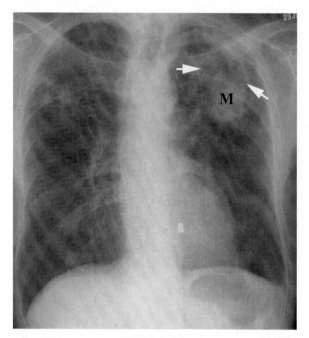

FIGURE 9.10.1

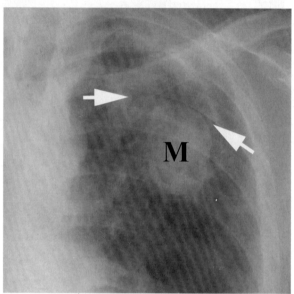

FIGURE 9.10.2

**FINDINGS:** A frontal chest radiograph (Fig. 9.10.1) reveals fibrocavitary changes in the upper lobes with a dependent soft-tissue mass in the left upper lobe cavity. A detail of the left upper lobe reveals a rounded mass (*M*) with well-defined superior border and thin rim of surrounding gas (Fig. 9.10.2, *arrows*).

**DIAGNOSIS:** Aspergilloma

**DISCUSSION:** Aspergillomas occur as a result of colonization of a preexisting cavitary lesion that may be produced by tuberculosis, fibrocavitary sarcoidosis, histoplasmosis, emphysema, or bronchiectasis (16). Pleural thickening adjacent to the cavity may precede visualization of the fungus ball, especially true in fibrocavitary sarcoidosis (17). In cavities resulting from tuberculosis, the incidence of aspergilloma may be as high as 10% (25). The aspergilloma itself consists of a mass of hyphae mixed together with mucus and cellular debris and as such represent a saprophytic form of infection. Although typically found in the upper lobes, aspergillomas can occur anywhere a cavity exists.

Although mild hemoptysis occurs within the majority of affected individuals, bleeding can be severe and life-threatening massive hemoptysis may require embolization (25). This is typically because of erosion into a bronchial artery, in particular with massive hemoptysis, but may also occur as a result of erosion into a pulmonary artery.

Treatment of aspergilloma is limited owing to the lack of blood supply. In most cases, no specific therapy is warranted and treatment is aimed at complications (such as bronchial artery embolization). In selected cases intracavitary instillation of amphotericin has been performed with variable results. In rare cases, surgery is necessary for control of recurrent hemoptysis and is associated with a relatively high rate of morbidity and mortality (25).

## Aunt Minnie's Pearls

The saprophytic form of *Aspergillus* infection is recognized as a fungus ball (aspergilloma) within a preexisting cavity.

Common causes of the preexisting cavity include tuberculosis, sarcoidosis, and emphysema.

**HISTORY:** A 72-year-old man with a history of recurrent ventricular tachycardia, now with exertional dyspnea and nonproductive cough

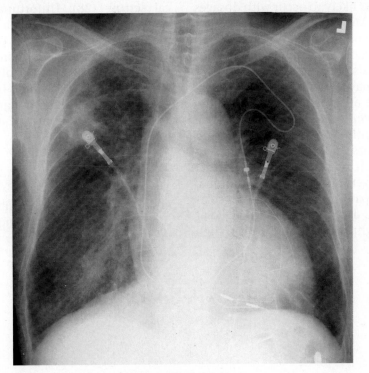

FIGURE 9.11.1

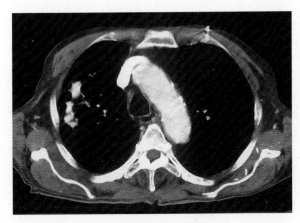

FIGURE 9.11.2

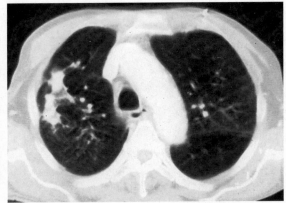

FIGURE 9.11.3

**FINDINGS:** Chest radiograph (Fig. 9.11.1) shows cardiomegaly and a transvenous pacemaker as well as automatic implantable cardioverter defibrillator (AICD) patches. Focal areas of increased opacity in the right upper lobe are better seen on the CT images (Figs. 9.11.2 and 9.11.3) as areas of high attenuation (almost as high as the contrast-enhanced aorta).

**DIAGNOSIS:** Amiodarone pulmonary toxicity

**DISCUSSION:** Amiodarone is an anti-arrhythmic agent that can cause pulmonary toxicity in 1% to 15% of treated individuals (26). Pulmonary toxicity may manifest within days of starting the medication and most cases will develop within 1 to 1.5 years after initiation of therapy. Toxicity appears to be dose-dependent with pulmonary symptoms manifesting more rapidly at higher doses and amiodarone pneumonitis is less likely to occur with dosages of ≤400 mg/day (26). Most often, patients present with a subacute course of dyspnea and nonproductive cough, but a more acute onset that mimics pulmonary infection can also be seen.

Chest radiographs may show focal areas of interstitial disease or dense areas of alveolar consolidation that are often asymmetric. The CT appearance may be quite varied with interstitial, alveolar, and mixed patterns of disease. Most often the presentation is similar to that of nonspecific interstitial pneumonitis or cryptogenic organizing pneumonia, whereas fibrosis (UIP pattern) and diffuse alveolar damage are rare (27). High attenuation alveolar consolidation is thought to be related to the high iodine content (37% by weight) of amiodarone and its prolonged half-life within the lung and is considered to be pathognomonic in the appropriate clinical setting (28). Unfortunately, high-attenuation pulmonary opacities are a relatively uncommon manifestation of disease. Attenuation of the liver and spleen is also often increased from iodine accumulation and is a marker of amiodarone use rather than toxicity. This feature, however, can be helpful when nonspecific pulmonary opacities are present and raise the possibility of amiodarone pulmonary toxicity.

## Aunt Minnie's Pearl

Amiodarone pulmonary toxicity is dose-related and may produce high-attenuation lung consolidation on CT.

**HISTORY:** A 28-year-old asymptomatic man, routine chest radiograph

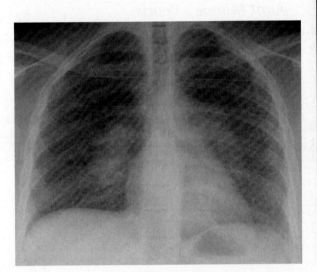

FIGURE 9.12.1

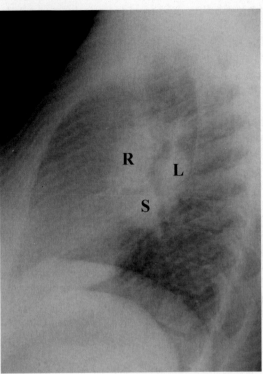

FIGURE 9.12.2

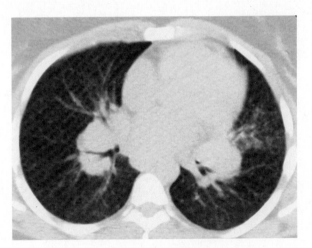

FIGURE 9.12.3

**FINDINGS:** Bilateral hilar (*R* and *L*), right paratracheal, aortopulmonary window, and subcarinal (*S*) lymphadenopathy are present on PA and lateral views of the chest with faint reticulonodular opacities in both lungs (Figs. 9.12.1 and 9.12.2). Axial CT (Fig. 9.12.3) confirm the adenopathy as well as reveal small subpleural, peribronchovascular, and perilymphatic nodules.

**DIAGNOSIS:** Sarcoidosis

**DISCUSSION:** Sarcoidosis is a systemic disease of unknown etiology characterized by formation of noncaseating epithelioid granulomata within lymph nodes, lungs, liver, and other organs (29).

The clinical and radiological manifestations of sarcoidosis are predominantly related to pulmonary involvement, and pulmonary involvement is present in approximately 90%. The most common radiographic finding in sarcoidosis is bilateral hilar, subcarinal, and right paratracheal lymphadenopathy (30). The chest x-ray may be normal in up to 10% even with nodal or lung parenchyma involvement. CT often reveals enlarged lymph nodes within the aortopulmonary window and the left paratracheal region as well. The interstitial pattern is often reticulonodular with small nodules located along bronchovascular bundles (29). Pulmonary parenchymal involvement in fact can be quite varied with patterns ranging from miliary nodules, to air-space opacities, to end-stage fibrosis and cavitation. With chronic pulmonary disease, fibrosis and bullae may predominate, typically with an upper lobe distribution.

Sarcoidosis can be staged by chest radiographs as stage 0 (no chest radiographic involvement), stage I (disease limited to mediastinal nodes), stage II (lung parenchyma and lymph node involvement), stage III (lung parenchyma involvement only), and stage IV (end-stage pulmonary fibrosis). In most cases the initial disease presentation regresses (with or without treatment), but when clinical progression of sarcoidosis occurs it often follows this radiographic continuum.

## Aunt Minnie's Pearls

Classic HRCT findings include well-defined nodules along the interlobular septa, peribronchovascular bundles, and pleural surfaces and smooth or nodular peribronchovascular thickening.

Subpleural and peri-fissural nodules are important in distinguishing sarcoidosis from the centrilobular nodules of hypersensitivity pneumonitis.

## Case 9.13

**HISTORY:** A 34-year-old male with acute dyspnea and pleuritic chest pain 3 days after suffering major lower extremity trauma

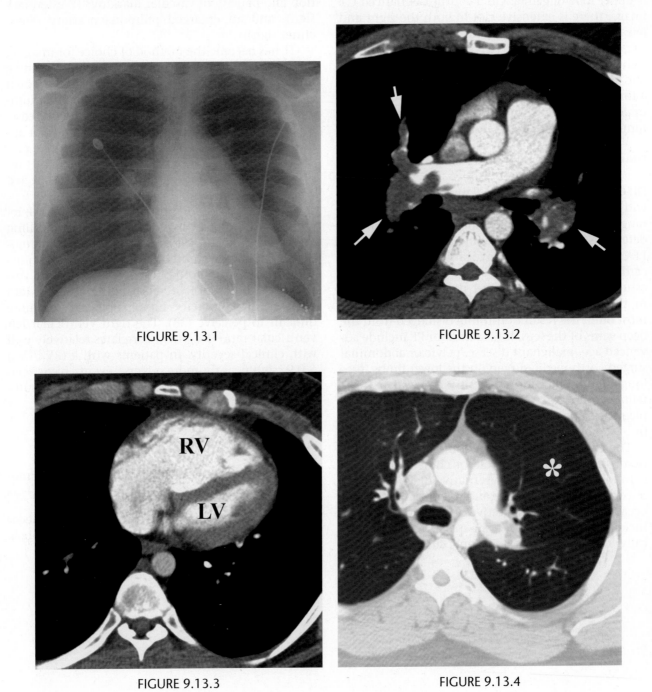

FIGURE 9.13.1

FIGURE 9.13.2

FIGURE 9.13.3

FIGURE 9.13.4

**FINDINGS:** On the chest radiograph (Fig. 9.13.1), the central pulmonary arteries are enlarged and there is upper lobe oligemia. On a contrast-enhanced CT image, there is extensive clot in both the right and left pulmonary arterial system (Fig. 9.13.2, *arrows*). In addition, there is relative enlargement of the right ventricle (*RV*) compared with the left (*LV*) and shift of the interventricular septum to the left, a finding of right heart strain (Fig. 9.13.3). The left upper lobe oligemia can be better appreciated with lung windows (Fig. 9.13.4, *asterisk*).

**DIAGNOSIS:** Acute pulmonary embolism (PE)

**DISCUSSION:** Acute PE is a relatively common event with a wide spectrum of clinical presentation that ranges from small asymptomatic and incidentally detected subsegmental PE to life-threatening central PE causing hypotension, myocardial infarction, and cardiogenic shock. The overall incidence has been estimated at approximately 1 per 1,000 population in the United States (31). Pulmonary emboli are most often the result of thrombi dislodged from the deep veins of the legs. Risk factors for PE include advanced age, malignant disease, pelvic or abdominal surgery, orthopedic surgery in the lower limbs, prolonged immobilization, obesity, congestive heart failure, and trauma. Dyspnea and chest pain, often pleuritic in nature, are the only symptoms reported by >50% of patients with PE.

The chest radiograph is seldom, if ever, diagnostic of PE, and the main role of chest radiography is to identify important alternative diagnoses such as congestive heart failure and pneumonia. On rare occasions, findings suggestive of PE may be present including wedge shaped air-space opacities typically located at the costophrenic sulci (pulmonary infarcts aka Hampton hump), regional hypoperfusion evident as areas of decreased lung attenuation and paucity of vascular markings (Westermark sign), and an enlarged pulmonary artery (Fleischner sign).

CT has become the method of choice for imaging PE in clinical routine in most institutions. Negative predictive value of CT has consistently been shown to surpass 96% both with single-detector and multidetector techniques (32). Underlying lung disease, inpatient status, and results of V/Q scan do not appear to have appreciable effects of the negative predictive value. A clear benefit of CT is the depiction of alternative diagnoses not otherwise suspected when pulmonary embolus is absent.

The diagnosis of PE is usually straightforward, relying on the direct observation of a central filling defect surrounded by a rim of contrast in a pulmonary artery. Often emboli lodge at bifurcation points and continue into both branch vessels. A sharp vessel cutoff or absence of vessel filling also provides evidence of pulmonary embolus but may be more difficult to perceive (33). The right ventricular/left ventricular ratio ($RV_D/LV_D$) correlates relatively well with clinical severity. In patients with a ($RV_D/LV_D$) > 0.9, significantly more adverse events have been observed, and a ratio of >1.5 appears to be sufficiently diagnostic of "massive" PE (34).

## Aunt Minnie's Pearls

RV/LV ratio can be used to predict severity of pulmonary thromboembolism.

Owing to a very high negative predictive value, a negative CT reliably excludes significant pulmonary emboli.

HISTORY: A 67-year-old man with dyspnea who has worked as a concrete driller for many years

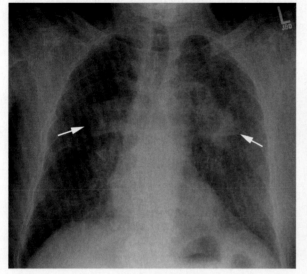

FIGURE 9.14.1

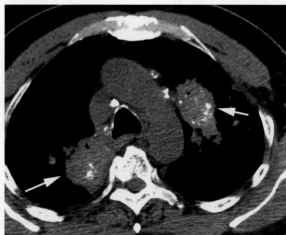

FIGURE 9.14.2

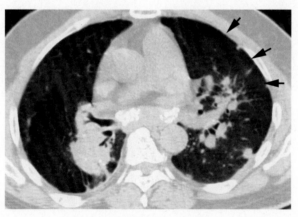

FIGURE 9.14.3

FINDINGS: A PA view of the chest (Fig. 9.14.1) shows reticulonodular interstitial opacities in the upper lobe and mass-like consolidation surrounding the hila (*arrows*). A transverse CT image mediastinal windows confirms the presence of perihilar masses with "eggshell" calcifications (Fig. 9.14.2, *arrows*). Transverse CT image in lung windows shows scattered tiny nodules seen best in posterior left lung as well as peripheral emphysema (*arrows*) related to progressive massive fibrosis causing the mass-like opacities on radiograph through the lower lobes (Fig. 9.14.3).

DIAGNOSIS: Complicated silicosis

DISCUSSION: Silicosis results from the inhalation of fine particles of silicon dioxide, which is commonly found in quartz (35). Affected individuals are often exposed through their occupation, typically mining, sandblasting, and quarrying. In the acute setting, a condition called acute silicoproteinosis may develop as a result of massive exposure. The radiographic findings typically consist of perihilar ground glass and consolidation that may take on a "crazy-paving" pattern (36).

Classic silicosis tends to be more indolent and present with chronic symptomatology. Radiographically there is both a simple and complicated form. Simple silicosis comprises punctate nodular opacities with predominant upper lobe involvement. Complicated silicosis, or progressive massive fibrosis, refers to the coalescence of small nodules into masses at least 1 cm in diameter. Lesions then tend to be pulled toward the hila resulting in distal emphysema and are seen to better advantage at CT. These large opacities are often surrounded by small nodules (36).

Peripheral (eggshell) calcification of hilar and mediastinal lymph nodes may also be present in silicosis but is not specific for the disease as they may also be seen with coal workers' pneumoconiosis, sarcoidosis, and treated lymphoma.

## Aunt Minnie's Pearl

Silicosis causes upper lobe nodules and conglomerate masses.

**HISTORY:** A 72-year-old World War II veteran with abnormal chest radiography results

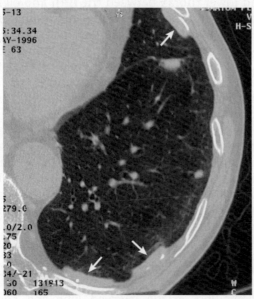

FIGURE 9.15.1

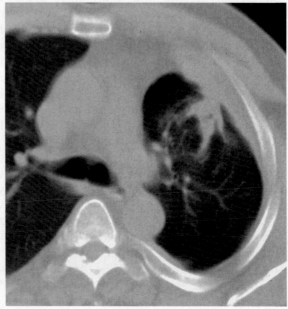

FIGURE 9.15.2

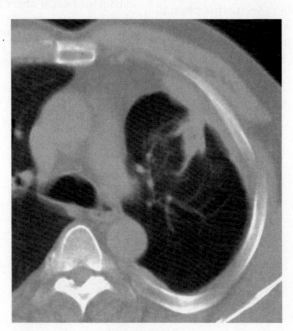

FIGURE 9.15.3

## Case 9.15 (Continued)

**FINDINGS:** An HRCT image shows pleural thickening and partially calcified pleural plaques (Fig. 9.15.1, *arrows*). Subpleural arcuate and short lines are faintly seen. Two CT images separated by 3 years (Figs. 9.15.2 and 9.15.3) show bronchi and vessels spiraling toward a mass in the left upper lobe. The mass is subtended by thickened pleura. No change in size or shape of the mass is seen over the 3 years.

**DIAGNOSIS:** Asbestosis and rounded atelectasis

**DISCUSSION:** Asbestos includes a group of crystalline, hydrated silica fibers that can be subdivided into six groups of which the most commonly used is chrysotile. The other 5 groups include the amphiboles of which crocidolite is the most important clinically (35). Manifestations of asbestos exposure include diseases of the pleura (pleural effusion, pleural plaques, and mesothelioma) and disease of the pulmonary interstitium (asbestosis). A secondary feature in the lung related to asbestos-related pleural plaques (although it can occur with pleural thickening of any cause) is helical atelectasis. In general the manifestation of disease is dependent on fiber burden with fewer fibers seen with pleural plaques than mesothelioma or asbestosis. In particular, increasing crocidolite burden is clearly associated with the development of asbestosis (35).

Pleural plaques are usually noted 20 to 30 years after the initial exposure, may be calcified or non-calcified and typically found along the diaphragm and lower thorax between the fifth and eighth ribs laterally and spare the costophrenic sulci (37). Pulmonary parenchymal abnormalities are required for the diagnosis of asbestosis and include curvilinear subpleural lines, parenchymal bands 2 to 5 cm long that traverse the lung at angles inconsistent with vessels, thickened short peripheral lines, and honeycombing (37).

Helical atelectasis occurs when an area of thickened pleura envelops adjacent lung. CT characteristics of helical atelectasis include a mass contiguous with an area of pleural thickening, with evidence of volume loss in the adjacent lung and a comet tail appearance of vessels and bronchi sweeping into the margin of the mass (37).

### Aunt Minnie's Pearls

Volume loss in the involved lobe and comet tail appearance of vessels and bronchi around the mass are classic for helical atelectasis.

Asbestosis = interstitial lung disease secondary to asbestos exposure.

HISTORY: Withheld

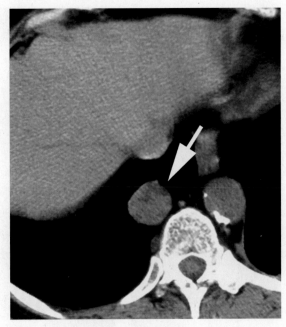

FIGURE 9.16.1

**FINDINGS:** An unenhanced CT scan (Fig. 9.16.1) shows a well-defined nodule in the right lower lobe with mixed soft tissue and fat density (*arrow*).

**DIAGNOSIS:** Pulmonary hamartoma

**DISCUSSION:** A hamartoma is a mass that contains tissues that are normally found in the organ of origin but are disorganized and in abnormal amounts. Because pulmonary hamartomas are of mesenchymal origin comprising mainly of fat and cartilage, they may not fit the true definition of a hamartoma. Pulmonary hamartoma is the most common benign tumor of lung, occurring in 0.25% of the population (38). The presence of characteristic "popcorn" calcification within the mass allows a highly specific plain-film diagnosis. Unfortunately, less than one-third of these masses will show calcification on plain films.

Either localized or generalized fat may be identified in up to 50% of hamartomas on CT. The presence of tissue with density of –40 HU to –120 HU is considered a reliable indicator of fat and therefore hamartomas (38). The observation of fat and calcium on thin-section CT images within a smoothly margin-ated mass <2.5 cm in size virtually excludes other neoplastic possibilities (39). These masses may grow slowly on follow-up chest radiographs, and there-fore management of these patients may still require surgical excision. The proper identification of a pulmonary hamartoma preoperatively, however, may allow conservative nonoperative management or wedge resection of the mass.

## Aunt Minnie's Pearl

The observation of fat and calcium on thin-section CT images within a smoothly marginated mass <2.5 cm in size virtually excludes other neoplastic possibilities.

**HISTORY:** Mild cough in a middle-aged man

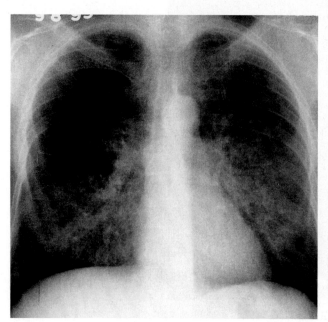

FIGURE 9.17.1

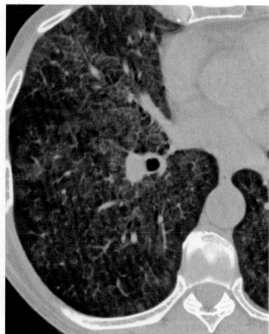

FIGURE 9.17.2

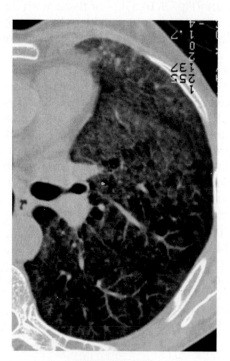

FIGURE 9.17.3

**FINDINGS:** PA view of the chest (Fig. 9.17.1) reveals small ill-defined opacities that approximate the size of a pulmonary acinus (6–10 mm). Kerley B lines are faintly seen in the periphery of the lung, and subpleural edema is identified as thickening of the minor fissure. Two views from an HRCT scan of the lungs (Figs. 9.17.2 and 9.17.3) show ground-glass opacification of the secondary pulmonary lobule, which is outlined by smooth, mild thickening of the interlobular septa.

**DIAGNOSIS:** Alveolar proteinosis

**DISCUSSION:** Pulmonary alveolar proteinosis (PAP) is a condition in which lipoproteinaceous material accumulates in the end air spaces (40). There are three distinct forms of disease: congenital (e.g., mutations in surfactant proteins), secondary (e.g., inhalation of inorganic dusts), and acquired which is considered idiopathic and may be an autoimmune disease against GM–CSF (40). PAP most commonly affects middle-aged males, who may present with mild symptoms of dyspnea, cough, and fatigue and is strongly associated with smoking. Chest radiographs reveal ill-defined acinar opacities with relative sparing of the extreme lung periphery. HRCT is helpful in establishing the diagnosis by demonstrating a characteristic "crazy-paving" pattern comprising ground-glass opacity of the secondary pulmonary lobule surrounded by smooth thickening of the interlobular septa (caused by superimposed edema) that border the lobule (41). The final diagnosis is confirmed by bronchoscopy with bronchoalveolar lavage. The lavage fluid returns opaque or milky white and contains foamy macrophages that stains positive with periodic acid–Schiff.

Patients are treated by whole lung lavage under general anesthesia. This procedure is curative in some patients; other patients will experience relapse and progressive worsening of the disease. PAP carries an increased risk of pulmonary infections, in particular by *Nocardia* species.

## Aunt Minnie's Pearls

The patchwork quilt or crazy paving appearance of the secondary pulmonary lobule on HRCT is characteristic of, but not specific for PAP.

The treatment for symptomatic PAP is whole lung lavage.

HISTORY: A 55-year-old man with subacute onset of high fever and chills

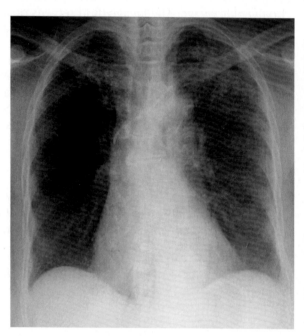

FIGURE 9.18.1

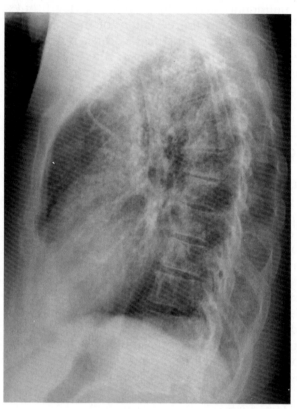

FIGURE 9.18.2

FINDINGS: Frontal and lateral radiographs (Figs. 9.18.1 and 9.18.2) show numerous miliary nodules diffusely throughout both lungs with somewhat more confluent and coalescent nodular opacities in upper lobes. Furthermore, note malpositioned central venous catheter with tip in azygous vein.

DIAGNOSIS: Miliary tuberculosis

DISCUSSION: Miliary tuberculosis (so-called because of the resemblance of the nodules to millet seeds) results from hematogenous dissemination of either primary or postprimary infection. Typical miliary lesions may not be visible on chest radiograph until 3 to 6 weeks after hematogenous dissemination (42). The characteristic findings of miliary TB consist of innumerable, 1- to 3-mm well-marginated nodules scattered diffusely through the lung parenchyma with mild basilar predominance. The nodules reside within the pulmonary interstitium, and the radiographic abnormality is the result of the summation of multiple nodules. Although the nodules are relatively uniform in size, the nodules in the upper lung zone tend to be larger than those in the lower lung zone and without therapy can coalesce. With appropriate treatment radiographic clearing may be extremely rapid. Miliary disease per se is not diagnostic of tuberculosis and may be seen in sarcoidosis and metastatic papillary thyroid carcinoma among other conditions.

## Aunt Minnie's Pearl

Miliary tuberculosis = hematogenous dissemination of infection to the lungs.

**HISTORY:** A 67-year-old female with dyspnea

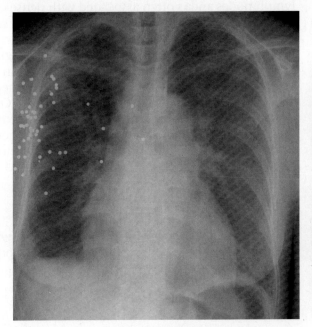

FIGURE 9.19.1

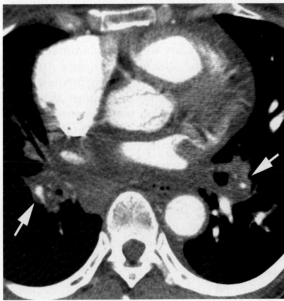

FIGURE 9.19.2

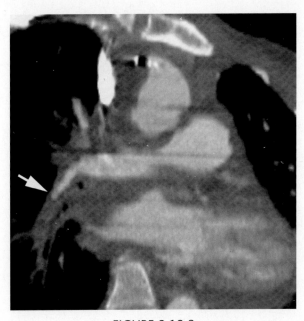

FIGURE 9.19.3

**FINDINGS:** Frontal radiograph (Fig. 9.19.1) shows enlargement of the right ventricle and hila. Axial CT (Fig. 9.19.2) shows soft-tissue attenuation throughout middle and posterior mediastinum with focal narrowing of the lower lobe pulmonary arteries (*arrows*). A coronal reformatted image (Fig. 9.19.3) shows the narrowing and obstruction to flow in the right lower lobe artery to better advantage (*arrow*).

**DIAGNOSIS:** Fibrosing mediastinitis

**DISCUSSION:** Fibrosing mediastinitis is a rare disease characterized by excessive production of fibrous tissue within the mediastinum. Although in many cases the cause remains obscure, many believe that most cases are secondary to fibro-inflammatory response to *Histoplasma capsulatum* antigens. Approximately 40% of patients with fibrosing mediastinitis are asymptomatic and come to medical attention when a chest roentgenogram incidentally reveals a mediastinal mass. Symptoms occur when the fibrous response constricts vital structures and patients may present with superior vena cava syndrome, esophageal obstruction, cough, dyspnea, hemoptysis, or pulmonary venous or arterial obstruction.

Radiographs may be normal or near normal in symptomatic patients. In these cases CT is quite helpful in documenting the extent of disease. Two types of fibrosing medistianitis have been described at CT: focal and diffuse. The focal type most commonly involves right paratracheal and subcarinal lymph nodes and is often associated with dense calcification. In the diffuse form, there is extensive soft tissue throughout the mediastinum with narrowing of bronchial and vascular structures. MR imaging may reveal low T2 signal indicating calcification or dense fibrosis and help differentiate fibrosing mediastinitis from more cellular infiltrative lesions. One neoplasm, sclerosing non-Hodgkin lymphoma, frequently produces fibrosis and may be very difficult to distinguish from fibrosing mediastinitis without large amounts of tissue (43).

## Aunt Minnie's Pearl

Symptomatic involvement of the mediastinum with calcified lymph nodes is most often the sequela of prior histoplasmosis infection.

**HISTORY:** A 68-year-old ship worker with vague chest pain, dry cough, and dyspnea

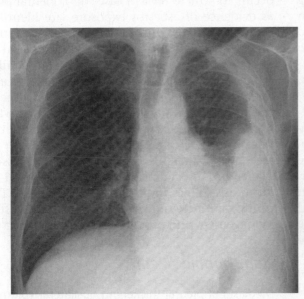

FIGURE 9.20.1

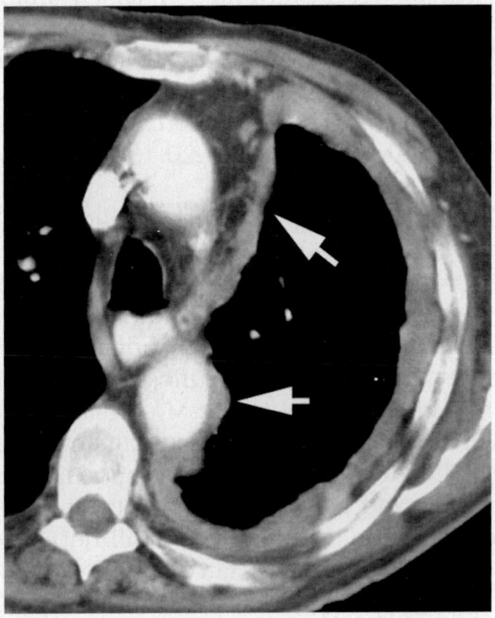

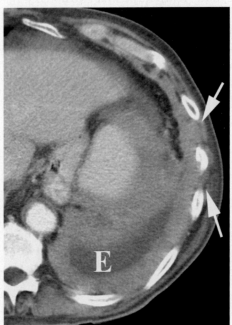

FIGURE 9.20.2

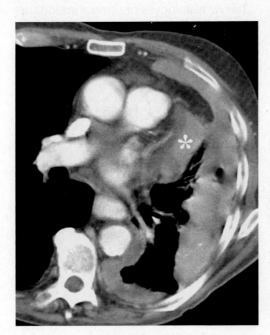

FIGURE 9.20.3

FIGURE 9.20.4

**FINDINGS:** Frontal radiograph (Fig. 9.20.1) shows large partially loculated left pleural effusion with volume loss of left hemithorax. Axial CT images show circumferential pleural thickening including the mediastinal pleura (Fig. 9.20.2, *arrows*), invasion of parietal pericardium (Fig. 9.20.3, *asterisk*) and chest wall invasion (Fig. 9.20.4, *arrows*). Note also loculated pleural effusion (Fig. 9.20.4, *E*).

**DIAGNOSIS:** Malignant pleural mesothelioma

**DISCUSSION:** Mesothelioma is a malignant neoplasm of serosal membranes of the body cavities. Approximately 80% of mesotheliomas originate in the pleural space and represents the most common primary tumor of the pleural cavity. Mesothelioma can be divided into epithelioid, sarcomatoid, and mixed variants. Epithelioid mesotheliomas tend to have the best prognosis and are more likely to be amenable to surgical resection. Most surgeons will not undertake resection in those with sarcomatoid elements. A history of exposure to asbestosis can be obtained from >50% of subjects in most series of patients with mesothelioma. The presenting complaints are chest pain, dyspnea, and recurrent pleural effusions.

Malignant mesothelioma may be suspected on chest radiographs demonstrating irregular, nodular, peripheral pleural opacities with associated ipsilateral pleural effusion. In many cases, encasement of the lung by tumor results in ipsilateral volume loss. Tumor extension into interlobar fissures occurs in 40% to 86% of cases (44). Pleural plaques, as evidence of asbestos exposure, are identified in only 20% of cases of mesothelioma. CT can demonstrate discrete pleural lesions, which would otherwise be obscured by pleural fluid on standard chest radiographs. Pleural lesions range from a focal mass to diffuse, nodular thickening involving the chest wall and mediastinal pleural surfaces. Chest wall and transdiaphragmatic involvement is important to delineate to determine resectability and often evaluated by MR imaging (44). In particular, loss of fat planes and direct extension into extrapleural fat are taken as a direct indication of invasion. PET/CT is gaining an increasing important role in the staging, management and prognosis of mesothelioma (45).

## Aunt Minnie's Pearls

Mediastinal pleural thickening, ipsilateral volume loss, and unilateral pleural effusion should raise the suspicion of mesothelioma.

Tumor histology is of utmost importance in determining resectability of mesotheliomas.

# Case 9.21

**HISTORY:** A 28-year-old HIV+ male with CD4 count of 120 cells/mm$^3$ and nonproductive cough

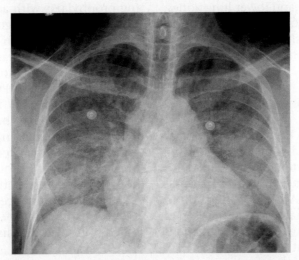

FIGURE 9.21.1

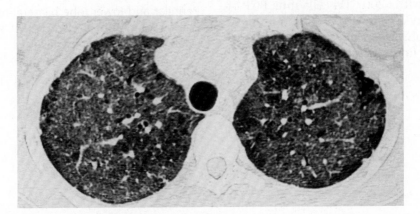

FIGURE 9.21.2

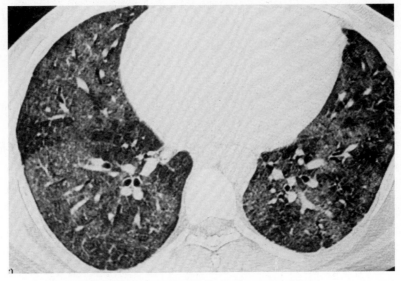

FIGURE 9.21.3

**FINDINGS:** Frontal chest radiograph (Fig. 9.21.1) shows bilateral, symmetrical ground-glass opacities mainly involving middle and lower lung zones. HRCT at the level of the aortic arch and diaphragms (Figs. 9.21.2 and 9.21.3) shows diffuse central ground-glass attenuation without significant interlobular septal thickening.

**DIAGNOSIS:** *Pneumocystis jirovecii* pneumonia

**DISCUSSION:** *Pneumocystis jirovecii* (formerly *P. carinii*) pneumonia (PCP) is one of the leading causes of morbidity and mortality in patients with AIDS and still the most common opportunistic pulmonary infection in patients with HIV infection in the United States. Approximately 25% of cases of pneumonia in HIV patients are related to PCP, and it is important to recognize that 25% of cases of HIV-associated PCP occur in patients who have not yet been diagnosed with HIV (46). In general, PCP develops in patients with >200 CD4 cells/mm. PCP often presents as a dry cough with fever and dyspnea.

Chest radiographs often reveal a perihilar or diffuse symmetric fine reticular pattern or a more granular/"ground-glass" appearance. Predominantly upper lobe disease may be seen in patients undergoing prophylaxis with aerosolized pentamidine (47). It is important to recognize that the chest radiograph in PCP associated with severe immune compromise may be entirely normal and HRCT may be required to confirm the diagnostic impression. The typical HRCT appearance of PCP is extensive ground-glass attenuation that may be patchy or geographic. In addition, there may be superimposed interlobular septal thickening giving the "crazy-paving" appearance. In more advanced disease, parenchymal cysts may be present. Of note, pleural effusions and adenopathy are absent both with chest radiographs and CT, and their presence should raise the possibility of a coexisting separate infection or other superimposed noninfectious disease (46).

## Aunt Minnie's Pearl

Perihilar and lower lobe bilateral reticular opacities on chest radiograph in HIV patient with CD4 count of >200 cells/mm$^3$ suggests PCP.

**HISTORY:** A 38-year-old female with dysphagia and dyspnea

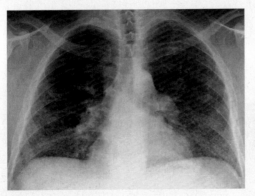

FIGURE 9.22.1

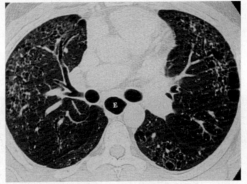

FIGURE 9.22.2

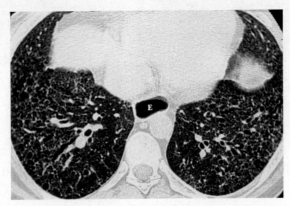

FIGURE 9.22.3

**FINDINGS:** Frontal chest radiograph (Fig. 9.22.1) shows lower lobe predominate basilar and peripheral reticular opacities associated with diminished lung volumes. Also note enlarged central pulmonary arteries from pulmonary arterial hypertension, presumably related to underlying interstitial lung disease. HRCT images at the level of carina and domes of diaphragms (Figs. 9.22.2 and 9.22.3) show predominately basilar and peripheral interlobular septal thickening honeycombing and traction bronchiectasis associated with dilated esophagus (*E*).

**DIAGNOSIS:** Progressive systemic sclerosis

**DISCUSSION:** Progressive systemic sclerosis is characterized by atrophy and sclerosis of many organ systems, including the skin, musculoskeletal system, and heart as well as the lungs. The basic pulmonary lesion is interstitial fibrosis, which may take the form of a fine reticular pattern that becomes more coarse and dense as the disease progresses, eventually producing a reticulonodular pattern. Characteristically, lung volumes are diminished with a basilar and peripheral distribution of disease with or without honeycombing.

HRCT is the method of choice for evaluating early parenchymal involvement and include ground-glass opacity, honeycombing, bronchiectasis, septal and pleural thickening, and subpleural cysts (48). The radiographic pattern is often that of usual interstitial pneumonitis, although histopathologic patterns of usual interstitial pneumonitis or nonspecific interstitial pneumonitis may be found. Although interstitial lung disease is the most common complication of PSS, occurring in up to 75% of cases, the disease is often subclinical and may be asymptomatic in the early stages (49). Esophageal dilatation may be seen on CT in up to 80% of patients with progressive systemic sclerosis. When the esophagus is involved, aspiration into the basal segments of lung may also account for the radiographic abnormalities.

### Aunt Minnie's Pearl

A usual interstitial pneumonitis or nonspecific interstitial pneumonitis pattern of interstitial disease associated with esophageal dilatation should suggest the diagnosis of scleroderma.

HISTORY: A 70-year-old woman with chronic cough

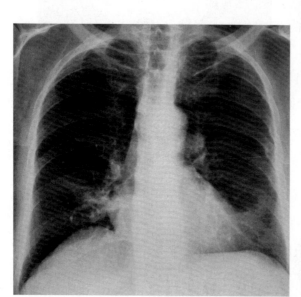

FIGURE 9.23.1

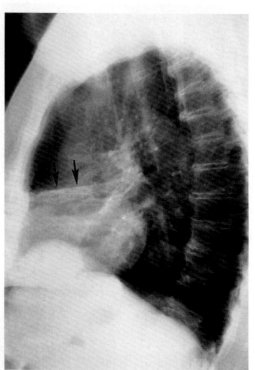

FIGURE 9.23.2

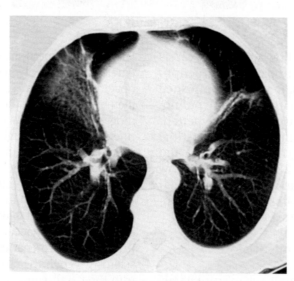

FIGURE 9.23.3

**FINDINGS:** Frontal chest radiograph (Fig. 9.23.1) shows faint opacity obscuring the right and left heart borders. Lateral radiograph (Fig. 9.23.2) shows course reticular opacities (*arrows*), suggestive of bronchiectasis. CT (Fig. 9.23.3) confirms varicoid bronchiectasis confined to the right middle lobe and lingula

**DIAGNOSIS:** Nonclassical *Mycobacterium avium–intracellulare*

**DISCUSSION:** The nontuberculous mycobacteria (NTMB) are a heterogeneous group of organisms that are ubiquitous within the soil. Although it is difficult to distinguish colonization from clinical infection, pulmonary NTMB disease is increasing in prevalence and is most commonly caused by *Mycobacterium avium–intracellulare* (MAI). The best criteria for NTMB pulmonary disease are repeated positive sputum or bronchoalveolar lavage fluid cultures combined with clinical and radiographic signs of infection. MAI can take several forms within the lung. Perhaps the most distinctive appearance is the nonclassic form that typically affects middle-aged White females. Also termed "Lady Windermere Syndrome," the radiographic findings include mild-to-moderate cylindrical bronchiectasis involving the right middle lobe and lingual (50). The spectrum of disease is felt to be related to relatively poor clearance of secretions from these regions followed by colonization of the organism. Chest wall deformities including pectus excavatum and severe scoliosis are thought to predispose individuals to the disease. Centrilobular nodules are often seen in association with bronchiectasis on CT and generally have a "tree-in-bud" appearance reflecting airways spread of disease.

## Aunt Minnie's Pearl

Right middle lobe and lingular bronchiectasis is characteristic of the nonclassical form of MAI.

HISTORY: Withheld

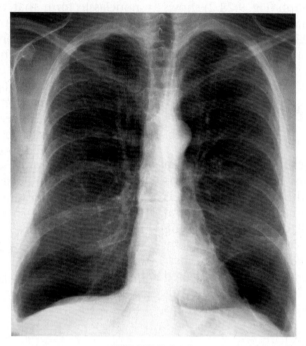

FIGURE 9.24.1

FINDINGS: Frontal chest radiograph (Fig. 9.24.1) shows large lower lobe bullae

DIAGNOSIS: Alpha-1-antitrypsin deficiency (AAT)

DISCUSSION: Emphysema is defined as abnormal permanent enlargement of the airspaces distal to the terminal bronchial caused by alveolar wall destruction with minimal fibrosis. AAT is a hereditary disease encompassing various genetic defects leading to diminished or absent activity of the most prevalent protease inhibitor in serum (51). The imbalance of protease/antiprotease concentration in the lung leads to breakdown of elastin and extracellular matrix leading to lung destruction (51). Radiologists should consider AAT in the differential diagnosis of emphysema in patients under the age of 45, those without emphysema risk factors and basilar predominant emphysema.

AAT is the prototype for panacinar emphysema involving the pulmonary acinus in a uniform and diffused manner, resulting in marked lung destruction. Radiographic findings within the lungs include overinflation and attenuation of bronchovascular markings. These findings predominantly involve lower lobes as opposed to upper lobe distribution traditionally associated with smoking-related emphysema. The main observations on CT scans in AAT are widespread areas of decreased lung attenuation without visible walls and a decrease in the diameter and number of pulmonary vessels in the region of the emphysema (52). As liver disease also occurs in relation to AAT, cirrhosis and its related findings may be revealed at CT. Treatment consists of cessation of smoking, bronchodilators, correcting the deficiency state, and in the most severe cases, lung transplantation (51).

## Aunt Minnie's Pearl

Emphysema in a young individual should raise the suspicion of AAT.

**HISTORY:** A 67-year-old smoker with chest pain, left arm pain and ptosis

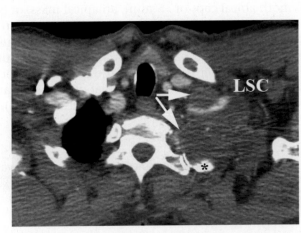

FIGURE 9.25.1

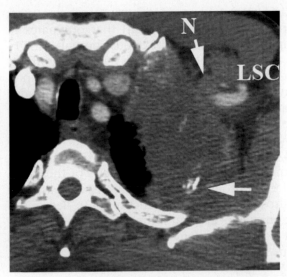

FIGURE 9.25.2

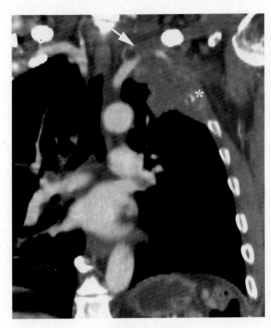

FIGURE 9.25.3

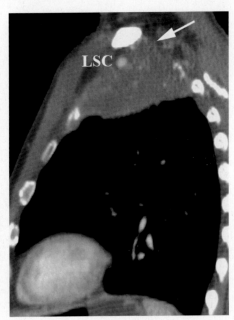

FIGURE 9.25.4

**FINDINGS:** Axial contrast-enhanced CT scan (Fig. 9.25.1) shows left superior sulcus tumor, which invades the chest wall surrounding the left subclavian artery (*LSC, arrows*) and destruction of left second rib (*asterisk*). More inferiorly (Fig. 9.25.2) there is gross chest wall involvement (*arrow*), extension along the left subclavian artery (*LSC*) and enlarged subpectoral lymph node (*N, arrow*). A coronal reformatted image (Fig. 9.25.3) gives a better appreciation for the extent of tumor including relationship to left subclavian artery (*arrow*) and rib destruction (*asterisk*). A sagittal reformatted CT image (Fig. 9.25.4) demonstrates growth posterior to the left subclavian artery (*LSC*) along the expected course of the brachial plexus (*arrow*).

**DIAGNOSIS:** Pancoast tumor

**DISCUSSION:** A pancoast tumor describes a mass lesion (usually lung neoplasm) that originates in the apex of the lung and extends through the visceral and parietal pleura to involve the sympathetic nerve trunks including the stellate ganglion, producing symptoms. The initial description included characteristic signs and symptoms associated with these tumors, including pain in the shoulder or arm (along the distribution of the eighth cervical trunk and first and second thoracic nerve trunks), weakness and atrophy of the muscles of the hand, Horner syndrome (ipsilateral ptosis, miosis, and anhidrosis), and bone destruction (53). Because of their unique location and their involvement of the chest wall, these tumors are generally defined as T3 lesions, but with invasion of the brachial plexus, mediastinal structures, or vertebral bodies these lesions can also be T4 lesions.

At PA and lateral chest radiography, a superior sulcus tumor may manifest as an apical cap or thickening (unilateral apical cap of >5 mm or asymmetry of both apical caps of >5 mm), an apical mass, or bone destruction. MR imaging is preferable to CT in the evaluation of suspected pancoast tumor because it can provide coronal and sagittal images of the tumor and can better demonstrate the relationship of the tumor to the chest wall, brachial plexus, subclavian vessels, and cervical and thoracic vertebrae (53).

## Aunt Minnie's Pearl

A tumor in the superior sulcus of the lung with invasion into the chest wall and involves the brachial plexus is termed a pancoast tumor.

**HISTORY:** A 27-year-old male with dyspnea and chest pain

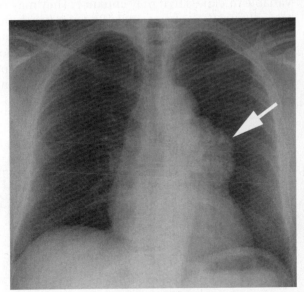

FIGURE 9.26.1

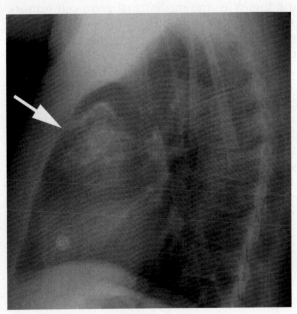

FIGURE 9.26.2

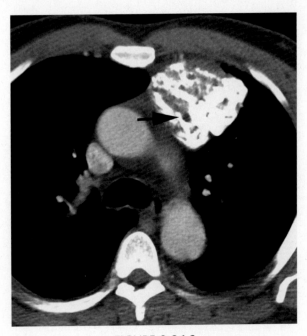

FIGURE 9.26.3

**FINDINGS:** PA and lateral views (Figs. 9.26.1 and 9.26.2) reveal partially calcified anterior mediastinal mass (*arrows*). Axial CT image (Fig. 9.26.3) through mediastinum demonstrates an anterior mediastinal mass with striated calcifications mixed with soft-tissue density and small focus of fat (*arrow*).

**DIAGNOSIS:** Mature teratoma

**DISCUSSION:** Germ cell tumors occur most frequently in the gonads but can occur in extragonadal location in rare instances, most commonly in anterior mediastinum. During embryogenesis, the primitive germ cells descend along the midline from the yolk sac endoderm to the gonads. The prevailing theory is that mediastinal germ cell tumors are felt to arise from multipotent germ cells that have become "misplaced" or arrested in their migration, most often near the thymus (54). Teratomas are a specific category of germ cell neoplasms and can be subdivided into mature (well-differentiated), immature (containing immature mesenchymal tissue or neuroepithelial tissue, and those with malignant components (55). Mature teratoma is the most common histologic type of mediastinal germ cell tumor.

At radiography teratomas usually appear as a sharply marginated, round or lobulated anterior mediastinal mass that extends to one side of the midline.

Calcification, ossification, or even teeth may be visible on chest radiographs (54). At CT, these tumors are heterogeneous, well-defined masses with walls of variable thickness that may enhance. They may contain all four tissue types, including soft tissue, fluid, fat, and calcium, but fluid-containing cystic components are usually prominent (54). On rare occasions, mature teratomas may rupture into the pleural space resulting in a pleural effusion and mimic the malignant germ cell varieties.

### Aunt Minnie's Pearl

Presence of fat and calcification within an anterior mediastinal mass is consistent mature teratoma.

HISTORY: A 47-year-old female with acute myelogenous leukemia

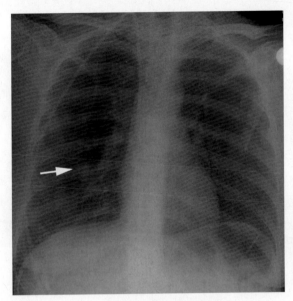

FIGURE 9.27.1

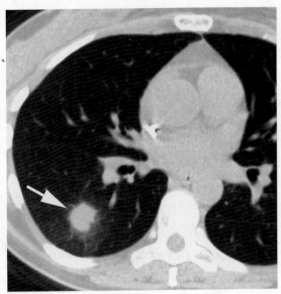

FIGURE 9.27.2

FINDINGS: Chest radiograph (Fig. 9.27.1) demonstrates ill-defined nodule in right mid lung (*arrow*). Transverse chest CT image (Fig. 9.27.2) confirms the presence of nodule will ill-defined borders and a ground-glass halo (*arrow*).

DIAGNOSIS: Invasive aspergillosis

DISCUSSION: Aspergillus can cause broad spectrum of pulmonary diseases, usually occurring in patients who have preexisting lung disease or some degree of immunological abnormality. The classification of pulmonary aspergillosis includes aspergilloma, allergic bronchopulmonary aspergillosis, chronic necrotizing aspergillosis, and invasive aspergillosis. Invasive aspergillosis is characterized by the involvement of normal lung tissue by *Aspergillus* organisms usually resulting in significant tissue damage and necrosis. It almost always occurs in immunosuppressed patients, particularly in neutropenic patients. Infiltration of lung tissue by fungus occurs with invasion of small arteries, vascular occlusion, and often infarction of involved lung (23).

Radiographic evaluation, although nonspecific, may reveal poorly defined pulmonary nodules or air-space consolidation early in the disease process. Characteristic CT findings comprise nodules surrounded by a halo of ground-glass attenuation ("halo sign") or pleura-based, wedge-shaped areas of consolidation. These findings correspond to hemorrhagic infarcts or adjacent hemorrhage (23). Typical findings occur during the healing process when nodules cavitate and air crescent characteristically develops. The presence of air crescent reflects lung necrosis where the sequestrum representing necrotic lung within the cavity. This finding should not be confused with mycetoma within the preexisting cavity, as the two entities are unrelated.

## Aunt Minnie's Pearls

Nodule surrounded by a halo of ground glass in a patient with severe neutropenia is consistent with invasive *Aspergillus*.

The presence of necrotic tissue in invasive aspergillosis is a different entity than a mycetoma that develops within preexisting cavity.

**HISTORY:** A 35-year-old smoker with cough and chest pain

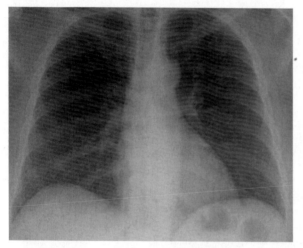

FIGURE 9.28.1

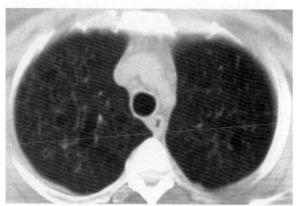

FIGURE 9.28.2

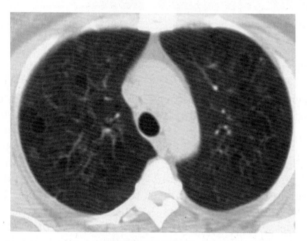

FIGURE 9.28.3

**FINDINGS:** PA radiograph (Fig. 9.28.1) reveals subtle upper lung zone predominant reticular opacities with questionable cystic lucencies. Axial CT images (Figs. 9.28.2 and 9.28.3) confirm presence of multiple cysts of various shapes and sizes. Some cysts coalesce into larger, more irregular structures with bizarre shapes.

**DIAGNOSIS:** Pulmonary Langerhans Cell Histiocytosis (PLCH)

**DISCUSSION:** Pulmonary Langerhans cell histiocytosis (PLCH) is a rare pulmonary disorder that typically affects young adults and is associated with cigarette smoking (56). Common presenting symptoms include cough and dyspnea. Most patients with PLCH exhibit chest radiographic abnormalities (57). Early in the disease, the most common radiographic manifestation is that of small nodules that are usually bilateral and symmetric in distribution. The nodules are predominantly distributed in the upper and middle lung zones with sparing of the lung bases near the costophrenic sulci, likely resulting from the inhalational component of the disease. As the disease progresses, reticulonodular abnormalities may predominate. Further progression may result in a predominance of cystic changes. As cysts become more numerous, nodules tend to occur less frequently. Lung volumes are normal or increased in most patients.

Chest CT, HRCT in particular, is superior to radiography in demonstrating the morphology and distribution of lung abnormalities. In most patients the main imaging feature is a combination of nodular and cystic lesions (57). Cystic lesions are the most common HRCT feature of PLCH and usually measure <10 mm in diameter but may be as large as 20 mm. Cyst walls may be thin and barely perceptible or may appear thick and nodular on HRCT scans. Although they may manifest as round or ovoid cystic spaces, they may also exhibit bizarre configurations. Cysts are often seen in association with nodules but may be the only HRCT finding. The nodules are characteristically irregular and follow a centrilobular distribution. The nodules may be few or innumerable, and they typically measure 1 to 5 mm in diameter but may be larger. Some authors have postulated that the natural history of PLCH is a progression from early-stage nodules to cavitary nodules, to thick-walled cysts, and finally to thin-walled cysts.

## Aunt Minnie's Pearl

Bilateral pulmonary nodules with predilection for the middle and upper lung zones and relative sparing of the lung bases are highly suggestive of PLCH, particularly if the patient is a cigarette smoker.

**HISTORY:** A 74-year-old male with bloody sputum, cough, and night sweats

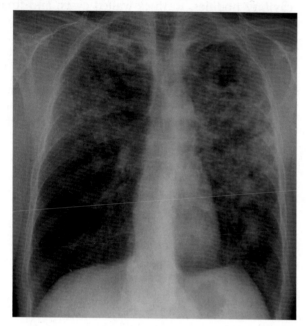

FIGURE 9.29.1

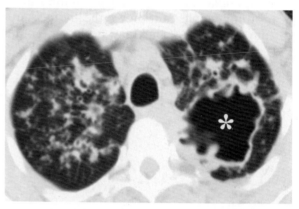

FIGURE 9.29.2

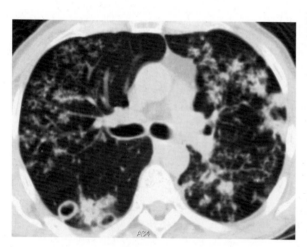

FIGURE 9.29.3

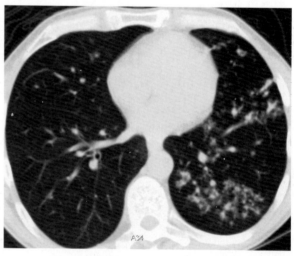

FIGURE 9.29.4

**FINDINGS:** Frontal view of the chest (Fig. 9.29.1) show cavitary lesion in left upper lobe associated with multiple ill-defined nodular opacities in both lungs. Axial CT images (Figs. 9.29.2 to 9.29.4) demonstrate the thick-walled cavity in the apical–posterior segment of the left upper lobe (Fig. 9.29.2, *asterisk*) with multiple small, centrilobular nodules connected to linear branching opacities (tree-in-bud) in both lungs as a result of endobronchial spread of disease.

**DIAGNOSIS:** Postprimary pulmonary tuberculosis—cavitary tuberculosis with endobronchial spread of infection

DISCUSSION: Pulmonary tuberculosis is classically divided into primary and postprimary (reactivation) tuberculosis. Primary tuberculosis typically involves middle and lower lobes and manifests radiologically as parenchymal disease, lymphadenopathy, pleural effusion, miliary disease, or atelectasis. Postprimary disease occurs in 5% to 10% of subjects with prior tuberculosis and results from "reactivation" of a previously dormant infection in 90% of cases; in a minority of cases, it represents continuation of the primary disease (so-called progressive primary disease) (58). The earliest radiologic finding in postprimary tuberculosis is the development of patchy, ill-defined segmental consolidation with a predilection for the apical or posterior segment of the upper lobes or the superior segment of the lower lobes. Tuberculous cavitation most commonly occurs within areas of consolidation and indicates a high likelihood of activity. Cavitation, the hallmark of postprimary tuberculosis, affects approximately 50% of patients (59). The cavities typically have thick, irregular walls. If left untreated, the disease progresses to lobar or complete lung opacification and destruction. Residual thin-walled cavities may be seen in both active and inactive disease.

Endobronchial spread is the most common complication of tuberculous cavitation and represents a chronic granulomatous infection in which active organisms spread via airways after caseous necrosis of bronchial walls (58). HRCT is sensitive in the detection of early endobronchial spread of disease, which manifests as small, poorly defined centrilobular nodules and branching centrilobular areas of increased opacity ("tree-in-bud" appearance) (59). Up to 40% of patients with postprimary tuberculosis have a marked fibrotic response, which manifests as atelectasis of the upper lobe, retraction of the hilum, compensatory lower lobe hyperinflation, and mediastinal shift toward the fibrotic lung.

## Aunt Minnie's Pearl

Nodules with tree-in-bud appearance in association with thick-walled cavity are seen in active tuberculosis with endobronchial spread of infection.

# Case 9.30

**HISTORY:** A 33-year-old female with pneumothorax following ultrasound-guided thoracentesis

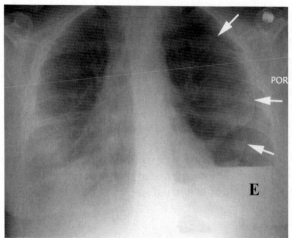

FIGURE 9.30.1

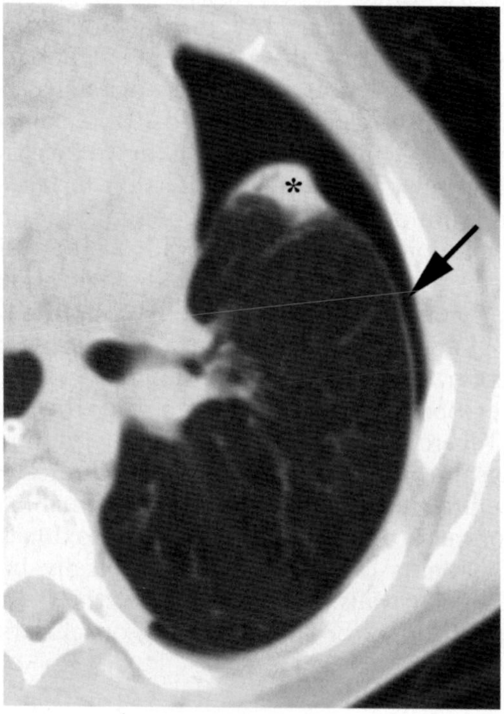

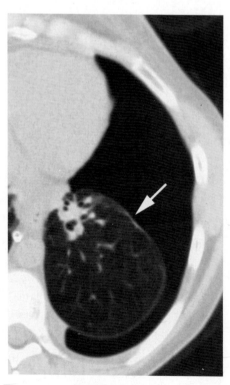

FIGURE 9.30.2

FIGURE 9.30.3

**FINDINGS:** Frontal view of the chest (Fig. 9.30.1) following ultrasound-guided thoracentesis shows a large left pneumothorax (*arrows*) without mediastinal shift and residual left pleural effusion (*E*). Axial CT images (Figs. 9.30.2 and 9.30.3) demonstrate thickening of the visceral pleura (*arrows*) as well as focal region of subpleural atelectasis (*asterisk*).

**DIAGNOSIS:** Trapped lung

**DISCUSSION:** Pneumothorax is the most common complication following thoracentesis. In some cases it can be related to the choice of needle, operator technique, or presence of underlying lung disease. Ultrasound guidance has been shown to limit the incidence of post-thoracentesis pneumothorax, presumably by reducing the risk of puncturing through the visceral pleura. If meticulous technique is used to prevent the entry of outside air and the visceral pleura is not transgressed, gas may still be found on occasion within the pleura in the setting of nonexpandable lung (60). This may either be the result of a central obstructing lesion or be the result of the restriction of the visceral pleura.

A trapped lung occurs when there is visceral pleural restriction in the absence of active pleural disease (61). This can be then be distinguished from an entrapped lung where there is active pleural disease as may be seen with an empyema or malignant effusion. In either case, negative intrapleural pressures can be seen with pleural manometry. Because of pleural restriction and adhesions, the pneumothorax related to visceral pleural restriction can be loculated on conventional radiography. At CT, visceral pleura thickening can be detected when there is residual air in the pleural space (61).

Ultimately, the pleural space will reaccumulate fluid in the absence of other intervention. Chest tube drainage is generally ineffective at re-expanding the lung and treatment needs to be directed at the underlying cause or with removal of the pleural peel via decortication.

## Aunt Minnie's Pearl

A pneumothorax following thoracentesis is usually diagnostic information, not a complication.

HISTORY: A 75-year-old man with progressive shortness of breath and nonproductive cough over the last year

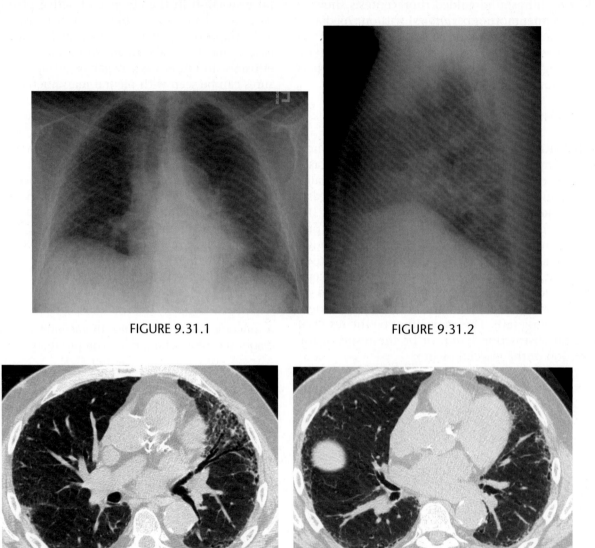

FIGURE 9.31.1                    FIGURE 9.31.2

FIGURE 9.31.3                    FIGURE 9.31.4

FINDINGS: PA and lateral chest radiographs show basal and peripheral predominant subpleural reticular opacities (Figs. 9.31.1 and 9.31.2). Axial CT images (Figs. 9.31.3 and 9.31.4) reveal subpleural reticular opacities, honeycombing, and traction bronchiectasis with a basal and peripheral distribution.

DIAGNOSIS: Usual interstitial pneumonia (UIP)

DISCUSSION: UIP is a histologic lung injury pattern resulting from disordered lung repair. The pathologic hallmarks are temporal and spatial heterogeneity (i.e., areas of mature and immature collagen admixed with regions of normal lung) and the presence of fibroblastic foci (62). This pattern of lung injury can also be seen in many other conditions, including collagen vascular diseases, drug reactions, asbestosis, and chronic hypersensitivity pneumonitis. After all other causes of UIP have been excluded, the disease is considered to be idiopathic pulmonary fibrosis (IPF).

UIP has a substantially worse prognosis than the other forms of interstitial pneumonitis such as nonspecific interstitial pneumonitis and cryptogenic organizing pneumonia. The median survival from the time of diagnosis of IPF is between 2.5 and 3.5 years.

Because the disease is one of fibrosis, treatment with steroids or other antiinflammatory agents is not efficacious.

The classic chest radiograph pattern includes low lung volumes and course reticular or reticulonodular interstitial disease with a basal and peripheral predominance. At HRCT, UIP can be confidently diagnosed when subpleural reticular opacities, honeycombing, and traction bronchiectasis with a basal and peripheral distribution are present, any ground-glass opacity present is less than the corresponding fibrosis, and key features such as centrilobular nodules or extensive emphysema are absent (63). In these cases, and in the context of an appropriate clinical examination, open lung biopsy is not necessary to confirm the diagnosis. In the absence of honeycomb change, the pattern is compatible with but not diagnostic of UIP and in such cases lung biopsy should be contemplated.

## Aunt Minnie's Pearl

The presence of UIP, as seen in the clinical entity IPF, can be confidently diagnosed when subpleural reticular opacities, honeycombing, and traction bronchiectasis are present with a basal and peripheral distribution, and atypical features are absent.

HISTORY: A 47-year-old man with sinusitis and renal insufficiency.

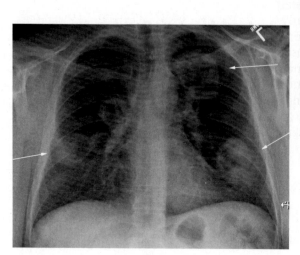

FIGURE 9.32.1

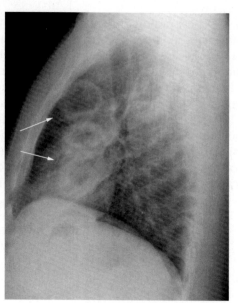

FIGURE 9.32.2

FINDINGS: PA and lateral chest radiographs show multiple thick-walled cavitary masses (*arrows*) in both lungs (Figs. 9.32.1 and 9.32.2).

DIAGNOSIS: Wegener granulomatosis

DISCUSSION: Wegener granulomatosis is a necrotizing vasculitis of mainly small and medium-sized vessels, which clinically presents as the triad of upper airway disease (e.g., sinusitis, otitis, nasal mucosa ulcers, bone deformities, subglottic stenosis), lower airway involvement (cough, chest pain, hemoptysis), and glomerulonephritis. Up to 90% of patients with active disease have elevated cytoplasmic–antineutrophil cytoplasmic antibody or c-ANCA titers.

The most common pulmonary radiologic manifestation of Wegener granulomatosis is waxing and waning pulmonary nodules and masses, which can be single or multiple and range in size from a few millimeters to >10 cm (64). Central cavitation occurs in approximately half of cases and is more common in larger nodules and masses >2 cm in diameter.

Thick- and thin-walled cavities may be seen. Occasionally, the dominant pulmonary finding may be ground-glass opacification and consolidation, which is suggestive of hemorrhage or possibly pulmonary edema related to underlying renal failure. Upper airway involvement is difficult to appreciate on chest radiographs but may be demonstrated as smooth or nodular circumferential tracheobronchial thickening. Pleural effusions and mediastinal lymphadenopathy may also be seen.

## Aunt Minnie's Pearls

Wegener granulomatosis classically presents as the triad of upper airway disease, lung involvement, and glomerulonephritis.

The most common pulmonary radiologic manifestation of Wegener granulomatosis is waxing and waning pulmonary nodules and masses up to 10 cm in diameter, with central cavitation.

**HISTORY:** A 69-year-old woman with history of adenocarcinoma of the upper lobe of the right lung

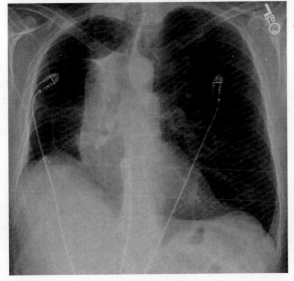

FIGURE 9.33.1

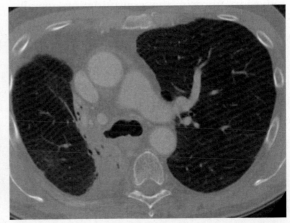

FIGURE 9.33.2

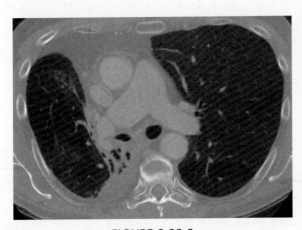

FIGURE 9.33.3

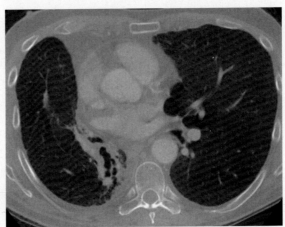

FIGURE 9.33.4

**FINDINGS:** PA radiograph (Fig. 9.33.1) and axial CT images of the chest (Figs. 9.33.2 to 9.33.4) demonstrate right-sided volume loss, dense consolidation, and bronchiectasis with adjacent pleural thickening. There is a sharp border between the consolidation and the more normal-appearing lung parenchyma, which does not correspond to a normal anatomic boundary.

**DIAGNOSIS:** Radiation fibrosis

**DISCUSSION:** Radiation-induced lung disease (RILD) owing to radiation therapy has many manifestations that are confined to the radiation field and are dependent on the interval after completion of therapy (22). In the acute phase, RILD appears as ground-glass opacity, consolidation, or nodular opacities ("radiation pneumonitis," occurring 4 to 12 weeks after completion of therapy), but in the late phase, it characteristically appears as traction bronchiectasis, volume loss, linear scarring, and consolidation ("radiation fibrosis", occurring 6 to 12 months after completion of therapy and possibly progressing for up to 2 years prior to stability). In some cases radiation pneumonitis may resolve, without progressing to fibrosis.

In radiation fibrosis, the consolidation usually coalesces and has a sharp interface corresponding to the radiation field, with more normal-appearing lung parenchyma adjacent to the affected area. These boundaries correspond to the radiation field rather than anatomic boundaries. Associated pleural thickening and effusion may occur. Ipsilateral displacement of the mediastinum and elevation of the ipsilateral hemidiaphragm are the result of volume loss on the affected side.

## Aunt Minnie's Pearl

Late manifestations of radiation fibrosis include volume loss and bronchiectasis with a sharp interface between normal and abnormal lung corresponding to the radiation field that usually becomes evident 6 to 12 months after completion of therapy. Progression is possible for up to 2 years prior to stability.

# Case 9.34

HISTORY: A 39-year-old man with long-standing asthma

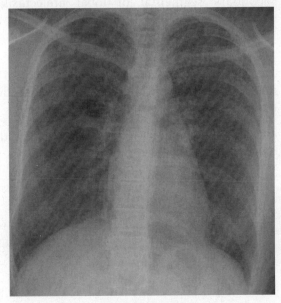

FIGURE 9.34.1

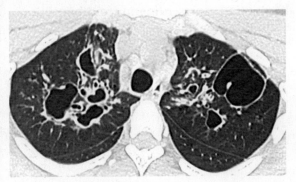

FIGURE 9.34.2

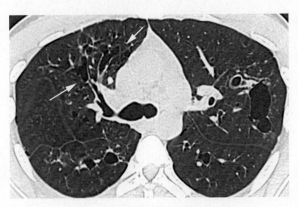

FIGURE 9.34.3

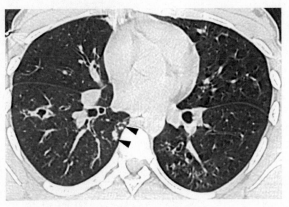

FIGURE 9.34.4

FINDINGS: PA radiograph (Fig. 9.34.1) shows areas of bronchiectasis predominantly in a central and upper lobe distribution. Axial CT images (Figs. 9.34.2 to 9.34.4) demonstrate areas of bronchial wall thickening, saccular bronchiectasis (Fig. 9.34.3, *arrows*), and mucoid impaction involving the segmental and subsegmental bronchi (Fig. 9.34.4, *arrowheads*).

DIAGNOSIS: Allergic bronchopulmonary aspergillosis (ABPA)

DISCUSSION: ABPA is on the spectrum of pulmonary disease caused by *Aspergillus* species and is characteristically seen in patients with a history of long-standing asthma and occasionally cystic fibrosis. A complex hypersensitivity reaction to the *Aspergillus* organisms, including a type I hypersensitivity reaction (IgE and IgG release) and type III hypersensitivity reaction (formation of antigen–antibody immune complexes) results in the attraction of eosinophils and mast cells leading to vasodilation and bronchoconstriction (65). The end result is plugs of inspissated mucus containing eosinophils and rare *Aspergillus* organisms in the segmental and subsegmental bronchi, with bronchial wall damage and bronchiectasis with mucoid impaction occurring as a result of excessive mucus production and abnormal ciliary function.

Radiographic and CT findings in ABPA include bronchiectasis (especially saccular), bronchial wall-thickening, and tubular opacities in a bronchial distribution representing mucoid impaction in the abnormally dilated bronchi ("finger-in-glove" opacities). These findings predominate in the upper and central airways. The impacted, inspissated mucus may have high attenuation (66). Secondary segmental or lobar atelectasis may occur.

## Aunt Minnie's Pearls

ABPA rather than true infection is a hyperreactive immune response to *Aspergillus* species.

Although uncommon, radiographically high-density mucus plugs can help to suggest the diagnosis.

HISTORY: A 62-year-old man with splenomegaly and pancytopenia

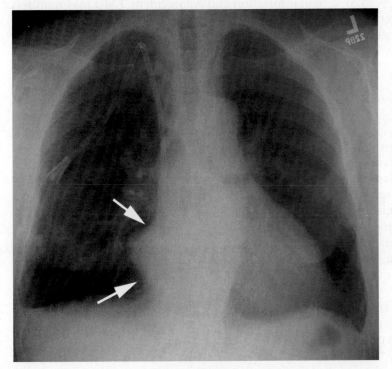

FIGURE 9.35.1

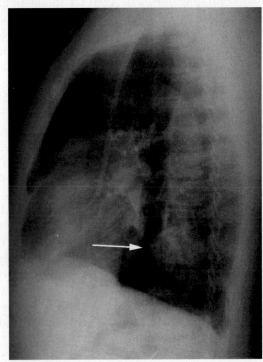

FIGURE 9.35.2

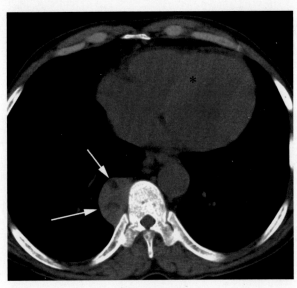

FIGURE 9.35.3

FINDINGS: PA and lateral chest radiographs (Figs. 9.35.1 and 9.35.2) show a lobulated right paravertebral mass (*arrows*). Axial CT image (Fig. 9.35.3) demonstrates well-demarcated right paravertebral soft tissue mass containing fat (*arrows*). Note also the presence of anemia as noted by visibility of intraventricular septum (*asterisk*).

DIAGNOSIS: Extramedullary hematopoiesis (EMH) associated with idiopathic myelofibrosis

DISCUSSION: EMH is the result of insufficient bone marrow hematopoiesis and can occur with various disorders, most commonly congenital anemias (e.g., sickle cell disease, thalasemmia, hereditary spherocytosis) and myeloproliferative disorders (chronic myelogenous leukemia, polycythemia vera, essential thrombocytosis, myelofibrosis). It can also occur in any disease that results in diffuse bone marrow replacement, such as lymphoma or metastatic disease.

EMH has been reported in various organs and organ systems, including the thyroid, prostate, pericardium, kidneys, and lungs. However, it typically involves the reticuloendothelial system, including the liver and spleen, where there is often diffuse organ infiltration and enlargement. EMH may manifest as pseudotumors, most classically in the paravertebral region of the chest, where the masses are slow-growing and do not cause erosion of the adjacent vertebral bodies (67). The typical appearance is that of unilateral or bilateral, sharply delineated, often lobulated paravertebral masses along the lower thoracic spine, which on CT appear as heterogeneous masses with or without macroscopic fat and enhancement. Long-standing manifestations may result in fatty replacement or iron deposition but do not typically calcify. Technetium-99m sulfur colloid imaging may be helpful in diagnosis. Fine-needle aspiration can confirm the diagnosis in equivocal cases if necessary.

## Aunt Minnie's Pearl

EMH should be considered in cases of long-standing anemias (e.g., sickle cell disease, thalasemmia) and myeloproliferative disorders as a cause of paravertebral masses.

# REFERENCES

1. Barnes NA, Pilling DW. Bronchopulmonary foregut malformations: Embryology, radiology and quandary. Eur Radiol 2003;13(12):2659–2673.
2. Petersen G, Martin U, Singhal A, et al. Intralobar sequestration in the middle-aged and elderly adult: Recognition and radiographic evaluation. J Thorac Cardiovasc Surg 2003; 26(6):2086–2090.
3. Glazer CS, Rose CS, Lynch DA. Clinical and radiologic manifestations of hypersensitivity pneumonitis. J Thorac Imaging 2002;17(4):261–272.
4. Silva CI, Churg A, Müller NL. Hypersensitivity pneumonitis: spectrum of high-resolution CT and pathologic findings. AJR Am J Roentgenol 2007;188(2):334–344.
5. Fliegauf M, Benzing T, Omran H. When cilia go bad: Cilia defects and ciliopathies. Nat Rev Mol Cell Biol 2007;8(11): 880–893.
6. Kennedy MP, Noone PG, Leigh MW, et al. High-resolution CT of patients with primary ciliary dyskinesia. AJR Am J Roentgenol 2007;188(5):1232–1238.
7. Pedicelli G, Ciarpaglini LL, De Santis M, et al. Congenital bronchial atresia (CBA). A critical review of CBA as a disease entity and presentation of a case series. Radiol Med 2005; 110(5–6):544–553.
8. Zylak CJ, Eyler WR, Spizarny DL, et al. Developmental lung anomalies in the adult: Radiologic–pathologic correlation. Radiographics 2002;22(suppl):25–43.
9. Berrocal T, Madrid C, Novo S, et al. Congenital anomalies of the tracheobronchial tree, lung, and mediastinum: Embryology, radiology, and pathology. Radiographics 2004;24(1):e17.
10. Gaeta M, Vinci S, Minutoli F, et al. CT and MRI findings of mucin-containing tumors and pseudotumors of the thorax: Pictorial review. Eur Radiol 2002;12(1):181–189.
11. Fazel A, Moezardalan K, Varadarajulu S, et al. The utility and the safety of EUS-guided FNA in the evaluation of duplication cysts. Gastrointest Endosc 2005;62(4):575–578.
12. Abbott GF, Rosado-de-Christenson ML, Frazier AA, et al. Lymphangioleiomyomatosis: Radiologic–pathologic correlation. Radiographics 2005;25:803–828.
13. Esther Pallisa, Pilar Sanz, Antonio Roman, et al. Lymphangioleiomyomatosis: Pulmonary and abdominal findings with pathologic correlation. Radiographics 2002;22:185.
14. Gossage JR, Kanj G. Pulmonary arteriovenous malformations. A state of the art review. Am J Resp Crit Care Med 1998;158:643–661.
15. White RI Jr, Mitchell SE, Barth KH, et al. Angioarchitecture of pulmonary arteriovenous malformations: An important consideration before embolotherapy. AJR Am J Roentgenol 1983;140:681–686.
16. Remy J, Remy-Jardin M, Giraud F, et al. Angioarchitecture of pulmonary arteriovenous malformations: Clinical utility of three-dimensional helical CT. Radiology 1994;191:657–664.
17. Golden R. The effect of bronchostenosis upon the roentgen ray shadows in carcinoma of the bronchus. AJR Am J Roentgenol 1925;13:21–30.
18. Woodring JH, Reed JC. Radiographic manifestations of lobar atelectasis. J Thorac Imaging 1996;11:109–144.
19. Kattan KR, Eyler WR, Felson B. The juxtaphrenic peak in upper lobe collapse. Radiology 1980;134:763–765.
20. Groskin SG. Heitzman's The lung: Radiologic–pathologic correlations, 3rd ed. St. Louis, MO; Mosby, 1993;419–428.
21. Honda O, Johkoh T, Ichikado K, et al. Comparison of high resolution CT findings of sarcoidosis, lymphoma, and lymphangitic carcinoma: Is there any difference of involved interstitium? J Comput Assist Tomogr 1999;23:374–379.
22. Choi YW, Munden RF, Erasmus JJ, et al. Effects of radiation therapy on the lung: Radiologic appearances and differential diagnosis. Radiographics 2004;24:985–998.
23. Franquet T, Müller NL, Giménez A, et al. Spectrum of pulmonary aspergillosis: Histologic, clinical, and radiologic findings. Radiographics 2001;21:825–837.
24. Libshitz HI, Atkinson GW, Israel HL. Pleural thickening as a manifestation of Aspergillus superinfection. AJR Am J Roentgenol 1974;120:883–886.
25. Soubani AO, Chandrasekar PH. The clinical spectrum of pulmonary aspergillosis. Chest 2002;121:1988–1999.
26. Camus P, Martin WJ, Rosenow EC. Amiodarone pulmonary toxicity. Clin Chest Med 2004;25:65–75.
27. Rossi SE, Erasmus JJ, McAdams P, et al. Pulmonary drug toxicity: radiologic and pathologic manifestations. Radiographics 2000;5:1245–1259.
28. Kuhlman JE, Teigen C, Ren H, et al. Amiodarone pulmonary toxicity: CT findings in symptomatic patients. Radiology 1990;177:121–125.
29. Iannuzzi MC, Rybicki BA, Teirstein AS. Sarcoidosis. N Engl J Med 2007;357(21):2153–2165.
30. Vagal AS, Shipley R, Meyer CA. Radiological manifestations of sarcoidosis. Clin Dermatol 2007;25:312–325.
31. Goldhaber SZ, Elliott CG. Acute pulmonary embolism: Part I: Epidemiology, pathophysiology, and diagnosis. Circulation 2003;108(22):2726–2729.
32. Quiroz R, Kucher N, Zou KH, et al. Clinical validity of a negative computed tomography scan in patients with suspected pulmonary embolism: A systematic review. JAMA 2005;293(16):2012–2017.
33. Ravenel JG, Kipfmueller F, Schoepf UJ. CT angiography with multidetector-row CT for detection of acute pulmonary embolus. Sem Roentgen 2005;40:11–19.
34. Quiroz R, Kucher N, Schoepf UJ, et al. Right ventricular enlargement on chest computed tomography: Prognostic role in acute pulmonary embolism. Circulation 2004;109(20): 2401–2404.
35. Mossman BT, Churg A. Mechanisms in the pathogenesis of asbestosis and silicosis. Am J Respir Crit Care Med 1998; 157:1666–1680.
36. Chong S, Lee KS, Chung MJ, et al. Pneumoconiosis: Comparison of imaging and pathologic findings. Radiographics 2006;26:59–77.
37. Roach HD, Davies GJ, Attanoos R, et al. Asbestos: When the dust settles an imaging review of asbestos-related disease. Radiographics 2002;22(suppl):167–184.
38. Gaerte SC, Meyer CA, Winer-Muram HT, et al. Fat-containing lesions of the chest. Radiographics 2002;22(suppl):61–78.
39. Siegelman SS, Khouri NF, Scott WW Jr, et al. Pulmonary hamartoma: CT findings. Radiology 1986;160:313–317.
40. Trapnell BC, Whitsett JA, Nakata K. Pulmonary alveolar proteinosis. N Engl J Med 2003;349(26):2527–2539.
41. Rossi SE, Erasmus JJ, Volpacchio M, et al. "Crazy-paving" pattern at thin-section CT of the lungs: Radiologic–pathologic overview. Radiographics 2003;23:1509–1519.
42. Leung AN. Pulmonary tuberculosis: The essentials. Radiology 1999;210:307–322.
43. Rossi ER, McAdams HP, Rosado-de-Christenson ML, et al. Fibrosing mediastinits. Radiographics 2001;21:737–757.
44. Wang ZJ, Reddy GP, Gotway MB, et al. Malignant pleural mesothelioma: Evaluation with CT, MR imaging, and PET. Radiographics 2004;24:105–119.
45. Truong MT, Marom EM, Erasmus JJ. Preoperative evaluation of patients with malignant pleural mesothelioma: Role of integrated CT-PET imaging. J Thorac Imaging 2006;21: 146–153.

46. Aviram G, Fishman JE, Boiselle PM. Thoracic infections in human immunodeficiency virus/acquired immune deficiency syndrome. Semin Roentgenol 2007;42(1):23–36.

47. Boiselle PM, Crans CA, Kaplan MA. The changing face of *Pneumocystis carinii* pneumonia in AIDS patients. AJR Am J Roentgenol 1999;172:1301–1309.

48. Franquet T. High resolution CT of lung disease related to collagen vascular disease. Radiol Clin North Am 2001;39:1171–1187.

49. Arroliga AC, Podell DN, Mathay RA. Pulmonary manifestations of scleroderma. J Thorac Imaging 1992;7:30–45.

50. Erasmus JJ, McAdams HP, Farrell MA, et al. Pulmonary nontuberculous mycobacterial infection: Radiologic manifestations. Radiographics 1999;19:1487–1505.

51. American Thoracic Society; European Respiratory Society. American Thoracic Society/European Respiratory Society statement: Standards for the diagnosis and management of individuals with alpha-1 antitrypsin deficiency. Am J Respir Crit Care Med 2003;168:818–900.

52. Shaker SB, Stavngaard T, Stolk J, et al. Alpha1-antitrypsin deficiency. 7: Computed tomographic imaging in alpha1-antitrypsin deficiency. Thorax 2004;59:986–991.

53. Rusch VW. Management of Pancoast tumours. Lancet Oncol 2006;7:997–1005.

54. Rosado-de-Christenson ML, Templeton PA, Moran CA. Mediastinal germ cell tumors: radiologic and pathologic correlation. Radiographics 1992;12:1013.

55. Moran CA, Suster S. Primary germ cell tumors of the mediastinum. Analysis of 322 cases with special emphasis on teratomatous lesions and a proposal for histopathologic classification and clinical staging. Cancer 1997;80:681–690.

56. Vassallo R, Ryu JH, Colby TV, et al. Pulmonary Langerhans'-cell histiocytosis. N Engl J Med 2000;342:1969–1978.

57. Abbott GF, Rosado-de-Christenson ML, Franks TJ, et al. Pulmonary Langerhans cell histiocytosis. Radiographics 2004;24:821–841.

58. Beigelman C, Sellami D, Brauner M. CT of parenchymal and bronchial tuberculosis. Eur Radiol 2000;10:699–709.

59. Harisinghani MG, McLoud TC, Shepard JO, et al. Tuberculosis from head to toe. Radiographics 2000;20:449–470

60. Heidecker J, Huggins JT, Sahn SA, et al. Pathophysiology of pneumothorax following ultrasound-guided thoracentesis. Chest 2006;130(4):1173–1184.

61. Huggins JT, Sahn SA, Heidecker J, et al. Characteristics of trapped lung: Pleural fluid analysis, manometry, and air-contrast chest CT. Chest 2007;131:206–213.

62. Katzenstein AL, Myers JL. Idiopathic pulmonary fibrosis: Clinical relevance of pathologic classification. Am J Respir Crit Care Med 1998;157:1301–1315.

63. Lynch DA, Travis WD, Muller NL, et al. Idiopathic interstitial pneumonias: CT features. Radiology 2005;236:10–21.

64. Allen SD, Harvey CJ. Imaging of Wegener's granulomatosis. BJR 2007;80:757–765.

65. Patterson K, Strek ME. Allergic bronchopulmonary aspergillosis. Proc Am Thorac Soc 2010;7:237-44.

66. Ward S, Heyneman L, Lee MJ, et al. Accuracy of CT in the diagnosis of allergic bronchopulmonary aspergillosis in asthmatic patients. AJR Am J Roentgenol 1999;173:937–942.

67. Castelli R, Graziadei G, Karimi M, et al. Intrathoracic masses due to extramedullary hematopoiesis. Am J Med Sci 2004;328:299–303.

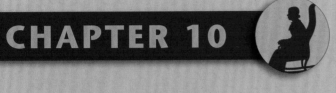

# CHAPTER 10

# CARDIAC RADIOLOGY

**Pal Suranyi / Yeong Shyan Lee / U. Joseph Schoepf**

**HISTORY:** A 57-year-old man with known history of triple vessel disease

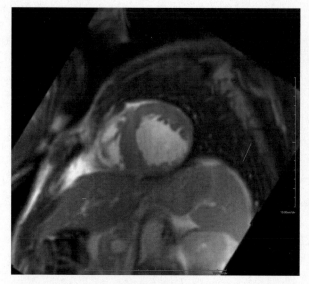

FIGURE 10.1.1

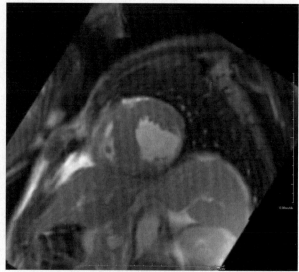

FIGURE 10.1.2

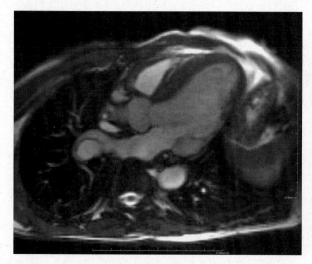

FIGURE 10.1.3

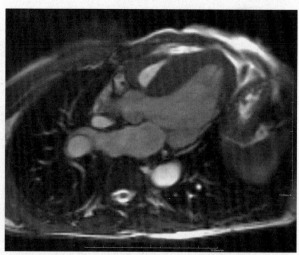

FIGURE 10.1.4

**FINDINGS:** Diastolic (Fig. 10.1.1) and systolic (Fig. 10.1.2) short axis steady-state free precession (SSFP) MRI images show focal akinesis and wall thinning of the lateral–inferolateral wall of left ventricle. These findings are confirmed on three-chamber long axis (left atrium, left ventricle, and aorta) diastolic and systolic views (Figs. 10.1.3 and 10.1.4). The short axis first-pass perfusion image (Fig. 10.1.5) shows hypoenhancement (*arrows*) in these segments of the left ventricular wall, compatible with hypoperfusion. Phase-sensitive inversion recovery (PSIR) image shows corresponding delayed transmural hyperenhancement (Fig. 10.1.6, *arrows*) 15 minutes following gadolinium-based contrast agent injection.

**DIAGNOSIS:** Chronic myocardial infarct at the left circumflex artery territory with scarring and associated wall thinning and focal segmental wall akinesis

**DISCUSSION:** Both myocardial ischemia and myocardial infarction appear hypointense on first-pass perfusion images. The viability of the region at question can be evaluated by delayed enhancement imaging (DE-MRI), where the signal from viable myocardium is minimized (nulled) by selecting an appropriate delay following an inversion recovery pulse. Hyperenhancement occurs in both acute infarction and chronic scarring. Hyperenhancement

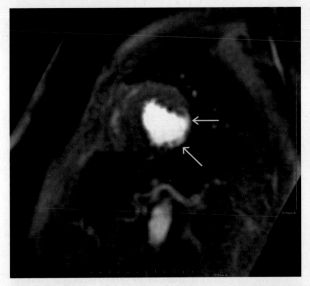

FIGURE 10.1.5

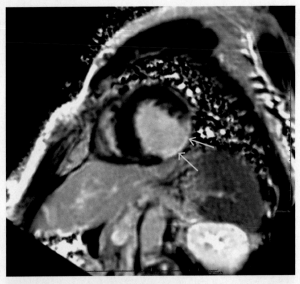

FIGURE 10.1.6

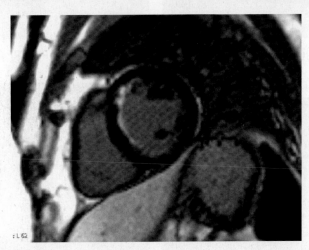

FIGURE 10.1.7

can range from subendocardial (Fig. 10.1.7), suggesting better prognosis owing to residual epicardial viable tissue, to transmural, indicating the absence of residual (salvageable) viable myocardium. The extent of transmurality has been shown to be a strong prognostic indicator for recovery of contractility following revascularization and medical therapy in patients with ischemic heart disease and left ventricular systolic dysfunction (1).

Localization of the infarct to specific coronary artery distribution is also made possible by demonstrating the wall motion abnormality in the cine MRI, although resting function by itself is not a reliable indicator of viability or the lack thereof.

## Aunt Minnie's Pearls

Both ischemic and infarcted myocardium may present as hypoenhanced regions on a perfusion scan with wall motion abnormality in the same region. The presence or absence of delayed enhancement decides viability.

The greater the transmurality of delayed enhancement, the worse the outcome following revascularization.

# Case 10.2

**HISTORY:** Two patients, with chest pain and abnormal Q waves and ST segment elevation on the ECG, a few weeks posttrauma. Figures 10.2.1A, B are MRI images of the first patient, whereas Figures 10.2.2A, B are CT images of the second patient.

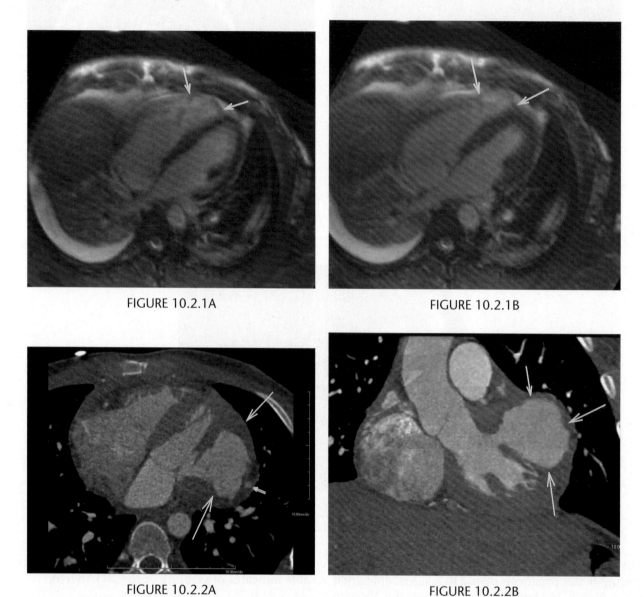

FIGURE 10.2.1A

FIGURE 10.2.1B

FIGURE 10.2.2A

FIGURE 10.2.2B

**FINDINGS:** Four-chamber SSFP cine MR images in diastolic and systolic phases (Figs. 10.2.1A, B) show an abnormal bulge (*arrows*) at the right ventricular anterior wall, which is accentuated in the systolic phase. The pericardium is well separated from this abnormal ventricular bulge. Right pleural effusion and left basilar lung collapse are also demonstrated in these two MR images.

Axial and reformatted coronal CT scans of the second patient show a large abnormal bulge that is lined by a thin layer of myocardium in the free wall of the left ventricle (Figs. 10.2.2A, B, *arrows*). Also noted is

focal dilatation of a coronary artery (*double arrows*) within the injured myocardium, suggesting the presence of traumatic coronary artery pseudoaneurysm.

**DIAGNOSIS:** Posttraumatic ventricular aneurysm

**DISCUSSION:** A true ventricular aneurysmal sac is lined by three layers of the heart wall, that is, the endocardium, the myocardium (and/or scar), and the epicardium, whereas a pseudoaneurysm sac comprises the epicardium and/or the pericardium containing blood from a ruptured ventricle. Both types may present as rare complications of myocardial infarction and may contain mural thrombi. Ventricular pseudoaneurysms may also be caused by chest trauma, cardiac surgery, or endocarditis. It is traditionally believed that a false aneurysm has a higher risk of delayed rupture. A correct diagnosis and differentiation between the two conditions is therefore important as surgery is the definite treatment of choice for cardiac pseudoaneurysm.

A true ventricular aneurysm is commonly located in the anterolateral or apical wall and has a wide ostium connecting the sac to the ventricle, whereas a pseudoaneurysm is more commonly located in the posterolateral wall with a wide mouth.

Injured, contused, and edematous myocardium lining a true aneurysm may show delayed enhancement, although pseudoaneurysms have also been shown to demonstrate marked delayed pericardial enhancement on MRI (2).

## Aunt Minnie's Pearls

True aneurysms are lined by endocardium, scarred myocardium, and epicardium and have wide ostia.

Pseudoaneurysms are lined by epicardium or pericardium and usually have narrow ostia.

# Case 10.3

**HISTORY:** CT scan of a 26-year-old man following left internal mammary artery to left anterior descending artery (LAD) bypass grafting at age 11 owing to LAD-territory ischemia

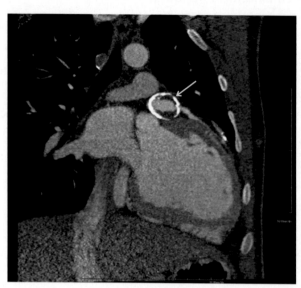

FIGURE 10.3.1A

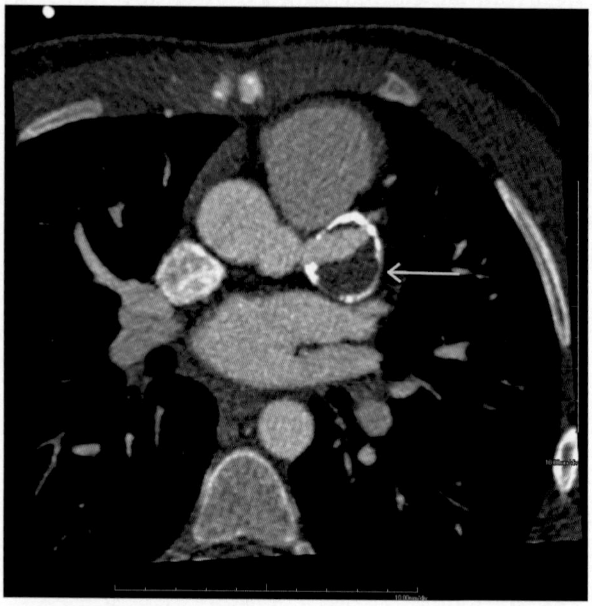

FIGURE 10.3.1B

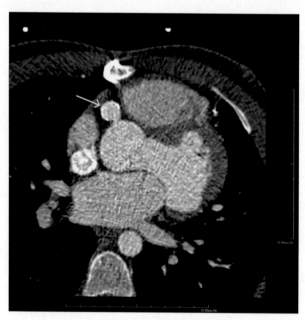

FIGURE 10.3.2

**FINDINGS:** Figures 10.3.1A, B show a large calcified aneurysm (*arrows*) with mural thrombus in the proximal left main coronary artery. Figure 10.3.2 shows another large calcified aneurysm in the proximal right coronary artery (*arrow*).

**DIAGNOSIS:** Kawasaki disease with coronary artery aneurysms

**DISCUSSION:** The major cause of coronary artery aneurysms in children and young adults is Kawasaki disease (mucocutaneous lymph node disease), an acute vasculitis of unknown etiology, affecting medium-sized arteries. It was first described by Dr. Tomisaku Kawasaki in 1967 (3). Most cases occur between 6 months and 8 years of age. These patients present with fever and swollen cervical lymph nodes and may have ischemic chest pain and ECG abnormalities.

Coronary aneurysms are believed to occur in 25% of children with Kawasaki disease (4). The coronary artery aneurysms generally occur within 3 to 6 months of the onset of the acute illness.

Small (<5 mm) and medium-sized coronary aneurysms (5–8 mm) may regress, but giant aneurysms (>8 mm) remain unchanged or may even progress to thrombosis, stenosis, and myocardial infarction. Early treatment of Kawasaki disease with aspirin and high-dose intravenous gamma globulin is effective in reducing the formation of coronary artery aneurysms.

## Aunt Minnie's Pearls

Coronary artery aneurysms are believed to occur in 25% of Kawasaki disease.

Giant aneurysms have lower rate of regression, higher risks of stenosis, and strongest association with myocardial infarction.

Always keep Kawasaki disease in the back of your mind when you do imaging for symptoms of ischemic heart disease in a child.

**HISTORY:** A 50-year-old asymptomatic adult with mid-systolic murmur that alters with position

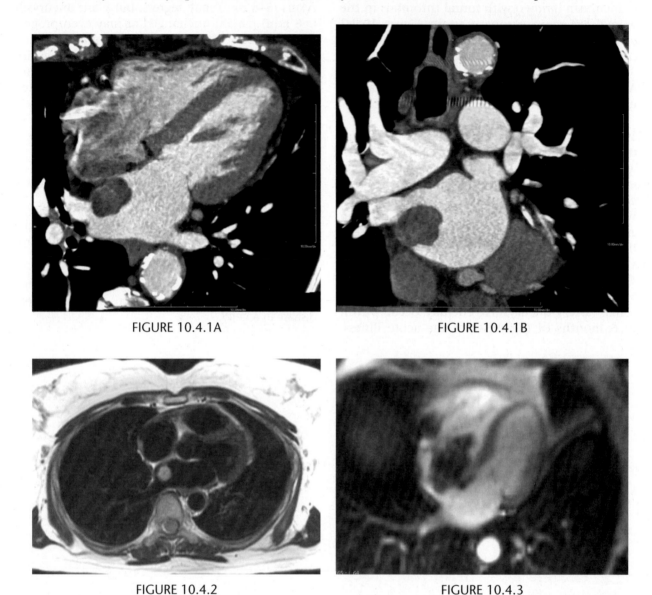

FIGURE 10.4.1A                    FIGURE 10.4.1B

FIGURE 10.4.2                    FIGURE 10.4.3

**FINDINGS:** Figures 10.4.1A, B show an ovoid hypodense mass with well-defined, slightly lobulated margin and mild contrast enhancement in the left atrium, adjacent to the interatrial septum.

**DIAGNOSIS:** Cardiac myxoma

**DISCUSSION:** Cardiac myxomas are the most frequent primary benign tumors of the heart. There is slight female predominance (5:4), and they usually occur between the age of 30 and 60 years. Patients may present with symptoms of mitral valve obstruction (cardiac failure or malaise), central embolism, and constitutional symptoms (fever, weight loss, or symptoms resembling connective tissue disorder owing to cytokine secretion) (5).

Most cardiac myxomas are sporadic but up to 7% of cases are familial. The so-called Carney complex is an autosomal dominant (AD) syndrome, characterized by multiple cardiac myxomas, spotty skin pigmentation, endocrine hyperactivity, and non-myxomatous extracardiac tumors.

Cardiac myxomas are commonly located in the left atrium (75%–80%) and usually arise from the fossa ovalis region of interatrial septum. The tumors are often gelatinous in appearance owing to the abundance of myxoid matrix. They could either be broadly based or have a narrow stalk (pedunculated).

On CT scan, myxomas are usually well-defined, smooth or lobulated, intracavitary cardiac masses and typically contain calcifications. They are usually of lower density than the myocardium and show heterogeneous contrast enhancement. Sometimes cardiac myxomas may mimic thrombi.

On MRI, myxomas are generally isointense with the myocardium in T1-weighted and hyperintense in T2-weighted images (Fig. 10.4.2). They might show areas of low-signal intensity on T2-weighted images owing to intralesional calcifications or hemosiderin.

Post-gadolinium, the lesion often show heterogeneous enhancement (Fig. 10.4.3). Most often they are in the left atrium where they often have round, smooth contours (Fig. 10.4.2). Less commonly myxoma may present as a right atrial mass, which is more likely to be lobulated (Fig. 10.4.3).

## Aunt Minnie's Pearls

Multiple myxomas + Spotty skin pigmentation + endocrine hyperactivity + nonmyxomatous extracardiac tumors = Carney complex (AD).

Myxoma may mimic thrombus. Lack of contrast enhancement makes thrombus more likely, especially given the low incidence of primary cardiac tumors.

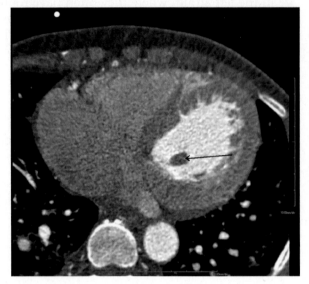

FIGURE 10.5.1A

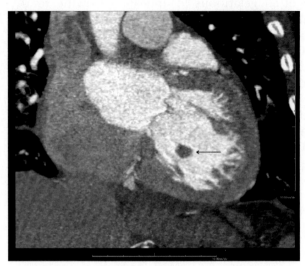

FIGURE 10.5.1B

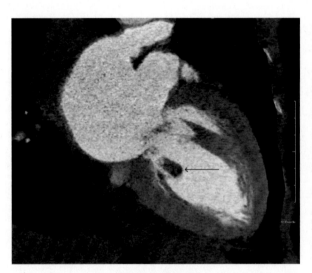

FIGURE 10.5.2

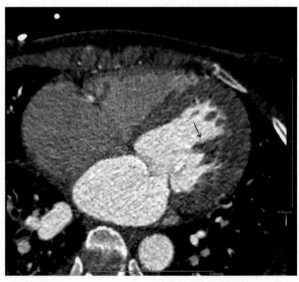

FIGURE 10.5.3

**FINDINGS:** Axial and reformatted coronal cardiac CT images (Figs. 10.5.1A, B, *arrow*) show a nodular mass in the left ventricle. It shows similar (although slightly lower) attenuation to the myocardium and is better demonstrated with a reconstructed oblique coronal MinIP (minimum intensity projection) image (Fig. 10.5.2, *arrow*). By careful examination of the cardiac anatomy, one can easily identify it as a disrupted posteromedial papillary muscle that is now contracted. The normal anterior lateral papillary muscle is demonstrated in the axial image (Fig. 10.5.3).

**DIAGNOSIS:** Ruptured papillary muscle

**DISCUSSION:** Acute rupture of the papillary muscle is uncommon. The causes of rupture of the papillary muscle include acute myocardial infarction (AMI) and cardiac contusion.

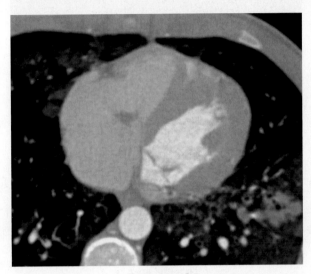

FIGURE 10.5.4A

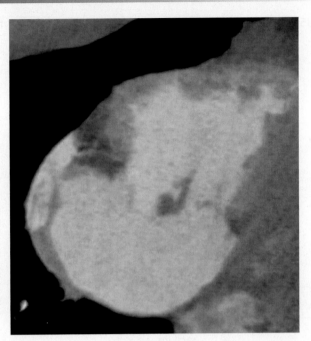

FIGURE 10.5.4B

Acute papillary muscle rupture usually occurs 2 to 7 days following AMI, and it accounts for 5% of mortality of AMI (6). Acute papillary muscle rupture usually occurs with inferior wall myocardial infarction, and the posteromedial papillary muscle is generally involved owing to the posterior descending coronary artery being its single blood supplying vessel (7). The anterolateral papillary muscle has dual blood supply from both the left anterior descending and left circumflex coronary arteries. Patients usually present with acute, severe mitral regurgitation and might be hemodynamically unstable. In rare instances, papillary muscle rupture can happen in the right ventricle as well, causing severe acute tricuspid regurgitation (Figs. 10.5.4A, B) Prompt recognition

of papillary muscle rupture is important as surgical repair could be lifesaving.

## Aunt Minnie's Pearls

Acute papillary muscle is uncommon but a potentially fatal complication of AMI.

High index of suspicion, early detection, and prompt surgical repair could be lifesaving.

MinIP helps visualize low-attenuation structures (chordae tendineae, papillary muscles, valves, dissection membranes).

HISTORY: A 32-year-old man with chest pain and abnormal myocardial perfusion SPECT

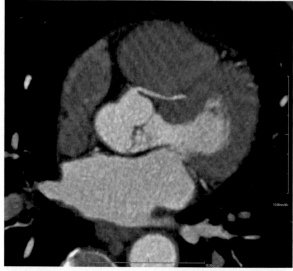

FIGURE 10.6.1

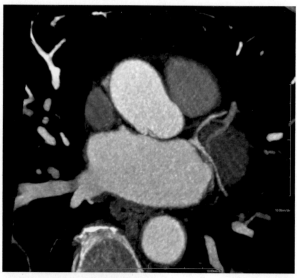

FIGURE 10.6.2

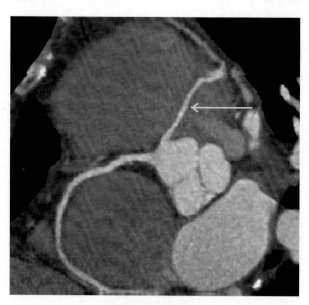

FIGURE 10.6.3

FINDINGS: Axial cardiac CT scans (Figs. 10.6.1 to 10.6.3) show both right and left (*arrow*) main coronary arteries arising from the anterior sinus of Valsalva. The main coronary artery then courses between the pulmonary artery and the aortic root and later bifurcates into the left anterior descending and left circumflex arteries. The circumflex artery makes a loop back and runs along the left atrioventricular groove. Otherwise the coronary arteries show neither luminal stenosis nor atherosclerotic plaques.

DIAGNOSIS: Malignant anomalous origin of the left main coronary artery

DISCUSSION: Anomalous coronary arteries are unusual and found in slightly <1% of the population (8). Anomalies of the coronary arteries may be associated with Klinefelter syndrome, trisomy 18, and Bland–White–Garland Syndrome. Clinically, anomalies of the coronary arteries may be divided into "malignant" or "nonmalignant" forms dependent on the origin and course. The nonmalignant forms are more common. Malignant forms of the anomalous coronary arteries are recognized cause of myocardial ischemia and sudden cardiac death. Examples of the malignant forms also include coronary fistulae, origin of the coronary arteries from the pulmonary artery (Figs. 10.6.4A, B)

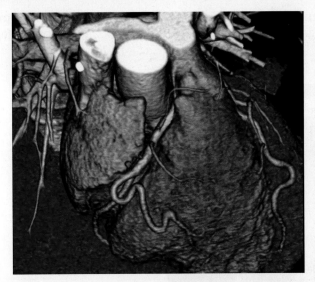

FIGURE 10.6.4A

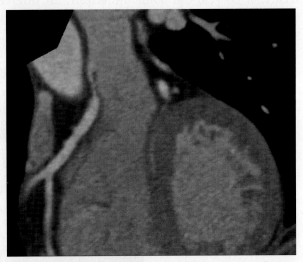

FIGURE 10.6.4B

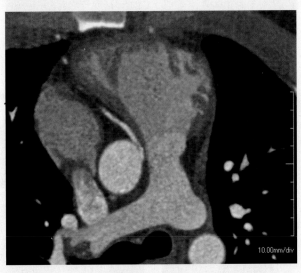

FIGURE 10.6.5

and origin of the coronary arteries from the contra-lateral sinus of Valsalva with interarterial (meaning between the aorta and pulmonary artery) or septal course. Arteries with an interarterial course may become kinked and compressed during exercise as blood pressure rises and the orientation of the great vessels change. Additional important features to note are takeoff at a very acute angle, slit-like opening, and elliptical cross section, which raise the possibility of intramural course (9). An example of this is shown in (Fig. 10.6.5), from a 28-year-old man with acute chest pain, who was found to have an RCA with intramural course. In some of these cases surgeons may be able to "unroof" the artery without the need for reimplanting.

Coronary artery anomalies following a course anterior to the pulmonary artery or having a retro-aortic course are not usually associated with ischemia or sudden cardiac death.

## Aunt Minnie's Pearls

Malignant forms of anomalous coronary arteries may cause myocardial ischemia or sudden cardiac death.

Anomalous origins of the coronary arteries from contralateral coronary sinus of Valsalva, not showing interarterial or septal course, are benign.

**HISTORY:** A 60-year-old adult underwent an interventional procedure for treatment of atrial fibrillation a few months ago. The initial follow-up CT scan (Fig. 10.7.1) and CT scans (Figs. 10.7.2A, B) done a few months after the first follow-up CT scan are shown.

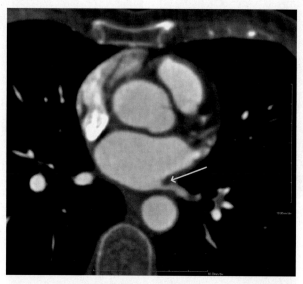

FIGURE 10.7.1

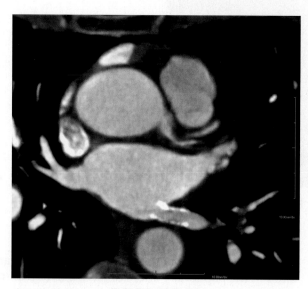

FIGURE 10.7.2A

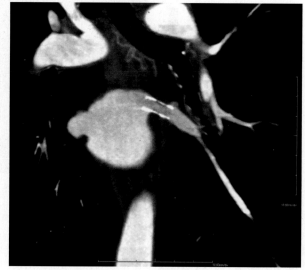

FIGURE 10.7.2B

**FINDINGS:** The initial CT scan (Fig. 10.7.1) reveals significant stenosis of the left inferior pulmonary vein (*arrow*). This pulmonary vein stenosis was later treated with stenting. The subsequent axial and reformatted coronal CT images (Figs. 10.7.2A, B) show significant improvement in the luminal diameter of this pulmonary vein with a patent stent that shows mild intimal hyperplasia.

**DIAGNOSIS:** Left inferior pulmonary vein stenosis treated with stenting

**DISCUSSION:** Atrial fibrillation is a common medical problem. It was traditionally treated with rate and rhythm control medications and anticoagulation. The discovery of the atrial arrhythmias often originating in the pulmonary veins has led to a new approach to treatment using pulmonary vein ablation, also called pulmonary vein antrum isolation.

Pulmonary vein stenosis is a recognized complication of this procedure. Other complications include left atrial perforation, atrial hematoma, pericardial effusion, and cardiac tamponade (10). The patient may be asymptomatic if the pulmonary vein stenosis is mild but may lead to veno-occlusive syndrome and present with hemoptysis if the stenosis is severe. Both MRI and multidetector CT scan are useful noninvasive modalities for preprocedural planning of pulmonary vein ablation and postprocedural follow-up of potential complications (11,12). Treatment of pulmonary vein stenosis is angioplasty with stenting, which can be followed up by CT.

## Aunt Minnie's Pearls

Pulmonary vein stenosis is a recognized complication of pulmonary vein ablation.

Before stenting, both MRI and CT are capable for assessment of pulmonary veins. Following stenting, CT is preferred.

**HISTORY:** A 1-year-old girl with diagnosis of congenital heart disease prenatally, who has just had an ungated cardiac CT scan for preoperative assessment. On clinical examination, she is cyanotic and auscultation reveals a systolic murmur with single second heart sound.

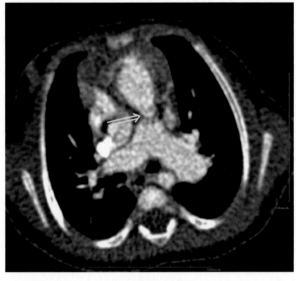

FIGURE 10.8.1

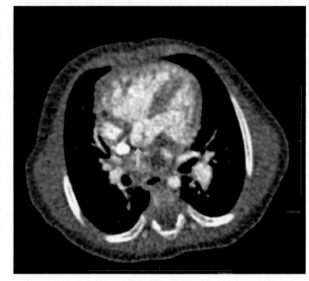

FIGURE 10.8.2

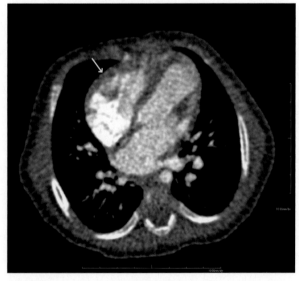

FIGURE 10.8.3

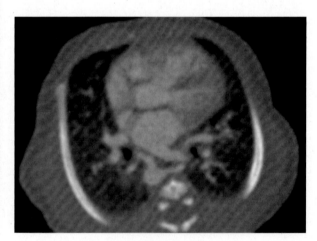

FIGURE 10.8.4

**FINDINGS:** Non-ECG gated axial CT images show supravalvular pulmonary artery stenosis (Fig. 10.8.1, *double arrow*), subvalvular ventricular septal defect (Fig. 10.8.2, *arrow*), an overriding aorta (Fig. 10.8.2, *double arrow*), and mild right ventricular hypertrophy (Fig. 10.8.3, *arrow*).

**DIAGNOSIS:** Tetralogy of Fallot (TOF)

**DISCUSSION:** TOF is one of the commonest cyanotic heart diseases where survival into adulthood is well-known (13,14). It accounts for approximately 10% of cases of congenital heart disease. TOF is really a spectrum of disease owing to anterior malalignment of the outflow septum, causing varying degrees of right ventricular outflow tract obstruction (RVOTO), subaortic ventricular septal defect (VSD) with overriding aorta, and right ventricular hypertrophy. Its most severe form is pulmonary atresia. It may be associated with other anomalies such as right-sided aortic arch, persistent left-sided superior vena cava, and anomalies of the coronary or pulmonary arteries and veins. TOF may be associated with chromosomal abnormalities, such as 22q11 deletion syndrome (also called velocardiofacial syndrome, DiGeorge syndrome).

The patient usually presents in the first few weeks of life with cardiac murmur or cyanosis that becomes more obvious after the ductus arteriosus closes in the first few days of life. On chest x-ray, the heart is often not enlarged, and there is oligaemia (decreased vascularity) of the lung fields. Hypoplasia of the main pulmonary artery and right ventricular hypertrophy may produce the classical *coeur en sabot* (boot-shaped heart) configuration of the cardiac silhouette (15).

Transesophageal echocardiography is the initial imaging modality of choice but CT and MRI are also widely used to detect associated extracardiac abnormalities. Tomographic imaging is also useful in finding multiple aortopulmonary collateral arteries (MAPCA) that are present in severe cases (Fig. 10.8.4). Initial treatment may be by a temporary systemic to pulmonary shunt (Blalock–Taussig shunt) to provide adequate blood supply to the lung followed by a series of operations to definitively correct the anomalies.

### Aunt Minnie's Pearls

Tetralogy of Fallot = VSD + overriding aorta + RVOTO and right ventricular hypertrophy.

Coeur en sabot (boot-shaped heart) + reduced pulmonary vasculature = suspect TOF.

# Case 10.9

**HISTORY:** A 15-year-old boy with previous balloon valvuloplasty for pulmonary stenosis as an infant

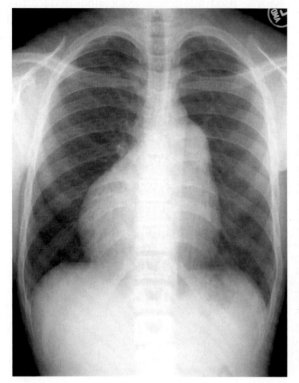

FIGURE 10.9.1A

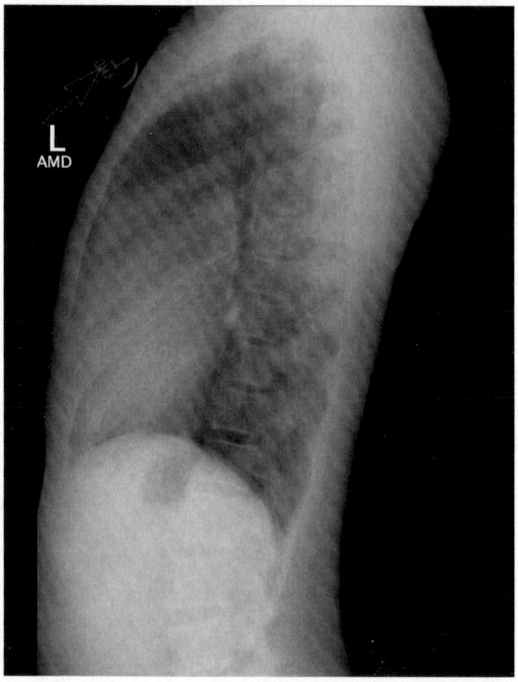

FIGURE 10.9.1B

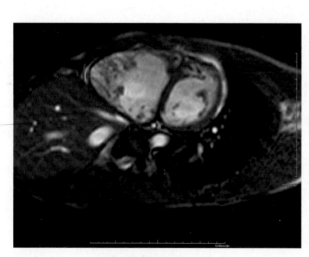

FIGURE 10.9.2A

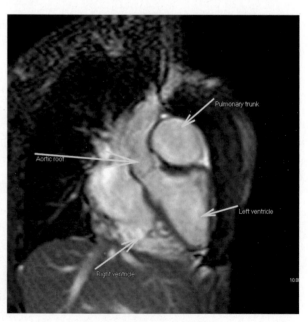

FIGURE 10.9.2B

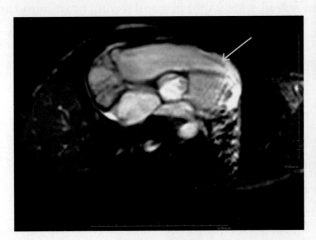

FIGURE 10.9.3A

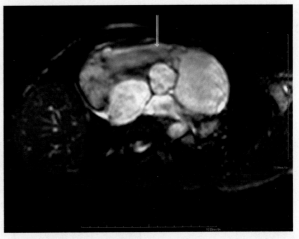

FIGURE 10.9.3B

**FINDINGS:** The frontal and lateral chest radiographs show enlargement of the right ventricle and dilatation of the pulmonary trunk (Figs. 10.9.1A, B). ECG-gated SSFP coronal and axial MR cardiac images show dilatation of the right ventricle, mild right ventricular wall thickening, and post-stenotic dilatation of the pulmonary trunk (Fig. 10.9.2A, B, *arrows*). Figure 10.9.3A shows ejection jet (*arrow*) from the pulmonary valve into the dilated pulmonary trunk and opening of the aortic valve in the systolic phase. Note also the consequent "flow artifact" vertically at the area of highest velocities. Turbulent retrograde flow (Fig. 10.9.3B, *double arrow*) is depicted in the pulmonary outflow tract in the diastolic phase owing to insufficiency of the balloon-dilated valve.

**DIAGNOSIS:** Pulmonary valve stenosis and regurgitation.

**DISCUSSION:** Pulmonic stenosis could occur either at the valvular, subvalvular, or supravalvular levels. It accounts for 5% to 7% of all congenital cardiac defects. Up to 95% of the cases are congenital. Other causes include carcinoid syndrome and rheumatic heart disease. It may also be associated with Noonan syndrome, TOF, and congenital rubella syndrome.

Classical chest radiographic findings of valvular pulmonary stenosis include post-stenotic dilatation of the pulmonary trunk and left pulmonary artery. The right pulmonary artery is usually normal. The right ventricle shows muscular hypertrophy and is usually only mildly enlarged until right ventricular failure develops. The aortic arch is less prominent than usual as it tends to be rotated by the hypertrophied right ventricle. Calcification in the pulmonary valve is rare. In pulmonary stenosis resulting from carcinoid syndrome, there is usually no post-stenotic dilatation of the pulmonary trunk as opposed to the congenital cause.

MRI allows quantitative measurement of the flow pattern, using phase encoded velocity mapping, which enables us to measure the peak velocity and quantify the regurgitant fraction. MRI is also capable of assessing right ventricular function (using multislice cine SSFP images). It has the advantage over echocardiography of not depending on a good acoustic window.

## Aunt Minnie's Pearls

Pulmonary stenosis = dilatation of the pulmonary trunk and left pulmonary artery + less prominent aortic arch + right ventricular enlargement.

Pulmonary stenosis without post-stenotic dilatation = carcinoid syndrome.

# Case 10.10

**HISTORY:** Cyanosis and dyspnea. Physical examination reveals widely split first and second heart sound and a systolic murmur

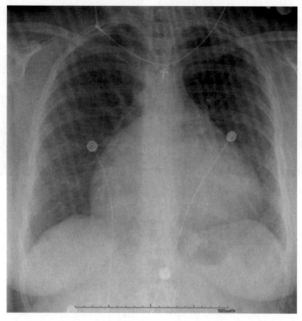

FIGURE 10.10.1

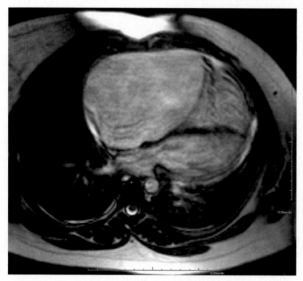

FIGURE 10.10.2A

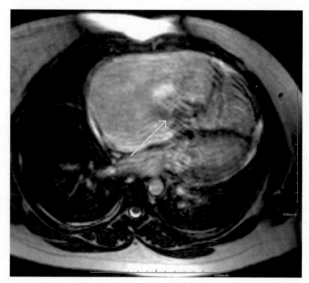

FIGURE 10.10.2B

**FINDINGS:** The chest radiograph (Fig. 10.10.1) reveals cardiomegaly with a box-like cardiac configuration, small ascending aorta and no enlargement of the pulmonary vasculature. Bright blood four-chamber cardiac cine MR images (Figs. 10.10.2A, B) reveal cardiomegaly with partial atrialization of the right ventricle. Tricuspid regurgitation with turbulent flow is also demonstrated in the systolic MR image of the four-chamber view of the heart (Fig. 10.10.2B, *arrow*).

**DIAGNOSIS:** Ebstein's anomaly

**DISCUSSION:** Ebstein's anomaly accounts for 0.5% to 0.7% of cases of congenital heart disease. It is characterized by the downward displacement of the septal and posterior tricuspid leaflets from the atrioventricular or AV junction into the right ventricular cavity, resulting in atrialization of the right ventricular inlet and tricuspid regurgitation. There is an association reported between this abnormality and maternal oral lithium intake (16).

Classic radiographic findings are a square or box-like cardiac configuration with a narrow vascular pedicle and a small aortic arch segment. The ascending aorta tends to be smaller than usual and is usually not appreciable in the frontal projection (17). This anomaly is often associated with an atrial septal defect with right-to-left shunting leading to cyanosis.

## Aunt Minnie's Pearls

Cyanosis + square-like cardiac silhouette + small pulmonary trunk and aorta = think of Ebstein's anomaly.

Ebstein's anomaly is associated with severe tricuspid valve regurgitation and severe right atrial enlargement.

**HISTORY:** A 36-year-old lady presents with acute chest pain and equivocal cardiac enzymes. Echocardiogram and CT scan were performed

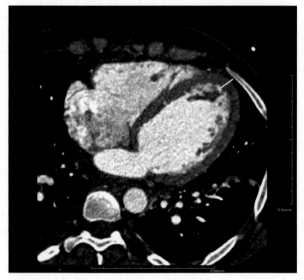

FIGURE 10.11.1A

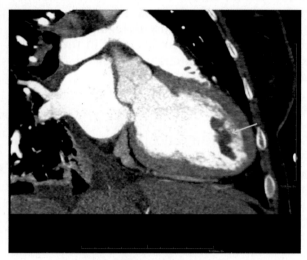

FIGURE 10.11.1B

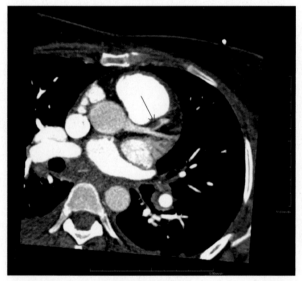

FIGURE 10.11.2

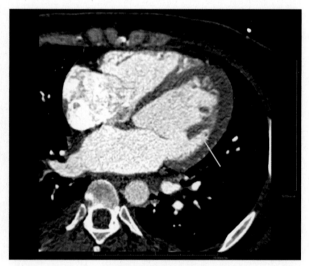

FIGURE 10.11.3

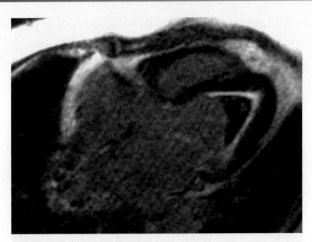

FIGURE 10.11.4

**FINDINGS:** Axial and reformatted coronal ECG-gated cardiac CT images (Figs. 10.11.1A, B, *arrows*) show an elongated left ventricular filling defect that is hypodense compared with the myocardium, suspicious of a ventricular thrombus. A filling defect with similar attenuation in the proximal left anterior descending artery is also seen (Fig. 10.11.2, *arrow*), which likely also represents thrombus rather than noncalcified plaque, considering the lack of atherosclerotic changes in the rest of the coronary arteries. Note that the normal papillary muscle is isoattenuating with the myocardium (Fig. 10.11.3, *arrow*), contrary to the ventricular thrombus, which is hypodense.

**DISCUSSION:** Cardiac thrombus is most frequently a complication of AMI. It usually occurs by 2 weeks after AMI. The incidence of left ventricular (LV) thrombus formation increases with the size of the infarct and the severity of myocardium dysfunction. It more commonly occurs with large anterior ST elevation infarctions. In different studies, the incidence of LV thrombi reported varies from 28% to 54% (18). Other causes of intracardiac thrombi include hypercoagulable states, nonrheumatic atrial fibrillation, rheumatic mitral stenosis, prosthetic valves, or Loeffler's endocarditis (Fig. 10.11.4). LV thrombus may lead to stroke or peripheral emboli if no anticoagulation treatment is given.

Echocardiogram, MRI and CT angiography can all detect cardiac thrombus but MRI has been shown to be the most sensitive examination (19). In equivocal cases, cine-MRI, first-pass perfusion imaging and delayed contrast-enhanced MRI will be helpful for further evaluation (19,20). With delayed contrast-enhanced MRI (DE-MRI), using an inversion recovery pulse sequence with a carefully selected inversion time, the signal from the normal myocardium will be suppressed (nulled). With DE-MRI, the intracavitary thrombus also appears dark and is usually surrounded by a strongly enhancing ring, and the adjacent acutely infarcted or scarred myocardium (or the inflamed subendocardium in Loeffler's endocarditis), if present, will also appear hyperintense (Fig. 10.11.4). The differentiation of Loeffler's endocarditis is relatively simple as the subendocardial hyperenhancement is more diffuse, not confined to a vascular territory and patients show marked hypereosinophilia.

## Aunt Minnie's Pearls

Risks of cardiac thrombus increases with infarction size, presence of poor cardiac function (i.e., ejection function <40%) and anterior myocardial infarct.

Thrombus can occur without myocardial infarction.

Contrast-enhanced MRI is helpful in equivocal cases and it is a sensitive modality for detecting small mural or intracavitary thrombi.

**HISTORY:** A 65-year-old man with history of ischemic heart disease, now presents with central chest pain

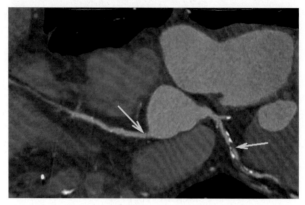

FIGURE 10.12.1

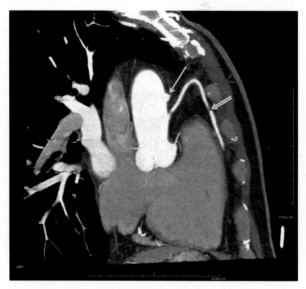

FIGURE 10.12.2A

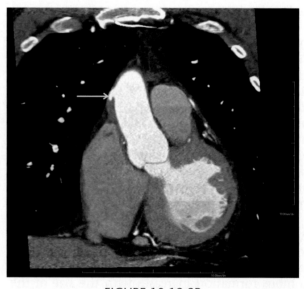

FIGURE 10.12.2B

**FINDINGS:** Reformatted CT image of the native coronary arteries shows significant right coronary artery ostial stenosis and proximal left anterior descending coronary artery stenosis (Fig. 10.12.1, *arrows*). Diffuse calcified plaques in both native coronary arteries are also demonstrated. The reformatted coronal CT images show complete occlusion of two venous bypass grafts that appear as small nipples on the aortic root (Figs. 10.12.2A, B, *arrows*). A third bypass graft with significant stenosis in its midsegment owing to noncalcified plaque is also demonstrated (Figs. 10.12.2A and 10.12.3, *double arrows*).

**DIAGNOSIS:** Occluded and stenosed coronary bypass grafts

**DISCUSSION:** CT coronary angiography has become an established modality for the assessment of suspected coronary artery bypass graft occlusion. ECG-gated multidetector-row cardiac CT yields high sensitivities and specificities in the 90% range while it saves the patient from the risks of conventional coronary angiography (21). The proximal anastomoses are easily found with CT, and the entire course of the bypass grafts can all be demonstrated

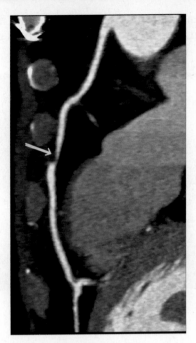

FIGURE 10.12.3

along with the status of the native coronary arteries, internal mammary arteries, and the subclavian arteries. The obtained information is crucial for planning interventions (stent sizing and planning approachability) or redo surgery.

Assessment of coronary artery graft patency requires knowledge of coronary artery graft procedures and anatomy. Current bypass techniques are free graft, in situ graft, sequential bypass graft, and Y or T graft. Free graft includes excised arterial or venous grafts, where the proximal end is anastomosed with the ascending aorta and the distal end to the coronary artery. In situ grafts are arterial grafts (usually the left internal mammary) with their native origin from the subclavian artery intact and the distal portion harvested from the chest wall and anastomosed to the coronary artery. Most surgeons use clips to secure the side branches, leading to streak artifacts along the graft. Sequential bypass grafts can be venous or arterial grafts used to supply two or more adjacent vessels. They are also anastomosed to the aorta proximally and have side-to-side anastomoses with the "jumped" vessel(s) along their course and are finally anastomosed end to side to another coronary artery. Y or T grafts are created using two bypass grafts, one of is an in situ or free graft and a second free graft is anastomosed to it resulting in a shape of an inverted Y or T.

For evaluation of the patency of free bypass grafts, the coronary CT angiogram can be performed starting at the level of the mid ascending aorta covering the entire heart. If, however, an in situ graft is present, or there is a possibility of redo surgery where the left or right internal mammary artery may potentially be utilized, the scan range needs to include the level of the extrathoracic origins of the internal mammary arteries to assess for atherosclerotic disease. If stents or extensive calcifications are present, sharper reconstruction kernels and thin maximum intensity projections (MIP) may be helpful for better visualization.

## Aunt Minnie's Pearls

For assessment of bypass graft patency, CT coronary angiograms should include the level of the extrathoracic internal mammary artery origin particularly if there is an in situ graft present or the utilization of the internal mammary arteries is planned.

Occluded venous grafts appear as small nipples on the aortic root.

**HISTORY:** A 70-year-old man with heart failure and membrane-like finding in the left atrium on echocardiography during preoperative evaluation for coronary artery bypass grafting

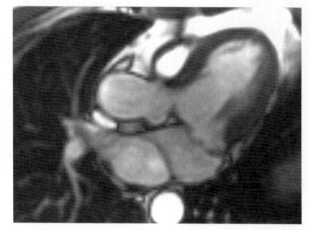

FIGURE 10.13.1A

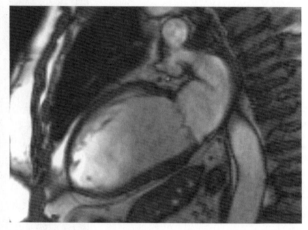

FIGURE 10.13.1B

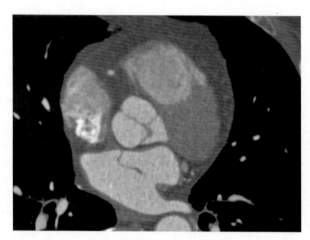

FIGURE 10.13.2A

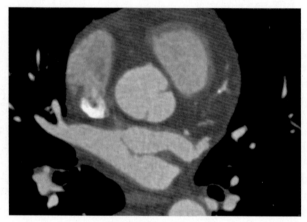

FIGURE 10.13.2B

**FINDINGS:** Bright blood cine MRI images demonstrate a thin membrane that divides the left atrium into two chambers. A proximal chamber that receives the pulmonic veins, and a more anteriorly located distal chamber that empties into the mitral valve (Figs. 10.13.1A, B).

**DIAGNOSIS:** Cor triatriatum

**DISCUSSION:** Cor triatriatum is a rare congenital malformation of the left atrium, occurring in 0.1% of all patients with congenital cardiac disease (22). In fact, it is a spectrum of abnormalities, that may or may not cause hemodynamically significant obstruction of pulmonary venous inflow into the anterior chamber and thus into the left ventricle. Symptoms are therefore very similar to those of mitral stenosis. Cor triatriatum is often associated with atrial septal defect (70%) and in some cases with partial anomalous pulmonary venous return. Identification is possible using CT as well, but only on gated images, as the membrane is usually very thin and moves during the cardiac cycle (Figs. 10.13.2A, B)

Evaluation should include velocity mapping in the pulmonary veins to assess for hemodynamic evidence of obstruction (23). A complication of severe obstruction may be thrombus formation or secondary pulmonary hypertension.

## Aunt Minnie's Pearls

Cor triatriatum is a congenital heart defect where the left atrium (cor triatriatum sinistrum) or right atrium (cor triatriatum dextrum) is subdivided by a thin membrane, resulting in three atrial chambers.

Cor triatriatum does no always cause hemodynamic compromise as long as the fenestration is large enough.

**HISTORY:** A 31-year-old man without significant prior medical history presenting with chest pain and dyspnea. For about 4 weeks prior to his presentation he had fevers, myalgia, fatigue, and night sweats. He was treated with antibiotics but symptoms worsened and he developed a friction rub; echocardiography found a small pericardial effusion.

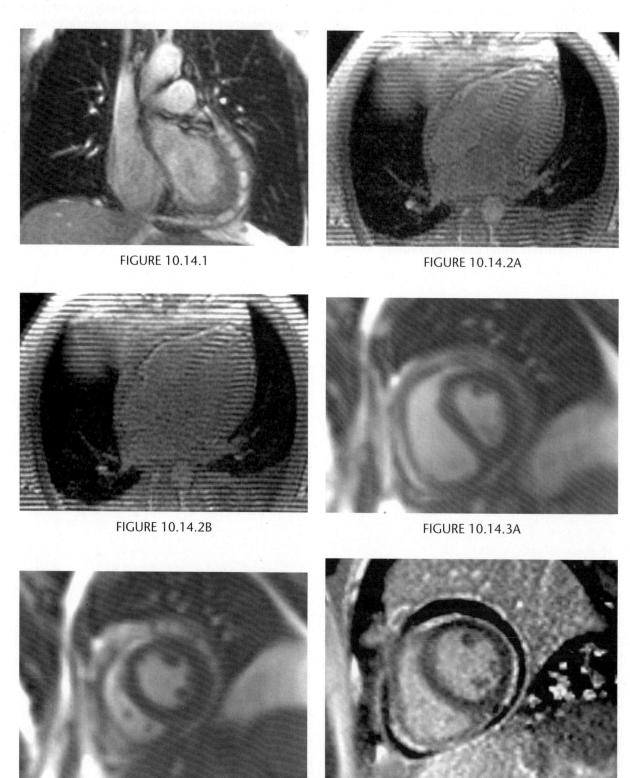

FIGURE 10.14.1

FIGURE 10.14.2A

FIGURE 10.14.2B

FIGURE 10.14.3A

FIGURE 10.14.3B

FIGURE 10.14.4

**FINDINGS:** Coronal bright blood image (Fig. 10.14.1) demonstrates a small pericardial effusion with multiple strands, suggestive of adhesions, within the pericardial sac. Myocardial tagging images (Figs. 10.14.2A, B) show persisting continuity between pericardial and myocardial tag lines in systole, consistent with absence of "slippage," confirming adhesion of the pericardium to the epicardium. Real-time cine MRI during deep inspiration shows flattening of the interventricular septum that is visible only during active inspiration (Fig. 10.14.3A), but not during expiration or at rest (Fig. 10.14.3B), consistent with ventricular interdependence, which is a hallmark of constrictive physiology. Delayed contrast-enhanced image (Fig. 10.14.4) demonstrates thickening and avid enhancement of the pericardium involving both the parietal and visceral layers.

**DIAGNOSIS:** Effusive-constrictive pericarditis.

**DISCUSSION:** A frequently encountered diagnostic dilemma for cardiologists is differentiation of whether a patient experiencing diastolic dysfunction is suffering from a myocardial process, that is, restrictive cardiomyopathy, or from extrinsic constrictive pericarditis. MRI is a unique modality in that it provides excellent soft tissue contrast and also has the ability to obtain moving images with high temporal resolution to assess physiology without the need for ionizing radiation (24).

Acute effusive-constrictive pericarditis is usually caused by a viral infection. Other infectious agents, such as pyogenic bacteria and tuberculosis may also cause constriction.

Constrictive pericarditis most often results from a chronic process. Calcifications may or may not be present, and it is important to note that the presence of pericardial calcifications is not pathognomonic for constriction. The etiology of chronic constriction encompasses a wide range of diseases such as uremia, connective tissue diseases, trauma, sarcoidosis, myocardial infarction (Dressler syndrome), and neoplasms. Among the iatrogenic causes are prior cardiac surgery, radiation, and drug reactions.

The management of chronic cases is usually surgical with pericardial stripping. Acute cases that are mildly or moderately symptomatic may be treated medically (colchicine), and MRI can play a crucial role in the follow-up of these patients.

## Aunt Minnie's Pearls

Best modality to visualize the pericardium and to differentiate constrictive versus restrictive processes is MRI.

Ventricular interdependence is a hallmark of constrictive physiology.

Constrictive pericarditis may develop acutely.

# REFERENCES

1. Choi KM, Kim RJ, Gubernikoff G, et al. Transmural extent of acute myocardial infarction predicts long-term improvement in contractile function. Circulation 2001;104(10):1101–1107.

2. Konen E, Merchant N, Gutierrez C, et al. True versus false left ventricular aneurysm: Differentiation with MR imaging—initial experience. Radiology 2005;236(1):65–75.

3. Kawasaki, T. [Acute febrile mucocutaneous syndrome with lymphoid involvement with specific desquamation of the fingers and toes in children]. Arerugi 1967;16(3):178–222.

4. Kato H, Sugimura T, Akagi T, et al. Long-term consequences of Kawasaki disease: A 10- to 21-year follow-up study of 594 patients. Circulation 1996;94(6):1379–1385.

5. Kato H, Ichinose E, Yoshioka F, et al. Fate of coronary aneurysms in Kawasaki disease: Serial coronary angiography and long-term follow-up study. Am J Cardiol 1982;49(7):1758–1766.

6. Pinede L, Duhaut P, Loire R. Clinical presentation of left atrial cardiac myxoma. A series of 112 consecutive cases. Medicine (Baltimore) 2001;80(3):159–172.

7. Reeder GS. Identification and treatment of complications of myocardial infarction. Mayo Clin Proc 1995;70(9):880–884.

8. Engel HJ, Torres C, Page HL Jr, et al. Major variations in anatomical origin of the coronary arteries: Angiographic observations in 4,250 patients without associated congenital heart disease. Cathet Cardiovasc Diagn 1975;1(2):157–169.

9. Miller CD, Hwang W, Case D et al. Stress CMR imaging observation unit in the emergency department reduces 1-year medical care costs in patients with acute chest pain: A randomized study for comparison with inpatient care. JACC: Cardiovasc Imaging. 2011;4:862–870.

10. Echahidi N, Philippon F, O'Hara G, et al. Life-threatening left atrial wall hematoma secondary to a pulmonary vein laceration: An unusual complication of catheter ablation for atrial fibrillation. J Cardiovasc Electrophysiol 2008;19(5):556–558.

11. Preis O, Digumarthy SR, Wright CD, et al. Digumarthy et al. Atrioesophageal fistula after catheter pulmonary venous ablation for atrial fibrillation: Imaging features. J Thoracic Imaging 2007;(3):283–285.

12. Wood MA, Wittkamp M, Henry D, et al. A comparison of pulmonary vein ostial anatomy by computerized tomography, echocardiography, and venography in patients with atrial fibrillation having radiofrequency catheter ablation. Am J Cardiol 2004;93(1):49–53.

13. Higgins CB, Mulder DG. Tetralogy of Fallot in the adult. Am J Cardiol 1972;29(6):837–846.

14. Marquis RM. Longevity and the early history of the tetralogy of Fallot. Br Med J 1956;1(4971):819–822.

15. Ferguson EC, Krishnamurthy R, Oldham SA, et al. Classic imaging signs of congenital cardiovascular abnormalities. Radiographics 2007;27(5):1323–1334.

16. Goldberg HL. Psychotropic drugs in pregnancy and lactation. Int J Psychiatry Med 1994;24(2):129–147.

17. Deutsch V, Wexler L, Blieden LC, et al. Ebstein's anomaly of tricuspid valve: critical review of roentgenological features and additional angiographic signs. Am J Roentgenol Radium Ther Nucl Med 1995;125(2):395–411.

18. Vecchio C, Chiarella F, Lupi G, et al. Left ventricular thrombus in anterior acute myocardial infarction after thrombolysis. A GISSI-2 connected study. Circulation 1991;84(2):512–519.

19. Srichai MB, Junor C, Rodriguez LL, et al. Clinical, imaging, and pathological characteristics of left ventricular thrombus: A comparison of contrast-enhanced magnetic resonance imaging, transthoracic echocardiography, and transesophageal echocardiography with surgical or pathological validation. Am Heart J 2006;152(1):75–84.

20. Mollet NR, Dymarkowski S, Volders W, et al. Visualization of ventricular thrombi with contrast-enhanced magnetic resonance imaging in patients with ischemic heart disease. Circulation 2002;106(23):2873–2876.

21. Stanford W, Brundage BH, MacMillan R, et al. Sensitivity and specificity of assessing coronary bypass graft patency with ultrafast computed tomography: Results of a multicenter study. J Am Coll Cardiol 1988;12(1):1–7.

22. Ostmann-Smith I, Silverman NH, Oldershaw P, et al. Cor triatriatum sinistrum: Diagnostic features on cross sectional echocardiography. Br Heart J 1984;51:211.

23. Grosse-Wortmann L, Al-Otay A, Goo HW, et al. Anatomical and functional evaluation of pulmonary veins in children by magnetic resonance imaging. J Am Coll Cardiol 2007;49(9):993–1002.

24. Zurick AO, Bolen MA, Kwon DH, et al. Pericardial delayed hyperenhancement with CMR imaging in patients with constrictive pericarditis undergoing surgical pericardiectomy. JACC Cardiovasc Imaging 2011;4(11):1180–1191.

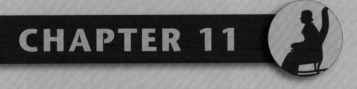

# CHAPTER 11

# BREAST IMAGING

**Michelle McDonough / Thomas L. Pope Jr. / Jennifer Cranny**

*The authors and editors acknowledge the contribution of the Chapter 9
authors from the second edition: Lisa F. Baron, MD, and Elizabeth W. Greer
and of Dr. Elizabeth DePeri and Dr. Beata Panzegrau from the third edition.*

# Case 11.1

**HISTORY:** Bilateral craniocaudal (CC) mammograms of three male patients complaining of breast tenderness and fullness

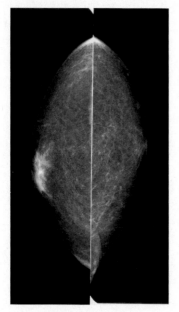

FIGURE 11.1.1

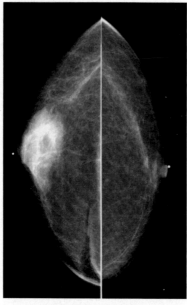

FIGURE 11.1.2

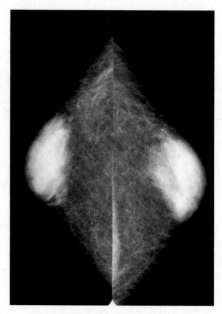

FIGURE 11.1.3

**FINDINGS:** Bilateral film-screen mammograms demonstrate varying degrees of gynecomastia. Figure 11.1.1 demonstrates mild, asymmetric glandular tissue in a flame-shaped distribution behind the right nipple. The contralateral breast is nearly completely fatty, containing a negligible amount of glandular breast tissue. Figure 11.1.2 depicts a greater degree of asymmetric ductal tissue in the retroareolar area, right greater than left. Figure 11.1.3 illustrates bilateral, symmetric gynecomastia—resembling the normal parenchymal distribution in a female.

**DIAGNOSIS:** Various mammographic presentations of gynecomastia

**DISCUSSION:** Gynecomastia is the development of ductal and stromal tissue elements within the male breast without true acinar lobule formation (e.g., fibroadenomas do not occur in men). The causes of gynecomastia can be physiologic, nonphysiologic, or idiopathic. The physiologic form of gynecomastia has a trimodal distribution: neonatal hypertrophy owing to maternal influence of estrogen, pubertal hypertrophy owing to high estradiol levels, and senescent hypertrophy owing to a decline in serum testosterone levels. These peaks are related to a relative increase in estrogen or an overall decrease in testosterone. Underlying disease processes can result in relative estrogen excess and may contribute to the development of gynecomastia: testicular and nontesticular tumors (e.g., lung, liver, adrenal), cirrhosis, nutritional deprivation, androgen deficiency, and systemic disorders. Nonphysiologic causes of gynecomastia include estrogenic active drugs (e.g., anabolic steroids, marijuana, digitalis), drugs that reduce testosterone action or production (e.g., cimetidine, phenytoin, methotrexate, diazepam), Klinefelter syndrome (e.g., elevated estrogen levels), and ambiguous genitalia syndromes. Nonphysiologic gynecomastia may result from cirrhosis, chronic renal failure, malnutrition, or drugs (1). However, the cause in 40% of these cases is idiopathic (2).

The usual clinical presentation of gynecomastia in a man is a complaint of breast tenderness with an associated soft retroareolar tissue mass. The diagnostic workup includes clinical examination and mammography with bilateral CC and mediolateral oblique (MLO) views. Mammography can be useful in differentiating benign from malignant breast disease (3). Gynecomastia has a variable pattern on the mammogram but usually appears as a fan-shaped, triangular density emanating from the nipple. Breast cancer tends to appear as an irregular, eccentric mass with possible calcifications. Ultrasound can be useful in the workup for possible malignancy (4).

## Aunt Minnie's Pearl

Soft, mobile, tender subareolar tissue (unilateral or bilateral) in a man = gynecomastia.

HISTORY: Withheld

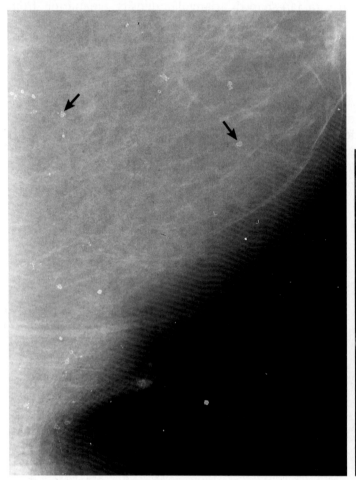

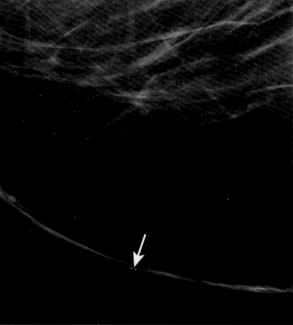

FIGURE 11.2.1                    FIGURE 11.2.2

FINDINGS: There are numerous, scattered, ring-shaped calcifications (Fig. 11.2.1, *arrows*) measuring 0.5 to 1 mm in diameter on the CC view of the medial breast. Their superficial location is best appreciated in the cleavage area in this case. The calcifications are mostly single, but some are clustered. Their centers are low density or lucent. The distinguishing feature is the less-than-perfect shape of the calcified ring, which often has a flattened side, giving it a polygonal appearance. Figure 11.2.2 is a supplemental view used to confirm this finding.

DIAGNOSIS: Dermal calcification of sebaceous glands

DISCUSSION: Sebaceous glands occur in the skin in association with hair follicles. When calcified, they are differentiated from fat necrosis by the location in the skin and by their polygonal shape. Their size corresponds to that of skin pores, whereas fat necrosis may have larger rings. Typical dermal calcifications are always benign and do not require biopsy (5). If the classic features are not present, however, the suspected location in the skin can be confirmed with tangential views, thereby avoiding biopsy of atypical skin calcifications that may mimic carcinoma (6).

## Aunt Minnie's Pearls

Polygonal calcified rings in a superficial location = dermal calcifications.

Tangential views confirm the diagnosis.

# Case 11.3

HISTORY: Palpable finding in medial left breast

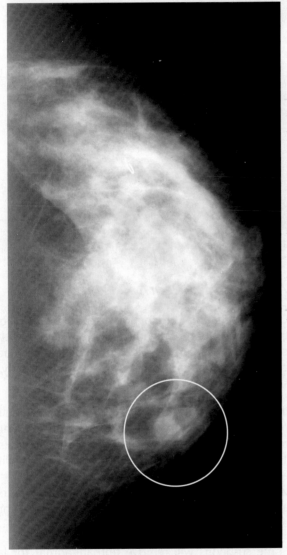

FIGURE 11.3.1

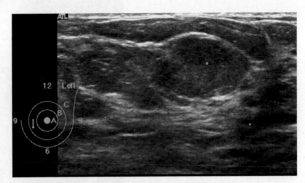

FIGURE 11.3.2

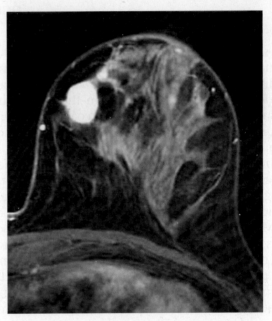

FIGURE 11.3.3

FINDINGS: Partially circumscribed mass medial left breast on mammography CC view (circled Fig 11.3.1) and incidental note of radiopaque marker in lateral aspect of breast. Ultrasound (Fig. 11.3.2) demonstrates a circumscribed mass with macrolobulations, mild internal heterogeneity, and acoustic enhancement correlating with the mammogram and palpable concern. A medial, circumscribed, ovoid mass intensely enhances on gadolinium-enhanced axial T1-weighted MR image (Fig. 11.3.3), on MR examination performed for contralateral breast concern.

DIAGNOSIS: Fibroadenoma

DISCUSSION: A fibroadenoma is a common benign tumor, occurring frequently in young women. Their growth is stimulated by estrogen, and peak incidence is between the ages of 25 and 35 years, decreasing around 40 years. The juvenile fibroadenoma occurs during puberty and has a tendency to grow to larger sizes. Therefore, complete surgical excision may be indicated. The adult variety typically occurs in young women and is usually smooth, rubbery, and clinically mobile and cannot be reliably distinguished from a circumscribed carcinoma (such as medullary or colloid/mucinous carcinoma) on the first mammogram. The absence of growth

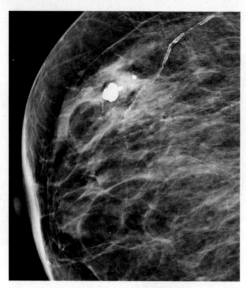

FIGURE 11.3.4

over several years is typical although some fibroadenomas increase in size over time. With advancing age and during menopause, the fibroadenoma usually degenerates with a decrease in the size of the mass while showing an increase in coarse, popcorn-like calcifications (Fig. 11.3.4 shows classic fibroadenoma course calcifications (7).

Fibroadenomas are classically ovoid or almond-shaped with smooth borders, internal homogeneous echogenicity, and acoustic enhancement. They can be incidental or evaluated because they are palpable. Multiplicity is often seen. In the majority of patients, in particular if there are any unusual features present, histologic confirmation of fibroadenoma with postbiopsy clip placement is chosen. Some clinicians will choose short-term follow-up imaging in young patients with typical findings of fibroadenoma because the risk of malignant transformation or associated malignancy is extremely low (8). Finally, some patients may prefer to have the lesion removed; ultrasound-guided percutaneous excision or cryoablation are two minimally invasive techniques to remove this benign tumor (9,10).

## Aunt Minnie's Pearls

Classic-appearing fibroadenomas can fluctuate slightly in size, by some reports up to 20% in volume, without concern. If they are atypical in appearance, imaging characteristics change, or they grow more rapidly, tissue diagnosis should be considered (11).

If palpable, they can then be followed up clinically. If not palpable, they can be followed with imaging. A reasonable plan is follow-up at 6-month intervals for 1 year and then annual imaging after size stability is established. If the patient is younger than 40 years and would not otherwise be imaged annually, excision is a reasonable option to eliminate the need for annual exams.

Some surgeons will remove fibroadenomas for large size rather than clinical or imaging follow-up. The size criteria for excision will vary, ranging from 20 to 30 mm.

**HISTORY:** A 34-year-old lactating woman 4 months postpartum with a palpable nontender lump

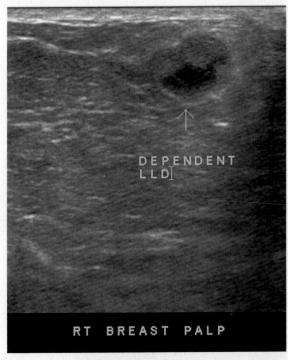

FIGURE 11.4.1

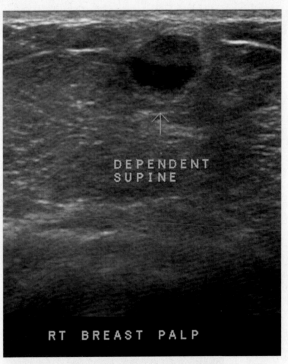

FIGURE 11.4.2

**FINDINGS:** Complex cystic mass with position-dependent eccentric echogenicity (Figs. 11.4.1 and 11.4.2).

**DIAGNOSIS:** Galactocele

**DISCUSSION:** A galactocele is a milk- or fat-containing cystic mass that results from cystic dilation of a duct during or after lactation. It occurs in women of childbearing age and is often palpable. It is most commonly nontender. The galactocele is diagnosed by visualization of a fat-fluid level, either on upright lateral mammogram or ultrasound, where they are usually well-circumscribed (12). All fat-containing masses in the breast are benign; therefore, the identification of fat within the mass may eliminate the need for definitive diagnosis.

If ambiguous imaging characteristics are present, such as acoustic shadowing, aspiration might be considered for diagnosis. Within the aspirate, a fat-fluid level may be visible within the syringe, or the fat component of the aspirate may float if the aspirate is added to a liquid phase fixative (13).

## Aunt Minnie's Pearls

If a lesion is thought to represent a galactocele, image the mass sonographically with the patient in different positions to demonstrate the mobility of the fat-containing portion of the mass and to confirm a fat-fluid level that makes the diagnosis.

Any fat-containing breast mass is benign.

# Case 11.5

**HISTORY:** Right breast mammogram obtained in a 63-year-old woman during annual examination

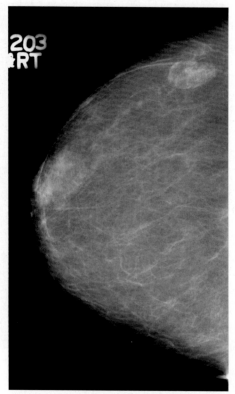

FIGURE 11.5.1

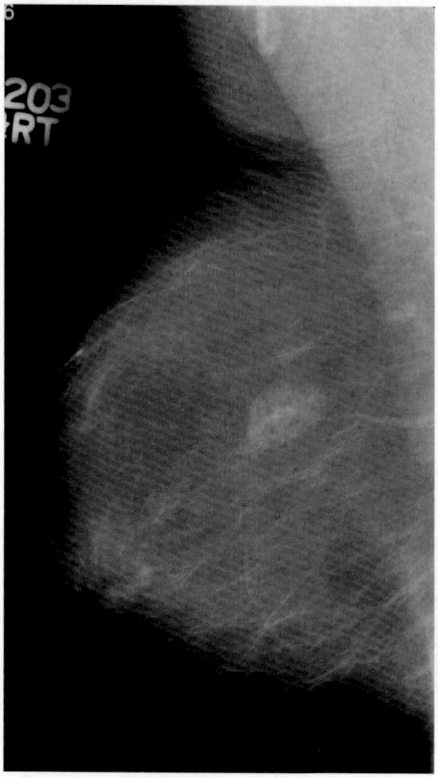

FIGURE 11.5.2

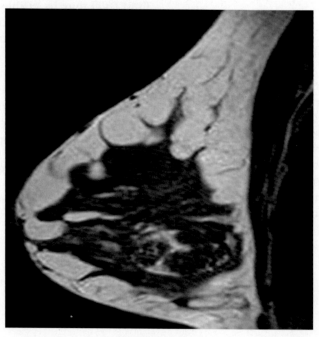

FIGURE 11.5.3

# Case 11.5 (Continued)

**FINDINGS:** Unilateral right breast film screen mammogram in CC and MLO projections (Figs. 11.5.1 and 11.5.2). Images show a 2-cm mixed density fat containing ovoid mass in the upper outer quadrant. T2 nonfat suppressed sagittal MRI (Fig. 11.5.3) shows a well-circumscribed 4.5-cm mass with visible fat and glandular elements contained within a visible capsule.

**DIAGNOSIS:** Hamartoma (fibroadenolipoma)

**DISCUSSION:** Hamartomas, also known as fibroadenolipomas, are a benign proliferation of fibrous, glandular, and fatty tissue elements surrounded by a thin pseudocapsule of connective tissue (11). On mammography, these masses have a typical round to oval configuration and contain visible soft-tissue density and fatty elements. The appearance of the fatty internal elements indicates a benign lesion that requires no additional workup or biopsy. These lesions may be palpable on physical examination. They are typically soft and freely mobile. Size can vary considerably from a few millimeters to several centimeters (12).

Risk for developing breast cancer is the same as the surrounding breast tissue and therefore is not increased over baseline. However, breast cancer can develop in any location that contains glandular elements, so assessment for interval change is always warranted (13).

Diagnosis is typically made by mammography alone and ultrasound is not usually required owing to its classic appearance. They can be found inadvertently on MRI with expected T1 and T2 elements of fat, fibrous tissue, and a pseudocapsule (14).

## Aunt Minnie's Pearls

Include in the differential diagnosis of fat-containing masses on mammography along with lymph nodes, lipomas, fat necrosis, and galactoceles.

These masses are almost always benign; however, as they do contain glandular elements, evaluation for interval growth or suspicious change is required.

**HISTORY:** A 50-year-old woman with a palpable mass in the upper outer quadrant of the left breast

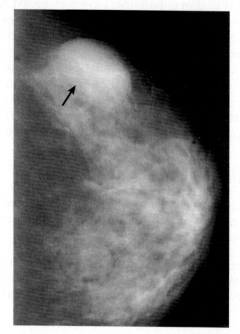

FIGURE 11.6.1

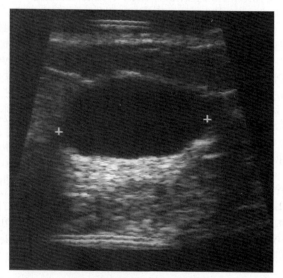

FIGURE 11.6.2

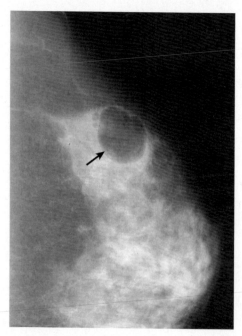

FIGURE 11.6.3

**FINDINGS:** A CC view of the left breast (Fig. 11.6.1) demonstrates a 3.5-cm oval mass located in the lateral portion of the breast with well-circumscribed margins (*arrow*). Breast tissue is visible "through" the lesion, indicating that it is a low-density, radiopaque mass. Sonography (Fig. 11.6.2) shows a completely anechoic, smooth-walled structure with a sharp back wall and enhanced through-transmission (between cursors). A postultrasound aspiration pneumocystogram (Fig. 11.6.3) reveals a well-demarcated, air-filled structure with a smooth inner wall (*arrow*).

**DIAGNOSIS:** Simple breast cyst

**DISCUSSION:** Mammograms do not detect breast cysts; instead, they show a mass that requires characterization with ultrasound. Ultrasonography classifies a mammographic lesion as a simple cyst when the mass has the following characteristics: smooth thin wall, completely anechoic pattern, and distal acoustic enhancement. Complicated cysts have a benign appearance but may contain a few internal echoes. This is likely owing to improved ultrasound technology. These can often be considered benign if there are no other concerning features. Complex cysts are lesions that lack the characteristics of a simple cyst and may contain one or more of the following features: irregular or thick wall, internal echoes, and diminished acoustic enhancement. Percutaneous aspiration or biopsy of complex cysts is frequently recommended.

Patients may present with a palpable mass, prompting the clinician to request mammography. In general, the definitive diagnosis requires both mammography and ultrasonography. Only when all criteria exhibited in Figure 11.6.2 are met can a simple cyst be diagnosed with confidence. Historically, pneumocystography could be performed to demonstrate a smooth inner wall by using air as the contrast medium. This procedure was performed mainly to exclude an intracystic mass and to correlate with mammographic findings (15,16).

### Aunt Minnie's Pearls

Ultrasound findings of smooth thin wall, anechoic signal, and distal acoustic enhancement = benign breast cyst.

Complex cysts should be aspirated and/or biopsied if they are not typical of a simple cyst.

HISTORY: Mammogram and ultrasound images from two patients with the same diagnosis

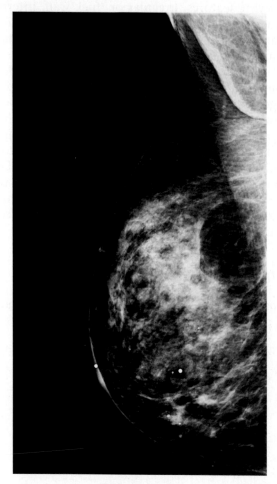

FIGURE 11.7.1

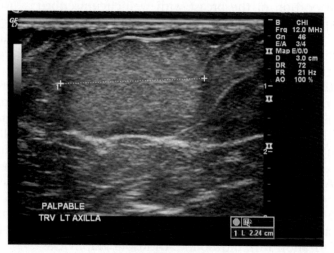

FIGURE 11.7.2

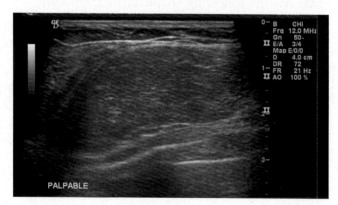

FIGURE 11.7.3

FINDINGS: MLO view of the right breast (Fig. 11.7.1) demonstrates a large, well-circumscribed, lucent lesion with thin capsule in the upper breast. Ultrasound image (Fig. 11.7.2) demonstrates well-circumscribed, homogeneous, hyperechoic lesion corresponding to mammographic abnormality. The second image figure (Fig. 11.7.3) demonstrates well-circumscribed, homogeneous, hypoechoic lesion in a different patient with the same pathology.

DIAGNOSIS: Lipoma

DISCUSSION: The lipoma is a common, asymptomatic, benign breast lesion, which is typically radiolucent on mammographic imaging. It is usually superficially located and has well-defined borders with very thin capsule. It may distort surrounding tissue by displacing adjacent breast parenchyma. When necrosis occurs, calcifications may be present. On physical examination, lipomas are typically soft, freely movable masses (17). Sonographic appearance may vary from hypoechoic to hyperechoic, but well-circumscribed margins and homogenous appearance are typical.

## Aunt Minnie's Pearl

Radiolucent lesion with thin capsule is diagnostic of lipoma.

**HISTORY:** Images of the right breast in a woman with prior history of benign breast biopsy

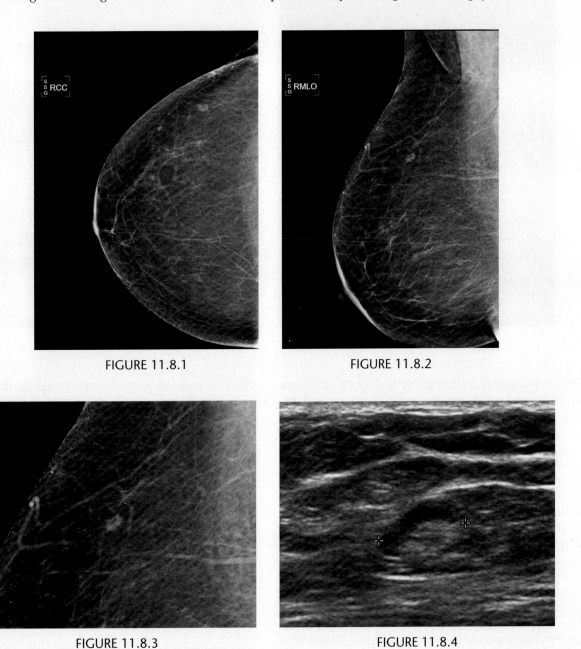

FIGURE 11.8.1

FIGURE 11.8.2

FIGURE 11.8.3

FIGURE 11.8.4

**FINDINGS:** Mammographic images in the CC and MLO projections (Figs. 11.8.1 and 11.8.2 and pictographic magnification Fig. 11.8.3) show a 10-mm ovoid mass in the upper outer quadrant with a fatty hilum. Ultrasound examination confirms a mass with central increased echogenicity consistent with a fatty hilum and a hypoechoic but thin cortex (Fig. 11.8.4). Sagittal T2-weighted MRI image without fat saturation shows the same ovoid mass with peripheral low-signal intensity and central fat signal adjacent to a blood vessel with visible chemical shift artifact (Fig. 11.8.5, *arrow*). Same sagittal MRI slice with T1-weighted imaging, fat saturation, and contrast. The ovoid mass shows fatty notch of the central aspect with enhancement of the cortical rim (Fig. 11.8.6).

**DIAGNOSIS:** Intramammary lymph node

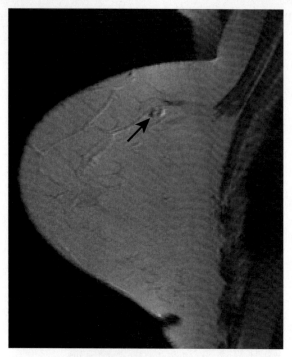

FIGURE 11.8.5

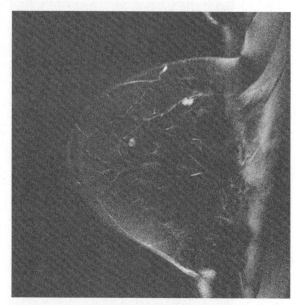

FIGURE 11.8.6

**DISCUSSION:** Intramammary lymph nodes are commonly found in the upper outer quadrant and axillary tail of the breast but can be found anywhere in the breast. They can vary in size but are typically ovoid or reniform in shape. The single best distinguishing feature on mammogram is a notch or central area of radiolucency corresponding to the fatty hilum. If this finding can be identified with certainty, additional imaging can be avoided (18). However, if a fatty hilum cannot be established at mammogram, ultrasound may be performed for further evaluation. Ultrasound can be used as an adjunct to mammography or as a primary method of evaluation in patients under the age of 30. At ultrasound, the mass is well-circumscribed with a peripheral hypoechoic rim or cortex and a central area of increased echogenicity corresponding to the fatty hilum. Blood flow to the central echogenic aspect of the mass can often be established with color Doppler exam (19). MR imaging is not typically done to evaluate lymph nodes, but they may often be seen as incidental findings for other indications. On T2-weighted images without fat saturation, the fatty hilum with its central high-signal intensity can often be established. Peripheral cortical rim is of low-signal intensity.

On T1-weighted post-contrast imaging, the peripheral cortical rim will often enhance. If fat saturation has been used to improve lesion conspicuity, the central fatty hilus will "disappear," will be suppressed. Lymph nodes can often be found immediately adjacent to a feeding vessel. Although mammogram, ultrasound, and MRI cannot determine metastatic disease within lymph nodes, certain features can suggest an increased likelihood of malignant involvement including increased size and density of the node on mammography, loss of the fatty hilum, increased cortical thickness, ill-defined or spiculated margins, and intranodal microcalcifications (20).

## Aunt Minnie's Pearls

Well-circumscribed reniform mass with central radiolucency, "notch," often in the upper outer quadrant/axillary tail of the breast. Ultarsound and MRI may show a central feeding vessel.

Suspect metastatic involvement if there is increased size and density, loss of the fatty hilum, or irregular margins.

**HISTORY:** Several cases are shown; histories are withheld

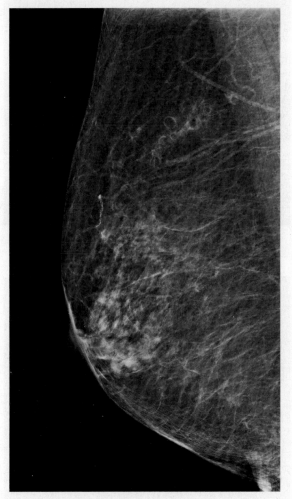

FIGURE 11.9.1

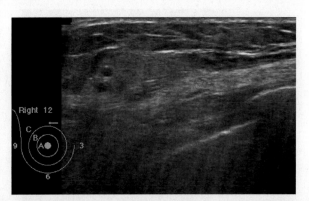

FIGURE 11.9.2

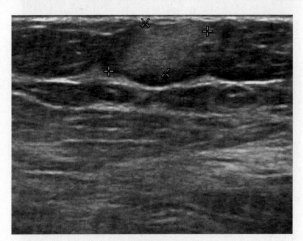

FIGURE 11.9.3

**FINDINGS:** Mammogram mediolateral (ML) view demonstrates an elongated mass superiorly with several rounded lucencies (Fig. 11.9.1). Ultrasound of the corresponding area shows increased echogenicity masses with cystic components (Fig. 11.9.2). In a different patient, ultrasound demonstrates a uniformly hyperechoic superficial mass (Fig. 11.9.3). A third patient has a fat-density mass with rim calcifications, sometimes called eggshell calcifications, in the anterior breast, shown here on an MLO view (Fig. 11.9.4). Corresponding MR images with T2-weighting (Fig. 11.9.5) and T1-weighting (Fig. 11.9.6) with contrast demonstrate fat signal–containing masses with a thin enhancing anterior wall and slight irregularity with enhancement posteriorly as well as a second low T2-enhancing irregular mass superiorly in the anterior breast, which corresponds well to dystrophic calcifications on the mammogram.

**DIAGNOSIS:** Fat necrosis

**DISCUSSION:** Fat necrosis has many appearances and can be a mimicker of tumor on all imaging modalities. A fat-containing mass with eggshell calcifications is a classic description for fat necrosis (21). However, depending on the age of the process and the inflammatory reaction that it incites, the findings can vary and include spiculated masses and irregular enhancing masses on MR, where fat signal can sometimes be obscured. Ultrasound typically shows hyperechoic masses, but in a more inflammatory state, findings can be more equivocal, with ill-defined masses of lower echogenicity.

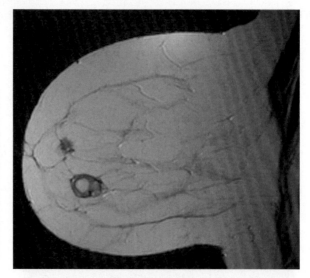

FIGURE 11.9.5

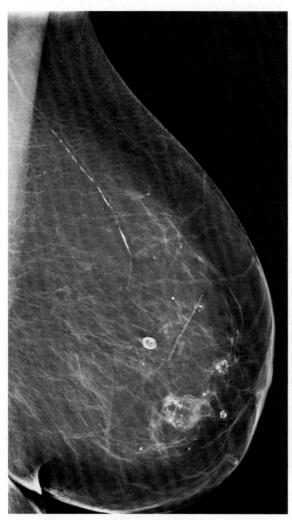

FIGURE 11.9.4

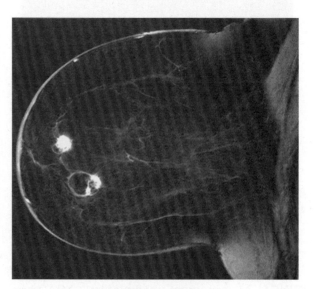

FIGURE 11.9.6

## Aunt Minnie's Pearls

Fat necrosis can be a mimicker of tumor. Without definitive findings and correlative history, biopsy should be considered (22).

MR is helpful to identify fat within a mass, particularly in a scar where overlying density makes fat less apparent on mammography or fibrosis within the scar shadows on ultrasound.

Fat necrosis will enhance on T1-weighted MR. If a recognizable oil cyst is not present, enhancement of the vascularized pseudocapsule can simulate malignancy (23,24).

Fat necrosis can be severely delayed, occurring 10 years or more after surgery.

**HISTORY:** Asymptomatic breast evaluated in a patient with contralateral cancer

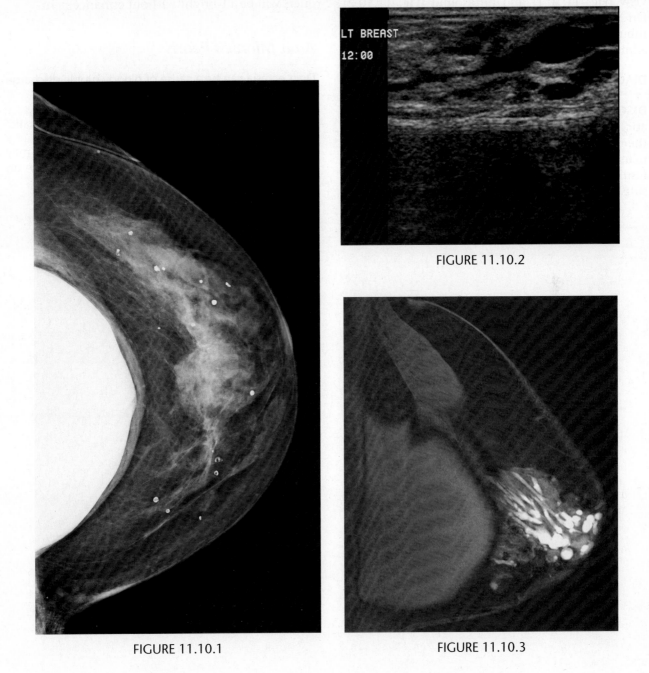

FIGURE 11.10.2

FIGURE 11.10.1

FIGURE 11.10.3

**FINDINGS:** Numerous dilated tubular structures in the retroareolar region on the mammogram CC view (Fig. 11.10.1) and ultrasound (Fig. 11.10.2). On MR (Fig. 11.10.3), linear and cystic dilations of tubular ductal structures are T1-bright prior to the administration of contrast.

**DIAGNOSIS:** Duct ectasia

**DISCUSSION:** Duct ectasia is most often asymptomatic. It sometimes presents as a palpable concern in the retroareolar region or a focal asymmetry on the mammogram (25). Occasionally, nipple discharge results, which can be heme-positive. Other more sinister causes of bloody nipple discharge should be excluded prior to attributing bloody discharge to ectasia. Inspissated proteinaceous secretions in the ducts will be T1-bright without enhancement.

## Aunt Minnie's Pearls

Duct ectasia can be a cause of bloody nipple discharge but should be a diagnosis of exclusion.

Duct ectasia is common and most often asymptomatic.

Ectasia can occur focally and peripherally and may sometimes explain a new mass or asymmetry on mammogram.

**HISTORY:** A 72-year-old for screening mammogram

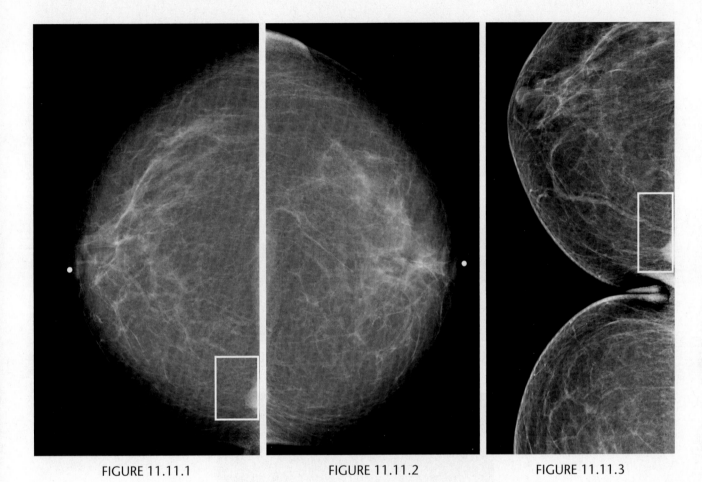

FIGURE 11.11.1     FIGURE 11.11.2     FIGURE 11.11.3

**FINDINGS:** Bilateral mammographic CC views (Figs. 11.11.1 and 11.11.2) show a focal triangular soft tissue "mass" in the far posterior medial aspect of the right breast, marked. Cleavage view shows similar finding (Fig. 11.11.3).

**DIAGNOSIS:** Sternalis muscle

**DISCUSSION:** Description and recognition of this anatomic variant on mammogram was first described in 1996 (26). The sternalis muscle runs longitudinally along the medial aspect of the sternum and is an anatomic variant in approximately 8% to 10% of individuals. Mammographically, this is typically seen only in the CC view and, although it can occur bilaterally, is most often unilateral. Mammographic images show a triangle or flame-shaped soft-tissue mass along the far posterior medial aspect of the breast measuring typically 1 to 2 cm. This variant is important to include in the differential diagnosis of unilateral posterior medial masses to decrease recall, workup, and biopsy. If however uncertainty persists, ultrasound can be performed in this region with an expected normal examination.

## Aunt Minnie's Pearl

Triangular density in the posterior medial aspect of the breast.

**HISTORY:** A 48-year-old woman with right breast pain

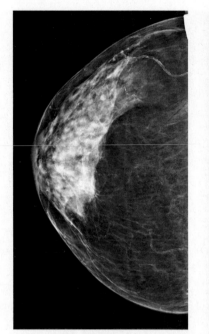

FIGURE 11.12.1

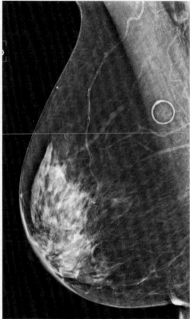

FIGURE 11.12.2

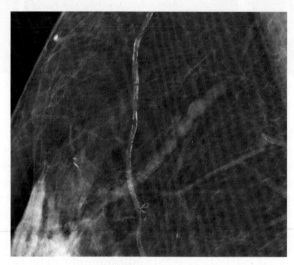

FIGURE 11.12.3

**FINDINGS:** In the lateral right breast on the CC projection (Fig. 11.12.1) just superficial to the skin is a "beaded" ropelike density. There is a corresponding elongated tubular density on the MLO projection in the superior posterior aspect of the breast consistent with a vessel (Fig. 11.12.2). Photographic magnification confirms a ropey beaded appearance (Fig. 11.12.3).

**DIAGNOSIS:** Mondor's disease, thrombophlebitis of a superficial vein (in this case the lateral thoracic vein)

**DISCUSSION:** This condition was described by the French surgeon Henry Mondor as thrombophlebitis of the superficial veins in the breast and may include the lateral thoracic vein, the thoracoepigastric vein, and the superior epigastric vein (27). Although the patient may have no symptoms, the most common presentation is a palpable tender breast mass. Mammographic evaluation may show the classic presentation of an elongated beaded vessel and be sufficient for diagnosis, but ultrasound can also be performed to show the extent of thrombosed vessel and exclude other underlying abnormalities (28).

This is typically a benign self-limited process that may or may not be associated with acute pain or symptomatology. Treatment is usually conservative with anti-inflammatory and analgesic medication as necessary for pain and discomfort. Etiology is often unclear but several suspected risk factors include prior trauma, breast surgery or biopsy, and cancer (29).

## Aunt Minnie's Pearls

Elongated beaded tubular density, representing the affected vessel, often corresponding to a palpable cord-like mass on physical examination.

Benign self-limiting condition often requiring little or no treatment.

**HISTORY:** New cancer diagnosis

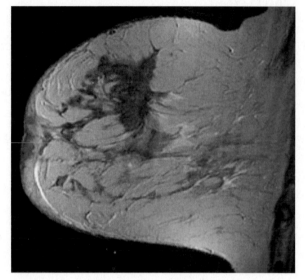

FIGURE 11.13.1

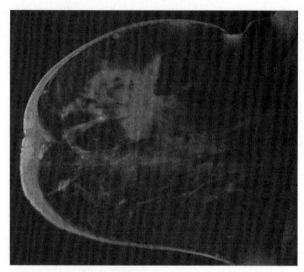

FIGURE 11.13.2

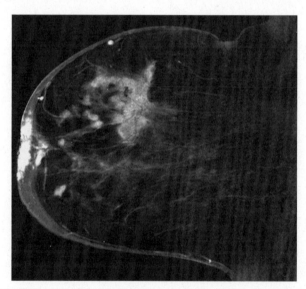

FIGURE 11.13.3

**FINDINGS:** MR images demonstrate nodules within thickened periareolar skin: (a) On T2-weighted image (Fig. 11.13.1), nodules are low signal. (b) On T1 pre-contrast image (Fig. 11.13.2), discrete masses are more difficult to visualize. (c) On T1 post-contrast image (Fig. 11.13.3), the nodules within the skin enhance intensely.

**DIAGNOSIS:** Metastatic skin nodules

**DISCUSSION:** Breast cancer can metastasize to the skin, either as inflammatory cancer with tumor cells occluding dermal lymphatics and causing lymphedema of the breast or with tumor masses as shown here (30,31).

## Aunt Minnie's Pearl

Skin metastases will enhance as discrete lesions on MR. This may occur within a background of mildly enhancing thickened skin, but skin without tumor should not enhance significantly.

**HISTORY:** CC screening mammogram of the right breast in an elderly woman

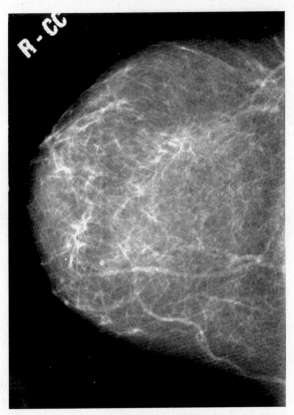

FIGURE 11.14.1

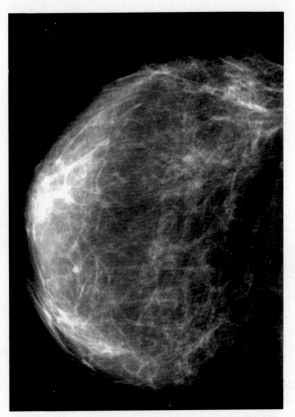

FIGURE 11.14.2

**FINDINGS:** Figure 11.14.1 demonstrates a normal appearance to the right breast parenchyma. Figure 11.14.2, taken 2 years after Figure 11.14.1, shows diffuse skin and trabecular thickening. No definite mass or microcalcification is identified.

**DIAGNOSIS:** Interval development of diffuse skin thickening related to congestive heart failure

**DISCUSSION:** Congestive heart failure (CHF) may be associated with unilateral breast edema and skin thickening, findings that are similar to those of inflammatory breast cancer (32). Inflammatory breast cancer has a poor prognosis, and the median overall survival with treatment is 13 months (33). It may be difficult to distinguish CHF from inflammatory breast cancer. A punch biopsy of the skin can help to accurately establish the diagnosis of inflammatory breast cancer (32,33).

### Aunt Minnie's Pearl

Skin and trabecular thickening in the setting of CHF and unremarkable skin biopsy = mammographic findings of congestive heart failure.

**HISTORY:** A 55-year-old patient for screening mammogram. Breast implants placed more than 15 years prior

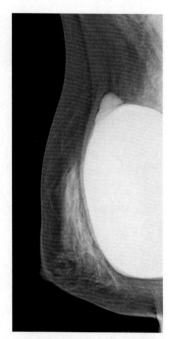

FIGURE 11.15.1

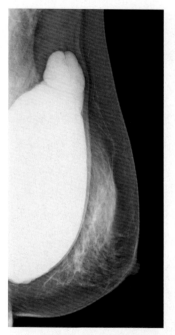

FIGURE 11.15.2

**FINDINGS:** Bilateral mammographic nonimplant displaced MLO views (Figs. 11.15.1 and 11.15.2) show retropectoral silicone implants with focal superior bulging and loss of normal implant contour. Silicone appears contained within the implant pocket, and there is no sign of free silicone.

In a different patient, MRI of the left breast on sagittal non-contrast T2-weighted imaging without fat saturation (Fig. 11.15.3) shows a classic "linguini sign" representing the free-floating collapsed elastomer shell/capsule and numerous water droplets seen as multiple T2-bright objects. Non-contrast axial T2-weighted short inversion time inversion recovery (STIR) with water suppression (Fig. 11.15.4) shows a linguini sign and multiple keyhole or "noose" signs demonstrating silicone on both sides of the capsule. In addition, in the far medial aspect there is a tiny amount of free silicone suggesting silicone outside the fibrous capsule consistent with extracapsular rupture as well.

**DIAGNOSIS:** Silicone implant rupture

**DISCUSSION:** To fully understand implant rupture, one must know the appropriate definitions. Implants have an elastomer shell/capsule encasing the silicone. In addition, the body forms a fibrous capsule around the entire implant. When a rupture occurs, we describe them as either intracapsular, contained within the body's fibrous capsule, or extracapsular, when silicone escapes the fibrous capsule into the surrounding breast parenchyma. Although implant rupture can be diagnosed on mammography and ultrasound, false-negative exams are high. MRI has the best sensitivity and specificity for diagnosing implant rupture at approximately 87% and 89%, respectively (34). Multiple-sequence types can be done to improve the sensitivity of detecting silicone rupture. Two commonly used are (a) T2-weighted fast-spin echo that shows silicone to be bright, fat to be moderate, and water to be very bright, and (b) STIR, with fat suppression showing silicone to be bright, fat to be dark, and water to be very bright (35).

The two most sensitive signs to suggest implant rupture are the linguini sign and the keyhole/

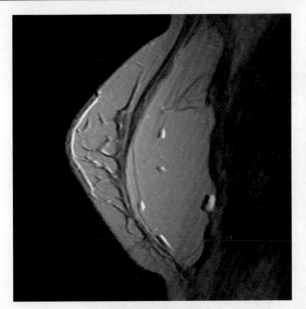

FIGURE 11.15.3

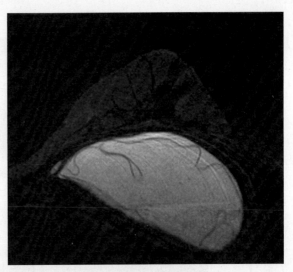

FIGURE 11.15.4

teardrop or noose sign. The linguini sign is the visualization of the elastomer shell as multiple low-signal lines within the silicone gel. This is considered the most reliable finding to predict implant rupture. The appearance of silicone on both sides of a radial fold is often an early sign of implant rupture and has been called the keyhole, notch, noose, or teardrop sign. Any silicone extending beyond the fibrous capsule, within the breast tissue, pectoralis muscle, or lymph nodes, is considered extracapsular rupture. Intracapsular rupture should also be seen concurrently, unless patient has had prior implant rupture (36).

## Aunt Minnie's Pearls

Silicone contained within the body's fibrous capsule but has leaked through the elastomer shell represents intracapsular rupture, whereas silicone outside the body's fibrous shell indicates extracapsular rupture.

MRI is the most sensitive, whereas mammography is the least sensitive method to detect implant rupture.

Visualization of linguini sign on MRI is consistent with implant rupture.

**HISTORY:** A 52-year-old woman seen at time of annual examination. No personal or family history of breast cancer

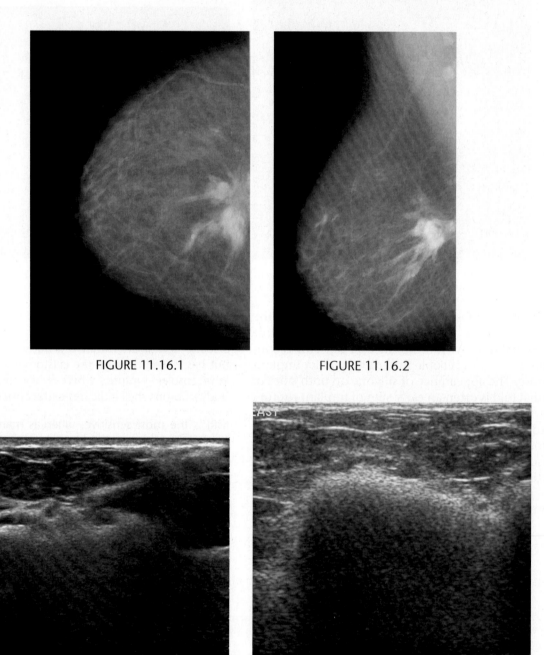

FIGURE 11.16.1                    FIGURE 11.16.2

FIGURE 11.16.3                    FIGURE 11.16.4

**FINDINGS:** Mammographic images of the right breast seen in CC and MLO projections (Figs. 11.16.1 and 11.16.2) show a large irregular mass of marked increased density in the posterior medial aspect of the breast.

Ultrasound (Figs. 11.16.3 and 11.16.4) shows a large hypoechoic mass with echogenic margins and distal shadowing, "snowstorm." Questioning of patient reveals a history of explanation for implant rupture several years ago.

**DIAGNOSIS:** Silicone granulomas consistent with free silicone from previous implant rupture with fibrous reaction

**DISCUSSION:** Silicone granulomas may appear on mammography as irregular masses. As free silicone in the breast tissue is of markedly increased density compared with normal breast parenchyma, suspicion for implant rupture can be entertained even if no implant remains. However, if silicone granulomas are mistaken on mammogram as breast malignancies, ultrasound may be performed. At ultrasound, a hyperechoic margin or border with posterior echogenic noise is often described. The echogenic margin is felt to represent fibrous reaction and the classic "snowstorm" appearance posterior to the mass is due to loss of sound transmission. Multiple conglomerates may be noted (37,38).

## Aunt Minnie's Pearl

Mammographic masses of marked increased density with snowstorm pattern on sonography = free silicone with history of extracapsular implant rupture.

**HISTORY:** A 45-year-old woman with "lumpy" breasts at clinical examination

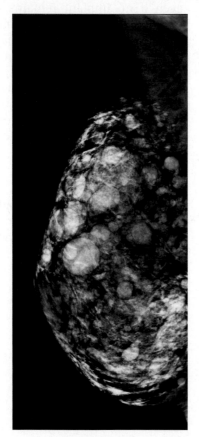
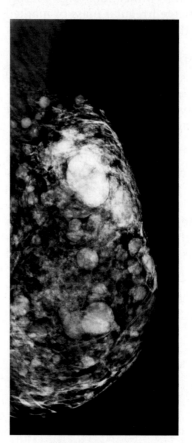

FIGURE 11.17.1                    FIGURE 11.17.2

**FINDINGS:** Bilateral MLO views (Figs. 11.17.1 and 11.17.2) show multiple high-density rounded masses throughout the two breasts with near complete obscuration of breast tissue. Bilateral non-contrast T1 fat-suppressed axial image (Fig. 11.17.3) and bilateral contrast-enhanced T1 fat-suppressed axial image (Fig. 11.17.4) show multiple bright and intermediate signal superficial round and oval masses corresponding to masses seen on mammogram. Patient gives a history of prior silicone injections for breast augmentation. Underlying breast parenchyma is clearly visible and evaluation is not affected by silicone.

**DIAGNOSIS:** Free silicone injection for breast augmentation

**DISCUSSION:** Injection of foreign material including free silicone for the purpose of breast augmentation was seen primarily in the 1950s and 60s. This procedure is now illegal in the US, although illicit use is still performed and still seen occasionally in patients from outside the US. Free silicone injection may be associated with silicone pulmonary embolism and respiratory distress (37). When injected into the breast tissue, silicone remains coalescent and generates a granulomatous or inflammatory reaction leading to firm palpable masses difficult to differentiate from malignancy. Owing to the high density of the material and diffuse nature of the injections, evaluation of the underlying breast parenchyma for breast cancer on mammogram is difficult if not impossible. In recent years, MRI has

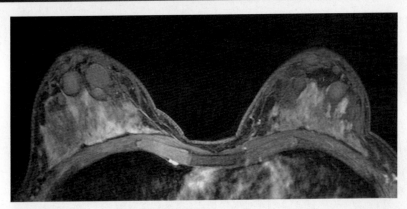

FIGURE 11.17.3

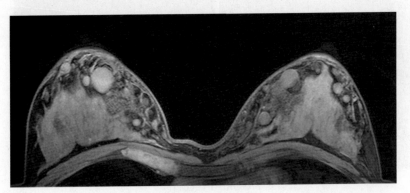

FIGURE 11.17.4

been used to screen women with silicone injections for breast cancer. MRI imaging shows siliconomas to be hyperintense on T2 imaging and are intermediate intensity with no contrast enhancement on T1 imaging allowing discrimination from breast malignancy (39).

## Aunt Minnie's Pearls

Multiple high-density round and oval masses obscuring the breast tissue on mammogram = injected silicone.

Breast tissue can be evaluated with MRI to exclude breast cancer in patients with silicone injections.

HISTORY: Screening mammogram

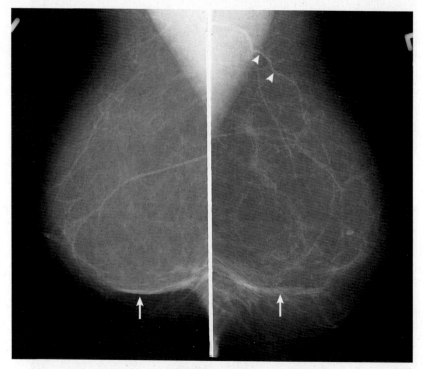

FIGURE 11.18.1

FINDINGS: Bilateral MLO views of the breasts (Fig. 11.18.1) show curvilinear opacities coursing across the inferior portions of both breasts (*arrows*). Minimal glandular tissue is identified above the level of the nipple. Notice the characteristic vascular calcifications that are tubular (*arrowheads*).

DIAGNOSIS: Bilateral reduction mammoplasty

DISCUSSION: Reduction mammoplasty is a common surgical procedure that often manifests characteristic changes on mammography. The surgical procedure involves an inframammary incision that is connected to a circumareolar incision by a third vertical incision. Glandular tissue and fat are removed from the breast in the regions of these incisions. This causes the remaining breast tissue to redistribute into the infraareolar portion of the breast on the MLO view. Nonanatomic curvilinear bands, often accompanied by dystrophic calcifications, are seen in the inferior breast, as in the index case. This combination of findings should allow the radiologist to recognize that the patient has undergone this surgical procedure (40).

## Aunt Minnie's Pearl

Altered bilateral architecture with curvilinear bands, dystrophic calcifications, and reduced glandular tissue = reduction mammoplasty.

HISTORY: Withheld

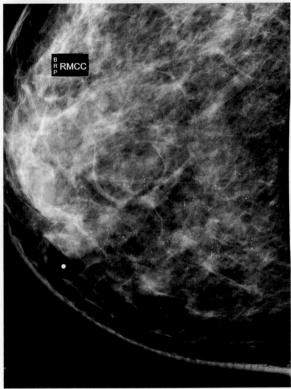

FIGURE 11.19.1

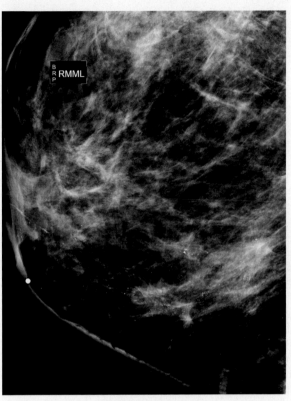

FIGURE 11.19.2

FINDINGS: Magnification views in the CC (Fig. 11.19.1) and ML (Fig. 11.19.2) projections demonstrate clustered pleomorphic calcifications in the low inner quadrant with linear and branching forms. The calcifications occupy the bulk of the quadrant and extend into the nipple. A mass is present within the anterior aspect of the calcifications and associated with a BB, marking a palpable concern. At least one additional mass is present more posteriorly within the region involved with the calcifications. Figures 11.19.3 and 11.19.4 are coned-down images of pleomorphic calcifications in two other patients, both with ductal carcinoma.

DIAGNOSIS: Pleomorphic calcifications

DISCUSSION: Pleomorphic, meaning many forms, is an ominous descriptor for calcifications. Pleomorphic calcifications should always undergo biopsy. They suggest intraductal tumoral necrosis with calcifications taking the form of the necrotic spaces, thus unpredictable and not conforming to an anatomic structure. When linear extensions and branching are present, the association with ductal processes is strongly suggested (41), raising concern for ductal carcinoma in situ (DCIS). It is very common for the patient to have no palpable correlate

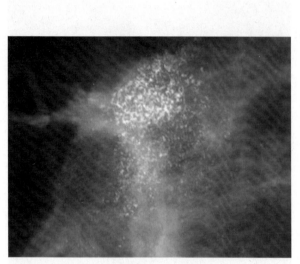

FIGURE 11.19.3

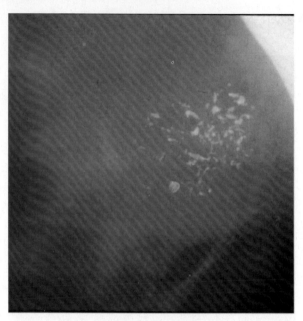

FIGURE 11.19.4

on physical examination and for calcifications to be found on routine screening mammography.

Although there are some benign processes that can potentially produce pleomorphic calcifications, such as fat necrosis, the high association of this finding with carcinoma warrants tissue diagnosis. If benign pathology is established and the pathology and the imaging findings are considered concordant, the calcifications can be followed as long as they remain stable. If they continue to change over time, the possibility of sampling error should be considered, and rebiopsy may need to be performed.

## Aunt Minnie's Pearls

Pleomorphic microcalcifications should always undergo biopsy.

Masses within areas of concerning calcifications should be targeted for biopsy, as they may represent invasive components of tumor and upgrade a tumor diagnosis preoperatively.

Linear and clustered distributions and branching of the calcifications are the most concerning features.

**HISTORY:** A 52-year-old patient presents for baseline mammogram

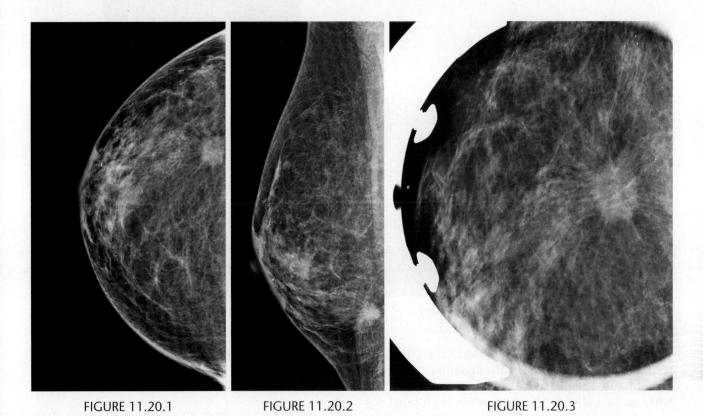

FIGURE 11.20.1       FIGURE 11.20.2       FIGURE 11.20.3

**FINDINGS:** Right breast mammogram with CC (Fig. 11.20.1) and MLO (Fig. 11.20.2) views show an irregular mass with increased density in the lower outer quadrant. Focal spot compression view (Fig. 11.20.3) of this area confirms a spiculated solitary mass. Ultrasound was performed to evaluate the mass (Fig. 11.20.4) and confirms a solid mass with angular margins that is taller than wide. Biopsy was performed due to the highly suspicious features and pathology confirmed invasive ductal carcinoma. Post-contrast T2 sagittal right breast MRI (Fig. 11.20.5) verified a solitary spiculated mass in the 7:00 position.

**DIAGNOSIS:** Breast carcinoma (invasive ductal carcinoma, NOS that is, not otherwise specified).

**DISCUSSION:** Although not all breast carcinomas appear the same, certain features should be considered malignant until proven otherwise. Features that suggest the mass/lesion is likely >95% certain to be malignant should be called BIRADS 5 (highly suspicious for malignancy) and require recommendation for biopsy (42). Mammographic features would include a spiculated or irregularly margin-ated mass, a focal area of increased or developing density or a mass associated with heterogeneous,

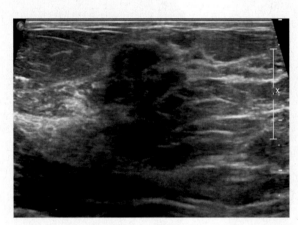

FIGURE 11.20.4

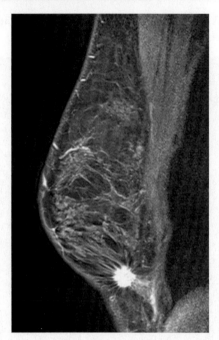

FIGURE 11.20.5

pleomorphic or linear calcifications (37). On ultrasound, features consistent with malignancy include a dominant irregular solid mass, often taller than wide (antiparallel to the chest wall), with posterior acoustic shadowing (43). The lesion will often have increase in color or Doppler blood flow. MRI has a multitude of obvious as well as subtle findings that suggest malignancy. Suspicion for malignancy may depend either on morphologic features or on kinetic enhancement pattern. Malignancy should always be considered for any mass that shows marked immediate enhancement with quick washout and/or morphologically appears similar to a suspicious mammographic mass with spiculated or irregular marginal features (44). Recommendation for biopsy should always be predicated on most suspicious features.

## Aunt Minnie's Pearls

Features highly suspicious for malignancy = BIRADS 5.

On mammogram, new irregular or spiculated mass with or without suspicious calcifications.

At ultrasound, solid mass with irregular, ill-defined, or angular borders, posterior acoustic enhancement and taller than wide.

On MRI, irregular, ill-defined or spiculated mass with or without marked enhancement and rapid washout.

# Case 11.21

**HISTORY:** Palpable right axillary mass

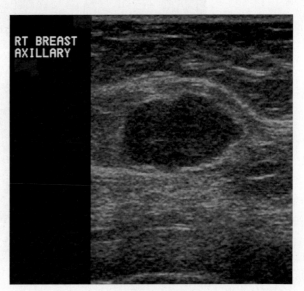

FIGURE 11.21.2

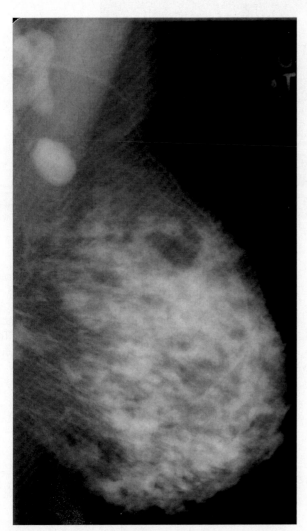

FIGURE 11.21.1

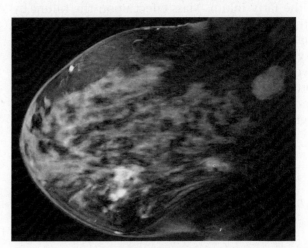

FIGURE 11.21.3

**FINDINGS:** Mammogram MLO view (Fig. 11.21.1) demonstrates dense breast tissue with a dense ovoid axillary mass suggestive of a pathologic lymph node, and several additional dense enlarged nodes can be partially visualized. On ultrasound (Fig. 11.21.2), an ovoid hypoechoic mass correlates with the palpable finding and mammogram. This is suspicious for tumor involving a lymph node. On the sagittal MR-enhanced T1 image (Fig. 11.21.3), an enlarged and enhancing lymph node is present posteriorly, with a replaced fatty hilum. In addition, a mammographically occult enhancing irregular mass is present within the breast. On the axial-enhanced T1

MR image (Fig. 11.21.4), enlarged lymph nodes are present in the axilla.

**DIAGNOSIS:** Pathologic axillary lymph node and enhancing suspicious irregular mass within the breast on MR that was mammographically occult and consistent with breast cancer primary

**DISCUSSION:** The appearance of lymph nodes on MR is most often indeterminate. Normal and reactive lymph nodes as well as metastatic nodes can enhance to varying degrees. The architecture of the node is the most specific indicator of likelihood of

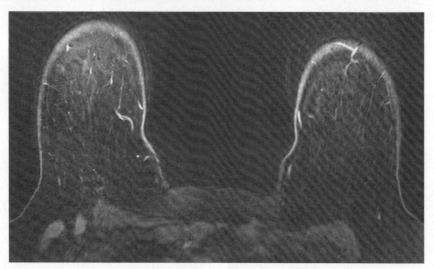

FIGURE 11.21.4

disease on all imaging modalities. The highest correlation with metastatic involvement of a lymph node is a round mass (45), with tumor replacement of the fatty hilum. Mass effect upon the hilum by a thickened cortex should be viewed as suspicious but can be seen with reactive nodes as well. Axillary lymph nodes can be normal while measuring several centimeters when a fatty hilum and a thin cortex are present (46). Metastatic axillary and locoregional nodes typically exhibit FDG uptake and therefore can be detected on PET scan.

## Aunt Minnie's Pearls

Lymph node enhancement on MR is indeterminate when lymph node has normal architecture (47).

The highest correlation with metastatic tumor to a node is obliteration of the fatty hilum or mass effect upon the hilum by a thickened cortex, particularly if the node is enlarged (48).

**HISTORY:** Palpable fixed mass with associated skin retraction in the inferior breast, difficult to visualize on mammography owing to deep location

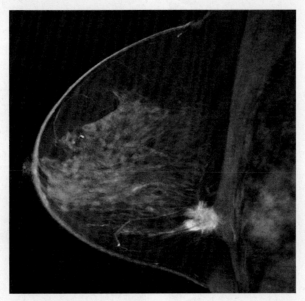

FIGURE 11.22.1

**FINDINGS:** Sagittal gadolinium-enhanced T1-weighted image (Fig. 11.22.1) demonstrates an enhancing spiculated mass inferiorly and posteriorly, with enhancement of the adjacent pectoralis muscle.

**DIAGNOSIS:** Pectoralis muscle invasion by tumor

**DISCUSSION:** No fat plane is visible between the mass and the pectoralis muscle, and there appears to be tenting of the muscle anteriorly toward the mass. There is enhancement of the pectoralis muscle fibers, which is the only confirmatory finding suggestive of pectoralis invasion. Tenting of the muscle is frequently seen, but without muscle enhancement, invasion of the muscle should not be suspected.

## Aunt Minnie's Pearl

Invasion of the pectoralis muscle should be suggested on MR imaging only when enhancement of the muscle is present (49).

HISTORY: A 51-year-old patient with new left breast swelling and nipple inversion

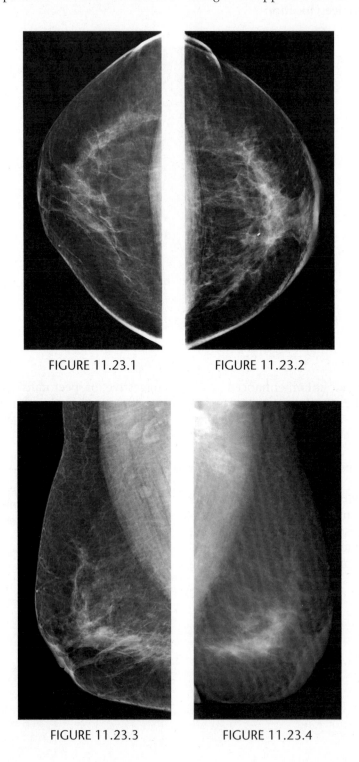

FIGURE 11.23.1          FIGURE 11.23.2

FIGURE 11.23.3          FIGURE 11.23.4

FINDINGS: Bilateral mammogram with CC (Figs. 11.23.1 and 11.23.2) and MLO (Figs. 11.23.3 and 11.23.4) views showing asymmetry in breast density, left greater than right, with visible skin thickening and nipple retraction on the left. There is an abnormal left axillary lymph node noted as well. Ultrasound of superior left breast (Fig. 11.23.5) confirms periareolar skin thickening with dominant solid irregular mass at the 11:30 to 12:00 position (Fig. 11.23.6). Percutaneous biopsy of the breast

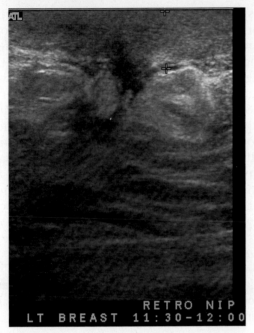

FIGURE 11.23.5

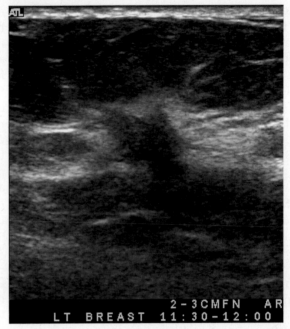

FIGURE 11.23.6

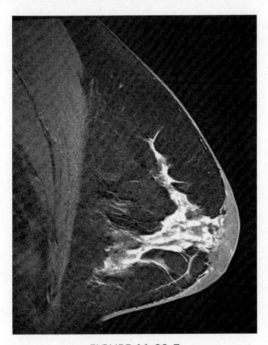

FIGURE 11.23.7

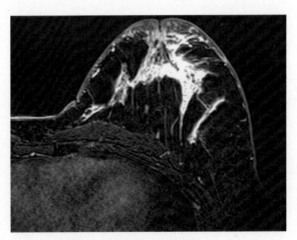

FIGURE 11.23.8

mass and punch biopsy of the skin confirm inflammatory breast cancer. Left breast T1-weighted fat saturation post-contrast sagittal image (Fig. 11.23.7) demonstrates marked skin thickening with large enhancing mass occupying the majority of the breast. Axial T1-weighted fat saturation post-contrast image (Fig. 11.23.8) shows a large central enhancing mass with nipple inversion.

**DIAGNOSIS:** Inflammatory right breast cancer with axillary metastasis

**DISCUSSION:** Inflammatory breast cancer is relatively rare, occurring in only 1% to 4% of all breast cancers but does have a higher incidence in the African American population (50). Diagnosis is often made based on clinical symptoms including erythema, breast swelling, induration, pain, and frequently *peau d'orange*. It can occasionally be confused with mastitis, and antibiotics may be given as a first line of treatment. Definitive pathologic diagnosis, is made by punch biopsy of the skin, and is based on the presence of tumor within the dermal lymphatics. Prognosis is poor with a high rate of morbidity. Punch biopsy should be performed in patients who do not respond to antibiotic treatment or if inflammatory breast cancer is suspected. Mammographic findings of inflammatory breast cancer are varied and may include any combination of skin thickening (92%), diffuse increased breast density (81%), trabecular thickening (62%), axillary adenopathy (58%), distortion or focal asymmetry (50%) and nipple retraction (38%). Discrete mass and suspicious calcifications are less common findings (51). Ultrasound is considered better than mammography at delineating a primary tumor and evaluating axillary contents (52,53). MRI can used to assess for pectoralis muscle involvement and documenting chemotherapeutic response (53).

## Aunt Minnie's Pearls

Clinical signs include erythema, induration, and *peau d'orange* and may be mistaken for mastitis . . . if uncertain punch biopsy of the skin for diagnosis.

Mammographic findings include skin thickening, increased asymmetric density, and trabecular thickening.

Ultrasound and MR can help delineate extent of disease and show treatment response.

**HISTORY:** A 53-year-old woman with a history of lumpectomy for invasive breast carcinoma and radiation treatment

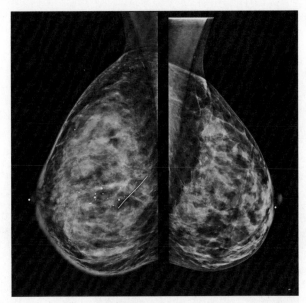

FIGURE 11.24.1

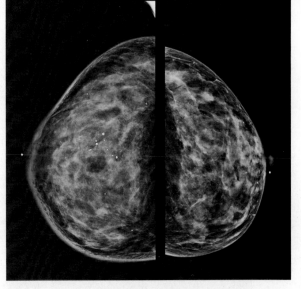

FIGURE 11.24.2

**FINDINGS:** MLO (Fig. 11.24.1) and CC views (Fig. 11.24.2) of the right breast demonstrates marked skin thickening, increased breast parenchyma density, and few coarse calcifications. Linear marker overlies site of prior lumpectomy. Normal left breast view for comparison.

**DIAGNOSIS:** Postradiation changes

**DISCUSSION:** Most women develop postradiation changes several weeks after the onset of treatment. Skin thickening and diffuse edema with trabecular thickening is present, which may resolve over weeks, months, or years or become permanent fibrosis. The apparent increased density on mammogram is because of lymphatic engorgement. In some cases this can also be affected by poor tolerance to compression related to breast sensitivity or diminished pliability of the breast tissue. Architectural distortion from lumpectomy may be present as well as scarring in the surgical bed secondary to irradiation treatment. As most postradiation changes are most prominent at 6 months after the start of irradiation, baseline mammograms are recommended at this time for future comparisons. Differential diagnosis of the skin thickening and increased parenchymal density includes congestive heart failure and inflammatory breast carcinoma. Clinical correlation helps to distinguish these entities from postradiation changes.

## Aunt Minnie's Pearl

Postradiation changes present as skin thickening and diffuse edema. A 6-month posttreatment mammogram is important to establish baseline for comparison for future screenings.

HISTORY: None given or needed. Figure 11.25.1 is a CC view and Figure 11.25.2 a ML view from a diagnostic mammogram for calcifications seen on patient's screening mammogram

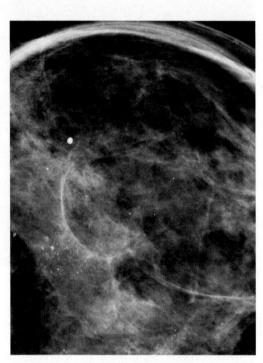

FIGURE 11.25.1

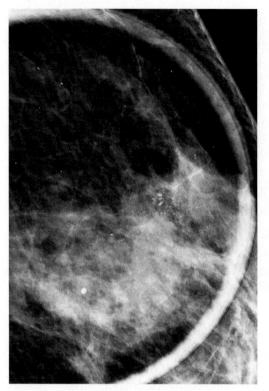

FIGURE 11.25.2

DIAGNOSIS: Milk of calcium calcifications

DISCUSSION: Calcifications may develop in small microcysts within the breast and on the standard MLO and CC views these calcifications may be mistaken for malignancy if not properly evaluated. This finding is estimated to occur in approximately 4% of mammograms (54–59). The standard workup of this finding is to have the woman return for coned-down CC (Figure 11.25.1) and 90° horizontal ML (Figure 11.25.2), or lateromedial views. It is imperative that magnification technique be used for this for better visualization.

On the CC view, the milk of calcium (MOC) calcifications will have a round and amorphous (smudged) appearance and on the horizontal beam image, the calcifications will layer in the bottom of the cyst to produce linear or crescent shapes (the "teacup"

appearance). When a workup reveals this classic appearance, the benign nature of the finding can be assured. No further imaging workup or intervention is warranted once this benign finding is seen.

## Aunt Minnie Pearls

Calcification of tiny microcysts (MOC) occurs approximately 4% of mammograms.

The smudged appearance on CC views and the "teacup" layering on horizontal vertical beam views (with magnification technique) is pathognomonic of MOC, a benign entity.

Once MOC calcifications have been shown on mammography, no further workup is necessary.

**HISTORY:** A 60-year-old patient concerned with a new palpable abnormality in the medial right breast. Prior history of left breast cancer

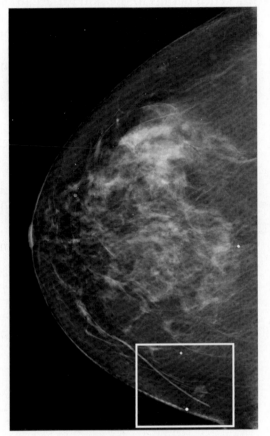

FIGURE 11.26.1

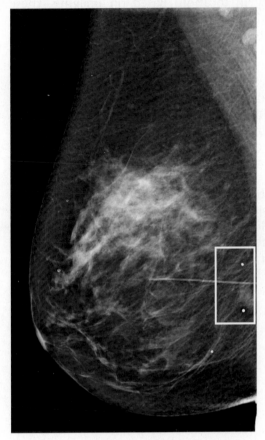

FIGURE 11.26.2

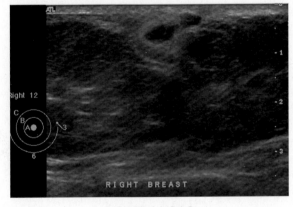

FIGURE 11.26.3

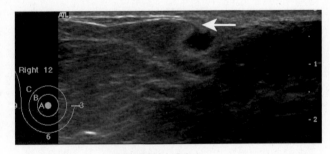

FIGURE 11.26.4

**FINDINGS:** Mammographic images in the CC and MLO projections show an ill-defined 1.5-cm mass in the medial aspect, 9:00 position, of the right breast. This area is marked with a BB marker to designate site of palpable concern (Figs. 11.26.1 and 11.26.2, area in box). Ultrasound examination demonstrates a subcutaneous cystic mass with low-level internal echoes (Fig. 11.26.3). A small pore can be seen extending to the skin surface (Fig. 11.26.4, pore marked with *arrow*).

**DIAGNOSIS:** Epidermoid/sebaceous cyst

DISCUSSION: Epidermoid cysts or sebaceous cysts can develop anywhere on the body. When they do occur on the breasts, they are often medial or inframammary in location. Based on imaging, these two entities are indistinguishable with the difference related to cell lining; epidermal for epidermal cysts and epithelial for sebaceous cysts. Although typically painless and asymptomatic, they can become red and painful when infected. Mammographically, these lesions are round or ovoid, often have an ill-defined margin and may be visibly close to the skin surface in at least one view (60). If a visible pore can be seen at the time of mammographic imaging additional studies may not be required. If however there is persistent concern, ultrasound examination can be performed. At ultrasound, these lesions are predominantly cystic but may contain low-level echoes related to the thick viscous material found within the obstructed gland/follicle. If in a cutaneous location, a "claw" sign can be seen showing the lesion to be visibly enclosed within the more hyperechoic skin; however, if the cystic mass is in a more subcutaneous location, a visible pore may be seen extending through the thickened dermis to the skin surface (61). As these lesions are related to the skin, they have no risk of breast malignancy and require no additional imaging or intervention unless they become infected. If this occurs, they can be treated with antibiotics, warm compresses, or occasionally require surgical/dermatological intervention with incision and drainage or removal (62).

## Aunt Minnie's Pearls

Mammographically round or ovoid with an ill-defined margin close to the skin surface. A visible pore may be seen on physical inspection of the breast.

Ultrasound will show a superficial cystic mass often with low-level echoes.

# REFERENCES

1. Cooper RA, Gunter BA, Ramamurthy L. Mammography in men. Radiology 1994;191:651–656.
2. Appelbaum AH, Evans GF, Levy KR, et al. Mammographic appearances of male breast disease. Radiographics 1999;19:559–568.
3. Evans GF, Anthony T, Turnage RH, et al. The diagnostic accuracy of mammography in the evaluation of male breast disease. Am J Surg 2001;181:96–100.
4. Yang WT, Whitman GJ, Yuen EH, et al. Mammographic appearances of male breast disease. AJR Am J Roentgenol 2001;176:413–416.
5. Homer MJ. Imaging features and management of characteristically benign and probably benign breast lesions. Radiol Clin North Am 1987;25:939–951.
6. Berkowitz JE, Gatewood OMB, Donovan GB, et al. Dermal breast calcifications: Localization with template-guided placement of skin marker. Radiology 1987;163:282.
7. Houlihan MJ. Fibroadenoma and hamartoma. In: Harris JR, Lippman ME, Morrow M, et al. (eds.). Diseases of the breast. Philadelphia, PA: Lippincott–Raven, 1993:45–47.
8. Dixon JM, Dobie V, Lamb J, et al. Assessment of the acceptability of conservative management of fibroadenoma of the breast. Br J Surg 1996; 83:264–265.
9. Sklair-Levy M, Sella T, Alweiss T, et al. Incidence and management of complex fibroadenomas. AJR Am J Roentgenol. 2008;190(1):214–218.
10. Mendelson EB. The breast. In: Rumack CM, Wilson SR, Charboneau JW (eds.). Diagnostic ultrasound, 2nd ed. St. Louis, MO: Mosby, 1998:775–776.
11. Arrigoni MG, Dockerty MB, Judd ES. The identification and treatment of mammary hamartoma. Surg Gynecol Obstet 1971;133:577–582.
12. Feder JM, de Paredes ES, Hogge JP, et al. Unusual breast lesions: Radiologic–pathologic correlation. RadioGraphics 1999; 19(90001):11–26.
13. Mester J, Simmons RM, Vasquez MF, et al. In situ and infiltrating ductal carcinoma arising in a breast hamartoma. AJR Am J Roentgenol 2000;175:64–66.
14. Harman, M Unal O, Ugras S, et al. Breast hamartoma: Radiologic appearances. Eastern Journal Medicine 2003;8(2):43–45.
15. Tabár L, Pentek Z, Dean PB. The diagnostic and therapeutic value of breast cyst puncture and pneumocystography. Radiology 1981;141:659–663.
16. Sickles EA. Breast imaging: From 1965 to the present. Radiology 2000;215:1–16.
17. Cardenosa G. Breast imaging companion, 2nd ed. Philadelphia, PA: Lippincott Williams & Wilkins, 2001.
18. Svane G, Franzén S. Radiologic appearance of nonpalpable intramammary lymph nodes. Acta Radiologica 1993; 34:577–580.
19. Shetty MK, Carpenter WS. Sonographic evaluation of isolated abnormal axillary lymph nodes identified on mammograms. J Ultrasound Med 2004;23(1):63–71.
20. Walsh R, Kornguth PJ, Soo MS, et al. Axillary lymph nodes: Mammographic, pathologic, and clinical correlation. AJR Am J Roentgenol 1997;168:33–38.
21. Magnant CM. Fat necrosis, hematoma, and trauma. In: Harris JR, Lippman ME, Morrow M, et al. (eds.). Diseases of the breast. Philadelphia, PA: Lippincott–Raven, 1993:62–63.
22. Jackson VP, Fu YS, Fu KL. Benign breast lesions. In: Bassett LW, Jackson VP, Fu YS, et al. (eds.). Diagnosis of diseases of the breast. Amsterdam, Netherlands: Elsevier, 2005:409–415.
23. Heywang SH, Hilbertz TH, Beck R, et al. Gd-DTPA enhanced MR imaging of the breast in patients with postoperative scarring and silicon implants. J Comput Assist Tomogr 1990; 14:348–356.
24. Rankin S. Benign breast disease. In: Warren R, Coulthard A (eds.). Breast MRI in practice, London, UK: Martin-Dunitz Ltd, 2002:92–93.
25. Cardenosa G. Major subareolar ducts. In: Breast imaging companion, 2nd ed. Philadelphia, PA: Lippincott Williams & Wilkins, 2001:184–187.
26. Bradley FM, Hoover HC, Hulka CA, et al. The Sternalis muscle: An unusual normal finding seen on mammogram. AJR Am J Roentgenol 1996;166:33–36.
27. Mondor H. Tronculite sous-cutane subaigue de la paroi thoracique anterio-laterale. Mem Acad Chir (Paris) 1939;65: 1271–1278.
28. Conant EF, Wilkes AN, Mendelson EB, et al. Superficial thrombophlebitis of the breast (Mondor's disease): Mammography findings. AJR Am J Roentgenol 1993;160:1201–1203.
29. Shetty MK, Watson AB. Mondor's Disease of the breast: Sonographic and mammographic findings Am J Roentgenol 2001;177(4):893–896.
30. Gilles R, Guinebretière JM, Shapeero LG, et al. Assessment of breast cancer recurrence with contrast-enhanced subtraction MR imaging: Preliminary results in 26 patients. Radiology 1993;188(2):473–478.
31. Ralleigh G, Walker AE, Hall-Craggs MA, et al. MR imaging of the skin and nipple of the breast: Differentiation between tumour recurrence and post-treatment change. Eur Radiol 2001;11(9):1651–1658.
32. Oraedu CO, Pinnapureddy P, Alrawi S, et al. Congestive heart failure mimicking inflammatory breast carcinoma: A case report and review of the literature. Breast J 2001;7:117–119.
33. Galmarini CM, Garbovesky C, Galmarini D, et al. Clinical outcome and prognosis of patients with inflammatory breast cancer. Am J Clin Oncol 2002;25:172–177.
34. Herborn CU, Marincek B, Erfman D, et al. Breast augmentation and reconstructive surgery: MR imaging of implant rupture and malignancy. Eur Radiol 2002;12:2198–2206.
35. Bassett LW, Jackson VP, Fu KL, et al. Diagnosis of diseases of the breast, 2nd ed. Philadelphia, PA: Elsevier Saunders, 2005:601–616.
36. Hallett RL. Breast, implant rupture. http://www.emedicine.com/radio/TOPIC112.HTM.
37. Radiological Society of North America (2006, November 30). Illicit Cosmetic silicone injections carry lethal consequences. *ScienceDaily*. Retrieved December 9, 2007, from http://www.sciencedaily.com/releases/2006/11/061129151526.htm
38. Caskey CI, Berg WA, Hamper UM, et al. Imaging spectrum of extracapsular silicone: Correlation of US, MR imaging, mammographic, and histopathologic findings. RadioGraphics 1999; 19:39–51.
39. Wang J, Shih TT, Li YQ, et al. Magnetic resonance imaging characteristics of paraffinomas and siliconomas after mammoplasty. J Formos Med Assoc 2002;101(2):117–123.
40. Mendelson EB. Evaluation of the postoperative breast. Radiol Clin North Am 1992;30:134–135.
41. Kopans DB. Breast imaging, 2nd ed. Philadelphia, PA: Lippincott–Raven, 1998.
42. American College of Radiology (ACR). ACR BI-RADS. In: ACR breast imaging reporting and data system, breast imaging atlas, 4th ed. Reston, VA. American College of Radiology; 2003.
43. Stavros AT, Thickman D, Rapp CL, et al. Solid breast nodules: Use of sonography to distinguish between benign and malignant lesions. Radiology 1995;196:122–134.
44. Kuhl CK. MRI of breast tumors. Eur Radiol 2000;10(1):46–58.
45. Yang WT, Ahuja A, Tang A, et al. High resolution sonographic detection of axillary lymph node metastases in breast cancer. J Ultrasound Med 1996;15(3):241–246.
46. Jackson VP, Fu YS, Fu KL. Benign breast lesions. In: Bassett LW, Jackson VP, Fu YS, et al. (eds.). Diagnosis of diseases of the breast. Amsterdam, Netherlands: Elsevier, 2005:407–408.

47. Hall-Craggs M, Ralleigh G. Magnetic resonance imaging of the normal breast. In: Warren R, Coulthard A (eds.). Breast MRI in practice. London, UK: Martin–Dunitz Ltd, 2002:79.

48. Lernevall A. Imaging of axillary lymph nodes. Acta Oncol 2000;39:277.

49. Morris EA, Schwartz LH, Drotman MB, et al. Evaluation of pectoralis major muscle in patients with posterior breast tumors on breast MR images: Early experience. Radiology 2000;214(1):67–72.

50. Chang S, Parker SL, Pam T, et al. Inflammatory breast carcinoma incidence and survival: The Surveillance, Epidemiology, and End Results Program of the National Cancer Institute, 1975–1992. Cancer 1998;82:2366–2372.

51. Kushwaha AC, Whitman GJ, Stelling CB, et al. Primary inflammatory carcinoma of the breast: Retrospective review of mammographic findings. AJR Am J Roentgenol 2000;174: 535–538.

52. Lee KW, Chung SY, Yang I, et al. Inflammatory breast cancer: Imaging findings. Clinical Imaging 2005;29;22–25.

53. Gunhan-Bilgen I, Ustun EE, Memis A. Inflammatory breast carcinoma: Mammographic, ultrasonographic, clinical, and pathological findings in 142 cases. Radiology 2002;223: 829–838.

54. Kopans DB. Breast imaging. New York, NY: Lippincott–Raven, 1998:328:361–362

55. Linden SS, Sickles EA. Sedimented calcium in benign breast cysts: The full spectrum of mammographic presentations. AJR Am J Roentgenol 1989;152:967–971.

56. American College of Radiology. Breast imaging reporting and data system (BI-RADS), 2nd ed. Reston, VA: American College of Radiology, 1995.

57. Homer MJ, Cooper AG, Pile-Spellman ER. Milk of calcium in breast microcysts: Manifestation as a solitary focal disease. AJR Am J Roentgenol 1988;150:789–790.

58. Imbriaco M, Riccardi A, Sodano A, et al. Milk-of-calcium in breast microcysts with adjacent malignancy. AJR Am J Roentgenol 1999;173:1137–1138.

59. Sickles EA, Abele JS. Milk of calcium within tiny benign breast cysts. Radiology 1981;141:655–658.

60. Cardenosa. Clinical breast imaging a patient focused teaching file. Philadelphia, PA: Lippincott Williams & Wilkins, 2007.

61. Scholl C. Sonographic features of benign breast masses: A case review http://www.eradimaging.com

62. Lam SY, Kashtoori JJ, Mun KS, et al. Epidermal inclusion cyst of the breast: A rare benign entity. Singapore Med J 2010; 51(12) :e191.

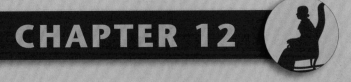

# CHAPTER 12

# GASTROINTESTINAL RADIOLOGY

**Melanie P. Caserta**

*The authors and editors acknowledge the contribution of the Chapter 9 authors from the second edition: Tara C. Noone, MD, and Sunil Kini, MD, and the Chapter 10 authors from the third edition: David J. Ott, MD, and John R. Leyendecker, MD. The author also acknowledges Michael Chen, MD, for assistance with image preparation.*

**HISTORY:** A 56-year-old man with a long history of heartburn

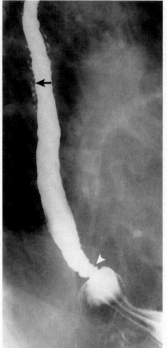

FIGURE 12.1.1

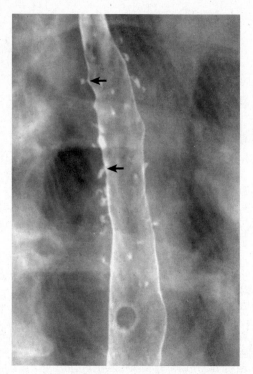

FIGURE 12.1.2

**FINDINGS:** Single-contrast (Fig. 12.1.1) and double-contrast (Fig. 12.1.2) esophagrams demonstrate innumerable, small, flask-shaped outpouchings projecting off the esophageal lumen (*arrows*). These outpouchings are several millimeters long and wide, and they have tiny ostia connecting them to the lumen of the esophagus. The distribution of the outpouchings is confined primarily to the midportion of the esophagus, although several are also seen in the distal esophagus. Demonstrated is also a sliding hiatal hernia with a stricture (Fig. 12.1.1, *arrowhead*) at the esophagogastric junction.

**DIAGNOSIS:** Esophageal intramural pseudodiverticulosis with hiatal hernia and peptic stricture

**DISCUSSION:** Esophageal intramural pseudodiverticulosis is a rare entity in which there is dilatation of the excretory ducts of submucosal mucous glands (1,2). Approximately 90% of patients have a long history of reflux esophagitis, and most have peptic strictures at the time of diagnosis. The condition is usually diagnosed by means of barium swallow, which reveals the numerous dilated excretory ducts. The distribution of pseudodiverticula may be diffuse or segmental. Although *Candida albicans* has been cultured from the esophagus in about one-half of affected patients, it is not thought to play any causal role in the development of pseudodiverticula and is likely just a secondary saprophyte. The condition itself is benign, and treatment should be directed toward the underlying reflux disease and stricture.

## Aunt Minnie's Pearls

Numerous, tiny, flask-shaped outpouchings from the esophagus = intramural pseudodiverticulosis.

This entity is associated with chronic esophagitis and peptic strictures.

HISTORY: Dysphagia and halitosis

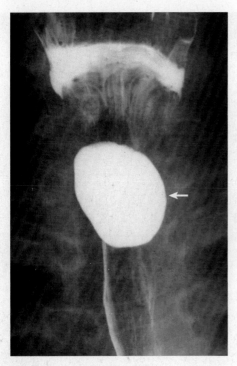

FIGURE 12.2.1

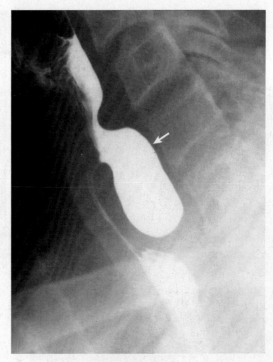

FIGURE 12.2.2

FINDINGS: Anteroposterior (Fig. 12.2.1) and lateral (Fig. 12.2.2) views of the neck obtained during a barium swallow study demonstrate a contrast-filled pouch (*arrow*) emanating from the posterior aspect of the esophagus just at the level of the pharyngoesophageal junction. The internal wall of the pouch is smooth, and the proximal esophageal folds are unremarkable. The proximal cervical esophagus is displaced anteriorly by the contrast-filled pouch.

DIAGNOSIS: Zenker's diverticulum

DISCUSSION: Zenker's diverticulum is a pulsion pseudodiverticulum at the pharyngoesophageal junction. The etiology is multifactorial but may relate to dysfunction of the upper esophageal sphincter or loss of tissue compliance in the same anatomic location (3,4). This produces elevated pressures in the hypopharynx and eventually leads to herniation of mucosa through a triangular defect in the posterior aspect of the inferior pharyngeal constrictor muscle known as Killian's dehiscence. These "diverticula" may become large, and patients frequently present with dysphagia, regurgitation, aspiration, pneumonia, weight loss, and halitosis.

## Aunt Minnie's Pearl

A Zenker's diverticulum is a pulsion pseudodiverticulum that occurs through Killian's dehiscence.

HISTORY: Epigastric pain

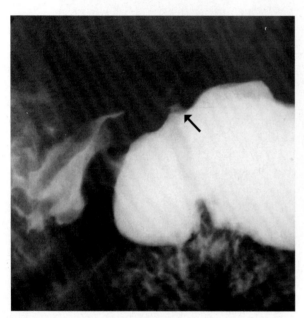

FIGURE 12.3.1

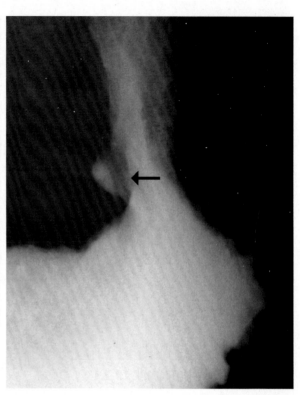

FIGURE 12.3.2

**FINDINGS:** Views from barium upper gastrointestinal series in two patients (Figs. 12.3.1 and 12.3.2) demonstrate small collections of contrast material along the lesser curvature of the stomach, consistent with gastric ulcers. At the base of each ulcer crater, a thin, radiolucent line (Fig. 12.3.1, *arrow*) and a thicker line (Fig. 12.3.2, *arrow*) are seen separating the ulcers from the gastric lumen (*arrows*).

**DIAGNOSIS:** Benign gastric ulcers, one with a thin Hampton's line; the other with a thicker ulcer collar

**DISCUSSION:** Numerous radiographic signs have been described to establish benignity of gastric ulcers (5). Smooth mucosal folds that extend to the edge of the ulcer crater are a reliable indicator of benignity. The smooth nature of the folds must be seen with certainty because nodular radiating folds may indicate an ulcerated malignancy. Other signs of a benign gastric ulcer are the ulcer collar, Hampton's line, and the penetration sign. The ulcer collar represents a rim of mucosa along the margin of the ulcer crater that is thickened by submucosal edema. A similar sign, the Hampton's line, is an extremely narrow, radiolucent line (1–2 mm) that separates the ulcer crater from the gastric lumen. This sign is rarely seen but virtually ensures the benign nature of the ulcer because a tumor mass is not be expected to preserve a thin band of normal mucosa at its margin. The penetration sign is seen when the ulcer crater, viewed in profile, projects beyond the gastric lumen. The single best sign of a benign ulcer is complete healing after a course of conservative medical therapy.

## Aunt Minnie's Pearls

Signs of a benign gastric ulcer include smooth, radiating mucosal folds; penetration sign; ulcer collar; and, especially, Hampton's line.

Complete ulcer healing with medical therapy is the most reliable sign of benignity.

# Case 12.4

HISTORY: Liver lesion identified on prior computed tomography (CT)

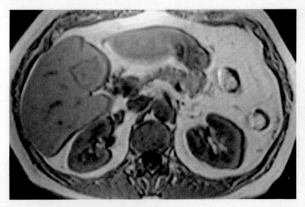

FIGURE 12.4.1

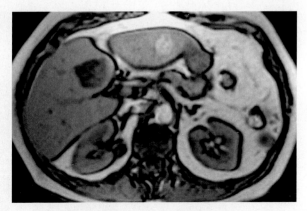

FIGURE 12.4.2

FINDINGS: Axial, in-phase spoiled-gradient-echo (SGE) (Fig. 12.4.1) and axial, out-of-phase SGE (Fig. 12.4.2) T1-weighted magnetic resonance (MR) images. The out-of-phase image demonstrates focal signal loss within the hepatic parenchyma adjacent to the ligamentum teres.

DIAGNOSIS: Focal fatty infiltration of the liver

DISCUSSION: Fatty infiltration of the liver (i.e., hepatic steatosis) results from the accumulation of triglycerides within hepatocytes. It occurs in various disease processes, including obesity, diabetes mellitus, and ethanol abuse. When the amounts of fat and water within a given voxel are similar, the transverse magnetization of the fat and water cancel out on opposed-phase gradient echo images. This phenomenon causes areas of fatty infiltration to lose signal on opposed phase images relative to in-phase images. Common locations for focal fatty infiltration include segment IV along the porta hepatis, near the fissure for the ligamentum teres, and along the gallbladder fossa (6).

Focal fatty infiltration must be distinguished from hepatic tumors that contain intracellular lipid. Examples of tumors that can contain lipid sufficient to lose signal on opposed-phase gradient echo images include hepatic adenoma and hepatocellular carcinoma. Focal fatty infiltration typically does not cause mass effect or displace or compress vessels (6).

## Aunt Minnie's Pearls

Loss of signal intensity within the hepatic parenchyma between in-phase and out-of-phase images occurs in the setting of fatty infiltration.

Common locations for focal fatty infiltration include the central tip of segment IV, along the ligamentum teres, and adjacent to the gallbladder.

Focal fatty infiltration does not typically displace vessels or cause mass effect.

HISTORY: Dysphagia

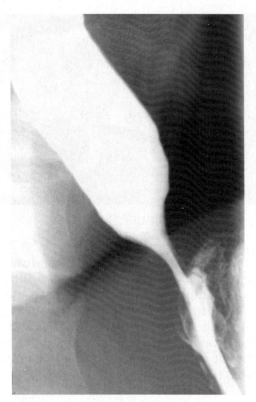

FIGURE 12.5.1

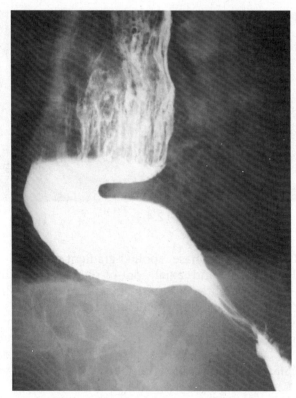

FIGURE 12.5.2

FINDINGS: An image of the lower esophagus (Fig. 12.5.1) demonstrates a smooth, tapered narrowing at the lower end; in another patient, a similar finding is seen but associated with esophageal dilatation and tortuosity (Fig. 12.5.2); both patients had esophageal aperistalsis on fluoroscopic observation.

DIAGNOSIS: Idiopathic achalasia

DISCUSSION: Idiopathic achalasia is a primary motility disorder of the esophagus of unknown etiology (7). On esophageal manometry, the two most important findings are a complete lack of esophageal peristalsis on all swallows observed and a failure of relaxation of the lower esophageal sphincter (LES); the radiographic features reflect these manometric abnormalities: Esophageal peristalsis is absent, and the "beaked" appearance of the lower esophagus results from the dysfunctional LES. With more chronic and severe disease, esophageal dilatation and retention of food and secretions are observed. The most important differential diagnosis is secondary achalasia, most often owing to an invasive adenocarcinoma at the esophagogastric junction, often arising from the gastric cardia. During fluoroscopy, look for periodic relaxation of the lower esophageal sphincter while drinking to distinguish primary achalasia from secondary achalasia. Secondary achalasia, also known as pseudoachalasia, will cause a fixed nonrelaxing obstruction (8).

Treatment consists of relieving the functional LES obstruction with a laparoscopic Heller myotomy or pneumatic dilatation; the use of botulinum toxin for temporary relief is another therapeutic option. Finally, patients with idiopathic achalasia are at higher risk for development of esophageal carcinoma.

## Aunt Minnie's Pearls

Idiopathic achalasia is easily diagnosed and is a treatable esophageal motility disorder.

Gastroesophageal junctional carcinoma is the most important differential diagnosis.

**HISTORY:** A 37-year-old, immunocompromised man with odynophagia

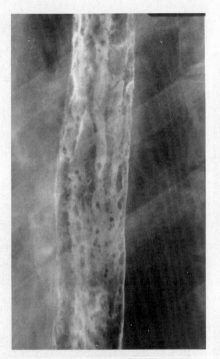

FIGURE 12.6.1

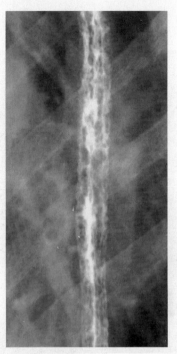

FIGURE 12.6.2

**FINDINGS:** Double-contrast (Fig. 12.6.1) and mucosal-relief (Fig. 12.6.2) esophagrams reveal diffuse and irregular, plaque-like filling defects.

**DIAGNOSIS:** Esophageal candidiasis

**DISCUSSION:** Infectious esophagitis is an increasingly common problem in patients with human immunodeficiency virus infection, malignancy, chronic immunosuppression for organ transplantation, or other illnesses that compromise the patient's immune status. Although various etiologic agents may be implicated in infectious esophagitis, the most common offending organism is *C. albicans*. Affected patients typically present with dysphagia, odynophagia, or chest pain. The radiographic appearance of candidal esophagitis is that of irregular, plaque-like filling defects that tend to be oriented along the long axis of the esophagus (9). With severe involvement, the plaques become coalescent and produce a "shaggy esophagus." Although this appearance is characteristic of candidal esophagitis, advanced herpetic esophagitis may have a similar appearance. The compromised immune status of these patients places them at increased risk for other infections that may be superimposed on the candidal esophagitis.

## Aunt Minnie's Pearls

Plaque-like filling defects = esophageal candidiasis.

Esophageal candidiasis is usually seen in immunocompromised patients.

**HISTORY:** Two patients with epigastric pain

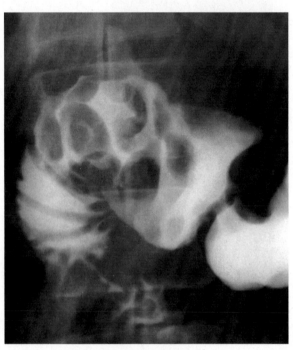

FIGURE 12.7.1

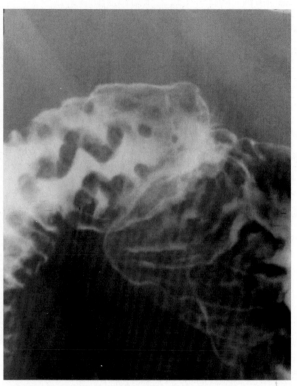

FIGURE 12.7.2

**FINDINGS:** A fluoroscopic spot film obtained during an upper gastrointestinal (UGI) examination (Fig. 12.7.1) shows multiple nodules within the duodenal bulb. A similar image in another patient (Fig. 12.7.2) demonstrates fold thickening and nodular erosions.

**DIAGNOSIS:** Duodenitis

**DISCUSSION:** Duodenitis is a common inflammatory process that predominately affects the duodenal bulb. The etiology is uncertain, but causative factors include excessive alcohol ingestion and the use of nonsteroidal anti-inflammatory drugs; although *Helicobacter pylori* has shown a near universal relationship (>90%) with duodenal ulcer, an association with duodenitis remains unproven. Radiographic detection of duodenitis is modest, and only the more severe forms are demonstrated; radiographic signs that suggest the disease include fold thickening, nodularity, and the presence of erosions; the sensitivity and specificity of these signs are inversely related with the finding of erosions being the most specific but least sensitive (10). Differential diagnosis is nearly nonexistent if multiple abnormalities are present; Brunner's gland hyperplasia was previously the main consideration but is likely a rare disorder; indeed, before the advent of UGI endoscopy, many radiographic diagnoses of Brunner's glands hyperplasia were likely patients with nonspecific duodenitis. Treatment initially involves cessation of potentially causative agents.

## Aunt Minnie's Pearls

Duodenitis is a common inflammation of the duodenal bulb.

Fold thickening with nodularity and erosions are specific findings.

HISTORY: UGI Bleeding

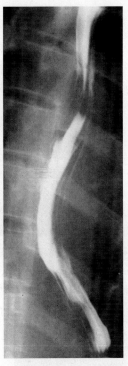

FIGURE 12.8.1

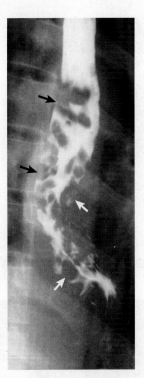

FIGURE 12.8.2

**FINDINGS:** The initial upright oblique full column esophagram film (Fig. 12.8.1) is unremarkable. The following film (Fig. 12.8.2), obtained with the patient in the recumbent position, demonstrates serpiginous, nodular filling defects (*arrows*).

**DIAGNOSIS:** Esophageal varices

**DISCUSSION:** Esophageal varices represent portal–systemic venous collateral pathways. They occur most commonly in the setting of portal hypertension in which venous blood from the splanchnic system is shunted through the esophageal or paraesophageal venous plexus into the azygous system and superior vena cava. Because of the cephalad direction of flow through the varices, they are referred to as "uphill" varices. Esophageal varices develop less commonly in the setting of superior vena cava (SVC) obstruction, in which venous blood from the head, upper extremities, and trunk is shunted through the esophageal or paraesophageal venous plexus and into the portal or azygous systems. These collaterals are referred to as "downhill" varices (11). The clinical relevance of esophageal varices lies in their tendency for rupture, with potentially severe UGI bleeding.

Varices may appear as nodular, serpiginous filling defects on barium esophagography. It is important to recognize the changing character of the filling defects during fluoroscopy because fixed defects may be encountered with varicoid carcinoma. Because the varices may be intermittently decompressed as a result of esophageal peristalsis and changing perfusion pressure during the examination, various provocative maneuvers have been proposed to increase the visualization of the varices. Common maneuvers used in radiology include prone and upright patient positioning and performance of respiratory maneuvers (11,12).

## Aunt Minnie's Pearls

Changing, serpiginous filling defects in the esophagus = varices.

Uphill varices result from portal hypertension.

Downhill varices result from SVC obstruction.

**HISTORY:** A 30-year-old woman with a history of a malignant skin lesion

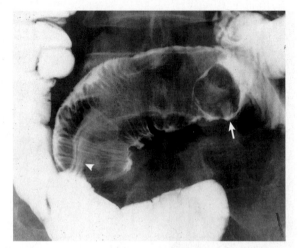

FIGURE 12.9.1

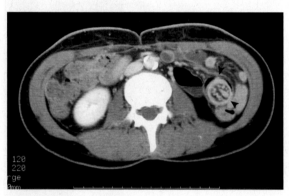

FIGURE 12.9.2

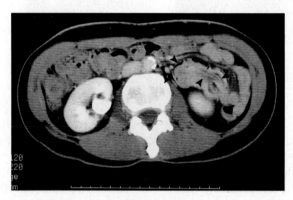

FIGURE 12.9.3

**FINDINGS:** A single view from a small bowel follow-through examination (Fig. 12.9.1) demonstrates a filling defect within the small bowel, surrounded by a coiled-spring pattern of mucosal folds. The leading edge of the filling defect looks like a mass (*arrow*). Barium extends into the central portion of the mass (*arrowhead*), which is a distinguishing feature of this case. CT confirms the abnormality and shows a filling defect in the small bowel, which has concentric bands of high and low attenuation (Figs. 12.9.2 and 12.9.3, *arrowheads*).

**DIAGNOSIS:** Small-bowel intussusception from metastatic melanoma

**DISCUSSION:** Idiopathic intussusception is a disease of the young. When intussusception is encountered in older individuals or neonates, a pathologic lead point is a primary consideration. In this case, the melanoma metastasis is seen leading the intussusceptum

into the intussuscipiens. Peutz–Jeghers syndrome, lymphoma, lipomas, or Meckel's diverticula may also present as lead masses. Causes of transient intussusception include scleroderma, sprue, and cystic fibrosis. The coiled-spring appearance is caused by a projection of inflamed and engorged mucosa into a barium pool that has retrograde filled the lumen of the intussuscipiens (13,14). The alternating bands of high and low attenuation demonstrated by CT result from intussuscepted mesenteric fat contrasted with mucosal–muscular interfaces (13).

## Aunt Minnie's Pearls

Coiled-spring appearance on small-bowel follow-through = intussusception.

Suspect a lead point in neonates, older children, and adults.

HISTORY: Follow-up after colectomy for colon cancer

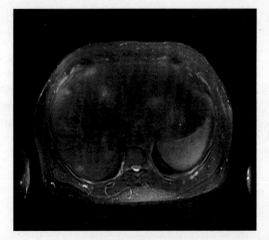

FIGURE 12.10.1

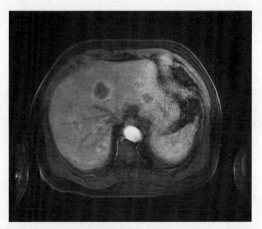

FIGURE 12.10.2

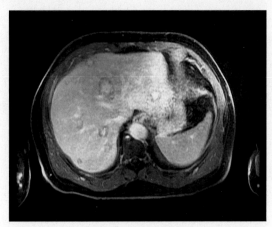

FIGURE 12.10.3

FINDINGS: Axial T2-weighted MR image (Fig. 12.10.1) through the liver shows multiple hepatic lesions that demonstrate mildly increased signal intensity relative to the liver. An arterial-phase T1-weighted MR image (Fig. 12.10.2) performed after administration of gadolinium-based contrast medium shows the lesions to initially enhance peripherally. An equilibrium-phase T1-weighted MR image (Fig. 12.10.3) shows that the lesions have enhanced centrally, whereas the lesion peripheries have relatively lower-signal intensity.

DIAGNOSIS: Liver metastases from carcinoma

DISCUSSION: Metastatic disease represents the most common type of malignant hepatic neoplasm. On MRI, liver metastases can have a highly variable appearance. However, the combination of multiple liver lesions demonstrating increased signal intensity on T2-weighted images, early peripheral enhancement, and central enhancement with peripheral low-signal intensity on delayed (equilibrium-phase) images is highly specific for metastatic carcinoma. The term *peripheral washout sign* has been coined to describe this particular enhancement pattern (15). Other types of malignant tumor (particularly cholangiocarcinoma) can produce a similar enhancement pattern, so the combination of clinical history and presence of multiple lesions is helpful in suggesting the diagnosis of metastases.

Hepatobiliary contrast agents, such as gadoxetic acid, allow for both dynamic contrast-enhanced imaging of lesions and increased lesion conspicuity on delayed T1-weighted images, which is a helpful feature in identifying metastases. Metastases are non-hepatocellular and thus will not retain the contrast on delayed imaging. Metastases appear hypointense compared with enhancing normal liver on hepatobiliary phase images (16).

## Aunt Minnie's Pearl

Multiple liver lesions demonstrating increased signal intensity on T2-weighted images, early peripheral enhancement, and prolonged central enhancement with lower-signal intensity periphery on delayed images suggests the diagnosis of metastatic carcinoma.

**HISTORY:** Patient who underwent laparoscopic adjustable band placement 3 years ago, now presents with abdominal pain after eating

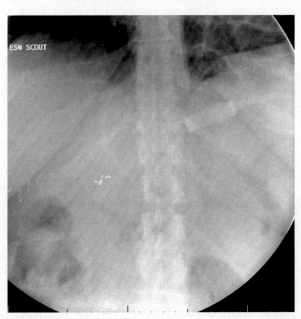

FIGURE 12.11.1

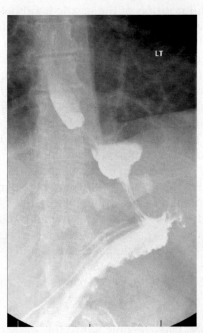

FIGURE 12.11.2

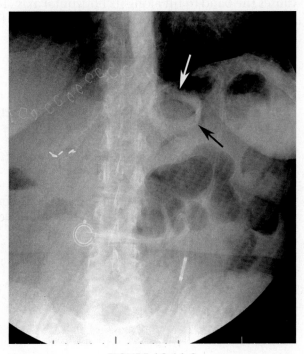

FIGURE 12.11.3

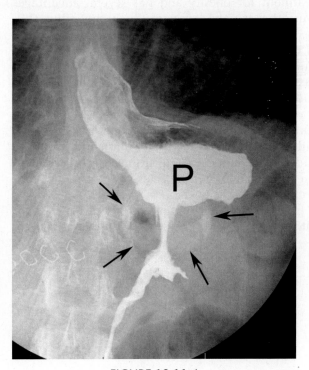

FIGURE 12.11.4

FINDINGS: The scout film (Fig. 12.11.1) and image from a contrast UGI examination (Fig. 12.11.2) were obtained one day after surgery. Note the appearance and position of the gastric band below the esophagogastric junction in the left upper quadrant (Fig. 12.11.1). The band appears disk-like, with the left lateral aspect directed toward the left shoulder. On the contrast UGI (Fig. 12.11.2), a small gastric pouch is seen above the band. Both images demonstrate the expected postoperative findings of the gastric band. Similar images, obtained 3 years later at the time of the patient's current presentation (Figs. 12.11.3 and 12.11.4) show alteration of the band position (*arrows*) and a larger gastric pouch (*P*) above the band. On the scout film (Fig. 12.11.3) the position of the band now has the configuration of the capital letter "O" (*arrows*), the so-called O sign. After the administration of oral contrast, the pouch is larger than expected (*P*), confirming downward slippage of the band.

DIAGNOSIS: Slipped gastric band exhibiting the O sign.

DISCUSSION: Laparoscopic adjustable gastric banding (LAGB) bypass is increasing in popularity as a treatment for obesity and has several advantages over other bariatric surgeries, including adjustability, reversibility, lack of anatomic alteration of the GI tract, and low surgical risk to the patient. In the immediate postoperative period, a limited UGI contrast study is often performed to evaluate for position of the band and any early complications such as obstruction or leak. The pouch size, band position and orientation, patency, size of gastric lumen within the band (normally 3–4 mm), and emptying into the remainder of the stomach are evaluated. The tubing and port are also assessed for intact connections and port position.

In addition to qualitative visual assessment with imaging, band position can be quantitatively evaluated with measurement of the "phi angle." The phi angle is constructed using the vertical axis of the spine and the long axis of the band, and it should range between 4° and 58°. The gastric pouch should be small, approximately 4 cm in diameter, when adequately filled (17). Contrast material should readily pass into the stomach, and it may be normal to see some delay in pouch emptying above the band. Periodically, the LAGB may need adjustments with initial adjustment typically performed 4 weeks after solids are introduced into the diet.

Complications related to LAGB can occur in the early postoperative period or later and can be considered in three categories: band-related, port-related (rare), and other. Band-related complications occur more commonly and include slippage, misplacement, stomal stenosis, pouch dilatation, and band erosion. Band slippage is a relatively common complication, which may result in stomal stenosis or obstruction necessitating acute surgical intervention. Slippage is defined as upward herniation of the distal stomach through the band, resulting in pouch enlargement (17). On scout imaging prior to UGI examination, a slipped band may assume an O-shaped configuration, the so-called O sign, which occurs when the weight of the herniated stomach causes the band to tilt along its horizontal axis (18). The band can then be seen partly en face and the phi angle will be increased.

## Aunt Minnie's Pearls

Normal position of the lap band is pointing toward the left shoulder with a phi angle between 4° and 58°.

A slipped gastric band may assume an "O" shape (the "O" sign).

Slippage of the gastric band can cause serious complications and may require acute surgical intervention.

**HISTORY:** Incidental finding on CT scan of the abdomen and MRI of the liver performed prior to and after intravenous administration of gadobenate dimeglumine

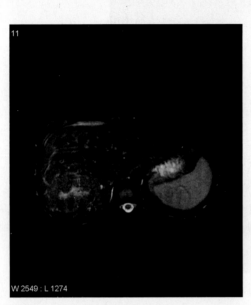

FIGURE 12.12.1

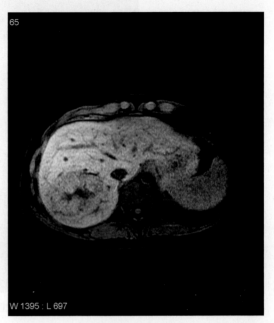

FIGURE 12.12.2

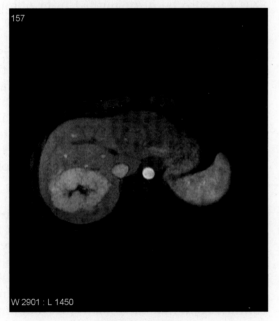

FIGURE 12.12.3

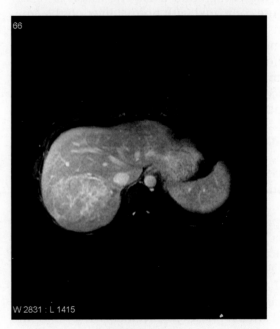

FIGURE 12.12.4

**FINDINGS:** Axial MR images through the liver demonstrate a lobulated lesion that is nearly isointense relative to liver on the fat-suppressed T2-weighted image (Fig. 12.12.1) and fat-suppressed T1-weighted image (Fig. 12.12.2). The center of the lesion (central scar) is bright on the T2-weighted image and relatively hypointense on the T1-weighted image. On the arterial phase gadolinium-enhanced image (Fig. 12.12.3), there is enhancement of the lesion (except for the central portion) well above

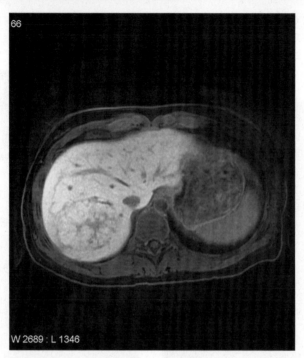

66

W 2689 : L 1346

FIGURE 12.12.5

that of the background liver. The lesion is nearly isointense compared with normal liver on the equilibrium phase image (Fig. 12.12.4), and there is enhancement of the central portion of the lesion. On the 1-hour delayed image (Fig. 12.12.5), the lesion has similar signal intensity to background liver with the exception of the center, which is once again hypointense.

DIAGNOSIS: Focal nodular hyperplasia (FNH)

DISCUSSION: FNH is a tumor comprising benign, but abnormally arranged, hepatocytes and fibrous stroma. A central fibrovascular scar and septa are often present. Bile ductules present within the lesion lack normal communication with the larger bile ducts. Kupffer cells of varying functionality are also present.

FNH is typically nearly isointense to liver on unenhanced CT and MR images and demonstrates marked arterial phase enhancement on CT and MRI after intravenous administration of extracellular contrast agents (19). Radiating hypointense septa are often visible on arterial phase images. The central stellate scar is slower to enhance than the main substance of the lesion but usually enhances within a few minutes of contrast administration (unlike the typical scar of fibrolamellar carcinoma, which tends

not to enhance even by the equilibrium phase). FNH can also be distinguished from fibrolamellar carcinoma on T2-weighted images, as the central scar is bright in FNH and typically dark in fibrolamellar carcinoma. On portal-phase images, typical FNH approximates the signal intensity of the normal liver or is mildly hyperintense. A central scar is absent in up to one-third of cases of FNH.

FNH can also be diagnosed with nuclear medicine techniques. FNH shows immediate uptake and delayed clearance of [99m]Tc HIDA in approximately 90% of cases and uptake of [99m]Tc sulfur colloid in approximately two-thirds of cases.

Hepatobiliary MR contrast agents have been used to improve lesion detection in the liver, and improve diagnostic certainty for lesions of hepatocellular origin, such as FNH. Hepatobiliary agents are taken up by functioning hepatocytes in varying degrees with a portion of excretion in the bile (16). Gadobenate dimeglumine is a gadolinium-based contrast agent that has a small (<5%) but important component of hepatobiliary clearance. As a result, typical FNH will retain gadobenate dimeglumine, appearing iso- to mildly hyperintense to liver on hepatobiliary phase images (1–3 hours after contrast administration; 20). A newer agent, gadoxetic acid, has 50% biliary clearance and 50% renal clearance, which provides excellent delayed hepatic and biliary tree imaging. FNH will appear iso- or more typically hyperintense to background liver on delayed hepatobiliary phase images (10–60 minutes after contrast administration) allowing for confident diagnosis of FNH (16).

### *Aunt Minnie's Pearls*

FNH resembles normal liver on unenhanced CT and MR images and demonstrates strong arterial phase enhancement with radiating septa after intravenous contrast administration.

The central scar of FNH is bright on T2-weighted images, low-signal intensity on T1-weighted images, and enhances after the arterial phase but within a few minutes of contrast administration.

FNH typically retains gadobenate dimeglumine or gadoxetic acid on hepatobiliary phase images.

**HISTORY:** Incidental finding on CT scan

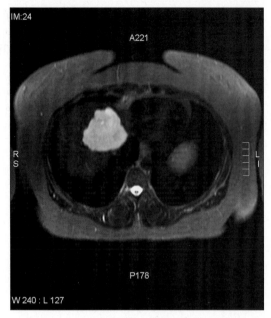

FIGURE 12.13.1

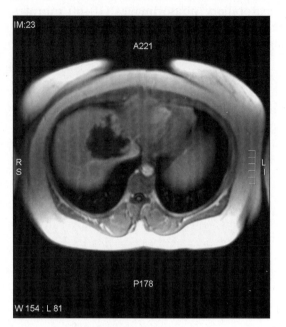

FIGURE 12.13.2

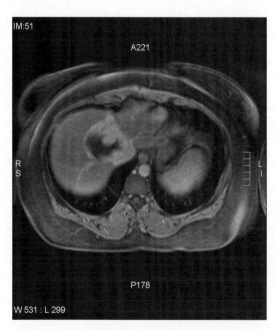

FIGURE 12.13.3

**FINDINGS:** A fat-suppressed T2-weighted image (Fig. 12.13.1) and early and delayed gadolinium-enhanced T1-weighted images (Figs. 12.13.2 and 12.13.3) demonstrate a large lesion in the dome of the liver. On the T2-weighted image, the lesion is very bright relative to the normal liver and has a lobulated, well-defined margin. On gadolinium-enhanced images, the lesion demonstrates early nodular, discontinuous peripheral enhancement that progresses in a centripetal manner. The enhancing portions of the lesion have similar signal intensity to the vascular blood pool.

**DIAGNOSIS:** Hepatic cavernous hemangioma

**DISCUSSION:** Cavernous hemangioma is the most common benign hepatic tumor and commonly presents as an incidental finding on CT or ultrasound. Pathologically, hemangiomas comprise blood-filled spaces with thin fibrous walls lined by endothelial cells. Prior to the widespread availability of MRI, the diagnosis of cavernous hemangioma (>2 cm) was confirmed with $^{99m}$Tc-labeled red blood cell scintigraphy. The diagnosis of hemangioma can also be suggested by ultrasound when a homogeneously hyperechoic lesion is identified within the liver in a patient with no risk factors for hepatocellular carcinoma or metastatic disease. Other typical sonographic features include an echogenic rim and a scalloped margin. When classic enhancement features are present, hemangiomas can be readily diagnosed by CT.

MRI is now commonly employed to confirm the diagnosis of hemangioma. Typical MRI features include a well-defined lobulated border and marked hyperintensity relative to liver on T2-weighted images. On dynamic gadolinium-enhanced images, typical hemangiomas demonstrate early nodular, discontinuous, peripheral enhancement that progresses centrally (centripetal enhancement). The degree of enhancement of a hemangioma parallels the enhancement of the hepatic vessels. On delayed post-contrast images, hemangiomas remain enhanced similar to the hepatic vessels. Complete filling-in of the lesion is typical of smaller lesions but not necessary to diagnose hemangioma, provided the lesion otherwise demonstrates classic features (21).

## Aunt Minnie's Pearls

Hemangiomas are the most common benign hepatic tumors.

Peripheral, nodular enhancement that progresses centrally and parallels the signal intensity of the vessels after administration of contrast material on CT and MRI is classic.

Hemangiomas are typically very bright on T2-weighted MR images.

HISTORY: Withheld

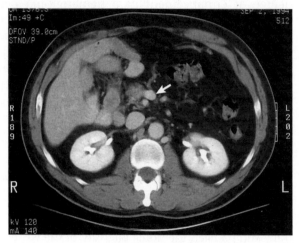

FIGURE 12.14.1

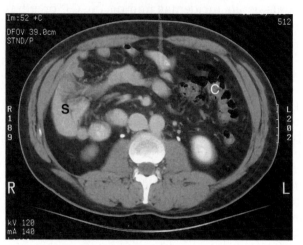

FIGURE 12.14.2

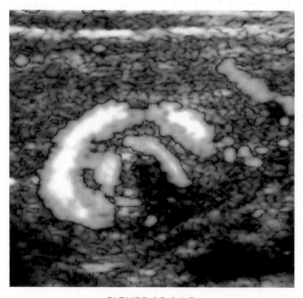

FIGURE 12.14.3

FINDINGS: View from a contrast-enhanced CT of the abdomen (Fig. 12.14.1) shows that the normal orientation of the superior mesenteric artery and vein is reversed with the larger vein (*arrow*) lying to the left of the artery. On an additional image (Fig. 12.14.2) the colon (*C*) is seen to lie only on the left side of the abdomen and the small intestine (*S*) only on the right. A Doppler ultrasound image in a second patient (Fig. 12.14.3) demonstrates the whirlpool sign.

DIAGNOSIS: Midgut malrotation (nonrotation)

DISCUSSION: The normal embryologic development of the intestines involves a complex sequence of events that results in the fixation of the cecum in the right lower quadrant of the abdomen and the duodenojejunal flexure in the left upper quadrant (22). Between these two points, the small intestine is anchored by the attachment of its mesentery. When abnormalities in this process occur, it may result in abnormal fixation of the small-bowel mesentery and predispose the midgut to volvulus. Patients with midgut malrotation also have an increased risk of small-bowel obstruction caused by peritoneal (Ladd's) bands. Nonrotation of the bowel may also occur and is diagnosed when the large intestine is located in the left hemiabdomen and the small bowel in the right hemiabdomen, as in the index case. On cross-sectional imaging studies, a reversal of the normal orientation of the superior mesenteric artery and vein is frequently seen in cases of midgut malrotation and nonrotation (23). An ultrasound whirlpool appearance is produced when the superior mesenteric vein wraps around the superior mesenteric artery, a relatively specific finding for malrotation with midgut volvulus.

## Aunt Minnie's Pearls

Reversal of superior mesenteric artery and vein orientation on cross-sectional imaging is seen in malrotation or nonrotation of the bowel.

Large intestine on the left and small intestine on the right = nonrotation.

There is an increased risk of midgut volvulus and small-bowel obstruction.

**HISTORY:** A 64-year-old woman with cirrhosis

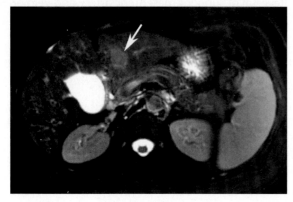

FIGURE 12.15.1

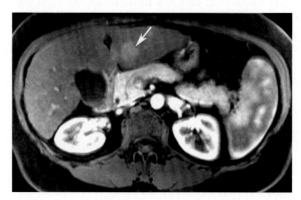

FIGURE 12.15.2

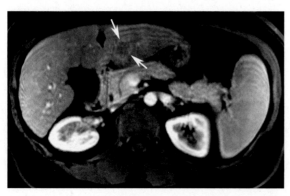

FIGURE 12.15.3

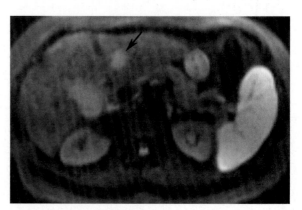

FIGURE 12.15.4

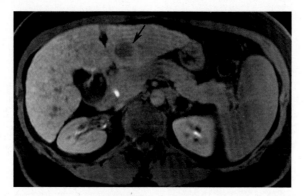

FIGURE 12.15.5

**FINDINGS:** Axial MR images through the liver demonstrate a mass (Fig. 12.15.1, *arrow*) in the left liver. The liver is noted to be cirrhotic with a nodular surface contour. The mass (*arrow*) demonstrates increased signal relative to background liver on T2-weighted image (Fig. 12.15.1). Dynamic gadoxetic acid–enhanced images show arterial enhancement (Fig. 12.15.2, *arrow*) and subsequent "washout" (mass becomes hypointense to liver) with a pseudocapsule (Fig. 12.15.3, *arrows*). Diffusion-weighted image (Fig. 12.15.4) shows increased signal (*arrow*) with low signal on the ADC map (not shown) indicating restricted diffusion within the mass. On the hepatobiliary phase image (Fig. 12.15.5) obtained at

20 minutes after contrast administration, the lesion is hypointense (*arrow*) relative to background liver.

**DIAGNOSIS:** Hepatocellular carcinoma

**DISCUSSION:** The incidence of hepatocellular carcinoma (HCC) continues to rise and worldwide is the third most common cause of death from cancer (24). However, with advances in detection and treatment, the prognosis of patients with HCC is no longer uniformly poor (25). A spectrum of hepatocellular nodules occur in cirrhosis, representing a continuum from regenerative nodules, to dysplastic nodules, to HCC. Vascularity patterns change from portal venous supply to predominantly arterial perfusion as the nodules progress to HCC (24). Characterization of small nodules in cirrhotic livers is difficult; however, the American Association for the Study of Liver Diseases has recently updated its guidelines to allow diagnosis of typical HCC in cirrhotic patients by imaging criteria alone without the need for biopsy. In nodules >1 cm in size, contrast-enhanced CT or MRI can confidently establish the diagnosis if the lesion demonstrates the typical imaging features of arterial enhancement followed by washout on subsequent dynamic phases (25). If the appearance is not typical on one imaging modality, there are two options: a second study could be performed with the other modality or biopsy could be performed.

A major advantage of MRI is the ability to perform multiple sequences that can help further characterize a lesion. Many, if not most, HCCs demonstrate restricted diffusion of water molecules, causing HCC to appear brighter than the background liver on diffusion-weighted imaging (DWI). DWI is particularly useful in distinguishing solid from cystic/necrotic components of tumors (26).

The use of hepatobiliary contrast agents can also help detect and characterize liver lesions in the setting of cirrhosis. Hepatobiliary specific agents, such as gadoxetic acid, are taken up by functioning hepatocytes and excreted in the bile. Typically, HCC will not retain the contrast agent and will appear darker than the background liver on hepatobiliary phase images, whereas regenerative nodules have normal hepatocellular functions and will typically retain hepatobiliary contrast similar to background liver. One must be careful not to rely on a single imaging characteristic to make the diagnosis of HCC, as some benign liver tumors can restrict diffusion, and some well or moderately differentiated HCCs can retain hepatobiliary contrast agents to a similar or greater degree than background liver. Other imaging features of HCC to look for on MRI include increased signal on T2-weighted image, portal vein invasion, pseudocapsule around the mass, internal mosaic architecture of the mass, and intralesional fat or lipid. The likelihood of a cirrhotic nodule representing HCC also increases with size (24).

## Aunt Minnie's Pearls

Cirrhotic nodules represent a spectrum. As nodules dedifferentiate, blood supply becomes progressively arterial.

---

In cirrhotic patient's, nodules >1 cm with imaging features typical for HCC (arterial enhancement and venous or delayed phase washout) on multiphase contrast-enhanced CT or MRI can be diagnosed as HCC by imaging alone.

---

In most cases, HCC should not retain hepatobiliary contrast on delayed images and will appear hypointense compared with the background enhancing liver.

HISTORY: Elderly diabetic woman with abdominal pain and fever

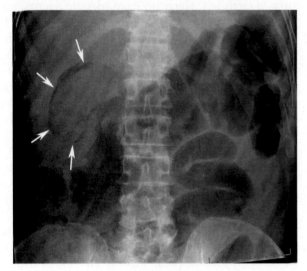

FIGURE 12.16.1

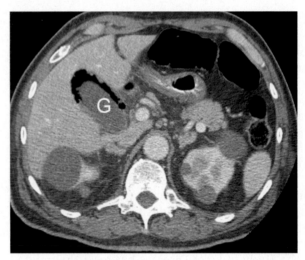

FIGURE 12.16.2

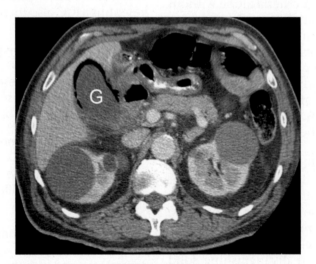

FIGURE 12.16.3

FINDINGS: A radiograph of the abdomen (Fig. 12.16.1) reveals abnormal collections of air in the expected location of the gallbladder (*arrows*). Two axial CT images of the upper abdomen (Figs. 12.16.2 and 12.16.3) confirm that gas is present in the wall of the gallbladder (*G*) and in the gallbladder fossa.

DIAGNOSIS: Emphysematous cholecystitis

DISCUSSION: Emphysematous cholecystitis is a severe form of acute cholecystitis in which cystic duct obstruction is followed by infection of the gallbladder by gas-producing organisms, usually *Escherichia coli*, *Clostridium* sp., or both. The condition is seen most frequently in diabetic patients and, unlike nonemphysematous acute cholecystitis, it is more frequent in men than in women (male-to-female ratio of 3:1). Emphysematous cholecystitis must be diagnosed early because of a high incidence of perforation and a high mortality rate. Percutaneous cholecystostomy is often performed as a temporizing measure until the patient is stable enough to undergo cholecystectomy. CT readily demonstrates air, which may be confined to the gallbladder lumen or may extend either intramurally or into the pericholecystic space (27).

## Aunt Minnie's Pearls

Emphysematous cholecystitis is caused by secondary infection by gas-producing organisms.

Emphysematous cholecystitis is more common in diabetics and in men.

There is a high risk of perforation and high mortality.

**HISTORY:** Abdominal distention

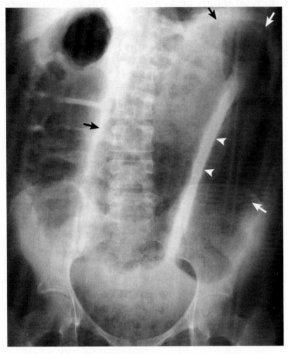

FIGURE 12.17.1

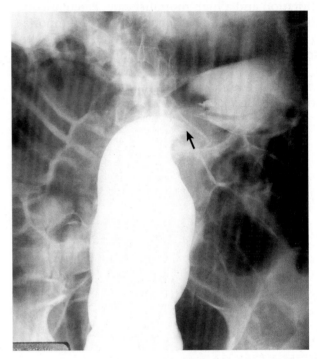

FIGURE 12.17.2

**FINDINGS:** A radiograph of the abdomen (Fig. 12.17.1) demonstrates a markedly distended loop of colon that projects superiorly from the pelvis to the level of the left hemidiaphragm (*black* and *white arrows*). A prominent stripe (*arrowheads*) is seen in the middle of the distended loop, which makes the loop mimic the appearance of a coffee bean. A fluoroscopic spot film from a contrast enema demonstrates tapered narrowing of the rectum at the rectosigmoid junction with a bird's beak deformity (Fig. 12.17.2, *arrow*). A small amount of contrast material is seen traversing the narrowed segment.

**DIAGNOSIS:** Sigmoid volvulus

**DISCUSSION:** Colonic volvulus is the third most common form of large intestine obstruction, after carcinoma and diverticulitis. A requisite condition for volvulus is the presence of a relatively redundant and mobile segment of bowel. The segments of the colon that are prone to volvulus include the sigmoid colon, cecum, and transverse colon. Sigmoid volvulus is more common in elderly patients and in populations that consume high-residue diets. Several findings on plain abdominal radiographs have been described with sigmoid volvulus, and some have been reported to be specific, such as the coffee-bean sign (i.e., dilated sigmoid loops with opposed walls that converge toward the lower left abdomen) (28). A more specific sign of sigmoid volvulus is the characteristic bird's beak deformity demonstrated on contrast enema near the rectosigmoid junction at the actual site of the volvulus. In some cases, the enema may actually reduce the volvulus, although sigmoidoscopy or tube decompression is usually the preferred treatment.

## Aunt Minnie's Pearls

Sigmoid volvulus occurs in patients with a redundant sigmoid colon.

Look for the coffee-bean sign on radiographs and the bird's beak deformity on contrast enemas.

HISTORY: Chronic abdominal pain

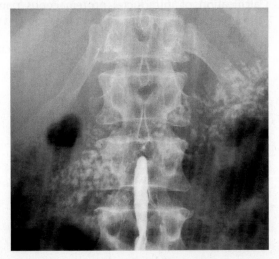

FIGURE 12.18.1

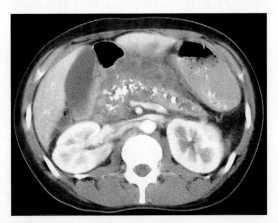

FIGURE 12.18.2

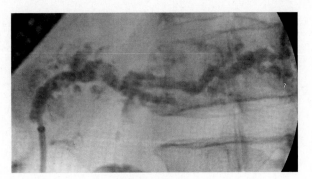

FIGURE 12.18.3

FINDINGS: A plain radiograph of the abdomen (Fig. 12.18.1) shows coarse calcification oriented obliquely in the upper abdomen in the expected position of the pancreas. Incidental note is made of retained myelographic contrast material. An axial CT image through the upper abdomen (Fig. 12.18.2) demonstrates calcification scattered diffusely throughout the pancreas, along with peripancreatic inflammatory changes.

DIAGNOSIS: Chronic calcific pancreatitis with superimposed acute pancreatitis

DISCUSSION: Although most cases of acute pancreatitis resolve without residual functional impairment or morphologic alteration, some patients go on to have recurrent episodes of acute pancreatitis. This is particularly true with alcohol-induced pancreatitis. These repeated episodes of pancreatitis result in progressive fibroinflammatory changes with reduction in the exocrine and endocrine functions of the pancreas (29). Morphologic alterations include diffuse or focal enlargement of the gland, pseudocyst or abscess formation, intraductal calcification, parenchymal atrophy, and ductal dilatation (30). The intraductal calcifications form by apposition of calcium carbonate onto intraductal proteinaceous concretions. In advanced cases, these calcifications are easily seen on plain abdominal radiographs and are virtually pathognomonic of chronic calcific

# Case 12.18 (Continued)

pancreatitis. With less advanced cases, the calcifications may not be evident on radiographs but are easily seen on CT. Findings of chronic pancreatitis on endoscopic retrograde cholangiopancreatography (ERCP) may also be specific, where the main duct is dilated and irregular, and marked dilatation of side branches or "side branch ectasia" occurs (Fig. 12.18.3).

## Aunt Minnie's Pearls

Calcification of intraductal proteinaceous pancreatoliths = calcific pancreatitis.

There is an increased incidence of chronic calcific pancreatitis with alcohol abuse.

# Case 12.19

**HISTORY:** A 58-year-old man with a history of pancreatitis

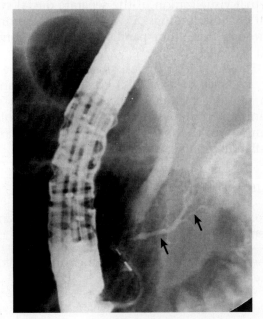

FIGURE 12.19.1

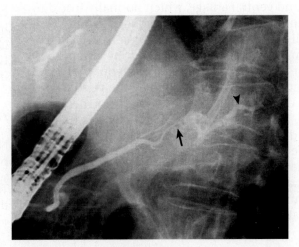

FIGURE 12.19.2

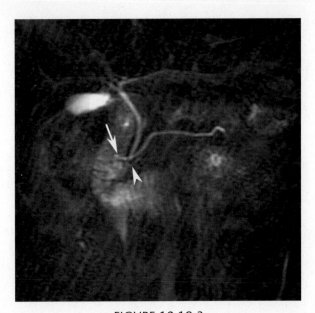

FIGURE 12.19.3

**FINDINGS:** An initial fluoroscopic ERCP spot film obtained during injection of major papilla (Fig. 12.19.1) demonstrates filling of a small ventral duct of the pancreas (*arrows*) and the common bile duct. The remainder of the pancreatic duct in the dorsal pancreas is seen after injection of the minor papilla (Fig. 12.19.2). Incidentally noted are a stricture (*arrow*) and duct enlargement with side branch ectasia in the tail (*arrowhead*). A coronal, T2-weighted magnetic resonance cholangiopancreatography (MRCP) image in a second patient (Fig. 12.19.3) demonstrates dominant drainage through the minor papilla (*arrow*) with a small ventral duct (*arrowhead*).

**DIAGNOSIS:** Pancreas divisum with changes of chronic pancreatitis in the dorsal pancreas

**DISCUSSION:** Pancreas divisum is a common congenital anomaly, occurring in up to 10% of the population. The embryonic pancreas develops from dorsal and ventral anlage, which normally fuse during fetal development. The two ductal systems also normally fuse. Failure of fusion results in pancreas divisum, in which two separate ductal systems persist. The uncinate process and the inferior portion of the pancreatic head are drained by the ventral pancreatic duct (i.e., duct of Wirsung) into the major papilla, and the remainder of the organ is drained by the dorsal accessory duct (i.e., duct of Santorini) into the minor papilla.

Standard ERCP injection into the major papilla reveals a short, tapering, ventral duct rather than the familiar long, undulating course of the main pancreatic duct. CT scans may reveal lobulation of the pancreatic head, separation of the ventral and dorsal portions of the pancreas by a cleft of fat, or actual visualization of the separate ductal systems. All of these findings, as well as dominant drainage through the minor papilla, may be demonstrated on MRI and MRCP.

Patients with pancreas divisum may have an increased risk for developing pancreatitis, especially in the dorsal pancreas, because the minor papilla cannot accommodate the normal volume of secretions from the major duct, resulting in stasis and inflammation (31).

## Aunt Minnie's Pearls

Nonfusion of ventral and dorsal pancreatic anlage = pancreas divisum.

There is an increased risk of pancreatitis, especially in the dorsal pancreas.

HISTORY: Intermittent abdominal pain in two patients

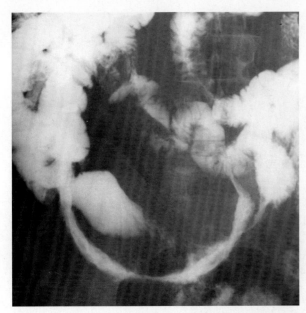

FIGURE 12.20.1

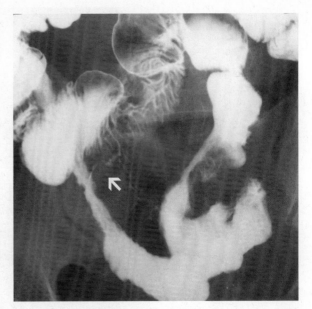

FIGURE 12.20.2

FINDINGS: Compression spot image from a small-bowel examination (Fig. 12.20.1) demonstrates multifocal narrowing of ileal bowel loops with mucosal ulceration; spot image in another patient showing similar findings with an enteric fistula (Fig. 12.20.2, *arrow*).

DIAGNOSIS: Crohn's disease of the small bowel

DISCUSSION: Crohn's disease is the most common inflammatory disease of the mesenteric small intestine and most often involves the ileal portion of the small bowel or the ileocecal region (32). The etiology of this disorder despite decades of investigation remains unknown. The disease most often affects younger adults and is a chronic, recurrent condition with a wide variety of symptoms and potential complications. The radiographic appearance is often specific; early erosive changes (i.e., aphthous ulcers) may be seen (which are difficult to detect on radiographic examination; the newer endoscopic modalities, especially videocapsule endoscopy, are much more sensitive techniques); with progression of disease, one or more loops of small bowel show narrowing, spasm, irregularity, ulceration, sinus tracts, and fistula formation, as manifested by the patients in the presentation. Depending on the appearance and extent of involvement, differential considerations include infections, such as *Yersinia enterocolitica*, and intrinsic neoplasms (e.g., lymphoma), but in most patients the appearance is often specific to suggest Crohn's disease.

## Aunt Minnie's Pearls

Crohn's disease presents with a wide variety of findings; however, a few other diseases of the small intestine have similar appearances.

Sinus tracts and fistula formation are often specific findings in this disorder.

**HISTORY:** Intermittent right upper quadrant pain and recent weight loss

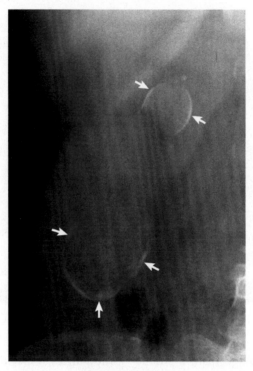

FIGURE 12.21.1

**FINDINGS:** Radiograph of the abdomen (Fig. 12.21.1) shows a thin, curvilinear calcification (*arrows*) that conforms to the expected shape of the gallbladder. The continuity of the calcification is disrupted abruptly, and a homogeneous soft-tissue mass spans the interval between the two calcifications.

**DIAGNOSIS:** Porcelain gallbladder with gallbladder carcinoma

**DISCUSSION:** The term *porcelain gallbladder* is derived from the appearance and texture of the gallbladder by gross pathologic examination (33). The affected gallbladder usually has a blue discoloration and brittle consistency. Radiographic examination demonstrates calcification of the gallbladder wall that may be extensive or patchy in distribution. The mural calcification may also be demonstrated by CT or ultrasonography. Cholelithiasis is present in most cases. Numerous theories have been proposed with respect to the pathogenesis of porcelain gallbladder, including chronic low-grade inflammation, intramural hemorrhage, and disorders of calcium metabolism. Most authorities believe that the condition represents a form of chronic cholecystitis. The entity is important from a clinical standpoint because of the association between porcelain gallbladder and gallbladder carcinoma, which is sufficiently frequent to warrant prophylactic cholecystectomy.

## Aunt Minnie's Pearl

There is an association between porcelain gallbladder and gallbladder carcinoma.

**HISTORY:** Right upper quadrant pain

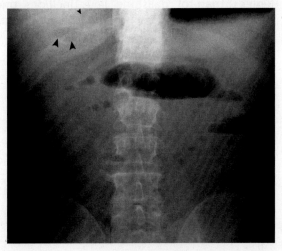

FIGURE 12.22.1

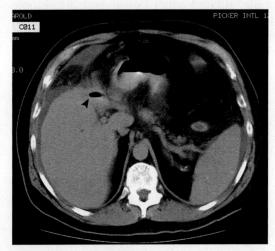

FIGURE 12.22.2

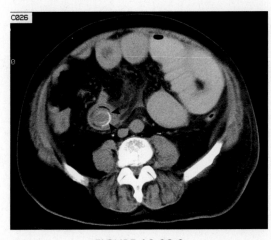

FIGURE 12.22.3

**FINDINGS:** An upright, plain radiograph of the abdomen (Fig. 12.22.1) shows a collection of air (*large arrowheads*) over the liver and air-filled, branching tubular structures (*small arrowhead*) in the liver. Demonstrated are also numerous dilated loops of small intestine with air-fluid levels and other signs of small-bowel obstruction. A CT scan through the upper abdomen reveals mild interstitial infiltration of the pericholecystic fat and air within the gallbladder (Fig. 12.22.2, *arrowhead*). An additional CT image through the lower abdomen demonstrates dilated loops of small intestine and a peripherally calcified structure (Fig. 12.22.3, *arrowheads*) contained within the lumen of the small intestine, consistent with an ectopic gallstone.

**DIAGNOSIS:** Gallstone ileus

**DISCUSSION:** Gallstone ileus develops after the erosion of a gallstone through the gallbladder wall and into a portion of the gastrointestinal tract. The fistulous tract usually forms between the gallbladder and duodenum, although fistulas to the stomach or colon may also occur. Small stones usually pass through the alimentary tract without consequence. Larger stones usually become impacted in the distal ileum, resulting in a mechanical small-bowel obstruction. The classic plain x-ray film findings of pneumobilia, dilated small bowel and an ectopic calcified gallstone (i.e., Rigler's triad) are considered pathognomonic of gallstone ileus; however, the complete triad is not seen in many cases (33,34).

### Aunt Minnie's Pearl

Rigler's triad of gallstone ileus includes pneumobilia, dilated small bowel, and an ectopic calcified gallstone.

**HISTORY:** A 34-year-old woman with history of mediastinal lymphoma

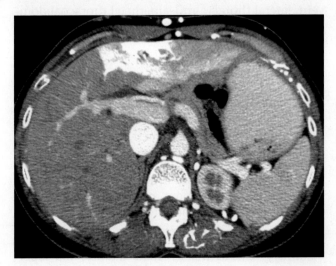

FIGURE 12.23.1

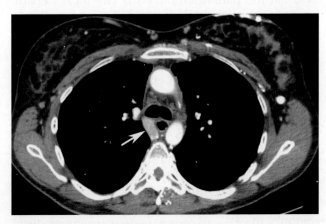

FIGURE 12.23.2

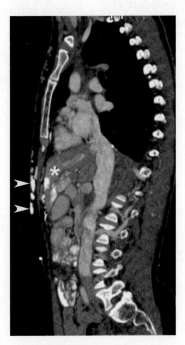

FIGURE 12.23.3

**FINDINGS:** Axial CT through the liver (Fig. 12.23.1) demonstrates early hyperenhancement in the left liver. Axial CT of the chest near the level of the carina (Fig. 12.23.2) shows an enlarged azygous vein (*arrow*) and the SVC is not visualized. Furthermore, note the collateral vessels in the left chest wall. Reformatted sagittal image of the chest/abdomen/pelvis (Fig. 12.23.3) demonstrates numerous superficial collateral veins in the upper abdomen (*arrowheads*).

Again seen is hyperenhancement of the left liver (*asterisk*) and the SVC is not seen in the chest.

**DIAGNOSIS:** SVC occlusion resulting in the CT equivalent of the "focal hepatic hot spot" sign clasically described on $^{99m}$Tc sulfur colloid scans

**DISCUSSION:** SVC obstruction results in collateral blood supply that can cause areas of focally increased blood flow to the left hepatic lobe via a systemic portal shunt. The typical collateral pathway resulting in this finding occurs between the internal mammary vein connecting to the left portal vein via the paraumbilical vein. The focal hepatic hot spot sign refers to an area of increased activity on $^{99m}$Tc sulfur colloid scans, classically in segment IV of the liver in the area formerly known as the quadrate lobe (35). The CT equivalent of this sign can be seen on contrast-enhanced CT with early contrast enhancement in this region. On CT, there is typically wedge-shaped hyperenhancement of segment IV of the liver on arterial phase imaging that often persists on portal venous phase imaging. This finding on abdominal CT should alert the radiologist to the probability of central venous occlusion in the chest. The diagnosis of SVC occlusion on CT requires two imaging findings: decreased or absent opacification of central venous structures distal to the site of obstruction and opacification of collateral venous channels (36). There are four main venous collateral pathways that carry blood around a central obstruction and back to the right heart: the azygous–hemiazygous system, internal mammary vein, lateral thoracic and superficial thoracoabdominal veins, and the vertebral venous plexus (36).

## Aunt Minnie's Pearls

The CT equivalent of the "focal hepatic hot spot" sign on abdominal CT is an important clue to the presence of central obstruction in the chest, which may be clinically unapparent owing to collateral formation.

The characteristic location in segment IV with wedge-shaped hyperenhancement on arterial and venous phase of imaging is an indicator of SVC obstruction.

The anterolateral collateral pathway from the internal mammary veins as well as lateral thoracic and superficial thoracoabdominal veins to the left portal vein via the paraumbilical vein is responsible for the focal hepatic hot spot sign.

HISTORY: Rectal bleeding in two different elderly patients

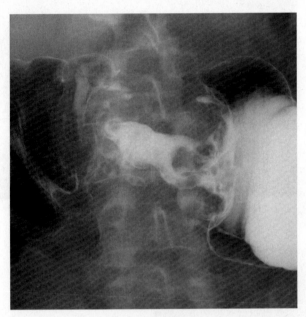

FIGURE 12.24.1

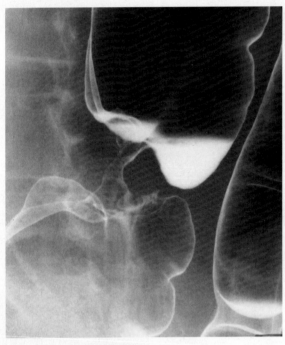

FIGURE 12.24.2

FINDINGS: Images from double-contrast barium enemas (Figs. 12.24.1 and 12.24.2) demonstrate annular narrowings in the transverse portion of the colon; the narrowings vary in appearance from a relatively smooth to a more irregular constriction in the two patients. This appearance is often referred to as the "apple-core lesion" and in the adult colon is invariably the result of an intrinsic malignancy.

DIAGNOSIS: Adenocarcinoma of the colon

DISCUSSION: Adenocarcinoma of the colon is one of the most common malignancies (>150,000 patients annually) in the United States and affects both women and men equally (37,38). Routine screening of the colon is recommended at age 50 in patients at average risk and earlier in individuals at higher risk (e.g., parent or sibling with a history of colon cancer). Adenomas are the precursors of colonic

carcinoma, and their detection and removal is an important aspect of periodic endoscopic surveillance. Adenocarcinomas vary in appearances from small, polypoid lesions, indistinguishable from benign polyps, to larger ulcerated, infiltrative, and annular malignancies. The "annular" carcinoma of the colon is an advanced malignancy with an appearance that is not mimicked by other focal colonic abnormalities in the adult large bowel.

## Aunt Minnie's Pearls

Adenocarcinoma of the colon is a common cancer that warrants screening in adults older than 50 who are at average risk.

Colonic narrowings with abrupt margins and irregular constriction are invariably carcinomas of the large bowel.

HISTORY: Multiple blood transfusions

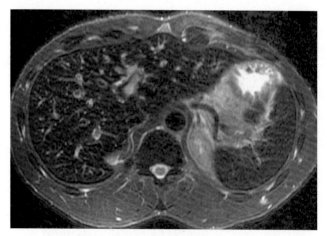

FIGURE 12.25.1

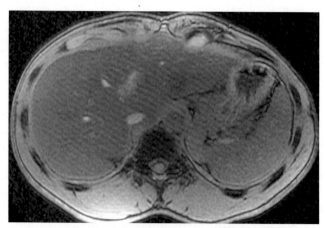

FIGURE 12.25.2

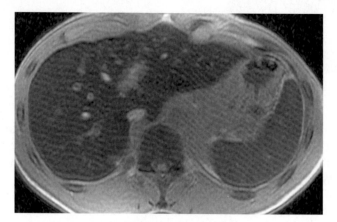

FIGURE 12.25.3

FINDINGS: An axial T2-weighted MR image through the liver and spleen (Fig. 12.25.1) demonstrates very low signal intensity of both organs. Gradient echo images performed with an opposed phase echo time of 2.1 msec (Fig. 12.25.2) and an in-phase echo time of 4.2 msec (Fig. 12.25.3) show relative signal loss of both the liver and spleen on the image with the longer echo time (Fig. 12.25.3).

DIAGNOSIS: Hemosiderosis

DISCUSSION: Excess iron deposition in the body can result from hereditary or acquired etiologies. Transfusional hemosiderosis describes excess iron deposition resulting from multiple blood transfusions. In this case, the excess iron is initially deposited within the reticuloendothelial (RE) cells of the liver, spleen, and bone marrow (39). On MR images, excess iron causes signal loss by creating local magnetic field heterogeneities around the iron particles (T2* effects). These effects are apparent on T2-weighted images and best seen on gradient echo images performed with a relatively long echo time (T2*-weighted).

Primary hemochromatosis is a hereditary abnormality resulting in excess iron absorption from the intestine (39). In primary hemochromatosis, the excess iron is deposited in parenchymal cells of various organs, such as the liver, pancreas, heart, and skin.

Transfusional hemosiderosis can be distinguished from primary (hereditary) hemochromatosis with MRI because the effects of the excess iron can be seen in the liver and spleen in the former case. The absence of excess iron deposition in the spleen and presence of excess iron resulting in signal loss within the liver and pancreas suggest the diagnosis of primary hemochromatosis rather than transfusional hemosiderosis. It should be noted that the RE system can eventually become saturated when a very large number of blood transfusions have been administered. In this case, iron can be deposited within the parenchyma of various organs including the liver, heart, and pancreas (39).

On T2-weighted images of the abdomen, the spleen is normally significantly brighter than the liver. In the case presented here, the liver and spleen are of similar low-signal intensity. This finding alone is sufficient to suggest the diagnosis of hemosiderosis. The diagnosis is confirmed on the gradient echo images because the liver and spleen lose signal intensity on the gradient echo image with longer echo time (Fig. 12.25.3 vs. Fig. 12.25.2) (40).

### Aunt Minnie's Pearls

Transfusional hemosiderosis results in low-signal intensity liver and spleen on T2-weighted and long TE gradient-echo images.

Primary (hereditary) hemochromatosis spares the spleen but can affect the pancreas when sufficiently severe.

Long TE gradient echo (T2*-weighted) images are useful for the detection of excess iron deposition.

HISTORY: Recurrent episodes of right upper quadrant pain

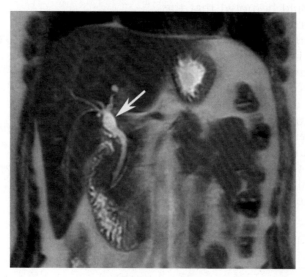

FIGURE 12.26.1

FINDINGS: A coronal, single shot fast spin echo (SS-FSE) image (Fig. 12.26.1) demonstrates focal dilatation of the extrahepatic bile duct (*arrow*) without evidence of distal stricture or proximal dilatation.

DIAGNOSIS: Choledochal cyst

DISCUSSION: Choledochal cysts result from congenital focal or diffuse dilatation of the bile ducts, and are more common in females (41). In some individuals, they may be acquired and possibly related to an anomalous pancreaticobiliary junction, with subsequent reflux of pancreatic secretions into the bile duct.

Choledochal cysts are classified into five major categories according to the Todani classification (41,42). Type I cysts (80%–90% of cases) are saccular or fusiform dilatations of the common bile duct. Type II cysts (2%) are true diverticula of the duct. Type III cysts (2%–5%), also called *choledochoceles*, result from dilatation of the terminal, intraduodenal portion of the common bile duct. Type IV cysts (19%) include a combination of both intrahepatic and extrahepatic bile duct cysts. Type V (i.e., Caroli's disease) refers to multiple cystic dilatations of the intrahepatic bile ducts and can be part of a general spectrum of cystic ectasia elsewhere, including medullary sponge kidney and autosomal recessive polycystic kidney disease (41,42). Choledochal cysts result in marked biliary stasis and therefore a predisposition to infection, inflammation, and stone disease. The risk of cholangiocarcinoma increases with age and occurs with a frequency of 3% to 28%. Treatment usually involves surgical resection.

## Aunt Minnie's Pearls

Choledochal cysts are categorized into five major types according to the Todani classification.

They result in biliary stasis with a predisposition for infection, inflammation, and stone disease.

HISTORY: Abdominal pain and jaundice

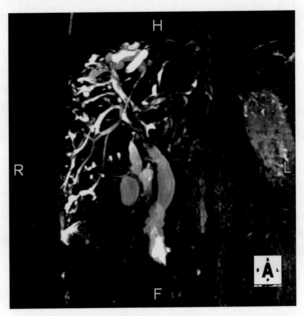

FIGURE 12.27.1

FINDINGS: Coronal maximum intensity projection image (Fig. 12.27.1) from a respiratory-triggered thin-section MRCP examination shows multiple cystic-appearing dilated intrahepatic bile ducts and fusiform dilatation of the extrahepatic bile duct.

DIAGNOSIS: Caroli disease

DISCUSSION: Caroli disease is an autosomal recessive disorder that manifests as multiple cystic dilatations of the intrahepatic bile ducts. It can be part of a general spectrum of cystic ectasia elsewhere, including medullary sponge kidney and autosomal recessive polycystic kidney disease (43). Despite the inclusion of Caroli disease in the Todani classification of choledochal cysts, it likely represents a distinct entity in the spectrum of ductal plate abnormalities (44,45).

Caroli disease results in biliary stasis and a predisposition to infection, inflammation, and stone formation (45). Patients are also at increased risk of cholangiocarcinoma (43,46). Caroli disease can mimic multiple hepatic cysts. In the case of Caroli disease, however, the "cysts" communicate with the bile ducts. In addition, portal triad structures are often engulfed by the dilated bile ducts in Caroli disease, creating a central "dot" within the central portions of the "cysts" as viewed on axial CT and MR images (47). Diffuse fusiform dilatation of the extrahepatic bile duct up to 3 cm is commonly present (43).

## Aunt Minnie's Pearls

Caroli disease manifests as multiple cystic dilatations of the intrahepatic bile ducts.

Patients with Caroli disease are predisposed to developing infection, inflammation, stone disease, and cholangiocarcinoma.

The "central dot" sign and communication with the bile ducts help distinguish Caroli disease from multiple hepatic cysts.

HISTORY: A 38-year-old man with hematochezia

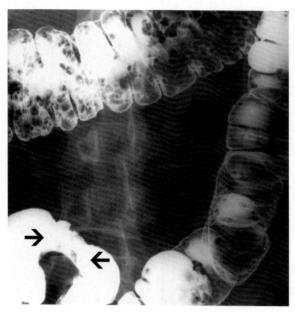

FIGURE 12.28.1

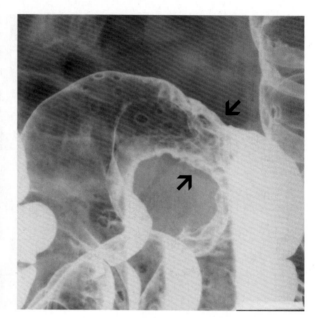

FIGURE 12.28.2

FINDINGS: Double-contrast barium enema images (Figs. 12.28.1 and 12.28.2) show innumerable filling defects in the visualized portions of the colon; these represent polyps of various sizes and shapes and are too numerous to count. In addition, a focal, infiltrative narrowing is present on both images (*arrows*) in the sigmoid colon, suspicious for a malignancy.

DIAGNOSIS: Familial polyposis coli with scirrhous carcinoma of the sigmoid colon

DISCUSSION: Familial polyposis coli is rare but is the most common of the adenomatous polyposis coli (APC) syndromes, which now encompass Gardner and Turcot syndromes (48). The APC gene on chromosome 5 has been identified, and depending on the mutations present, various organ-related presentations may be seen in the affected patients.

Individuals with this disorder will develop numerous adenomas throughout the colon, usually starting after puberty; these polyps will form in the rectum and the entire colon. The development of carcinoma of the colon is inevitable, usually by the middle decades of life; thus, early proctocolectomy is recommended. Although gene mutations are often spontaneous, early sigmoidoscopic screening and genetic mapping are necessary in affected families.

## Aunt Minnie's Pearls

Familial polyposis typically presents with numerous, diffuse colonic polyps.

Complicating carcinoma invariably occurs and is often fatal.

HISTORY: Right lower quadrant pain and fever

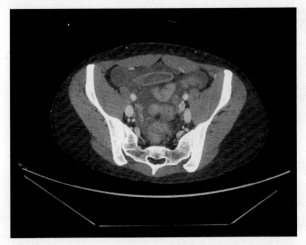

FIGURE 12.29.1

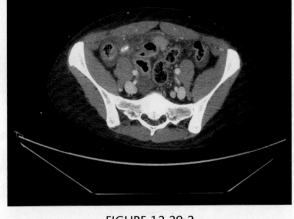

FIGURE 12.29.2

FINDINGS: An enhanced axial CT image through the lower abdomen (Fig. 12.29.1) demonstrates a blind-ending fluid-filled tubular structure with wall enhancement (dilated inflamed appendix) originating from the right lower quadrant. A slightly more cephalad image (Fig. 12.29.2) shows a calcification (appendicolith) at the site where the appendix joins the cecum. The appendiceal wall fails to enhance at the base (around the region of the appendicolith), and there is copious free fluid present in the pelvis.

DIAGNOSIS: Acute appendicitis (perforated)

DISCUSSION: Acute appendicitis represents inflammation of the appendix owing to obstruction of the lumen and subsequent infection. CT findings of acute appendicitis include a dilated appendix (diameter >6–10 mm), appendiceal wall thickening, thickening of the lateral conal fascia, and inflammation of the periappendiceal fat (fat stranding; 49).

In some cases, thickening of the cecal apex and/or a calcified appendicolith will be present. The presence of a calcified appendicolith on CT increases the likelihood of appendiceal perforation (49). When a portion of the appendiceal wall fails to enhance after intravenous contrast administration, perforation should be suspected (50,51). Other findings that support the diagnosis of perforated appendicitis include extraluminal air, extraluminal appendicolith, and abscess formation (51).

## Aunt Minnie's Pearls

A dilated appendix with periappendiceal inflammation suggests the diagnosis of appendicitis.

Additional CT findings of appendicitis include calcified appendicolith, cecal tip thickening, periappendiceal fluid, or abnormal appendiceal wall enhancement.

**HISTORY:** Sudden onset of left lower quadrant pain

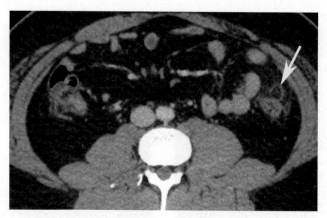

FIGURE 12.30.1

**FINDINGS:** Enhanced axial CT image of the left lower quadrant (Fig. 12.30.1) shows an ovoid fat-density paracolic mass (*arrow*) with a hyperattenuating rim and increased attenuation centrally. There is associated thickening of the lateral conal fascia.

**DIAGNOSIS:** Epiploic appendagitis

**DISCUSSION:** Epiploic appendages are fatty, finger-like structures that are attached to the serosal surface of the colon. When these appendages undergo torsion, the central draining vein thromboses. The inflamed visceral peritoneum of the torsed appendage appears as a hyperattenuating ring, whereas the thrombosed vein appears as a central high attenuation structure on CT (52,53). Eventually, an infarcted epiploic appendage can calcify and become detached from the colon. Because epiploic appendagitis is a self-limiting disease, the role of CT is to exclude more serious causes of acute abdominal pain.

## Aunt Minnie's Pearl

Epiploic appendagitis appears as a paracolic fatty mass with a hyperattenuating rim and central focus of increased density.

# REFERENCES

1. Plavsic BM, Chen MYM, Gelfand DW, et al. Intramural pseudodiverticulosis of the esophagus detected on barium esophagograms: Increased prevalence in patients with esophageal carcinoma. AJR Am J Roentgenol 1995;165:1381–1385.
2. Levine MS. Other esophagitides. In: Gore RM, Levine MS (eds.). Textbook of gastrointestinal radiology, 3rd ed. Philadelphia, PA: Saunders, 2008:394–397.
3. Cook IJ, Gabb M, Panagopoulos V, et al. Pharyngeal (Zenker's) diverticulum is a disorder of upper esophageal sphincter opening. Gastroenterology 1992;103:1229–1235.
4. Achkar E. Zenker's diverticulum. Dig Dis 1998;16:144–151.
5. Levine MS. Peptic ulcers. In: Gore RM, Levine MS (eds.). Textbook of gastrointestinal radiology, 3rd ed. Philadelphia, PA: Saunders, 2008:529–561.
6. Valls C, Iannacconne R, Alba E, et al. Fat in the liver: Diagnosis and characterization. Eur Radiol 2006;16:2292–2308.
7. Ott DJ. Motility disorders of the esophagus. In: Gore RM, Levine MS (eds.). Textbook of gastrointestinal radiology, 3rd ed. Philadelphia, PA: Saunders, 2008:323–335.
8. Johnson CD, Schmidt GD. Mayo Clinic gastrointestinal imaging review. Florence, KY: Mayo Clinic Scientific Press and Informa Healthcare USA, Inc., 2005:17–19.
9. Levine MS, Rubesin SE. Diseases of the esophagus: Diagnosis with esophagography. Radiology 2005;237:414–427.
10. Gelfand DW, Dale WJ, Ott DJ, et al. Duodenitis: Endoscopic–radiologic correlation in 272 patients. Radiology 1985;157:577–581.
11. Levine MS. Miscellaneous abnormalities of the esophagus. In: Gore RM, Levine MS (eds.). Textbook of gastrointestinal radiology, 3rd ed. Philadelphia, PA: Saunders, 2008:483–490.
12. Farber E, Fischer D, Eliakim R, et al. Esophageal varices: Evaluation with esophagography with barium versus endoscopic gastroduodenoscopy in patients with compensated cirrhosis—blinded prospective study. Radiology 2005;237:535–540.
13. Warshauer DM, Lee JKT. Adult intussusception detected at CT or MR imaging: Clinical-imaging correlation. Radiology 1999;212:853–860.
14. Gourtsoyiannis NC, Papakonstantinou O, Bays D, et al. Adult enteric intussusception: Additional observations on enteroclysis. Abdom Imaging 1994;19:11–17.
15. Mahfouz A-E, Hamm B, Wolf K-J. Peripheral washout: A sign of malignancy on dynamic gadolinium-enhanced MR images of focal liver lesions. Radiology 1994;190:49–52.
16. Seale MK, Catalano OA, Saini S, et al. Hepatobiliary specific MR contrast agents: Role in imaging the liver and biliary tree. Radiographics 2009;29:1725–1748.
17. Mehanna MJ, Birjawi G, Moukaddam HA, et al. Complications of adjustable gastric banding, a radiological pictorial review. AJR Am J Roentgenol 2006;186:522–534.
18. Pieroni S, Sommer EA, Hito R, et al. The "O" sign, a simple and helpful tool in the diagnosis of laparascopic adjustable gastric band slippage. AJR Am J Roentgenol 2010;195:137–141.
19. Hussain SM, Terkivatan T, Zondervan PE, et al. Focal nodular hyperplasia: Findings at state-of-art MR imaging, US, CT, and pathologic analysis. RadioGraphics 2004;24:3–19.
20. Grazioli L, Morana G, Federle MP, et al. Focal nodular hyperplasia: Morphologic and functional information from MR imaging with gadobenate dimeglumine. Radiology 2001;221:731–739.
21. Ros PR, Erturk SM. Benign tumors of the liver. In: Gore RM, Levine MS (eds.). Textbook of gastrointestinal radiology, 3rd ed. Philadelphia, PA: Saunders, 2008:1591–1622.
22. Rubesin SE. Miscellaneous abnormalities of the small bowel. In: Gore RM, Levine MS (eds.). Textbook of gastrointestinal radiology, 3rd ed. Philadelphia, PA: Saunders, 2008:933–943.
23. Pickhardt PJ, Bhalla S. Intestinal malrotation in adolescents and adults: Spectrum of clinical and imaging features. AJR Am J Roentgenol 2002;179:1429–1435.
24. Parente DB, Perez RM, Araujo AE, et al. MR imaging of hypervascular lesions in the cirrhotic liver: A diagnostic dilemma. RadioGraphics 2012;32:767–787.
25. Bruix J, Sherman M. Management of hepatocellular carcinoma: An update. Hepatology 2011;53(3):1020–1022.
26. Taouli B, Koh DM. Diffusion-weighted MR imaging of the liver. Radiology 2010;254:47–66.
27. Bennett GL. Cholelithiasis and cholecystitis. In: Gore RM, Levine MS (eds.). Textbook of gastrointestinal radiology, 3rd ed. Philadelphia, PA: Saunders, 2008:1411–1456.
28. Burrell HC, Baker DM, Wardrop P, et al. Significant plain film findings in sigmoid volvulus. Clin Radiol 1994;49:317–319.
29. Taylor AJ, Bohorfoush AG III. Pancreatic duct in inflammation of the pancreas. In: Interpretation of ERCP with associated digital imaging correlation. Philadelphia, PA: Lippincott-Raven, 1997:231–259.
30. Miller FH, Keppke AL, Balthazar EJ. Pancreatitis. In: Gore RM, Levine MS (eds.). Textbook of gastrointestinal radiology, 3rd ed. Philadelphia, PA: Saunders, 2008:1885–1914.
31. Mortelé KJ, Rocha TC, Streeter JL, et al. Multimodality imaging of pancreatic and biliary congenital anomalies. RadioGraphics 2006;26:715–731.
32. Gore RM, Masselli G, Caroline DJ. Crohn's disease of the small bowel. In: Gore RM, Levine MS (eds.). Textbook of gastrointestinal radiology, 3rd ed. Philadelphia, PA: Saunders, 2008:781–806.
33. Baker SR, Cho KC. Plain films of the liver, bile ducts, and spleen. In: The abdominal plain film with correlative imaging, 2nd ed. Stamford, CT: Appelton & Lange, 1999:369–452.
34. Friedman AC, Maurer AH. Cholelithiasis and cholecystitis. In: Friedman AC, Dachman AH (eds.). Radiology of the liver, biliary tract, and pancreas. St Louis, MO: Mosby, 1994:445–538.
35. Dickson AM. The focal hepatic hot spot sign. Radiology 2005;237:647–648.
36. Virmani V, Lal A, Ahuja CK, et al. The CT quadrate lobe hot spot sign. Ann Hepatol 2010;9(3):296–298.
37. Ott DJ. Barium enema: Colorectal polyps and carcinoma. Semin Roentgenol 1996;31:125–141.
38. Thoeni RF, Laufer I. Polyps and colon cancer. In: Gore RM, Levine MS (eds.). Textbook of gastrointestinal radiology, 3rd ed. Philadelphia, PA: Saunders, 2008:1121–1166.
39. Siegelman ES, Mitchell DG, Semelka RC. Abdominal iron deposition: Metabolism, MR findings, and clinical importance. Radiology 1996;199:13–22.
40. Merkle EM, Nelson RC. Dual gradient echo in-phase and opposed-phase hepatic MR imaging: A useful tool for evaluation more than fatty infiltration or fatty sparing. RadioGraphics 2006;26:1409–1418.
41. Carrico CWT, Bissett GS III. Diseases of the pediatric gallbladder and biliary tract. In: Gore RM, Levine MS (eds.). Textbook of gastrointestinal radiology, 3rd ed. Philadelphia, PA: Saunders, 2008:2305–2324.
42. Kim OH, Chung HJ, Choi BG. Imaging of the choledochal cyst. RadioGraphics 1995;15:69–88.
43. Levy AD, Rohrmann CA Jr, Murakata LA, et al. Caroli's disease: Radiologic spectrum with pathologic correlation. AJR Am J Roentgenol 2002;179:1053–1057.
44. Desmet VJ. Congenital diseases of intrahepatic bile ducts: Variations on the theme "ductal plate malformation." Hepatology 1992;16:1069–1083.
45. Brancatelli G, Federle MP, Vilgrain V, et al. Fibropolycystic liver disease: CT and MR imaging findings. RadioGraphics 2005;25:659–670.

46. Bloustein PA. Association of carcinoma with congenital cystic conditions of the liver and bile ducts. Am J Gastroenterol 1977;67:40.
47. Choi BI, Yeon KM, Kim SH, et al. Caroli disease: Central dot sign in CT. Radiology 1990;174:161–163.
48. Butler CL, Buck JL. Polyposis syndromes. In: Gore RM, Levine MS (eds.). Textbook of gastrointestinal radiology, 3rd ed. Philadelphia, PA: Saunders, 2008:1189–1201.
49. Pinto Leite N, Pereira JM, Cunha R, et al. CT evaluation of appendicitis and its complications: Imaging techniques and key diagnostic findings. AJR Am J Roentgenol 2005;185:406–417.
50. Tsuboi M, Takase K, Kaneda I, et al. Perforated and nonperforated appendicitis: Defect in enhancing appendiceal wall-depiction with multidetector row CT. Radiology 2008;246:142–147.
51. Horrow MM, White DS, Horrow JC. Differentiation of perforated from nonperforated appendicitis at CT. Radiology 2003;227:46–51.
52. Rioux M, Langis P. Primary epiploic appendagitis: Clinical, US, and CT findings in 14 cases. Radiology 1994;191:523–526.
53. van Breda Vriesman AC. The hyperattenuating ring sign. Radiology 2003;226:556–557.

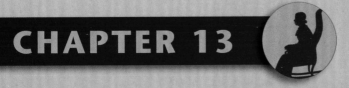

# CHAPTER 13

# GENITOURINARY RADIOLOGY

**Brian Dupree / Samuel Porter / Judson R. Gash**

*The authors and editors acknowledge the contribution of the Chapter 11 author from the third edition: Daniel J. Kirzeder, MD and Chapter 10 authors from the second edition: Tara C. Noone, MD, Norbert Burzynski, MD, Robert Bechtold, MD, and Raymond B. Dyer, MD.*

**HISTORY:** Patient with history of urinary tract infections.

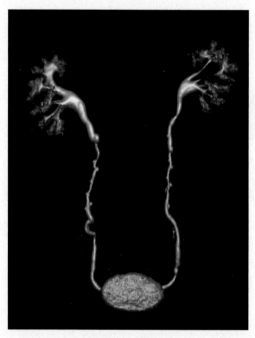

FIGURE 13.1.1

**FINDINGS:** Coronal volume rendered 3D image (Fig. 13.1.1) of the urinary tract during the excretory phase demonstrates multiple small ureteral outpouchings

**DIAGNOSIS:** Ureteral pseudodiverticulosis

**DISCUSSION:** Ureteral pseudodiverticula are small outpouchings of the ureteral lumen that are sharply demarcated and usually vary in size from 1 to 3 mm in width and length (1,2). Three to eight diverticula clustered over a distance of 2 to 6 cm in the midureter are commonly seen. The involved ureteral segment is often narrowed but is not usually obstructed. Bilateral ureteral involvement may be seen in up to 50% of cases. The outpouchings represent down-growth of the transitional epithelium into the ureteral wall, probably as a result of epithelial hyperplasia. Because the outpouchings do not contain all layers of the ureteral wall, they are pseudodiverticula (1,2). The hyperplastic response has been associated with urinary stone disease and obstruction, infection, and transitional cell carcinoma. Patients with pseudodiverticula therefore should be monitored closely for the development of transitional cell neoplasms, especially in the bladder (3).

## Aunt Minnie's Pearls

Small outpouchings of the ureter that do not contain all the layers of the ureteral wall = pseudodiverticula.

Patients with pseudodiverticulosis should be monitored for the development of transitional cell carcinoma.

**HISTORY:** A 32-year-old female undergoing infertility workup

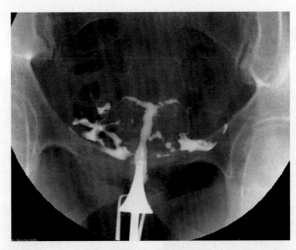

FIGURE 13.2.1

**FINDINGS:** Hysterosalpingogram (Fig. 13.2.1) shows a narrowed endocervical canal and a hypoplastic, small uterine cavity with a T-shaped configuration. Multiple irregularities consistent with fibrous scars (synechiae) are present.

**DIAGNOSIS:** Uterine hypoplasia secondary to in utero DES exposure

**DISCUSSION:** Diethylstilbestrol (DES) is a potent synthetic estrogen that was prescribed between the late 1940s until about 1970 for pregnant women to prevent recurrent spontaneous abortions, premature deliveries, and other pregnancy complications. The strong estrogen effects of DES disrupt the differentiation of estrogen-sensitive organs during organogenesis and can lead to structural fetal malformations of the uterus and fallopian tubes. Abnormalities of the uterine cavity are detected by hysterosalpingogram (HSG) in as many as 69% of DES-exposed women (4) and most commonly include uterine hypoplasia (a T-shaped uterine cavity), bands and synechiae, and irregular uterine margins (5). MR imaging has also been shown to adequately depict uterine abnormalities associated with DES exposure (6). The intrauterine abnormalities associated with DES exposure predispose women to menstrual dysfunction and pregnancy complications such as spontaneous abortions, ectopic pregnancy, and prematurity (7,8). In addition, clear cell carcinoma of the vagina is seen in 0.1% of patients with a history of DES exposure (9).

## Aunt Minnie's Pearls

Uterine hypoplasia with a T-shaped uterine cavity configuration is the classic imaging manifestation of previous in utero DES exposure.

The intrauterine abnormalities associated with DES exposure predispose women to pregnancy complications including spontaneous abortions, ectopic pregnancy, and prematurity.

HISTORY: A 72-year-old female with complaints of pneumaturia, fecaluria, and recurrent urinary tract infections

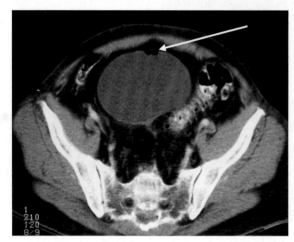

FIGURE 13.3.1

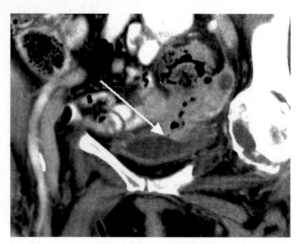

FIGURE 13.3.2

FINDINGS: Contrast-enhanced CT in the axial plane (Fig. 13.3.1) demonstrates air within the bladder lumen (*arrow*) and a reformatted coronal image (Fig. 13.3.2) demonstrates a direct communication from a sigmoid diverticulum to the bladder (*arrow*).

DIAGNOSIS: Colovesical fistula

DISCUSSION: A colovesical fistula is an abnormal internal connection between the colon and urinary bladder. The most common cause of colovesical fistula is sigmoid diverticulitis (10). Other etiologies include colorectal adenocarcinoma, inflammatory bowel disease, radiation therapy, pelvic surgery, and foreign bodies (11). Patients commonly present with nonspecific irritative symptoms of cystitis and have a positive urine culture. The classic symptoms of pneumaturia and fecaluria usually occur late in the disease process (12). In the CT evaluation of patients with suspected colovesical fistula, a scan should be performed with an enteric contrast agent but before the administration of intravenous contrast. The presence of enteric contrast within the bladder is diagnostic of a fistula. Additional CT findings of colovesical fistula include gas within the bladder lumen (in the absence of recent bladder catheterization) and thickened bladder or bowel wall adjacent to the fistula (11). In addition to documenting the fistula, CT also allows the evaluation of intraluminal and extraluminal pathologic conditions that may be helpful in planning surgical intervention (12). Cystoscopy and colonoscopy are useful in the evaluation of patients with colovesical fistula, particularly to exclude underlying neoplasm.

## Aunt Minnie's Pearls

The most common cause of colovesical fistula is sigmoid diverticulitis; however, underlying neoplasm must be excluded.

CT finding of colovesical fistula include gas within the urinary bladder lumen, thickening of the bladder or colon wall adjacent to the fistula, and a fistula tract opacified with air or enteric contrast.

Reformatted coronal imaging is often very valuable for demonstrating the fistula.

HISTORY: A 25-year-old male with history of seizures who presents with left flank pain

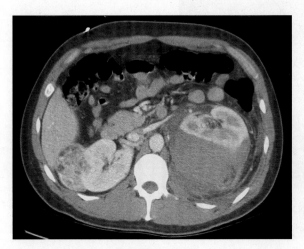

FIGURE 13.4.1

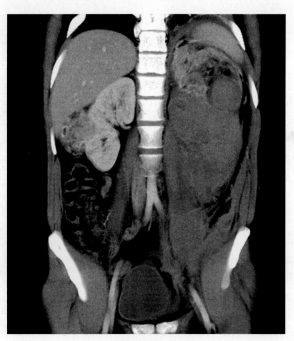

FIGURE 13.4.2

FINDINGS: Contrast-enhanced axial CT (Fig. 13.4.1) shows a large perinephric hematoma, which anteriorly displaces and deforms the left kidney. Coronal MPR image from the same CT scan (Fig. 13.4.2) shows, in addition to the large perinephric hemorrhage, bilateral fat-containing renal lesions.

DIAGNOSIS: Bilateral angiomyolipomas (AMLs) with left perinephric hematoma secondary to spontaneous left AML hemorrhage

DISCUSSION: Tuberous sclerosis complex (TSC), or Bourneville disease, is an autosomal dominant genetic disorder that is characterized by hamaratomatous tumors involving multiple organ systems. Hamaratomatous tumors comprise adipose tissue, thick-walled blood vessels, and sheets of smooth muscle in variable proportion. AMLs are renal hamaratomatous tumors present in up to 80% of patients with TSC. Of the three renal manifestations of TSC (AMLs, cysts, and rarely, renal cell carcinoma), AMLs are by far the most common, and they are often multiple and bilateral (13). Radiographically, AMLs present as fat-containing renal lesions, often diagnosed on CT or MRI. The larger the AML, the more likely to hemorrhage, and thus lesion >4 to 5 cm tend to be treated (excised or embolized), whereas smaller lesions are typically followed.

## Aunt Minnie's Pearls

Multiple bilateral renal angiomyolipomas are the most common renal manifestation of TSC.

Larger AMLs (>4 cm) are commonly treated secondary to threat of spontaneous hemorrhage.

**HISTORY:** A 5-day-old female infant with a history of prenatal cyst and a lower abdominal mass

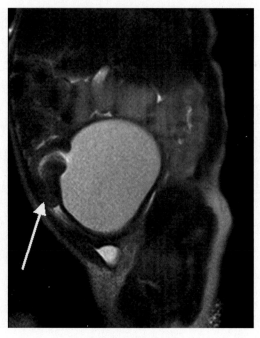

FIGURE 13.5.1

**FINDINGS:** Sagittal T2-weighted image of the pelvis (Fig. 13.5.1) demonstrates a severely dilated fluid-filled vagina that displaces the uterus (*arrow*) anteriorly and superiorly.

**DIAGNOSIS:** Hydrocolpos

**DISCUSSION:** The most common pelvic masses in neonates include hydrocolpos, hydrometro-colpos, and ovarian cysts. Hydrocolpos is defined as distension of the vagina. Both hydrocolpos and hydrometrocolpos can result from vaginal or cervical stenosis, hypoplasia, or agenesis (Meyer–Rokitansky–Kuster–Houser syndrome), which is often associated with additional congenital anomalies (14). Hydrocolpos in patients with a persistent urogenital sinus must be diagnosed and treated early in life to avoid potential complications. Some cases of hydrocolpos are identified on prenatal ultrasound. MRI has become an alternative and complementary method for the equivocal prenatal cases. It provides excellent anatomic detail and soft-tissue contrast with multiple reconstruction planes and a large field of view. Shorter MRI acquisition times reduce the effects of fetal motion and have expanded the role MRI in these settings (15). Trans-abdominal indwelling vaginostomy tube is the preferred approach for some pediatric surgeons. The most common complication is compression of the trigone, causing extrinsic ureterovesical obstruction, leading to megaureters and hydronephrosis, which can ultimately cause renal failure. Surgically draining the hydrocolpos may significantly improve the hydronephrosis (16).

## Aunt Minnie's Pearls

Hydrocolpos is a distended vagina filled with fluid that may present as a cystic mass on prenatal ultrasound or as a palpable mass on postnatal physical exam.

MRI has become a complementary modality for the equivocal prenatal ultrasound.

The most common associated complication is hydro-nephrosis secondary to extrinsic obstruction of the ureterovesical junction.

**HISTORY:** A 62-year-old female with complaint of "bladder spasms"

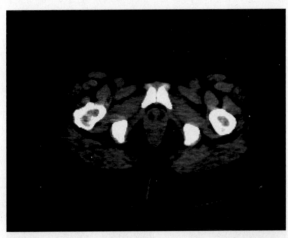

FIGURE 13.6.1

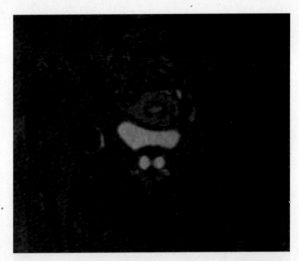

FIGURE 13.6.2

**FINDINGS:** Axial CT (Fig. 13.6.1) and coronal T2-weighted MR (Fig. 13.6.2) images through the pelvis in the same patient demonstrate a cystic collection "surrounding" the urethra.

**DIAGNOSIS:** Urethral diverticulum

**DISCUSSION:** Urethral diverticula are estimated to occur in 1% to 6% of women, most often between the third and sixth decades of life. Multiple nonspecific genitourinary symptoms predominate including repeated lower urinary tract infections, urinary incontinence, dysuria, frequency and urgency, urethral pain, dyspareunia, hematuria, and postvoid dribbling (17). The majority of urethral diverticula are located in the middle third of the urethra and often involve the posterolateral wall. Most urethral diverticula are the sequelae of periurethral gland infection that result in glandular dilatation and then progress to fistulization with the urethra (18). It should be noted that most urethral diverticula appear to "surround" the urethra, unlike most diverticula, that appear as outpouchings. Complications of urethral diverticulum include recurrent infection, urinary incontinence, calculus formation, and development of intradiverticular neoplasms. Urethral diverticula are associated with increased incidence—owing to urinary stasis—of stone formation and malignancy, especially urothelial carcinoma. Various diagnostic methods have been used to evaluate the female urethra including voiding cystourethrography, double-balloon urethrography, Ultrasound (US), CT, CT voiding urethrography and virtual urethroscopy, MR imaging, and fiberoptic urethroscopy. MRI has become the imaging study of choice with its multiplanar capabilities and excellent soft-tissue contrast (19). Transvaginal diverticulectomy is the most common surgical treatment.

## Aunt Minnie's Pearls

A urethral diverticulum appears as cystic lesion adjacent to or surrounding the midurethra.

A filling defect in a urethral diverticulum may represent calculus formation or intradiverticular neoplasm. Adenocarcinoma is the most common diverticular malignancy.

HISTORY: A 47-year-old man with history of adrenal mass

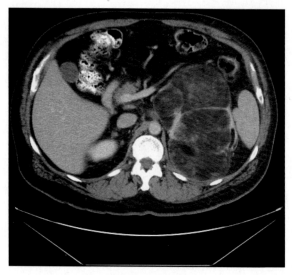

FIGURE 13.7.1

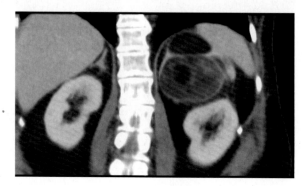

FIGURE 13.7.2

FINDINGS: An unenhanced, axial CT image of the abdomen (Fig. 13.7.1) shows a large, left adrenal mass with obvious low-attenuation fatty elements and several internal septations. Coned coronal reformatted CT image (Fig. 13.7.2) shows the mass displaces the left kidney inferiorly. A well-defined fat plane separates the mass form the left kidney, confirming that the mass arises from an extrarenal location.

DIAGNOSIS: Adrenal myelolipoma

DISCUSSION: Adrenal myelolipomas are benign tumors comprising variable amounts of mature adipose cells and hematopoietic tissue. This neoplasm is functionally inactive and is usually discovered incidentally during abdominal imaging or autopsy (20,21). Although most myelolipomas are asymptomatic, hemorrhage or necrosis can occur within the tumor, and adjacent structures may be compressed, especially by larger lesions. The demonstration of well-defined macroscopic fat within an adrenal mass on CT examination virtually confirms the diagnosis of adrenal myelolipoma. Other considerations in the differential diagnosis of a suprarenal fatty mass include an exophytic renal or extrarenal angiomyolipoma, a retroperitoneal teratoma, lipoma, or possibly a liposarcoma. Careful analysis of the lesion for exact location, margination, internal consistency, and CT attenuation values should allow a correct diagnosis. Tumors with irregular margins, internal heterogeneity, significant contrast enhancement, and attenuation values greater than that of normal fat should be considered suggestive of malignancy (21,22). Resection is recommended for symptomatic lesions, those that grow during surveillance intervals, or those that are >7 cm (because of increased risk of bleeding and rupture).

## Aunt Minnie's Pearls

Myelolipomas are benign, nonfunctioning tumors containing fat and marrow elements.

Precontrast CT scans or MR images are most useful to identify fat within adrenal lesions.

HISTORY: A 17-year-old female 8 days after severe trauma. CT without contrast in a different patient several months after trauma

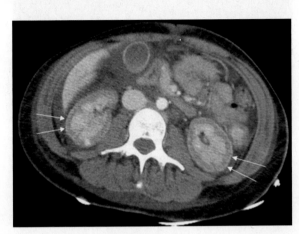

FIGURE 13.8.1

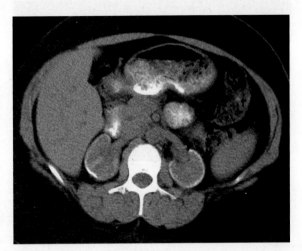

FIGURE 13.8.2

FINDINGS: Axial contrast-enhanced CT image (Fig. 13.8.1) shows lack of peripheral cortical contrast enhancement bilaterally, with normal enhancement of the renal medulla. A thin rim of enhancement of the very periphery of kidneys is seen bilaterally (*arrows*). A follow-up CT image (different patient) showing a thin rim of renal cortical calcification consistent with cortical nephrocalcinosis (Fig. 13.8.2).

DIAGNOSIS: Acute renal cortical necrosis

DISCUSSION: Acute renal cortical necrosis, results from ischemia of the renal cortex secondary to decreased arterial perfusion. On a contrast-enhanced CT immediately following the insult, acute cortical necrosis manifests as lack of enhancement of the peripheral renal cortex, with normal medullary enhancement (23). A thin rim of enhancing cortical tissue is classically visualized at the extreme periphery secondary to preservation of the renal capsular blood flow. With time (approximately 2 months later), the kidney will atrophy and cortical nephrocalcinosis may occur (24). Although the exact pathologic mechanism of acute cortical necrosis is not precisely known, intrarenal vascular spasm or intravascular thrombosis leading to cortical ischemia are possible explanations. Cortical necrosis may develop as a consequence of shock (trauma, etc.), obstetric complications (i.e., abruptio placentae, placenta previa, septic abortion, eclampsia), transfusion reaction, or other causes of hemolysis, endotoxins, and renal allograft rejection (25).

## Aunt Minnie's Pearls

Renal cortical necrosis manifests acutely as decreased enhancement of the renal cortices on contrast-enhanced CT.

Acute renal cortical necrosis is most commonly seen in the setting of hemorrhagic shock, in particular in the setting of obstetric complication.

Cortical nephrocalcinosis is a common sequela of acute renal cortical necrosis.

**HISTORY:** A 38-year-old female with a history of cervical carcinoma referred for a surveillance imaging PET/CT

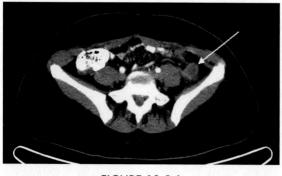

FIGURE 13.9.1

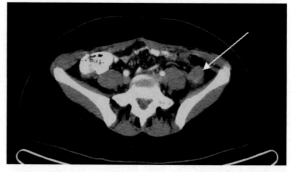

FIGURE 13.9.2

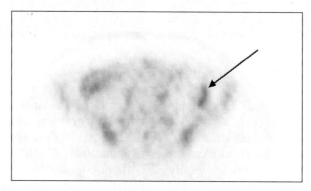

FIGURE 13.9.3

**FINDINGS:** Axial CT, PET, and fused images from a PET/CT (Figs. 13.9.1 to 13.9.3) demonstrate a 3-cm rounded cystic and solid mass (*arrows*) in the low left paracolic gutter with moderate FDG activity (SUV = 3.8)

**DIAGNOSIS:** Transposed ovary

**DISCUSSION:** Therapeutic irradiation of the pelvis for malignancy ruins the ovary, resulting in ovarian failure with menopausal symptoms. Thus in patients with midline malignancies such as cervical carcinoma requiring radiation treatment, who wish to preserve function and potential fertility options, the ovaries can be surgically transposed out of the anticipated radiation field. The procedure comprises severing the uterine and broad ligament attachments, and moving the ovary, along with its suspensory ligament and gonadal vascular pedicle, outward into the low paracolic gutter, just lateral to the cecum or descending colon (26). One or both ovaries may be transposed. This is all well and good until the uninitiated radiologist misdiagnoses the transposed ovary as a peritoneal metastatic deposit (27). This is particularly possible as the normal premenopausal ovary can demonstrate (even after hysterectomy) moderate hypermetabolic activity. Obviously being acquainted with this procedure is necessary to avoid this important pitfall. Surgical history can clinch the diagnosis, but as radiologists, to rely on having that, as we know, is even a bigger pitfall. Fortunately, there are imaging clues that can help us distinguish a transposed ovary from a metastasis. The morphology of the normal ovary is helpful. Usually the premenopausal ovary, comprising small cysts within a solid background, is recognizable, particularly on

MRI. However, the ovary may be devoid of cysts and look solid, or be full of cysts and look cystic. A second clue, often used to identify the ovary on CT in general, is following the gonadal veins from their superior origin (IVC on the right, renal vein on the left) down to the area in question. The gonadal veins, when the ovaries are transposed, deviate laterally over the psoas muscles, coursing laterally behind the colon directly to the ovary, and can be followed in most cases of transposition. Finally, a thoughtful surgeon will often place a surgical clip or two in the area of a transposed ovary allowing its identification (not so much for the diagnostic radiologist, but for the radiation oncologist) (28).

## Aunt Minnie's Pearls

Radiation therapy for pelvic malignancies results in ovarian failure, and to avoid this, the ovaries can be surgically transposed out of their normal location (and out of the radiation field).

The transposed ovary can mimic a peritoneal metastatic deposit.

Knowledge of typical ovarian appearance, following the gonadal vessels, and a surgical clip (along with history, of course) can be used to differentiate a normal transposed ovary from a metastasis.

HISTORY: A 19-year-old male with history of hypertension

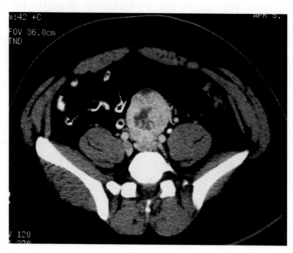

FIGURE 13.10.1

FINDINGS: Axial contrast-enhanced CT image of the lower abdomen (Fig. 13.10.1) shows a hypervascular mass arising just anterior to the bifurcation of the common iliac vessels. The mass demonstrates heterogeneous peripheral enhancement and a central hypodense region suggesting internal necrosis.

DIAGNOSIS: Pheochromocytoma at the organ of Zuckerkandl

DISCUSSION: Paragangliomas are tumors arising from chromaffin cells of the autonomic nervous system (29). Paragangliomas arising from the adrenal medulla are termed pheochromocytomas and the term *paraganglioma* is commonly used to refer to extra-adrenal tumors. Pheochromocytomas and paragangliomas often result in elevated serum catecholamine levels and the related clinical symptoms of hypertension, palpitations, tachycardia, diaphoresis, or headache. Pheochromocytomas are classically described according to the rule of 10s: 10% extra-adrenal, 10% malignant, 10% bilateral, 10% familial, and 10% are not associated with hypertension. However, recent studies suggest that as many as 25% of pheochromocytomas are extra-adrenal in location (30), originating within the sympathetic neural tissue outside the adrenal gland. One of the most common abdominal locations for extra-adrenal paragangliomas is the organ of Zuckerkandl, followed by the bladder and the sympathetic trunk (30). The organ of Zuckerkandl is the term given to the confluence of para-aortic sympathetic tissue just below the origin of the inferior mesenteric artery. Paragangliomas are usually heterogeneous in appearance on CT and intensely enhance after contrast administration. The typical hyperintense appearance on T2-weighted MR imaging sequences has been described as "light bulb" bright, although this is seen less commonly than a heterogeneous necrotic mass. Once diagnosed, treatment for paragangliomas arising from the organ of Zuckerkandl is surgical excision (31).

## Aunt Minnie's Pearl

Extra-adrenal paragangliomas commonly arise from the organ of Zuckerkandl, at the aortic bifurcation.

**HISTORY:** Two patients involved in motor vehicle accidents with blunt pelvic trauma

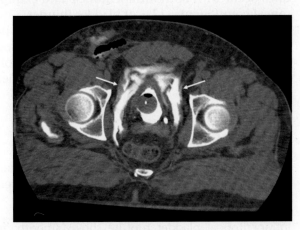

FIGURE 13.11.1

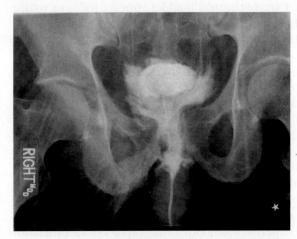

FIGURE 13.11.2

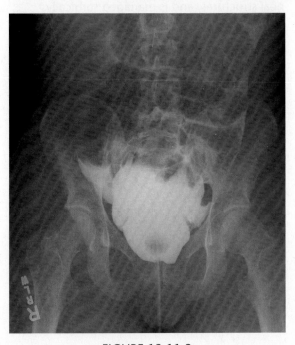

FIGURE 13.11.3

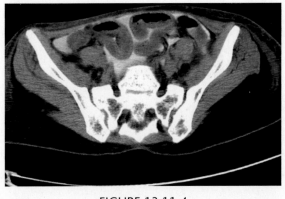

FIGURE 13.11.4

**FINDINGS:** Imaging evaluation of the first patient included CT cystogram image of the pelvis at the level of the acetabular roof (Fig. 13.11.1) and a pelvic radiograph. The axial CT image demonstrates rupture of the bladder wall with accumulation of contrast in the molar tooth-shaped prevesical extraperitoneal space (*arrows*). The anteroposterior pelvic radiograph (Fig. 13.11.2) demonstrates ill-defined flame-shaped contrast accumulation along both sides of the bladder; however no bowel is outlined by contrast. Frontal pelvic radiograph of the second patient performed after catheterization

of the bladder and instillation of contrast material (Fig. 13.11.3) shows contrast material outlining loops of bowel in the peritoneal space. Follow-up axial CT image (Fig. 13.11.4) confirms intraperitoneal location of contrast material.

**DIAGNOSIS:** Extraperitoneal bladder rupture (patient 1) and intraperitoneal bladder rupture (patient 2)

**DISCUSSION:** The possibility of bladder injury should be considered in all patients who suffer blunt or penetrating pelvic trauma. Gross hematuria occurs in up to 95% of cases of bladder rupture. Extraperitoneal bladder rupture (62% of major bladder injuries) is usually associated with pelvic fractures and is classified into simple and complex subtypes. In simple extraperitoneal rupture, contrast extravasation is limited to the pelvic extraperitoneal space. In complex extraperitoneal rupture, contrast extravasation extends beyond the prevesical space into the thigh, scrotum, or perineum, implying a fascial boundary injury (32,33). Treatment is usually nonsurgical catheter drainage. This approach is unlike intraperitoneal bladder rupture, which requires surgical management. With intraperitoneal rupture (25% of major bladder injuries), the irritative effect of urine exposed to the large surface area of the peritoneum can cause rapid development of chemical peritonitis, which complicates the patient's clinical management. Intraperitoneal bladder rupture is generally considered a surgical emergency

necessitating urgent primary repair of the bladder wall (32,33). Occasionally, combined bladder ruptures occur with both intraperitoneal and extraperitoneal components (12% of bladder injuries).

Although conventional cystography has been used to evaluate for bladder injury, CT cystography has been shown to be more accurate and often integrates more easily into the trauma patient's evaluation.

## Aunt Minnie's Pearls

Extraperitoneal bladder rupture demonstrates flame-like, infiltrating contrast extravasation and is generally managed conservatively.

Intraperitoneal bladder rupture shows smooth, free-flowing contrast outlining bowel and other intraperitoneal structures, and is managed surgically.

**HISTORY:** A 25-year-old African American male with sickle cell trait presents with hematuria and right flank pain

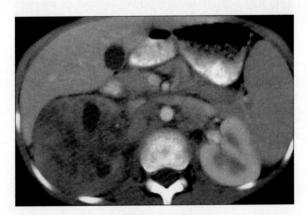

FIGURE 13.12.1

**FINDINGS:** A contrast-enhanced axial CT image of the abdomen (Fig. 13.12.1) demonstrates diffuse, ill-defined mass-like enlargement of the right kidney with heterogeneously decreased enhancement but no change in reniform shape.

**DIAGNOSIS:** Renal medullary carcinoma

**DISCUSSION:** Renal medullary carcinoma represents a very rare renal tumor that occurs almost exclusively in African American patients with sickle cell trait. The most common imaging presentation is a centrally located, infiltrative renal mass with preservation of normal renal contours. In addition, this particular renal tumor is extremely aggressive and commonly has metastatic involvement of lymph nodes, liver, and lungs at the time of presentation. As expected, prognosis is very poor with a majority of patients living <4 months after diagnosis. Thankfully, the diagnosis is rare with <100 documented cases in the US. (34,35).

## Aunt Minnie's Pearl

Although a rare diagnosis, the constellation of a young African American patient with sickle cell trait who presents with hematuria, flank pain, and a central, infiltrative renal mass highly suggests the diagnosis of renal medullary carcinoma.

**HISTORY:** A 62-year-old female with a history of diabetes mellitus presents with right flank pain and dysuria

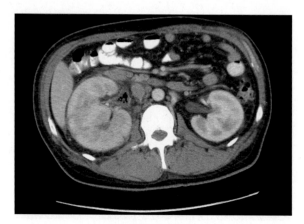

FIGURE 13.13.1

**FINDINGS:** Axial contrast-enhanced CT (Fig. 13.13.1) depicts gas in the right renal pelvis. The urothelium is thickened, and the right kidney is asymmetrically enlarged with decreased enhancement and a somewhat patchy nephrogram.

**DIAGNOSIS:** Emphysematous pyelitis (EP)

**DISCUSSION:** EP is defined as the presence of gas limited to the renal collecting system secondary to acute bacterial infection. EP affects women three times as often as men, and most patients have diabetes mellitus or obstructing stone disease (36). Pyuria is often present on urinalysis with *Escherichia coli* being the most common infecting organism (37). EP is considered a benign entity with an excellent prognosis. CT is the most reliable imaging modality for diagnosing EP and helps exclude potential complications such as perirenal fluid collections, abscess formation, or the presence of intraparenchymal gas representing the more serious emphysematous pyelonephritis (36). EP should be differentiated from other etiologies of air collecting systems including iatrogenic instrumentation, fistula between bowel, and reflux of air from the bladder or ileal conduit (38). EP usually responds well to intravenous antibiotic therapy in the absence of obstruction and surgical or percutaneous drainage is seldom necessary.

## Aunt Minnie's Pearls

EP has a much better prognosis than emphysematous pyelonephritis.

CT is the most sensitive imaging modality for depicting EP and excluding potential complications.

# Case 13.14

HISTORY: A 38-year-old man with left renal mass

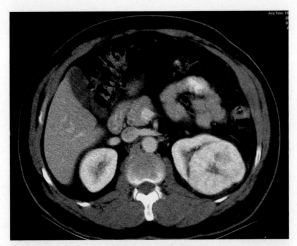

FIGURE 13.14.1

FINDINGS: Axial contrast-enhanced CT image (Fig. 13.14.1) shows a large left renal mass with a sharply marginated, central, stellate region of low attenuation. The right kidney is normal.

DIAGNOSIS: Renal oncocytoma

DISCUSSION: Renal oncocytomas are tumors that arise from the epithelial cells of the distal tubule or collecting ducts. Oncocytomas comprise approximately 5% of all renal tumors and are most often incidental findings even though they average >7 cm in diameter at diagnosis. The typical features of oncocytoma on CT and MRI are a solid cortical renal mass, central stellate scar, sharp margin with normal parenchyma, absence of necrosis and hemorrhage, and enhancement after intravenous contrast administration (24). On angiography, oncocytomas typically demonstrate a "spoke-wheel" pattern of vessels penetrating centrally into the tumor (25). Unfortunately, the imaging characteristics of oncocytomas do not allow confident differentiation from renal adenocarcinomas (39). Therefore, oncocytomas require surgical excision for definitive treatment. Even today, percutaneous biopsy is not generally recommended for diagnosing oncocytoma because oncocytomas and the closely related chromophobe type RCC have significant overlapping histologic features. Therefore, percutaneous biopsy is still considered unreliable for differentiation (40). When the imaging characteristics of a renal mass are consistent with oncocytoma, it is important to suggest such a diagnosis as oncocytomas may be amenable to nephron sparing surgery.

## Aunt Minnie's Pearls

The classic CT characteristics of renal oncocytoma are an enhancing solid renal cortical mass with central stellate scar.

The imaging characteristics of renal oncocytoma overlap with renal adenocarcinoma.

HISTORY: An 84-year-old male previously diagnosed with renal cell carcinoma

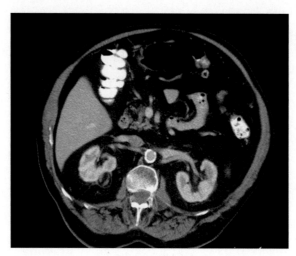

FIGURE 13.15.1

FINDINGS: Axial (Fig. 13.15.1) contrast-enhanced CT images through the kidneys demonstrate an exophytic thin curvilinear hyperattenuating halo in the perinephric fat and nonenhancing internal nodule

DIAGNOSIS: Renal halo sign after percutaneous radiofrequency ablation

DISCUSSION: The incidence of renal cell carcinoma (RCC) continues to increase as many tumors are detected earlier at cross-sectional imaging. Radiofrequency ablation (RFA) is now an established treatment options for stage T1aN0M0 RCC (41). Percutaneous image-guided tumor ablation is being used with increasing frequency as a minimally invasive treatment option, especially in patients who are poor candidates for surgical resection. The increasing use of percutaneous image-guided RFA requires familiarity with the appearance of an ablation site after successful treatment. An understanding of the normal expected temporal progression of an ablation cavity can help prevent unnecessary biopsy, repeated ablation, or even surgery. In successfully treated tumors, the tumor does not enhance after administration of intravenous contrast material (42). A curvilinear hyperattenuating

area, or halo, is often seen within the perinephric fat surrounding the ablated lesion. The renal halo sign is a common and benign imaging finding after percutaneous RFA, occurring in 75% of renal tumors treated with RFA (43). A change in lesion size is not a reliable indicator of treatment adequacy. The postablation lesion can be larger than the preablation tumor because a peripheral margin of normal renal tissue is also ablated. In one study, almost all small lesions (<3 cm before ablation) appeared larger on the 1- to 2-month follow-up with both CT and MRI (44). Multiphasic contrast-enhanced CTs or MRIs are necessary to assess the degree of enhancement. The most reliable sign of tumor relapse is an enlarging nodular or crescentic area that shows contrast enhancement (1).

## Aunt Minnie's Pearls

The renal halo sign is a benign imaging finding that is encountered on CT and MR images in 75% of patients after RFA.

The postablation renal halo should not be confused with tumor recurrence or angiomyolipoma.

**HISTORY:** A 65-year-old male with episodic dysuria

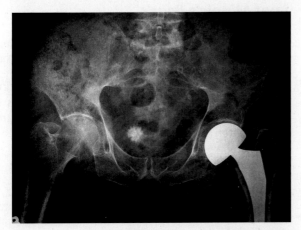

FIGURE 13.16.1

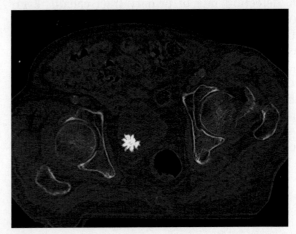

FIGURE 13.16.2

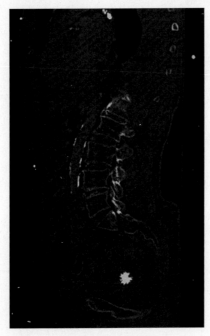

FIGURE 13.16.3

**FINDINGS:** An AP pelvic radiograph (Fig. 13.16.1) shows a calcific density in the rightward pelvis resembling the head of a morning star (medieval weapon). Contrast-enhanced axial CT image (Fig. 13.16.2) and sagittal multiplanar reformatted image (Fig. 13.16.3) demonstrate a spiculated calcific density, which rests in the dependent portion of the urinary bladder.

**DIAGNOSIS:** Jack stone (urinary tract calculus)

**DISCUSSION:** Urinary tract stones come in a wide variety of shapes and sizes. One such shape of urinary tract calculus has been likened to a child's jack toy, which describes its shape quite well. "Jack stones" (as they are now called) are most commonly found in the bladder, but they have also been described in the kidney (25). Like most urinary tract calculi, jack stones are composed of calcium oxalate. In fact, up to 80% of urinary tract calculi are calcium-based. The next most common components of these calculi include struvite, uric acid, and cystine. Despite variation in composition, CT yields >95% detection rate of urinary tract calculi. Even radiolucent stones caused by anti-HIV protease inhibitor drugs (i.e., indinavir) can be detected on occasion as many contain at least a small percentage of calcium. In addition, the radiologist can gain a detective advantage by looking at secondary signs of urinary obstruction (i.e., hydroureteronephrosis, perinephric/periureteral stranding, and soft-tissue rim sign) and by closely inspecting three areas of ureteral narrowing (ureteropelvic junction, pelvic brim, and ureterovesical junction) where stones are most commonly lodged (45).

## Aunt Minnie's Pearls

Urinary tract calculi take on myriad shapes and sizes, including the multi-spiculated "jack stone" configuration.

CT scans are very sensitive and specific for urinary tract calculus detection. Even radiolucent stones can be detected with a high index of suspicion and careful search pattern.

**HISTORY:** A 35-year-old male with flank pain

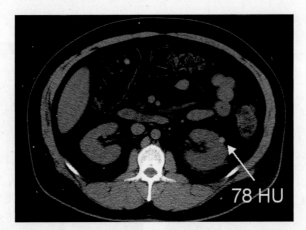

FIGURE 13.17.1

**FINDINGS:** Axial noncontrast CT (Fig. 13.17.1) demonstrates an exophytic hyperdense mass from the left lateral kidney with an internal density of 78 HU.

**DIAGNOSIS:** Hyperdense cyst

**DISCUSSION:** A hyperdense cyst contains fluid higher than water attenuation (>20 HU) with sharp, smooth margins and does not enhance with contrast media. Benign cysts are the most common type of hyperdense renal mass and are frequently found in patients with either acquired cystic renal disease or autosomal dominant polycystic renal disease (46). The attenuation of hyperdense renal cysts can be variable and is dependent on their content. Cysts that measure between 20 and 40 HU tend to be proteinaceous cysts and those with attenuations >40 to 50 HU are likely hemorrhagic cysts.

Bosniak II cysts are small (≤3 cm) homogeneously hyperdense, nonenhancing cystic masses that are considered benign and do not require additional evaluation (47). One recent study suggests that when a hyperdense renal lesion is encountered on an unenhanced CT scan, the probability of the mass being benign is >99.9% as long as the attenuation is 70 HU or higher and the mass is homogeneous (48). Therefore, if a hyperdense cyst has attenuation >70 HU, unnecessary imaging, surgical resection, or ablation can be avoided.

## Aunt Minnie's Pearl

A homogeneous renal mass measuring >70 HU at unenhanced CT has a >99.9% chance of representing a hyperdense renal cyst rather than RCC.

**HISTORY:** A 46-year-old female with hematuria

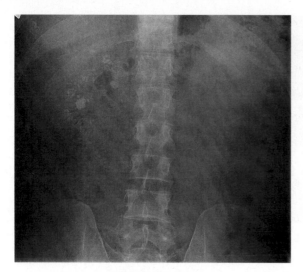

FIGURE 13.18.1

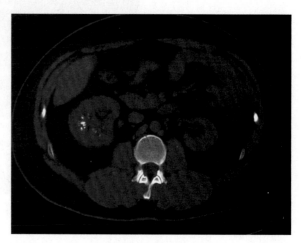

FIGURE 13.18.2

**FINDINGS:** Abdominal radiograph (Fig. 13.18.1) demonstrates innumerable calcifications projecting over the right kidney. Noncontrast CT (Fig. 13.18.2) of the same patient demonstrates medullary nephrocalcinosis in a somewhat enlarged right kidney. The left kidney is normal.

**DIAGNOSIS:** Medullary sponge kidney (MSK)

**DISCUSSION:** MSK represents a type of cystic renal disease characterized by congenital ectasia and cystic dilatation of the renal medullary terminal collecting ducts. Findings are often bilateral; however, MSK can be distinguished from systemic/metabolic causes of medullary nephrocalcinosis (hyperparathyroidism, renal tubular acidosis, etc.) when findings are asymmetric, in particular when unilateral. The prevalence of MSK is estimated as high as 1 in 5,000 in the general population (49). Multidetector CT urography may show the characteristic "paintbrush" appearance of papillary blush and associated calculi in the dilated collecting ducts.

Multidetector CT urography has greater sensitivity than intravenous urography for the detection of dilated medullary collecting ducts in patients with MSK (50). The kidneys may be mildly enlarged in medullary sponge, unlike other causes. MSK may be incidentally identified but often presents in patients owing to stone disease (hematuria, renal colic, fever, and dysuria; 50). Establishing the diagnosis of MSK has clinical value despite no specific available therapy because it identifies high-risk patients for stone formation and recurrent urinary tract infection (51). MSK usually follows a benign clinical course, although associated complications of obstruction and infection may rarely lead to chronic kidney disease and renal failure (49).

## Aunt Minnie's Pearl

MSK may be unilateral or involve a single a papilla unlike systemic/metabolic causes of medullary nephrocalcinosis like hyperparathyroidism or renal tubular acidosis.

HISTORY: A 17-year-old female with uterine anomaly detected on ultrasound

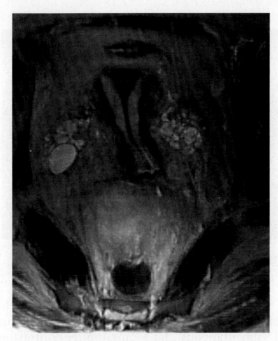

FIGURE 13.19.1

FINDINGS: Axial oblique T2-weighted image parallel to the long axis of the uterus (Fig. 13.19.1) demonstrates two endometrial cavities with a complete septum that extends to the cervical os. The fundal contour is flat to slightly convex, without indentation.

DIAGNOSIS: Septate uterus

DISCUSSION: Müllerian duct anomalies (MDAs) cause alterations in the normal uterine contour and potential etiology of female infertility. Septate uterus is the most common MDA, accounting for approximately 55% of all MDAs, and is associated with the poorest reproductive outcomes (52). Septate uterus results from a partial or complete failure of resorption of the uterovaginal septum after fusion of the Müllerian ducts. Accurate characterization of MDAs is imperative because reproductive outcomes and treatment options vary between the different classes of anomalies. If an MDA is suspected or incompletely characterized at hysterosalpingography, further evaluation is often performed with pelvic US, MR imaging, or both. MR imaging has the highest reported accuracy (nearly 100%) for the characterization of MDAs (53). Oblique imaging parallel to the long axis of the uterine body permits characterization of the uterine contour and septum, enabling differentiation from bicornuate uterus. The external uterine contour is usually convex, flat, or minimally indented by <1 cm with septate uterus, in contrast to that of a bicornuate uterus. The septum of a septate uterus may be a combination of both fibrous tissue and muscle. A thin fibrous septum is demonstrated as low signal intensity on T2-weighted MR images, whereas a thicker septum comprising abundant muscular tissue has intermediate signal intensity (54). The septum may be partial or complete, extending to the external cervical os. A septate uterus is often treated with hysteroscopic metroplasty of the septum with improved reproductive outcomes (9).

## Aunt Minnie's Pearls

Septate uterus is the most common MDA with the poorest reproductive outcomes.

MRI is very accurate for the characterization of MDAs.

HISTORY: A 29-year-old woman presents with abdominal pain. The patient provides a history of previous cesarean section and endometriosis

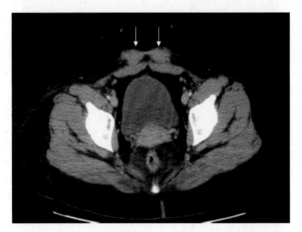

FIGURE 13.20.1

FINDINGS: An unenhanced CT image (Fig. 13.20.1) shows two small soft-tissue density masses within the ventral abdominal wall subcutaneous fat (*arrows*). The masses abut the underlying rectus musculature.

DIAGNOSIS: Incisional endometriosis

DISCUSSION: Endometriosis affects approximately 15% of menstruating women and is defined as the presence of functioning endometrial tissue outside the uterine endometrium and myometrium. Endometriosis most commonly occurs within the pelvis and involves the fallopian tubes, ovaries, and bladder. Unusual extrapelvic sites of endometrial implants have been reported, including subcutaneous implants within the anterior abdominal wall. Most cases of abdominal wall endometriosis are associated with prior cesarean section surgical scars (55). It is thought that surgical procedures that violate the uterine cavity, such as cesarean sections, may result in the direct transplant of endometrial tissue to the subcutaneous tissue. The classic symptoms of endometriosis include cyclic pain and discomfort associated with menses. However, incisional endometriosis frequently presents as an abdominal mass with noncyclical symptoms (56,57). The classic CT appearance includes ill-defined subcutaneous mass isodense to musculature with slight enhancement after contrast administration. On ultrasound, endometriosis appears as a hypoechoic heterogenous mass with internal vascularity (57), and MR depicts endometriosis as hypointense to muscle on T1-weighted images, hyperintense on T2-weighted images, with post-contrast enhancement. Imaging findings of a solid subcutaneous mass near a cesarean section scar strongly suggest the diagnosis of incisional endometriosis (57), although the differential diagnosis includes hematoma, suture granuloma, lipoma, abscess, cyst, incisional hernia, lymphoma, sarcoma, desmoid tumor, or metastasis. Ultrasound-guided fine-needle aspiration is often used for pathologic diagnosis and the definitive treatment is wide local excision.

## Aunt Minnie's Pearls

Imaging findings of a solid mass near a cesarean section incisional scar should raise the suspicion of incisional endometriosis.

Incisional endometriosis often presents with noncyclic symptoms.

**HISTORY:** A 50-year-old male with a history of a right renal cell carcinoma status post-partial right nephrectomy.

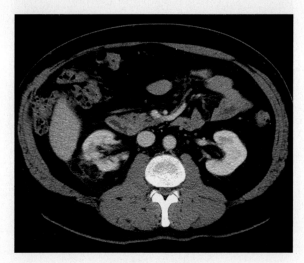

FIGURE 13.21.1

**FINDINGS:** Axial CT of the abdomen demonstrates a 4-cm "fatty" lesion along the lateral periphery of the right kidney (Fig. 13.21.1).

**DIAGNOSIS:** Right renal pseudolesion caused by fat packing from previous partial nephrectomy

**DISCUSSION:** A case such as this reminds the radiologists of the importance of clinical history, particularly prior surgical intervention. For patients who are status post-partial nephrectomy, the postoperative kidney typically has a wedge-shaped parenchymal defect, usually abuts and adheres to the dorsal abdominal wall, and shows adjacent fibrotic or reactive changes in the perinephric space. In some cases (as this one showed), the surgeon chooses to pack the surgical defect with fat to lower the possibility of postoperative bleeding. Over time, the adipose-rich packing material can take on a similar appearance to an AML and misdiagnosis can easily occur without a thorough investigation for any prior renal surgeries (58,59).

## Aunt Minnie's Pearls

Nephron sparing surgery is commonly used by urologists today, and radiologists should be familiar with the postoperative appearance of the kidney following partial nephrectomy.

Urologists commonly pack the partial nephrectomy surgical bed with fat for hemostatic purposes, and this "fatty mass" can be mistaken for AML on follow-up CT examinations.

Careful review of the patient's clinical history is crucial to help evade easily avoidable errors.

HISTORY: An 87-year-old male with hematuria

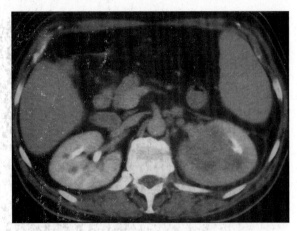

FIGURE 13.22.1

FINDINGS: Axial contrast-enhanced CT during urographic phase of contrast enhancement (Fig. 13.22.1) shows an infiltrating renal lesion with epicenter in the renal sinus.

DIAGNOSIS: Infiltrating urothelial carcinoma (formerly TCC)

DISCUSSION: Urothelial carcinoma (UC) can occur anywhere along the urinary urothelium and approximately 5% of urothelial tumors arise from the ureter or renal pelvis rather than the bladder. Not uncommonly, UC can be multifocal, thus the diagnosis of should prompt the evaluation of the entire urothelium to exclude synchronous disease and follow up for metachronous lesions. In fact, up to 40% of patients with UC of the collecting system may have carcinomas of the bladder diagnosed within a short time. Patients with an upper urinary tract tumor may present with gross or microscopic hematuria, and occasionally pain if the tumor is causing obstructive symptoms. Multidetector computed tomography urography, that is, MDCTU has been shown to be a useful technique in evaluating the urothelium and detecting urinary tract abnormalities (including UC) in the evaluation of patients with hematuria (60–63).

Renal UC, in late stage or when aggressive, may invade the adjacent kidney. When this occurs the growth pattern within the renal parenchyma tends to be infiltrating (maintaining the reniform shape) as opposed to exophytic and rounded. In addition to UC, some other neoplasms may be infiltrating including squamous cell carcinoma (primary or metastatic), lymphoma, and in rare cases RCC and other rare renal tumors. Renal infarcts and infection also have an infiltrating appearance. Epicenter in the renal pelvis, adenopathy, lack of significant inflammation, and clinical scenario often suggests the diagnosis with confidence.

## Aunt Minnie's Pearl

High-grade TCC should be considered first when encountering an infiltrating lesion centered at the renal pelvis.

**HISTORY:** A 32-year-old female with a history of pelvic infections presents with sharp stabbing pelvic pain and fever

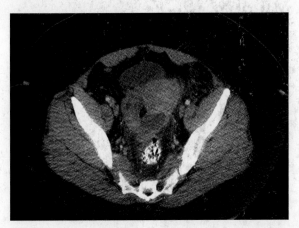

FIGURE 13.23.1

**FINDINGS:** Axial contrast-enhanced CT of the pelvis (Fig. 13.23.1) demonstrates a large multiloculated cystic mass with thickened septations in the right adnexa, adjacent inflammatory stranding, and mass effect on the uterus.

**DIAGNOSIS:** Tubo-ovarian abscess (TOA)

**DISCUSSION:** TOA is a well-recognized complication of pelvic inflammatory disease (PID). PID results from an ascending vaginal or cervical infection that progresses to endometritis followed by salpingitis. Inadequate treatment of PID can lead to infection of the ovary and TOA (65). *Neisseria gonorrhoeae* or *Chlamydia trachomatis* is the offending agent in up to two-thirds of cases. As many as 24% of visits to the emergency department for gynecologic pain are attributable to PID (66). Although US should be the initial diagnostic test if TOA is clinically suspected, familiarity with multidetector CT findings is important because CT may initially be obtained in the emergency setting in patients who present with nonspecific clinical symptoms. Previously described CT findings of TOA include a thick-walled mass in an adnexal location with fluid attenuation, septa, indistinct borders between the uterus and adjacent bowel loops, anterior displacement of the mesosalpinx, and gas bubbles within the mass (67). Imaging findings of endometriosis can mimic those of TOA. Treatment modalities include IV antibiotics, image-guided drainage, and surgical resection.

## Aunt Minnie's Pearls

US should be the initial diagnostic test if TOA is suspected clinically.

Internal gas bubbles are the most specific sign of TOA, but a rare finding.

Correctly identifying TOA on any modality is important as rupture can result in life-threatening peritonitis.

HISTORY: A 41-year-old patient with right upper quadrant pain

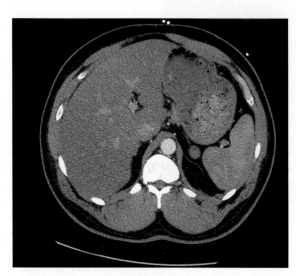

FIGURE 13.24.1

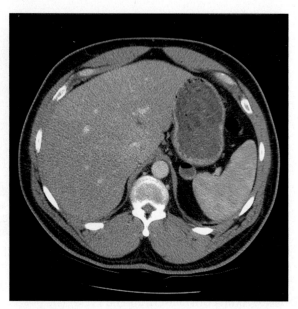

FIGURE 13.24.2

FINDINGS: Contrast-enhanced axial CT image of the upper abdomen (Fig. 13.24.1) incidentally noted a 1.5-cm nodular lesion in a left "adrenal" location. A second axial CT image (Fig. 13.24.2) demonstrates an air-fluid level. Additional imaging demonstrated a clear communication between this lesion and the gastric lumen as well as a separate adrenal gland with normal contours.

DIAGNOSIS: Gastric fundal diverticulum mimicking an adrenal lesion

DISCUSSION: A gastric fundal diverticulum is most commonly located along the posterior wall of the proximal stomach. Given this suprarenal location, gastric diverticula can often mimic a left retroperitoneal lesion (particularly an adrenal mass). Without a clear air-fluid level or connection to the stomach on the imaging study, it can be difficult to distinguish a gastric diverticulum from an adrenal lesion. In such cases, an imaging study using enteric contrast material can be helpful for establishing an accurate diagnosis. Additionally, the contents of the gastric diverticulum will not enhance on a CT with IV contrast (68).

## Aunt Minnie's Pearls

A gastric fundal diverticulum can mimic a retroperitoneal lesion.

Carefully separate the left adrenal gland from any lesions along the posterior wall of the proximal stomach. If not clearly separate, then consider an imaging study with enteric contrast for further delineation.

As gastric diverticula are most commonly incidental findings and rarely associated with complications, no additional follow-up is needed in the asymptomatic patient.

HISTORY: A 21-year-old man presents with abdominal pain

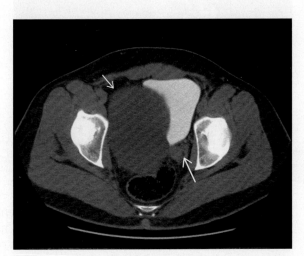

FIGURE 13.25.1

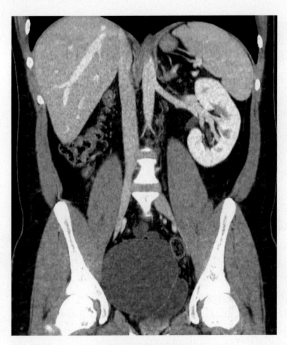

FIGURE 13.25.2

FINDINGS: Axial excretory phase contrast-enhanced CT through the pelvis (Fig. 13.25.1) shows a well-defined cystic mass (10 HU) occupying the bulk of the pelvis, with leftward displacement of the contrast-filled urinary bladder (*small arrow*). A normal enhancing left seminal vesicle is visualized (*large arrow*). Coronal reformation (Fig. 13.25.2) shows an absent right kidney with a normal left kidney.

DIAGNOSIS: Seminal vesicle cyst with ipsilateral renal agenesis

DISCUSSION: Cysts of the seminal vesicle are uncommon and can be either congenital or acquired. Approximately two-thirds of congenital seminal vesicle cysts are associated with abnormalities of the upper urinary tract, most commonly ipsilateral renal agenesis or dysplasia. The common embryologic origin of the genital and urinary tracts explains this association. During the 12th embryologic week, maldevelopment of the distal mesonephric duct and faulty ureteral budding leads to renal agenesis or dysplasia, and atresia of the ejaculatory duct leads to the formation of seminal vesicle cysts. Small seminal vesicle cysts (<5 cm) are often asymptomatic and identified incidentally, although they may present with symptoms related to voiding or chronic epididymitis or prostatitis (69). Patients with "giant" (>12 cm) seminal vesicle cysts may present with symptoms of bladder or colonic obstruction secondary to mass effect (69). Seminal vesicle cysts are accurately characterized by CT as near-water-attenuation retrovesicular masses that arise in the expected area of the seminal vesicle cephalic to the prostate gland (70). On MRI, seminal vesicle cysts are fluid signal intensity on T2-weighted images, variable signal intensity on T1-weighted images (owing to internal hemorrhagic or proteinaceous debris), and do not enhance after contrast administration (70).

## Aunt Minnie's Pearl

Congenital seminal vesicle cysts are often associated with ipsilateral renal anomalies owing to their common embryonic origin.

HISTORY: A 29-year-old female with right flank pain

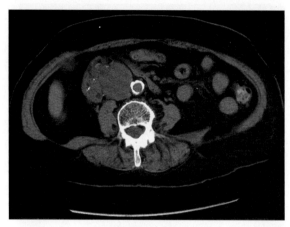

FIGURE 13.26.1

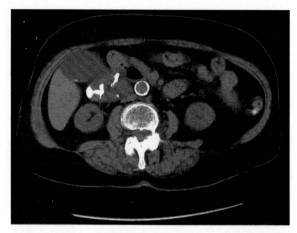

FIGURE 13.26.2

FINDINGS: An unenhanced axial CT of the abdomen (Figs. 13.26.1 and 13.26.2) shows a 6-cm right retroperitoneal mass that contains large soft-tissue component, large calcifications, and small foci of fat and proteinaceous fluid. The mass is separate from the right kidney.

DIAGNOSIS: Primary retroperitoneal teratoma

DISCUSSION: Primary retroperitoneal teratomas are rare entities that represent <12% of all primary retroperitoneal tumors. In addition, <20% of these lesions occur in adults (71). Primary retroperitoneal teratomas develop from germ cells that fail to migrate to their normal gonadal location. Once formed, these lesions may be solid or cystic and commonly contain mature tissues (i.e., teeth, skin, fat, cartilage, bone). Primary retroperitoneal teratomas can be benign or malignant, and the malignant type more commonly affects adults. On CT, teratomas are usually heterogeneous, well-defined, solid, or multiloculated cystic lesions that may contain calcifications, bony elements, teeth, protein, and fat. A fat-fluid level with nondependent fat layer is virtually pathognomonic of a teratoma. Imaging is helpful for surgical planning, especially anatomical relationships with adjacent abdominal viscera (72). Laboratory values can be helpful as alpha-fetoprotein levels are normal in the benign type and can be elevated in the malignant type. Benign lesions have an excellent prognosis if surgically excised, whereas malignant lesions frequently recur with <2 years survival after surgery (73).

## Aunt Minnie's Pearl

A retroperitoneal mass that contains soft tissue, calcification, and a fat-fluid level is virtually pathognomonic of a teratoma.

# Case 13.27

HISTORY: An 18-year-old female with low abdominal pain and cramping

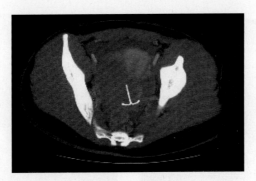

FIGURE 13.27.1

FINDINGS: Axial contrast-enhanced CT of the abdomen and pelvis (Fig. 13.27.1) demonstrates an abnormal extrauterine position of the intrauterine device (IUD). The IUD is posterior the uterine fundus surrounded by heterogenous free fluid and clot in the rectouterine pouch.

DIAGNOSIS: Migration of intrauterine device

DISCUSSION: When migration of an IUD is suspected, ultrasound is appropriate for initial evaluation. Ultrasound is widely available and can often provide answers to clinical questions related to the IUD. Uterine perforation is an uncommon but serious complication in females with an IUD, occurring in up to one of every 1,000 cases (74). Perforation is thought to be related to low estrogen levels leading to uterine shrinkage. A postpartum period <6 months, lactation, and amenorrhea may increase the risk of perforation. Uterine perforation is thought to occur frequently at the time of device insertion, and it should be suspected in patients with a missing IUD string and acute abdominal pain. CT is the best modality for the evaluation of complications associated with intraabdominal IUDs, such as visceral perforation (75). Management of uterine perforation by an IUD is controversial. Although it is agreed that all patients with perforation should receive empirical antibiotics, some data suggest that surgical treatment should be reserved for symptomatic patients (76). However, surgical removal of an intraabdominal IUD is recommended by the World Health Organization and is generally accepted as appropriate treatment (77).

## Aunt Minnie's Pearls

US is appropriate for initial evaluation of an IUD. Conventional radiography of the abdomen is used to locate an IUD when it is not visualized at US. CT is the best modality for identifying complications of an intraabdominal IUD.

Detection of IUD expulsion or displacement should be immediately communicated to the patient and the referring clinician, as they can decrease contraceptive efficacy and may require further management.

# Case 13.28

HISTORY: A 31-year-old female with a history of irregular menses

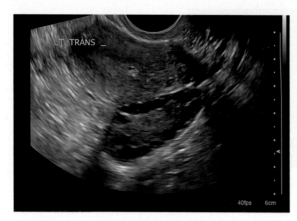

FIGURE 13.28.1

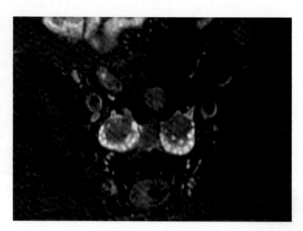

FIGURE 13.28.2

FINDINGS: Pelvic ultrasound and T2-weighted MRI demonstrates an enlarged ovary with >12 subcentimeter peripheral follicles surrounding a prominent hyperechoic (US) (Fig. 13.28.1) and hypointense (MRI) ovarian stroma (Fig. 13.28.2). No evidence of dominant follicle.

DIAGNOSIS: Polycystic ovary syndrome (PCOS)

DISCUSSION: Also known as Stein–Leventhal syndrome, PCOS is one of the most common causes of female infertility. PCOS is an endocrinologic disorder characterized by chronic anovulation and hyperandrogenism. Furthermore, PCOS has a classic triad of obesity, amenorrhea, and hirsutism; but only half of patients present with this combination. Therefore, imaging evaluation tends to follow to gain further information (78). In 2003, the Rotterdam consensus imaging criteria was revised and gave radiologists consensus diagnostic criteria for diagnosis of PCOS. Imaging criteria includes the following: ovarian volume >10 cm$^3$, >12 subcentimeter follicles per ovary, and no dominant follicle/corpus luteal cyst. The combination of these imaging findings and clinical signs/symptoms of PCOS will essentially confirm the diagnosis. Exclusion of other possible etiologies (congenital adrenal hyperplasia, androgen-secreting tumor, and Cushing syndrome) is important as well (79). Typical US/MRI findings include enlarged, rounded ovaries with numerous small, peripherally located follicles and stroma showing increased echogenicity (US) or decreased signal on T2-weighted imaging (MRI). Long-term follow-up should be recommended in such patients as PCOS patients have an increased risk of breast and uterine cancer secondary to unopposed high estrogen levels (56).

## Aunt Minnie's Pearls

Enlarged ovaries with multiple peripherally located small follicles around a abnormal stroma in a patient with oligomenorrhea and hyperandrogenism has PCOS until proven otherwise.

Increased risk of endometrial and breast cancer necessitates long-term follow-up in patients diagnosed with PCOS.

HISTORY: Two patients scanned for abdominal pain

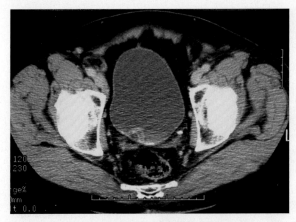

FIGURE 13.29.1

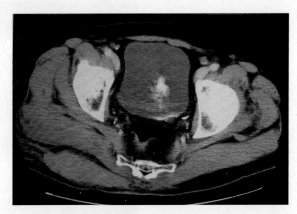

FIGURE 13.29.2

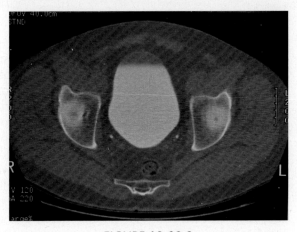

FIGURE 13.29.3

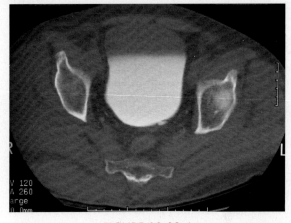

FIGURE 13.29.4

FINDINGS: Figure 13.29.1 demonstrates a rounded sessile mass like density along the rightward bladder base, whereas Figure 13.29.2 shows a papillary-like "lesion" in the mid-bladder. Delayed images (Figs. 13.29.3 and 13.29.4) in each patient demonstrate no abnormality.

DIAGNOSIS: Bladder pseudotumors owing to ureteral jets

DISCUSSION: Rather than a simple tube or conduit for urine flow, the ureter actively contracts in a complex, coordinated fashion to force urine into the bladder. Although the size and pressure created by peristalsis varies, the ureteral bolus is propelled through the ureteral vesicle junction into the bladder creating the so-called ureteral jet. This jet can be identified and interrogated on color Doppler ultrasound (80), the presence or absence (and perhaps waveform) used for diagnostic purposes, especially to diagnose ureteral

obstruction. Ureteral jets can also be seen on contrast-enhanced CT, especially when the bladder is scanned just as contrast is starting to enter the unopacified bladder. Although usually easily recognized, occasionally the appearance of the jet can mimic a bladder mass. A few clues can help, jets are usually created at that unique time when the contrast is just starting to reach the bladder. Furthermore, jets originate at the ureterovesical junction and project obliquely across the bladder. Despite being aware this pitfall, and using all clues, delayed images, ultrasound or even cystoscopy may be necessary to exclude a true bladder mass.

## Aunt Minnie's Pearls

A ureteral jet is created by urine (and contrast) being propelled into the bladder by ureteral peristalsis

On CT, the ureteral jet can mimic a bladder mass

HISTORY: A 57-year-old female imaged for pelvic discomfort

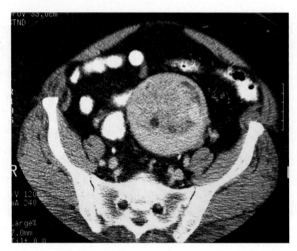

FIGURE 13.30.1

FINDINGS: Axial post-contrast CT (Fig. 13.30.1) demonstrates a heterogeneous pelvic mass, shown on additional images to be arising from the uterine fundus. Lower density areas measured fatty attenuation.

DIAGNOSIS: Lipoleiomyoma

DISCUSSION: Like all of us, the uterine fibroid tires of being ordinary and desires to be unique—to be different. Being calcified is old hat and does not cut it. Cystic, hemorrhagic or torsed is not even different enough for some. For a rare few, leiomyomas may contain fat, warranting the appellation lipoleiomyoma. As the myometrium does not contain fat, the presumed origin is some lipocytic transformation of immature mesenchymal tissues (81). Fat-containing fibroids are usually found in postmenopausal women, and clinically present (if symptomatic at all) and are managed like ordinary leiomyomas. On CT, lipoleiomyomas contain variable amounts of macroscopic fat ranging from nearly completely lipomatous to containing only small areas of fat, such as in our case. Identification of the uterine origin of the mass allows differentiation of other fatty pelvic masses, especially ovarian teratomas (81). This distinction is important as teratomas are generally resected, whereas lipoleiomyomas need not be. Finally, there has been at least one case of a lipoleiomyosarcoma reported; however this is so rare that unless there is evidence of direct invasion or metastasis, the fat-containing uterine mass can be confidently considered a benign lipoleiomyoma.

## Aunt Minnie's Pearls

In rare cases, uterine leiomyomas contain fat and are called lipoleiomyomas

Other than containing fat, these lesions are like other fibroids in regard to clinical presentation, course, and management

# Case 13.31

**HISTORY:** Two middle-aged asymptomatic patients

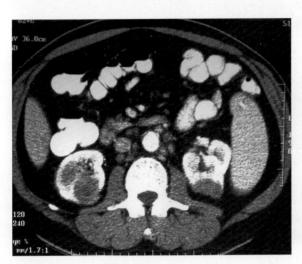

FIGURE 13.31.1

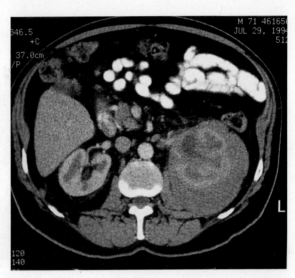

FIGURE 13.31.2

**FINDINGS:** Axial contrast-enhanced CT image of the first patient (Fig. 13.31.1) demonstrates bilateral homogeneous renal masses with minimal contrast enhancement on corticomedullary phase. Axial contrast-enhanced CT image of the second patient (Fig. 13.31.2) shows a perirenal soft tissue mass enveloping and infiltrating the left kidney.

**DIAGNOSIS:** Renal lymphoma

**DISCUSSION:** Lymphoma usually involves the kidney in a recognizable pattern. The most common manifestation of renal lymphoma is multiple masses, and most often affects both kidneys. This pattern (multiple masses) occurs in 40% to 60% of cases (82,83).

A second pattern of renal lymphoma is perirenal disease. Although the perirenal pattern is only seen in 10% of renal lymphoma cases, the imaging appearance is virtually pathognomonic. In addition, renal lymphoma is considered the most common perirenal mass. A key point to recognize is that

lymphomatous masses are mostly homogeneous and routinely enhance less than normal renal parenchyma. Additional clues for diagnosing lymphoma can be key for clinching the diagnosis, such as retroperitoneal adenopathy or splenomegaly (84,85).

## Aunt Minnie's Pearls

Lymphoma is a common disease process; therefore, recognition of common and pathognomonic features of renal lymphoma is a key skill for any radiologist.

Contrast-enhanced CT is considered the most efficient means of diagnosing renal mass patients who are suspected to have lymphoma.

Bilateral renal masses are the most common appearance of renal lymphoma.

A perirenal soft tissue mass is most commonly lymphoma.

**HISTORY:** A 27-year-old male who presents with perineal pain and blood at the urethral meatus following a bicycling injury

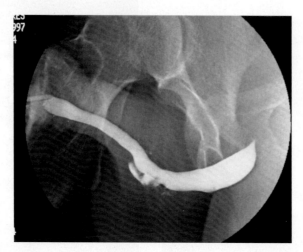

FIGURE 13.32.1

**FINDINGS:** Retrograde urethrogram (Fig. 13.32.1) demonstrates partial disruption of the anterior urethra with contrast extravasation from the ventral urethra.

**DIAGNOSIS:** Anterior urethral injury, incomplete rupture

**DISCUSSION:** Urethral injury is a common complication of trauma to the pelvis, occurring in up to 25% of adult patients with pelvic fractures. Isolated urethral injuries may not be life-threatening, but identification of injury is important as long-term morbidity is common (especially if proper treatment is delayed). If urethral injury is suspected clinically, then high-quality urethrography must be integrated into the imaging protocol prior to Foley catheter insertion (which could convert a partial urethral disruption to a complete disruption or contaminate a previously sterile pelvic hematoma).

During retrograde urethrography, the radiologist determines the absence or presence of urethral injury and then classifies the injury based on fluoroscopic appearance. The radiologist typically uses the American Association for Surgery of Trauma (AAST) and Goldman Systems for urethral injuries classification to describe the injury and guide therapy. One of the radiologist's most important tasks is to determine partial versus complete disruption, as therapy is significantly different for each (86).

Partial urethral rupture entails urethrographic documentation of contrast extravasation but maintenance of urethral continuity (i.e., extravasation from the urethra with bladder opacification). According to AAST, treatment of partial rupture includes conservative management with suprapubic or urethral catheterization.

However, complete urethral rupture shows disruption of urethral continuity and failure to opacify the proximal urethra. According to AAST, treatment of complete rupture includes endoscopic realignment or delayed graft urethroplasty. In addition, measurement of the defect length is important as longer defects require more extensive urethroplasty (87,88).

## Aunt Minnie's Pearls

Clinical suspicion of urethral injury warrants urethrography, which is the mainstay for identifying and classifying urethral injuries.

Abnormal stretching/elongation or contrast extravasation encountered on urethrography denotes urethral injury.

After identifying urethral injury location, classification of partial versus complete urethral transection is paramount, as treatments are different for each.

HISTORY: A 17-year-old male presents for scrotal ultrasound after trauma

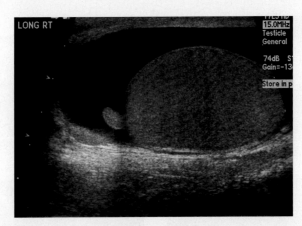

FIGURE 13.33.1

FINDINGS: The ultrasound reveals a 5-mm polypoid projection arising from the superior pole of an otherwise normal testis (Fig. 13.33.1). The projection is slightly hyperechoic to the testis. There is a moderate hydrocele.

DIAGNOSIS: Appendix Testis

DISCUSSION: The scrotum, perhaps jealous of all the attention garnered by the more famous GI tract appendix, decided to have five appendices (three are microscopic and not seen with imaging, and the fourth, the appendix of the epididymis, is pretty uncommon) (89). The appendix of the testis, however, deserves more attention than it gets as it is common and clinically important as it may torse. It was once suggested that the appendix testis was visible only if torsed; however this is clearly not the case, as it can frequently be seen normally (90). The normal appendix arises near the upper pole of the testis in the groove next to the head of the epididymis, is best seen in the setting of a hydrocele, ranges from 1 mm to 7 mm in size, and is typically of similar echogenicity to the epididymis. Morphologically they vary: most are finger-like and sessile, but can be "stalked" and more likely thus to torsion. The appendix can also appear cystic or calcified, usually secondary to prior torsion. Although occasional low blood flow may be seen with Doppler, color flow is not detected in the normal appendix. As stated, torsion of the appendix of the testis is a common cause of acute scrotal pain, particularly in boys younger than 13 years (91). On ultrasound, the torsed appendix testis appearance can overlap the normal appearance but is often enlarged (>6 mm), of variable echogenicity (hyperechoic mostly, but can be hypoechoic), rounded, and demonstrates a surrounding hyperemic reaction in the adjacent tissues, and often surrounded by a hydrocele.

## Aunt Minnie's Pearls

The appendix testis is a relatively common finding at scrotal ultrasound, especially in the presence of a hydrocele.

The normal appendix should not be confused for a mass.

Torsion of the appendix is a common cause of acute scrotal pain, particularly in younger boys.

HISTORY: Two -aged female patients with right flank and pelvic pain

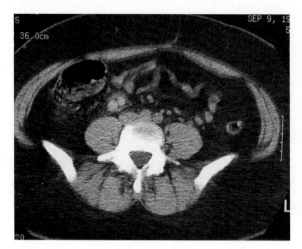

FIGURE 13.34.1

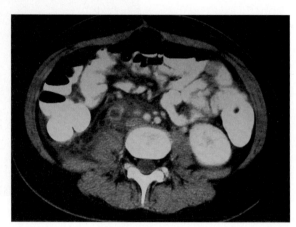

FIGURE 13.34.2

FINDINGS: Axial non-contrast CT image of the first patient (Fig. 13.34.1) demonstrates an enlarged right ovarian vein with hyperdense lumen and mild inflammatory changes at the vessel periphery. Axial contrast-enhanced CT image of the second patient (Fig. 13.34.2) shows an enlarged right ovarian vein with well-defined enhancing wall and a central low-attenuation filling defect. The image also depicts perivascular fat stranding suggestive of thrombophlebitis.

DIAGNOSIS: Ovarian vein thrombosis

DISCUSSION: Ovarian vein thrombosis, once considered rare, occurs more commonly than previously thought. Although most occur after childbirth, particularly in the setting of endometritis, it can occur in other settings including patients with PID, following gynecologic surgery and in oncology patients.

Although often asymptomatic or resulting in vague pain, the condition can be more serious including clot propagation, pulmonary embolism, and sepsis. CT is the mainstay of diagnosis. On noncontrast CT the thrombosed gonadal vein is often enlarged, hyperdense, and surrounded by inflammation. Contrast studies show the hypodense thrombus within an enlarged vein, with wall enhancement and adjacent inflammation. Once recognized, treatment typically consists of anticoagulation and NSAIDs (92).

## Aunt Minnie's Pearls

Ovarian vein thrombosis may occur following pregnancy, pelvic surgery, in patients with PID or malignancy.

The condition is serious and life-threatening.

# REFERENCES

1. Cochran ST, Walsman J, Barbaric ZL. Radiographic and microscopic findings in multiple ureteral diverticula. Radiology 1980;137:631–636.
2. Wasserman NF, La Pointe S, Posalaky IP. Ureteral pseudodiverticulosis. Radiology 1985;155:561–566.
3. Parker MD, Rebsamen S, Clark RL. Multiple ureteral diverticula: A possible radiographically demonstrable risk factor in development of transitional cell carcinoma. Urol Radiol 1989;11:45–48.
4. Kaufman RH, Adam E, Binder GL, et al. Upper genital tract changes and pregnancy outcome in offspring exposed in utero to diethylstilbestrol. Am J Obstet Gyencol 1980;137(3):299–308.
5. Kaufman RH, Noller K, Adam E, et al. Upper genital tract abnormalities and pregnancy outcome in diethylstilbestrol-exposed progeny. Am J Obstet Gyncol 1984;148:973–984.
6. Van Gils AP, Tham RT, Falke TH, et al. Abnormalities of the uterus and cervix after diethylstilbestrol exposure: Correlation of findings on MR and hysterosalpingography. AJR Am J Roentgenol 1989;153:1235–1238.
7. Swan SH. Intrauterine exposure to diethylstilbestrol: Long-term effects in humans. APMIS 2000;108(12):793–804.
8. Troiano RN, McCarthy SM. Mullerian Duct anomalies: Imaging and clinical issues. Radiology 2004;233(1):19–34. doi:10.1148/radiol.2331020777
9. Kaufman RH, Adam E, Hatch EE, et al. Continued follow-up of pregnancy outcomes in diethylstilbestrol-exposed offspring. Obstet Gynecol 2000;96(4):483–489.
10. Pickhardt PJ, Bhalla S, Balfe DM. Acquired gastrointestinal fistulas: Classification, etiologies, and imaging evaluation. Radiology 2002;224:9–23.
11. Yu NC, Raman SS, Patel M, et al. Fistulas of the genitourinary tract: A radiologic review. Radiographics 2004;24:1331–1352.
12. Jarret TW, Vaughan ED. Accuracy of computerized tomography in the diagnosis of colovesical fistula secondary to diverticular disease. J Urol 1995;153(1):44–46.
13. Winterkorn EB, Daouk GH, Anupinde S, et al. Tuberous sclerosis complex and renal angiomyolipoma: Case report and review of the literature. Pediatr Nephrol 2006;21:1189–1193.
14. Nalaboff KM, Pellerito JS, Ben-Levi E. Imaging the endometrium: Disease and normal variants. Radiographics 2001;21:1409–1424.
15. Adaletli I, Ozer H, Kurugoglu S, et al. Case report: Congenital imperforate hymen with hydrocolpos diagnosed using prenatal MRI. AJR Am J Roentgenol 2007; 189:W23–W25.
16. Bischoff A, Levitt MA, Breech L, et al. Hydrocolpos in cloacal malformations. J Pediatr Surg 2010;45(6):1241–1245.
17. Chou CP, Levenson RB, Elsayes KM, et al. Imaging of female urethral diverticulum: An update. Radiographics 2008 28:1917–1930.
18. Hahn WY, Israel GM, Lee VS. MRI of female urethral and periurethral disorders. AJR Am J Roentgenol 2004;182:677–682.
19. Dwarkasing RS, Dinkelaar W, Hop WCJ, et al. MRI evaluation of urethral diverticula and differential diagnosis in symptomatic women. AJR Am J Roentgenol 2011;197:676–682.
20. Musante F, Derchi LE, Zappasodi F, et al. Myelolipoma of the adrenal gland: Sonographic and CT features. AJR Am J Roentgenol 1988;151:961–964.
21. Dunnick NR. Adrenal imaging: Current status. AJR Am J Roentgenol 1990;154:927–993.
22. Daneshmand S, Quek ML. Adrenal myelolipoma: Diagnosis and management. Urol J 2006;3:71–74.
23. Sallomi DF, Yaqoob M, White E, et al. Case report: The diagnostic value of contrast-enhanced computed tomography in acute bilateral renal cortical necrosis. Clin Radiol 1995;50:126–127.
24. Dunnick NR, Sandler CM, Newhouse JH, et al. Textbook of uroradiology, 3rd ed. Philadelphia, PA: Lippincott Williams & Wilkins, 2001.
25. Dyer RB, Chen MY, Zagoria RJ. Classic signs in uroradiology. Radiographics. 2004;24(suppl 1):247–280.
26. Bashist B, Freidman WN, Killackey MA. Surgical transposition of the ovary: Radiologic appearance. Radiology 1989;173:857–860.
27. Ryan JG, Taylor AG, Christian MG. What this all is about. Rad Imaging Tenn 1989;31:5–30.
28. Saksouk F, Johnson, S. Recognition of the ovaries and ovarian origin of pelvic masses with CT. Radiographics 2004 (suppl.);24:133–146.
29. Blake MA, Kalra MK, Maher MM, et al. Pheochromocytoma: An imaging chameleon. Radiographics 2004; 24(suppl 1):87–99.
30. Madani R, Al-Hashmi M, Bliss R, et al. Ectopic pheochromocytoma: Does the rule of tens apply? World J Surg 2007;31:849–854.
31. Subramanian A, Maker VK. Organs of Zuckerkandl: Their surgical significance and a review of a century of literature. Am J Surg 2006;192:224–234.
32. McCallum RW. Lower urinary tract trauma. Appl Radiol 1993;22:15–20.
33. Sandler CM, Hall JT, Rodriguez MB, et al. Bladder injury in blunt pelvic trauma. Radiology 1986;158:633–638.
34. Khan A, Thomas N, Costello B, et al. Renal medullary carcinoma: Sonographic, computed tomography, magnetic resonance and angiographic findings. Eur J Radiol 2000;35(1):1–7.
35. Davidson AJ, Choyke PL, Hartman DS, et al. Renal medullary carcinoma associated with sickle cell trait: Radiologic findings. Radiology 1995;195(1):83–85.
36. Grayson DE, Abbott RM, Levy AD, et al. Emphysematous infections of the abdomen and pelvis: A pictorial review. Radiographics 2002;22:543–561.
37. Joseph RC, Amendola MA, Artze ME, et al. Genitourinary tract gas: Imaging evaluation. Radiographics 1996;16:295–308.
38. Roy C, Pfleger DD, Tuchmann CM, et al. Emphysematous pyelitis: Findings in five patients. Radiology 2001;218:647–650.
39. Davidson AJ, Hayes WS, Hartman DS, et al. Renal oncocytoma and carcinoma: Failure to differentiate with CT. Radiology 1993;186:693–696.
40. Morra MN, Das S. Renal oncocytoma: A review of histogenesis, histopathology, diagnosis and treatment. J Urol 1993;150(2, pt 1):295–302.
41. Patel U, Sokhi H. Imaging in the follow-up of renal cell carcinoma. AJR Am J Roentgenol 2012;198(6):1266–1276.
42. Kawamoto S, Permpongkosol S, Bluemke DA, et al. Sequential changes after radiofrequency ablation and cryoablation of renal neoplasms: Role of CT and MR imaging. Radiographics 2007;27:343–355.
43. Schirmang TC, Mayo-Smith WW, Dupuy DE, et al. Kidney neoplasms: Renal halo sign after percutaneous radiofrequency ablation—incidence and clinical importance in 101 consecutive patients. Radiology 2009;253(1):263–269.
44. Davenport MS, Caolili EM, Cohan RH, et al. MRI and CT characteristics of successfully ablated renal masses: Imaging surveillance after radiofrequency ablation. AJR Am J Roentgenol 2009;192(6):1571–1578.
45. Dyer BD, Chen MY, Zagoria RJ. Abnormal calcifications in the urinary tract. Radiographics 1998;18:1405–1424.
46. Silverman SG, Mortele KJ, Tuncali K, et al. Hyperattenuating renal masses: Etiologies, pathogenesis, and imaging evaluation. Radiographics 2007;27:1131–1143.
47. Silverman SG, Israel GM, Herts BR, et al. Management of the incidental renal mass. Radiology 2008;249:16–31.

48. Jonisch AI, Rubinowitz AN, Mutalik PG, et al. Can high-attenuation renal cysts be differentiated from renal cell carcinoma at unenhanced CT? Radiology 2007;243:445–450.

49. Mayall GF. The incidence of medullary sponge kidney. Clin Radiol 1970;21(2):171–174.

50. Katabathina VS, Kota G, Dasyam AK, et al. Adult renal cystic disease: A genetic, biological, and developmental primer. Radiographics 2010;30:1509–1523.

51. Maw AM, Megibow AJ, Grasso M, et al. Diagnosis of medullary sponge kidney by computed tomographic urography. Am J Kidney Dis 2007;50(1):146–150.

52. Robbins JB, Parry JP, Guite KM, et al. MRI of pregnancy-related issues: Müllerian duct anomalies. AJR Am J Roentgenol 2012; 198(2):302–310.

53. Steinkeler JA, Woodfield CA, Lazarus E, et al. Female infertility: A systematic approach to radiologic imaging and diagnosis. Radiographics 2009;29:1353–1370.

54. Imaoka I, Wada A, Matsuo M, et al. MR imaging of disorders associated with female infertility: Use in diagnosis, treatment, and management. Radiographics 2003;23:1401–1421.

55. Nirula R, Greaney GC. Incisional endometriosis: An under-appreciated diagnosis in general surgery. J Am Coll Surg 2000;190:404–407.

56. Blanco RG, Parithivel VS, Shah AK, et al. Abdominal wall endometriomas. Am J Surg 2003;185:596–598.

57. Hensen JH, Van Breda Vriesman AC, Puylaert JB. Abdominal wall endometriosis: Clinical presentation and imaging features with emphasis on sonography. AJR Am J Roentgenol 2006;186:616–620.

58. Pai D, Willatt JM, Korobkin M, et al. CT appearances following laparoscopic partial nephrectomy for renal cell carcinoma using rolled cellulose bolster. Cancer Imaging 2010;10(1):161–168.

59. Israel GM, Hecht E, Bosniak MA. CT and MR imaging of complications of partial nephrectomy. Radiographics 2006;26:1419–1429.

60. Caoili EM, Cohan RH, Korobkin M, et al. Urinary tract abnormalities: Initial experience with multi-detector row CT urography. Radiology 2002;222:353–360.

61. Anderson EM, Murphy R, Rennie ATM, et al. Multidetector computed tomography urography (MDCTU) for diagnosing urothelial malignancy. Clin Rad 2007;62:324–332.

62. Browne RFJ, Meehan CP, Colville J, et al. Transitional cell carcinoma of the upper urinary tract: Spectrum of imaging findings. Radiographics 2005;25:1609–1627.

63. Caoili EM, Inampudi P, Cohan RH, et al. Optimization of multi-detector row CT urography: Effect of compression, saline administration, and prolongation of acquisition delay. Radiology 2005;235:116–123.

64. Pickhardt P, Lonergan G, Davis C, et al. From the archives of the AFIP. Radiographics 2000;215–243.

65. Wilbur AC, Aizenstein RI, Napp TE. CT findings in tuboovarian abscess. AJR Am J Roentgenol 1992;158:575–579.

66. Potter AW, Chandrasekhar CA. US and CT evaluation of acute pelvic pain of gynecologic origin in nonpregnant premenopausal patients. Radiographics 2008;28:1645–1659.

67. Yitta S, Hecht EM, Slywotzky CM, et al. Added value of multiplanar reformation in the multidetector CT evaluation of the female pelvis: A pictorial review. Radiographics 2009;29:1987–2003.

68. Silverman PM. Gastric diverticulum mimicking adrenal mass: CT demonstration. J Comput Assist Tomogr 1986;10:709–710.

69. Heaney JA, Pfister RC, Meares EM. Giant cyst of the seminal vesicle with renal agenesis. AJR Am J Roentgenol 1987;149:139–140.

70. Arora SS, Breiman RS, Webb EM, et al. CT and MRI of congenital anomalies of the seminal vesicles. AJR Am J Roentgenol 2007;189:130–135.

71. Choi BI, Chi JG, Kim SH, et al. MR imaging of retroperitoneal teratoma: Correlation with CT and pathology. J Comput Assist Tomogr 1989;13:1083–1086.

72. Davidson AJ, Hartman DS, Goldman SM. Mature teratoma of the retroperitoneum: Radiologic, pathologic, and clinical correlation. Radiology 1989;172:421–425.

73. Gatcombe GH, Assikis V, Kooby D, et al. Primary retroperitoneal teratomas: A review of the literature. J Surg Oncol 2004;86(2):107–113.

74. Harrison-Woolrych M, Ashton J, Coulter D. Uterine perforation on intrauterine device insertion: Is the incidence higher than previously reported? Contraception 2003;67(1):53–56.

75. Boortz HE, Margolis DJA, Ragavendra N, et al. Migration of intrauterine devices: Radiologic findings and implications for patient care. Radiographics 2012;32:335–352

76. Markovitch O, Klein Z, Gidoni Y, et al. Extrauterine mislocated IUD: Is surgical removal mandatory? Contraception 2002;66(2):105–108.

77. World Health Organization. WHO mechanism of action, safety, and efficacy of intrauterine devices. Geneva, Switzerland: World Health Organization, 1987:48–63.

78. The Rotterdam ESHRE/ASRM-Sponsored PCOS consensus workshop group: Revised 2003 consensus on diagnostic criteria and long-term health risks related to polycystic ovary syndrome (PCOS). Hum Reprod 2004;19(1):41–47.

79. Balen AH, Laven JS, Tan SL, et al. Ultrasound assessment of the polycystic ovary: International consensus definitions. Hum Reprod Update 2003;9(6):505–514.

80. Leung VY, Chu WC, Yeung CK, et al. Doppler waveforms of the ureteric jet: An overview and implications for the presence of a functional sphincter at the vesicoureteric junction. Pediatr Radiol. 2007;37:417–425.

81. Prieto A, Crespo C, Pardo A, et al. Uterine lipoleiomyomas: US and CT findings. Abdom Imaging 2000;25:655–657.

82. Jafri SZH, Bree RL, Amendola MA, et al. CT of renal and perirenal non-Hodgkin lymphoma. AJR Am J Roentgenol 1982;138:1101–1105.

83. Sheth S, Ali S, Fishman E. Imaging of renal lymphoma: Patterns of disease with pathologic correlation. Radiographics 2006;26:1151–1168.

84. Urban BA, Fishman EK. Renal lymphoma: CT patterns of emphasis on helical CT. Radiographics 2000;20(1):197–212.

85. Cohan RH, Dunnick NR, Leder RA, et al. Computed tomography of renal lymphoma. J Comput Assist Tomogr 1990;14(6):933–938.

86. Ingram MD, Watson SG, Skippage PL, et al. Urethral injuries after pelvic trauma: Evaluation with urethrography. Radiographics 2008;28(6):1631–1643.

87. Moore EE, Cogbill TH, Malagoni MA, et al. Organ injury scaling. Surg Clin North Am 1995;75:293–303.

88. Goldman SM, Sandler CM, Corriere JN Jr, et al. Blunt urethral trauma: A unified, anatomical mechanical classification. J Urol 1997;157:85–89.

89. Sellars ME, Sidhu PS. Ultrasound appearances of the testicular appendages: Pictorial review. Eur Radiol 2003;13:127–135.

90. Yang DM, Lim JW, Kim JE, et al. Torsed appendix testis. J Ultrasound Med 2005;24:87–91.

91. Baldisserotto M, Ketzer de Souza JC, Pertence AP, et al. Color Doppler sonography of normal and torsed testicular appendages in children. AJR Am J Roentgenol 2005;184:1287–1292.

92. Karaosmanoglu, D, Karcaaltincaba, M, Karcaaltincaba D, et al. MDCT of the ovarian vein: Normal anatomy and pathology. AJR Am J Roentgenol 2009;192:295–299.

93. Goergen TG, Lindstrom RR, Tan H, et al. CT appearance of acute renal cortical necrosis. AJR Am J Roentgenol 1981;137:176–177.